Tumors of the Soft Tissues

AFIP Atlas
of
Tumor Pathology

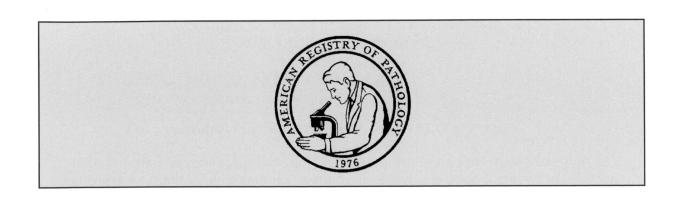

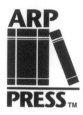

ARP PRESS

Silver Spring, Maryland

Editorial Director: Mirlinda Q. Caton
Production Editor: Dian S. Thomas
Editorial Assistant: Magdalena C. Silva
Editorial Assistant: Alana N. Black
Copyeditor: Audrey Kahn

Available from the American Registry of Pathology
Silver Spring, Maryland 20910
www.arppress.org
ISBN 1-933477-31-8
978-1-933477-31-2

AFIP ATLAS OF TUMOR PATHOLOGY

Fourth Series
Fascicle 20

TUMORS OF THE SOFT TISSUES

by

Markku Miettinen, MD

Senior Clinician, Head of Surgical Pathology
Laboratory of Pathology, National Institutes of Health
Former Chair, Department of Soft Tissue Pathology
Armed Forces Institute of Pathology
Washington, DC

John F. Fetsch, MD

Soft Tissue Pathology, The Joint Pathology Center
National Capital Region Medical Directorate
Silver Spring, Maryland

Cristina R. Antonescu, MD

Attending Pathologist
Director of Bone and Soft Tissue Pathology
Memorial Sloan-Kettering Cancer Center
New York, New York

Andrew L. Folpe, MD

Professor of Laboratory Medicine and Pathology
Mayo Clinic
Rochester, Minnesota

Paul E. Wakely, Jr., MD

Professor of Pathology, Department of Pathology
Wexner Medical Center, The Ohio State University
Columbus, Ohio

Published by the
American Registry of Pathology
Silver Spring, Maryland
2014

AFIP ATLAS OF TUMOR PATHOLOGY

EDITOR
Steven G. Silverberg, MD
Department of Pathology
University of Maryland School of Medicine
Baltimore, Maryland

EDITORS' NOTE

The Atlas of Tumor Pathology has a long and distinguished history. It was first conceived at a cancer research meeting held in St. Louis in September 1947 as an attempt to standardize the nomenclature of neoplastic diseases. The first series was sponsored by the National Academy of Sciences-National Research Council. The organization of this formidable effort was entrusted to the Subcommittee on Oncology of the Committee on Pathology, and Dr. Arthur Purdy Stout was the first editor-in-chief. Many of the illustrations were provided by the Medical Illustration Service of the Armed Forces Institute of Pathology (AFIP), the type was set by the Government Printing Office, and the final printing was done at the Armed Forces Institute of Pathology (hence the colloquial appellation "AFIP Fascicles"). The American Registry of Pathology (ARP) purchased the Fascicles from the Government Printing Office and sold them virtually at cost. Over a period of 20 years, approximately 15,000 copies each of nearly 40 Fascicles were produced. The worldwide impact of these publications over the years has largely surpassed the original goal. They quickly became among the most influential publications on tumor pathology, primarily because of their overall high quality, but also because their low cost made them easily accessible the world over to pathologists and other students of oncology.

Upon completion of the first series, the National Academy of Sciences-National Research Council handed further pursuit of the project over to the newly created Universities Associated for Research and Education in Pathology (UAREP). A second series was started, generously supported by grants from the AFIP, the National Cancer Institute, and the American Cancer Society. Dr. Harlan I. Firminger became the editor-in-chief and was succeeded by Dr. William H. Hartmann. The second series' Fascicles were produced as bound volumes instead of loose leaflets. They featured a more comprehensive coverage of the subjects, to the extent that the Fascicles could no longer be regarded as "atlases" but rather as monographs describing and illustrating in detail the tumors and tumor-like conditions of the various organs and systems.

Once the second series was completed, with a success that matched that of the first, ARP, UAREP, and AFIP decided to embark on a third series. Dr. Juan Rosai was appointed as editor-in-chief, and Dr. Leslie Sobin became associate editor. A distinguished Editorial Advisory Board was also convened, and these outstanding pathologists and educators played a major role in the success of this series, the first publication of which appeared in 1991 and the last (number 32) in 2003.

The same organizational framework applies to the current fourth series, but with UAREP and AFIP no longer functioning, ARP is now the responsible organization. New features include a hardbound cover and illustrations almost exclusively in color. There is also an increased emphasis on the cytopathologic (intraoperative, exfoliative, or fine needle aspiration) and molecular features that are important in diagnosis and prognosis. What does not change from the three previous series, however, is the goal of providing the practicing pathologist with thorough, concise, and up-to-date information on the nomenclature and classification; epidemiologic, clinical, and pathogenetic features; and, most importantly, guidance in the diagnosis of the tumors and tumorlike lesions of all major organ systems and body sites.

As in the third series, a continuous attempt is made to correlate, whenever possible, the nomenclature used in the Fascicles with that proposed by the World Health Organization's Classification of Tumors, as well as to ensure a consistency of style. Close cooperation between the various authors and their respective liaisons from the Editorial Board will continue to be emphasized in order to minimize unnecessary repetition and discrepancies in the text and illustrations.

Particular thanks are due to the members of the Editorial Advisory Board, the reviewers (at least two for each Fascicle), the editorial and production staff, and the individual Fascicle authors for their ongoing efforts to ensure that this series is a worthy successor to the previous three.

Steven G. Silverberg, MD
Ronald A. DeLellis, MD
William A. Gardner, MD
Leslie H. Sobin, MD

PREFACE AND ACKNOWLEDGMENTS

This book follows the long tradition of AFIP Atlases of Tumor Pathology. The text is aimed as a practical diagnostic aid for pathologists, cytopathologists and pathology trainees, but we hope that our clinical colleagues and others may also find it a useful source of information on soft tissue tumors and tumor-like lesions.

We put emphasis on diagnosis, so the presentation is generally concise, yet more comprehensive on key points. Site-specific soft tissue entities covered in other Fascicles are often excluded due to space constraints. We emphasize diagnostically important information on immunohistochemistry and genetics, but also include additional details when biologically significant.

We thank Mirlinda Caton and the staff of the American Registry of Pathology for help, guidance and patience, and Dr. William Gardner, former executive director of ARP, for entrusting the project to us. We also thank Dr. Florabel G. Mullick, Director of the AFIP, as well as our fellow staff members for their help. We were fortunate to draw insight for this project from the AFIP Soft Tissue Pathology Department files, built by Dr. Franz Enzinger, Dr. Sharon W. Weiss, and others over many decades. Additionally, we thank our families for their support and patience during the preparation of this Fascicle.

Markku Miettinen, MD
John F. Fetsch, MD
Cristina R. Antonescu, MD
Andrew L. Folpe, MD
Paul E. Wakely, Jr., MD

CONTENTS

1 SPECIMEN EVALUATION

The overall framework for the evaluation of a soft tissue specimen includes the use of clinical information, radiologic findings, and adjunct tests for tumor diagnosis (especially immunohistochemistry and molecular genetics). Discussed as well are the principles of tumor grading and reporting for a sarcoma specimen.

SPECIMEN TYPE

Needle core biopsy is a standard mode of preoperative evaluation of a deep mass since blind surgery for an unknown mass generally is not favored. The diagnosis is often possible based on a representative core (1). Tumors in which diagnostic findings are focal, however, such as atypia in atypical lipomatous tumor/well-differentiated liposarcoma, may be impossible to diagnose with this modality, and such a diagnosis can never be ruled out with a negative biopsy. Also, focal specific differentiation may be absent in a needle core specimen, and may result in a less specific diagnosis. Tumor grading is frequently difficult, as the criteria based on grading may not be observed in a small specimen. Although the presence of high-grade features allows for accurate grading, the lack of these features in a small sample does not necessarily mean a low grade; therefore, needle core biopsies can only give a minimum grade.

Fine needle aspiration biopsy as the first line of diagnosis is only feasible in centers with special expertise on the interpretation of such specimens. In general practice, it may help confirm recurrent or metastatic tumors (2,3). A special chapter in the end of this Fascicle discusses the fine needle aspiration of soft tissue tumors.

Incisional biopsy offers more abundant diagnostic material and also may more easily allow for partition of the specimen for special studies, such as molecular genetics. A definitive resection specimen allows for a complete view of the tumor, although post-treatment (chemotherapy, radiation) specimens can include alterations that preclude tumor grading or even histogenetic typing. In general, the pathologist is expected to provide assessment of margin status, so that these specimens have to be inked for accurate evaluation of margins. Close margins are best assessed in sections perpendicular to the tumor surface. Although the size of the sample remains arbitrary, 1 section/cm of maximum tumor diameter is a general guideline.

CLINICAL HISTORY

The clinical history can be a very useful aid in the specific diagnosis. The patient age and sex, the lesion site (including tissue plane), and clinical tumor size are the minimum requirements and may allow the formulation of the main diagnostic options. Additional factors include a history of previous tumors or radiation treatment, and the possible presence of a tumor syndrome, such as neurofibromatosis.

RADIOLOGIC CORRELATION

Radiologic studies provide information on tumor location, size, and tissue content. These factors are useful for a specific diagnosis, and such information can enhance the value of a small biopsy.

Examples of radiologic contributions to specific diagnoses include the use of radiographs and computerized tomography (CT) scans to observe tumor calcification for the diagnosis of synovial sarcoma and myositis ossificans, and magnetic resonance imaging (MRI) to determine the presence of a myxoid character and fatty components for the diagnosis of liposarcoma, especially the dedifferentiated variant (4).

SPECIAL STUDIES

Today, immunohistochemical tests are the most important special studies. These studies have largely replaced electron microscopy as a tool for tumor typing. Histochemical stains are still useful in certain cases.

Examples of the application of histochemical stains are the demonstration of glycogen

Table 1-1

NEWER IMMUNOHISTOCHEMICAL MARKERS[a]

ALK (CD246)	Anaplastic lymphoma kinase (in inflammatory myofibroblastic tumor)
ERG	ETS-related gene (a transcription factor), an endothelial marker
FLI1	Freund's leukemia integration 1 transcription factor (gene/protein name); gene usually rearranged and expressed in Ewing sarcoma
D240	Podoplanin (Clone designation of an antibody to podoplanin)
GFAP	Glial fibrillary acidic protein (intermediate filament subunit protein)
INI1	SWI/SNF-related matrix-associated actin-dependent regulation of chromatin sub family member 1; name of a chromatin remodeling protein lost in epithelioid sarcoma; also known as SMARCB1
KIT (CD117)	Receptor tyrosine kinase expressed in gastrointestinal stromal and some other tumors
MDM2	Murine double minute 2 homolog (marker of well-differentiated and dedifferentiated liposarcoma)
MITF	Microphthalmia transcription factor (marker for melanocytic neoplasms)
PROX1	Prospero homeobox 1 transcription factor (gene and protein name); marker of endothelial neoplasms, especially of lymphatic type endothelia
SMARCB1	See INI1
TFE3	Transcription factor E 3 (marker of alveolar soft part sarcoma)
TLE1	Transducin-like enhancer protein 1 (marker of synovial sarcoma)
VEGFR3	Vascular endothelial cell growth factor receptor 3 (endothelial marker)
WT1	Wilms tumor gene/protein; marker for mesothelial neoplasm, desmoplastic small round cell tumor, and others

[a]These are terms discussed or referenced in the text and/or figure legends of this Fascicle.

(periodic acid–Schiff [PAS] with diastase) in Ewing sarcoma, diastase-resistant PAS-positive crystals in alveolar soft part sarcoma, and elastic fibers in elastofibroma. Elastin stains may assess arterial structures adjacent to tumors (elastic laminae).

Immunohistochemistry

A variety of cell type-specific antigens are used as immunohistochemical markers (only newer immunohistochemical markers are listed in Table 1-1). They include cytoskeletal proteins, membrane receptors and other membrane antigens, and cytoplasmic proteins. Extracellular matrix proteins, such as collagen type IV and laminin, are sometimes useful for demonstrating cell types with prominent basement membranes, such as Schwann cells. Nuclear transcription factors (microphthalmia, Prox1) are part of a growing number of newer cell type markers (5). Vimentin, a general "mesenchymal" marker, has limited use because of its widespread expression and lack of cell type specificity.

A basic panel for the diagnosis of soft tissue tumors includes CD34, desmin, epithelial membrane antigen (EMA), keratin cocktail (AE1/AE3), smooth muscle actin, and S-100 protein. This panel should be expanded to cover the differential diagnostic possibilities. These are presented in detail in the following chapters with each entity, and only a summary of the most commonly used markers is presented here.

CD34 is expressed in many fibroblastic tumors, as well as in subsets of vascular endothelial cell tumors. Positive spindle tumors include dermatofibrosarcoma protuberans, solitary fibrous tumor, Kaposi sarcoma, spindle cell lipoma, well-differentiated and dedifferentiated liposarcomas, and variably, myxofibrosarcomas.

Desmin is usually detected in benign and malignant smooth muscle tumors and rhabdomyosarcoma. In addition, it is expressed in other tumors, for example, aggressive angiomyxoma, angiomatoid fibrous histiocytoma, and tenosynovial giant cell tumor (focally). Sarcomas positive for desmin, especially when negative for smooth muscle actin, should be tested for myogenic determination factors (MyoD1, myogenin), as these are expressed in rhabdomyosarcoma (as well as in any malignant tumor with heterologous skeletal muscle differentiation).

EMA is useful in assessing epithelial and perineurial cell tumors.

Keratin cocktail AE1/AE3 typically detects positive cells in synovial sarcoma, epithelioid sarcoma, mixed tumor/myoepithelioma, carcinomas, and mesothelioma. Although many unrelated tumors with no true epithelial differentiation may contain positive cells, this is usually only a focal finding. Such tumors include smooth muscle tumors (benign and malignant) and pleomorphic undifferentiated sarcoma/myxofibrosarcoma.

S-100 protein is typically strongly expressed in benign nerve sheath tumors and metastatic melanoma, and is very useful in differentiating between these and other entities. Nevertheless, some unrelated tumors can be moderately or even extensively positive, including synovial sarcoma. Nearly every tumor contains a variable number of S-100 protein–positive dendritic antigen-presenting cells. While these cells should not be considered as positive staining of the tumor, the presence of dendritic antigen-presenting cells constitutes a useful internal positive control verifying valid staining.

Alpha-smooth muscle actin (α-SMA) is expressed in both smooth muscle and myofibroblasts, and by virtue of the latter, many nonmyoid tumors contain positive cells, for example, myxofibrosarcoma and undifferentiated sarcoma. SMA positivity does not constitute evidence of specific smooth muscle differentiation in the setting of undifferentiated sarcoma.

Endothelial cell differentiation to detect angiosarcoma is usually successful with CD31, but histiocytes, plasma cells, and platelets (thrombi) are also positive. On the other hand, CD34 is expressed in only 50 percent of angiosarcomas. ERG (ETS-related gene) transcription factor, a new marker that is fairly restricted to endothelia and is conserved in malignant endothelia, is a promising new marker for angiosarcoma.

Proliferation markers (Ki67 and analogs) are useful, in some instances, to determine the proliferating fraction. The differential diagnostic criteria between benign and malignant tumors are not sufficiently developed, however, for a straightforward routine application (6,7).

Electron Microscopy

Today electron microscopy has limited use in tumor typing. The specific applications include detection of smooth muscle differentiation in leiomyosarcoma, skeletal muscle differentiation in rhabdomyosarcoma, prominent cell processes and layers of basement membranes in schwannoma, crystals with lattice-like structure with 100-angstrom periodicity in alveolar soft part sarcoma, and tall microvilli in mesothelioma (8,9). Some advocate electron microscopy in the diagnosis of small round cell tumors (10). In general, this method is unsuitable for the typing of undifferentiated and poorly differentiated tumors.

GENETICS

Cytogenetic evaluation requires unfixed tumor tissue. This modality not only gives specific diagnostic information but also enhances the scientific knowledge of tumor genetics. Most tumor translocations have been initially observed cytogenetically. Other characteristics of certain tumor types include losses or gains of chromosomal segments and the presence of abnormal chromosomes, such as ring chromosomes. The specimen should be submitted to the laboratory either as fresh tissue (if the laboratory is not distant), or immersed in a tissue culture medium for shipment to an outside facility (11).

Tumor-specific translocations and gene amplifications are observed with fluorescence in situ hybridization (FISH) techniques using specific probes, many of which detect the most common sarcoma translocations. Specific applications include the use of double-color break-apart probes for diagnosis of *SS18* gene rearrangements in synovial sarcoma translocation, *FOXO1* split rearrangement in alveolar rhabdomyosarcoma, and *ALK* gene rearrangement in inflammatory myofibroblastic tumor (12–14). These are discussed in detail with each entity in the following chapters.

EWSR1 (Ewing sarcoma) gene rearrangement is useful in the diagnosis of Ewing sarcoma and also other sarcomas that feature *EWSR1* gene translocations. Obviously this rearrangement is not specific for Ewing sarcoma, and additional probes for fusion partners are necessary for FISH studies.

The test for *MDM2* gene amplification can help diagnose atypical lipomatous tumor and well-differentiated and dedifferentiated liposarcoma. Chromogenic techniques (CISH) are potentially also useful, but they are more difficult to interpret and not generally recommended with the yet available reagents.

The new understanding of tumor genetics is also a rich source for the discovery for potential specific therapeutic targets (15).

RECOGNIZING NON-SOFT TISSUE TUMORS

The differential diagnosis of soft tissue tumors is not limited to specific soft tissue entities, but also includes metastatic tumors

Table 1-2

GENERAL PRINCIPLES OF TUMOR GRADING[a]

Differentiation
    1, 2, or 3 points (see Table 1-2)

Mitotic rate per 10 high-power fields
0-9	1 point
10-19	2 points
>19	3 points

Tumor necrosis
None	0 points
< 50%	1 point
≥50%	2 points

Total score of point and final grade
2-3	Low
4-5	Intermediate
6-8	High

[a]According to the updated version of the French Federation of Cancer Centers grading system. The grade is calculated as a sum of score points given by differentiation, mitotic rate, and extent of tumor necrosis.

Table 1-3

DIFFERENTIATION SCORES ASSIGNED TO VARIOUS SARCOMA TYPES [a]

Differentiation score 1
    Well-differentiated fibrosarcoma, liposarcoma, or leiomyosarcoma

Differentiation score 2
    Conventional fibrosarcoma
    Myxoid sarcomas (MFH[b], liposarcoma, chondrosarcoma)
    Storiform-pleomorphic MFH
    Conventional leiomyosarcoma
    Well-differentiated or conventional angiosarcoma
    Conventional MPNST

Differentiation score 3
    Poorly differentiated fibrosarcoma
    MFH/pleomorphic undifferentiated sarcoma with a nonstoriform pattern
    Round cell liposarcoma
    Pleomorphic sarcomas (liposarcoma, leiomyosarcoma)
    Rhabdomyosarcoma (embryonal, alveolar, pleomorphic)
    Poorly differentiated and epithelioid angiosarcoma
    Triton tumor, epithelioid MPNST
    Extraskeletal mesenchymal chondrosarcoma
    Mesenchymal chondrosarcoma
    Osteosarcoma
    Ewing family tumors/PNET
    Synovial sarcoma
    Clear cell sarcoma
    Epithelioid sarcoma
    Alveolar soft part sarcoma
    Malignant rhabdoid tumor
    Undifferentiated sarcoma

[a]According to the updated version of the French Federation of Cancer Centers grading system. Modified from reference 16.
[b]MFH = malignant fibrous histiocytoma; MPNST = malignant peripheral nerve sheath tumor; PNET = peripheral neuroectodermal tumor.

such as carcinomas, malignant mesothelioma, melanoma, and even some lymphomas. These possibilities should be considered in the differential diagnosis by including pertinent immunohistochemical testing of such alternatives (keratin, epithelial membrane antigen, calretinin, S-100 protein, lymphoid markers). Especially, metastatic carcinoma, mesothelioma, and melanoma should be considered in the differential diagnosis of epithelioid soft tissue malignancies.

GRADING AND PROGNOSTICATION OF SARCOMAS

Grading applies only to sarcomas; there are no grading systems for nonmalignant soft tissue tumors. The best-documented and most practical grading system is the one developed by the French Federation of Cancer Centers (16,17). This system divides sarcomas into three numeric grades of 1, 2, and 3, corresponding to low, intermediate, and high grades. The grade assignment is based on three factors: differentiation, mitotic activity, and tumor necrosis, each of which gives 0-3 points. The summary of the points establishes the grade, as shown in Table 1-2.

The differentiation (level) is determined by tumor type, as shown in Table 1-3. Based on this table, many tumor types are assigned a fixed differentiation number. For example, all synovial sarcomas receive 3 points for differentiation.

Well-differentiated liposarcomas and leiomyosarcomas receive 1 point for differentiation, while conventional (moderately differentiated) ones receive 2 points.

The mitotic rate is counted in an area of 10 standard high-power fields. Because the grading system has been developed using a microscopic field size smaller than in most current microscopes, adjustment has to be made (often 6-7 fields instead of 10).

Tumor necrosis implies coagulative necrosis, generally with visible shadows of tumor cells. Hyaline change and fibrosis are not counted as necrosis. The percentage of necrosis is based on gross assessment or by microscopy, although the latter may be less accurate if sampling is biased toward viable tissue.

The clinical value of grading is best demonstrated for common spindle cell sarcomas, such as myxofibrosarcoma/pleomorphic undifferentiated sarcoma, synovial sarcoma, and leiomyosarcoma. The grading has limited impact in rare tumors that show little variation from case to case (alveolar soft part sarcoma, clear cell sarcoma, epithelioid sarcoma). Such tumors are often considered nongradable. For some tumor types, the application of grading principles has not yielded clinically significant information (for example, malignant peripheral nerve sheath tumor, angiosarcoma). Some tumors are automatically high grade (Ewing sarcoma). Extensive treatment response (necrosis, fibrosis, paucicellularity) often renders tumors nongradable (18–20).

Recently, nomograms that incorporate tumor size, depth, site, histologic type, and patient age have been developed for more accurate prognostication (21–23). Tumor type-specific nomograms have been developed for tumors such as liposarcoma and synovial sarcoma (24,25). Other prognostication systems have used combinations of parameters such as tumor size, presence of vascular invasion, and extent of tumor necrosis (the "SIN system") (26).

Another recent development is the characterization of sarcomas by genomic complexity in the CINSARC project (complexity index in sarcoma). In this study, a panel of expression patterns of 67 genes was predictive of low or high risk for metastasis, and the prediction was more accurate than based on the French Federation of Cancer Centers grading system (27).

MANAGEMENT OF SPECIMEN AND REPORTING

Obtaining the tumor specimen fresh increases diagnostic options and is recommended, especially for larger specimens and any malignant tumors. The Association of Directors of Anatomic Pathology has published guidelines for the evaluation of soft tissue sarcoma specimens. Recommendations include reporting the type of specimen (procedure), histologic type, tumor size, closest resection margins, depth and involvement of anatomic layers, presence and quantity of tumor necrosis, and lymph node status if applicable. Additional descriptors may include mitotic rate, possible presence of vascular invasion, detailed characterization of the nature of invasion, and presence of an inflammatory component (28).

REFERENCES

1. Huang AJ, Kattapuram SV. Muskuloskeletal neoplasms: biopsy and intervention. Radiol Clin North Am 2011;49:1287-1305.
2. Domanski HA. Fine needle aspiration cytology of soft tissue lesions: diagnostic challenges. Diagn Cytopathol 2007;35:768-773.
3. Wakely PE Jr. Myxomatous soft tissue tumors: correlation of cytopathology and histopathology. Ann Diagn Pathol 1999;3:227-242.
4. Walker EA, Salesky JS, Fenton ME, Murphey MD. Magnetic resonance imaging of malignant soft tissue neoplasms in the adult. Radiol Clin North Am 2011;49:1219-q34; vi.
5. Miettinen M. Immunohistochemistry of soft tissue tumors. In: Miettinen M, ed. Modern soft tissue pathology. Cambridge/New York: Cambridge University Press; 2010:44-104.
6. Meister P. [Histological grading of soft tissue sarcomas: stratification of G2 sarcomas in low- or high-grade malignant tumors.] Pathologe 2005;26:146-148. [German]
7. Hoos A, Urist MJ, Stojadinovic A, et al. Validation of tissue microarrays for immunohistochemical profiling of cancer specimens using the example of human fibroblastic tumors. Am J Pathol 2001;158:1245-1251.
8. Erlandson RA, Woodruff JM. Role of electron microscopy in the evaluation of soft tissue neoplasms, with emphasis on spindle cell and pleomorphic tumors. Hum Pathol 1998;29:1372-1981.
9. Ordóñez NG, Mackay B. Electron microscopy in tumor diagnosis: indications for its use in the immunohistochemical era. Hum Pathol 1998;29:1403-1411.

10. Peydro-Olaya A, Llombart-Bosch A, Carda-Batalla C, Lopez-Guerrero JA. Electron microscopy and other ancillary techniques in the diagnosis of small round cell tumors. Sem Diagn Pathol 2003;20:25-45.

11. Bridge JA. Contribution of cytogenetics to the management of poorly differentiated sarcomas. Ultrastruct Pathol 2008;32:63-71.

12. Mertens F, Antonescu CR, Hohenberger P, et al. Translocation-related sarcomas. Semin Oncol 2009;36:312-323.

13. Romeo S, Dei Tos AP. Clinical application of molecular pathology in sarcomas. Curr Opin Oncol 2011;23:379-384.

14. Lasota J. Molecular genetics of soft tissue tumors. In: Miettinen M, ed. Modern soft tissue pathology. Cambridge/New York: Cambridge University Press; 2010:127-180.

15. Taylor BS. Barretina J, Maki RG, Antonescu CR, Singer S, Ladanyi M. Advances in sarcoma genomics and new therapeutic targets. Nat Rev Cancer 2011;11:541-557.

16. Coindre JM. Grading of soft tissue sarcomas: review and update. Arch Pathol Lab Med 2006;130:1448-1453.

17. Coindre JM, Nguyen BB, Bonichon F, de Mascarel I, Trojani M. Histopathologic grading in spindle cell soft tissue sarcomas. Cancer 1988;61:2305-2309.

18. Kilpatrick SE. Histologic prognostication in soft tissue sarcomas: Grading versus subtyping or both? A comprehensive review of the literature with proposed practical guidelines. Ann Diagn Pathol 1999;3:48-61.

19. Oliveira AM, Nascimento AG. Grading in soft tissue tumors: principles and problems. Skeletal Radiol 2001;30:543-559.

20. Deyrup AT, Weiss SW. Grading of soft tissue sarcomas: the challenge of providing precise information in an imprecise world. Histopathology 2006;48:42-50.

21. Kattan MW, Laung DH, Brennan MF. Postoperative nomogram for 12-year sarcoma-specific death. J Clin Oncol 2002;20:791-796.

22. Mariani L, Miceli R, Kattan MW, et al. Validation and adaptation of a nomogram for predicting the survival of patients with extremity soft tissue sarcoma using a three-grade system. Cancer 2005;103:402-408.

23. Eilber FC, Brennan MF, Eilber FR, Dry SM, Singer S, Kattan MW. Validation of the postoperative nomogram for 12-year sarcoma-specific mortality. Cancer 2004;101:2270-2275.

24. Dalal KM, Kattan MW, Antonescu CR, Brennan MF, Singer S. Subtype specific prognostic nomogram for patients with primary liposarcoma of the retroperitoneum, extremity, or trunk. Ann Surg 2006;244:381-391.

25. Canter RJ, Qin LX, Maki RG, Brennan MF, Ladanyi M, Singer S. A synovial sarcoma-specific preoperative nomogram supports a survival benefit to ifosfamide-based chemotherapy and improves risk stratification for patients. Clin Cancer Res 2008;14:8191-8197.

26. Gustafson P, Akerman M, Alvegård TA, et al. Prognostic information in soft tissue sarcoma using tumour size, vascular invasion and microscopic tumour necrosis—the SIN system. Eur J Cancer 2003;39:1568-1576.

27. Chibon F, Lagarde P, Salas S, et al. Validated prediction of clinical outcome in sarcomas and multiple types of cancer on the basis of a gene expression signature related to genomic complexity. Nat Med 2010;16:781-787.

28. Association of Directors of Anatomic and Surgical Pathology. Recommendations for the reporting of soft tissue sarcoma. Virchows Arch 1999;434:187-191.

2 NONMALIGNANT FIBROBLASTIC AND MYOFIBROBLASTIC TUMORS AND TUMOR-LIKE LESIONS

The lesions discussed in this chapter have fibroblastic and/or myofibroblastic differentiation. Some also have additional lines of differentiation, including cartilage, bone, or fat. While all these lesions are nonmetastasizing, there is considerable variation in the potential for recurrence and locally aggressive behavior. Diagnosis generally is based on a constellation of characteristic histologic findings, correlated with clinical observations. None of the lesions have a unique immunohistochemical profile, so immunohistochemical studies are largely used to narrow the differential diagnosis by excluding other types of differentiation (e.g., smooth muscle, skeletal muscle, and neural differentiation). Nuclear expression of β-catenin has special value in the diagnosis of desmoid-type fibromatosis and Gardner-associated fibroma. Histochemical stains are helpful for the diagnosis for elastofibroma and infantile digital fibromatosis but otherwise have only limited value.

Electron microscopy has largely been superseded by immunohistochemistry, and while it may still be of academic interest, it has no practical role in the diagnosis of these lesions. The ultrastructural features of myofibroblasts include a "wrinkled" (infolded/notched) nucleus, a prominent rough endoplasmic reticulum and Golgi apparatus, bundles of microfilaments with dense bodies, plasmalemmal attachment plaques, pinocytotic vesicles, partial investment by basal lamina, intercellular intermediate and gap junctions, and cell-to-stroma fibronexus attachments (1). There is a spectrum of differentiation for myofibroblasts, so some less-differentiated cells have ultrastructural findings that approach the appearance of fibroblasts and other better-differentiated cells and may be difficult to distinguish from smooth muscle cells. Additionally, not all cells that meet a histomorphologist's (somewhat loose) immunohistochemical definition of a myofibroblast fulfill the more strict electron microscopic definition.

Molecular genetic evaluation currently has only a limited role in the diagnosis and management of these fibroblastic/myofibroblastic tumors, but it may play a greater role in the near future.

NODULAR FASCIITIS

Definition. *Nodular fasciitis* is a benign, self-limiting, proliferation of fibroblasts and myofibroblasts featuring a monomorphic population of plump, "activated," spindle cells, characteristically arranged in a loose tissue culture–like growth pattern and punctuated with focal mucoid degeneration. *Intravascular fasciitis, cranial/parosteal fasciitis* (2), and *ossifying fasciitis* are closely related entities. Synonyms include *pseudosarcomatous fasciitis* and *pseudosarcomatous myofibroblastic proliferation.*

Nodular fasciitis continues to be a difficult diagnosis for the general surgical pathologist and is probably the most common benign soft tissue entity overinterpreted as sarcoma.

Clinical Features. Nodular fasciitis equally affects males and females and occurs in all age groups, but there is a peak incidence in young adulthood between the ages of 20 and 40 years (3–5). It is almost always solitary and typically exhibits rapid initial growth, with accompanying localized tenderness in half of the patients. The anatomic distribution is wide, but there is a predilection for the upper extremities (especially the forearm), followed in frequency by the trunk (4,6–9); the remainder of the cases is equally divided between the head and neck region and lower extremities. Most cases involve the subcutaneous tissue and underlying fascia, but some cases are intramuscular (often with some fascial involvement), periosteal, or dermal in location (10).

Intravascular fasciitis generally occurs in young individuals before the age of 30 years (11). It primarily affects the subcutaneous vessels of the upper extremities or head and neck region. Cranial fasciitis has a peak incidence in the first year of life but is also seen in early

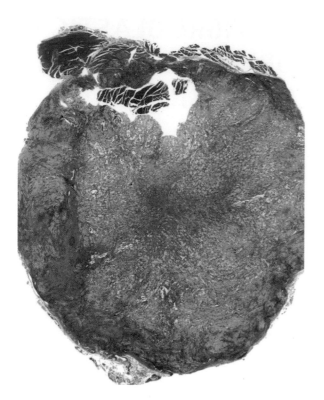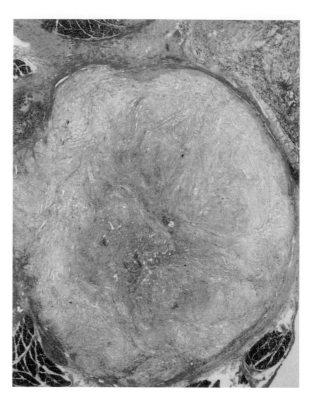

Figure 2-1

NODULAR FASCIITIS

The low-power view shows the well-demarcated, nodular growth pattern, whether fascial-based (left) or intramuscular (right).

childhood, and rarely, in patients 10 years of age or older (12–16). Males are affected more than twice as often as females. The process characteristically involves the outer table of the skull and adjacent soft tissue, but it can penetrate the inner table of bone and extend into the meninges.

Gross Findings. Nodular fasciitis is usually 3 cm or smaller in size, and examples larger than 4 cm are rare (4,7,17–19). The lesions vary from soft to firm, depending on the amount of accompanying myxoid matrix versus collagen. Some examples are grossly cystic. On cut section, the process forms a well-circumscribed nodular mass, or less commonly, has a stellate configuration, especially when epicentered on fascia.

Microscopic Findings. At low magnification, most examples have a nodular configuration (fig. 2-1), centered in the subcutis, but regardless of whether the process is superficial or deep in muscle, there is often some association with fascia. The lesions contain moderately cellular

proliferations of plump, "activated" fibroblasts and myofibroblasts, arranged in loose, C- and S-shaped fascicles and broad storiform arrays (fig. 2-2). Solid growth may predominate in some (often early) lesions, but even these commonly contain small foci with mucoid degeneration (fig. 2-3).

At the most easily recognizable stage, nodular fasciitis features increased myxoid matrix, imparting a characteristic "feathery," tissue culture-like growth pattern; over time, cystic foci and scattered bundles of hyalinized intralesional collagen may develop (figs. 2-2D, 2-3A). The lesional cells have lightly eosinophilic cytoplasm and elongated vesicular nuclei with small nucleoli. Cytologic atypia and pleomorphism are negligible. While mitotic figures may be numerous, atypical mitotic figures are exceptional. Extravasated red blood cells, scattered lymphocytes, and osteoclast-like giant cells are common (fig. 2-3B–D) (3,7).

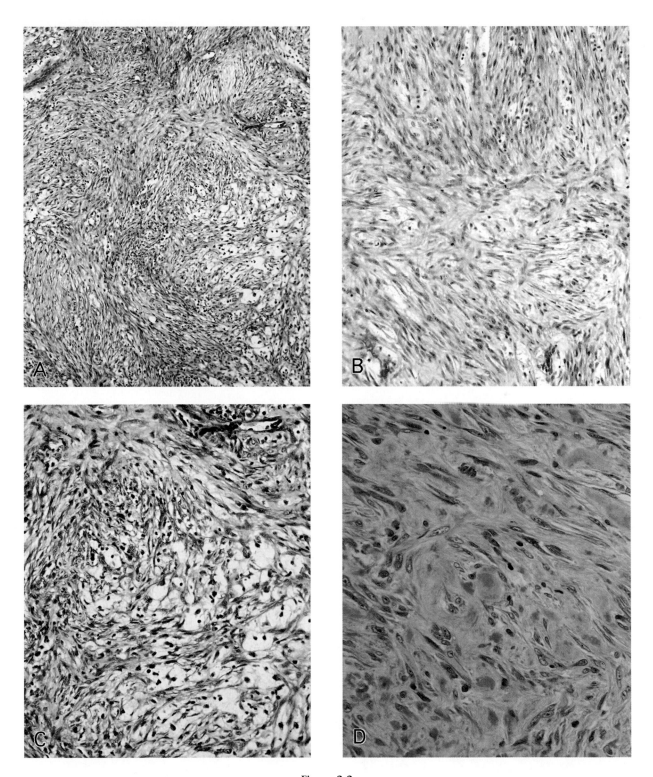

Figure 2-2

NODULAR FASCIITIS

Low (A), intermediate (B,C), and high (D) power views show a loosely organized, tissue culture-like proliferation of uniformly bland spindle cells (A,B) and scattered foci with mucoid degeneration (C). Areas with hyalinized, keloid-like collagen are present (D), especially in older lesions.

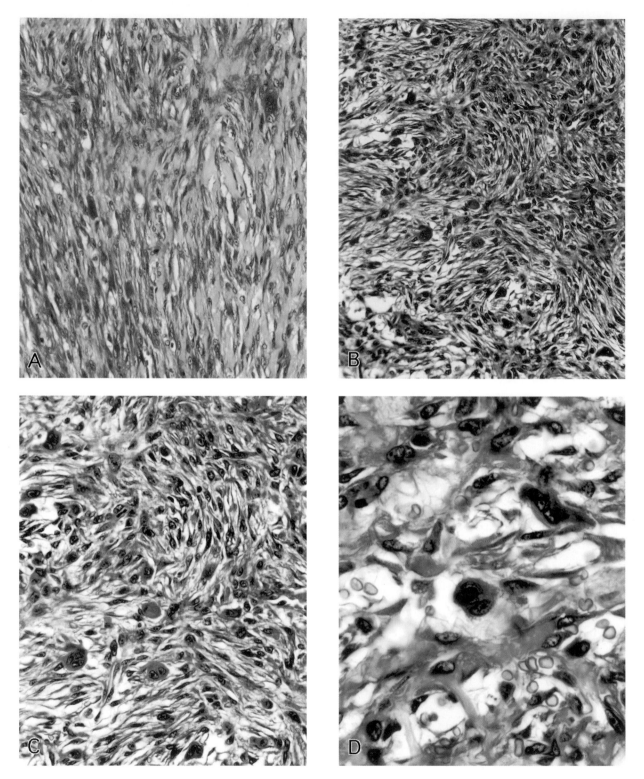

Figure 2-3

CELLULAR NODULAR FASCIITIS

Clues to the diagnosis include a lobular contour, uniformity of the lesional cells, focal collagen bundles (A), and small areas with early mucoid degeneration (B–D). The last may contain focal osteoclast-like giant cells (C,D).

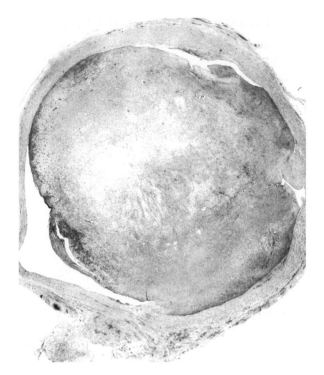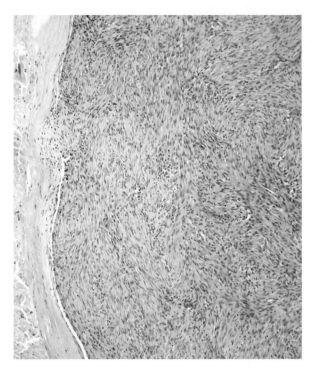

Figure 2-4

INTRAVASCULAR NODULAR FASCIITIS

Low (left) and intermediate (right) power views show the loose, tissue culture-like growth pattern of the spindle cells (right).

Intravascular fasciitis is a variant of nodular fasciitis that usually affects small to medium-sized vessels, usually veins (fig. 2-4). The process may be intraluminal, intramural, or involve both vessel and adjacent soft tissue. In some cases, special stains are needed to highlight the residual vessel wall. Because of vascular involvement, the lesions may exhibit a multinodular or plexiform growth pattern (11).

Cranial fasciitis is a variant of nodular fasciitis that affects the calvaria and adjacent soft tissues. Bone erosion is common and reactive new bone formation is often present. Some examples penetrate the calvaria and attach to the dura mater.

Special Studies. The spindle cells in nodular fasciitis are typically positive for smooth muscle actin, muscle-specific actin, and calponin (8,20). These cells are usually desmin negative, and do not express nuclear β-catenin (21), h-caldesmon (20), smooth muscle myosin (20), CD34 (17), and keratins or S-100 protein (8). CD68/CD163 highlights scattered osteoclast-like giant cells (8,17).

Genetics. Although the human androgen receptor (HUMARA) test has failed to demonstrate clonality (22), cytogenetic studies have documented karyotypic abnormalities, indicating that nodular fasciitis is a benign, self-limiting neoplasm rather that a reactive process (23–26). Reported clonal cytogenetic abnormalities include the 3q21 and 15q22–q26 chromosomal regions. *MYH9-USP6* gene fusion has been recently established as a recurrent genetic change in nodular fasciitis (26a).

Differential Diagnosis. Proliferative fasciitis and proliferative myositis feature plump ganglion cell-like myofibroblasts and tend to be more infiltrative, entrapping regional structures. Rare examples of nodular fasciitis contain foci with metaplastic ossification (e.g., ossifying fasciitis/fasciitis ossificans, panniculitis ossificans) (27–29). Up to 25 percent of fibromas of tendon sheath have areas indistinguishable from nodular fasciitis. Fibroma of tendon sheath, however, tends to have a more variable composition, with cellular foci juxtaposed to heavily collagenized paucicellular areas.

Desmoplastic fibroblastoma is typically less cellular than nodular fasciitis and features sparse stellate-shaped fibroblasts in a myxocollagenous matrix. Fibrous histiocytomas are generally more superficial than nodular fasciitis and typically lack an association with the fascia. These lesions characteristically have a stellate configuration and feature spindle cells with denser nuclei, a more heterogeneous composition including xanthoma cells and siderophages, and an absence of mucoid degeneration.

Desmoid-type fibromatoses typically form larger masses than nodular fasciitis. They are infiltrative and destructive, and feature spindle cells with slightly more atypical, darker-staining nuclei. They also have better-developed, broad storiform and fascicular growth patterns with evenly distributed, slightly dilated or slit-like vessels. In addition, they have a different gene expression signature than nodular fasciitis (30) and approximately 80 percent have nuclear immunoreactivity for β-catenin.

Myxofibrosarcoma is typically infiltrative, and even when low grade, features more nuclear atypia and pleomorphism than nodular fasciitis. Atypical mitotic figures may be encountered, and a curvilinear vascular pattern with focally increased cellularity around the vessels is common.

Myointimoma, as described in the corpus spongiosum of the glans penis (fig. 2-5), is a rare, indolent entity that warrants brief comment in the differential diagnosis of intravascular fasciitis (31–35). This process has also been confused with intravascular leiomyomatosis and myofibroma. It features multinodular intravascular growth of a homogeneous population of bland myofibroblasts and an immunohistochemical pattern similar to that of nodular fasciitis (31–33).

Treatment and Prognosis. Nodular fasciitis is a benign self-limiting process. Spontaneous resolution is well documented, and simple excision without attention to margins proves curative in almost all instances (more than 98 percent) (3,4,18). Recurrence is so uncommon that when this happens, a review of the initial histopathology is often recommended to confirm the accuracy of the original diagnosis (4). Recurrences are typically cured by simple re-excision and metastases do not occur.

PROLIFERATIVE FASCIITIS AND MYOSITIS

Definition. *Proliferative fasciitis* and *proliferative myositis* are benign, self-limiting proliferations of fibroblasts and myofibroblasts, including a subpopulation of cells with epithelioid, ganglion cell–like morphology. This process has a greater tendency for infiltration and entrapment of regional structures than nodular fasciitis. Older synonyms when nodular and proliferative fasciitis were lumped together were *pseudosarcomatous fasciitis* and *pseudosarcomatous myofibroblastic proliferation.*

General Considerations. Proliferative fasciitis and proliferative myositis are histologically similar and differ only by anatomic location (36–41). These lesions morphologically overlap with nodular fasciitis. Their demographics, growth pattern, and ganglion cell-like myofibroblasts are distinctive, however.

Clinical Features. Proliferative fasciitis and proliferative myositis usually affect middle-aged and older adults with no gender predilection (36, 37,40,42,43). Examples in childhood are rare. Like nodular fasciitis, these lesions tend to evolve over a short period of time and stabilize as masses almost always smaller than 5 cm (36,38). While tenderness is encountered in half of patients with proliferative fasciitis, proliferative myositis is usually asymptomatic. Proliferative fasciitis has a predilection for the upper extremity, especially the forearm, followed in frequency by the leg (usually thigh) and trunk (36). Proliferative myositis primarily affects the shoulder girdle/upper arm region, thigh, and trunk, with infrequent involvement of head and neck (38).

Gross Findings. Proliferative fasciitis and proliferative myositis form poorly circumscribed gray-white masses. Proliferative fasciitis generally predominates in the subcutis, extending along the fascial plane. Proliferative myositis involves skeletal muscle, and frequently, its overlying fascia (fig. 2-6). It often contains entrapped, reddish brown skeletal muscle fibers.

Microscopic Findings. Both proliferative fasciitis and proliferative myositis contain spindled cells similar to those of nodular fasciitis but additionally have variable numbers of large epithelioid cells with eccentric nuclei that have some resemblance to ganglion cells (figs. 2-7–2-11). These cells sometimes aggregate around a central paucicellular area of increased

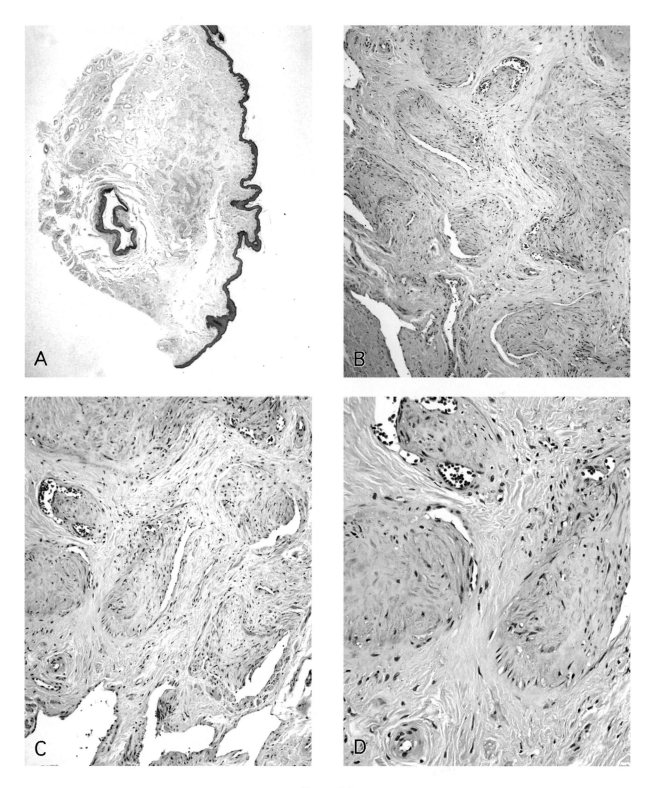

Figure 2-5

PENILE MYOINTIMOMA

A–D: This distinctive myointimal proliferation resides within the vasculature of the corpus spongiosum and is seen in the vascular lumens.

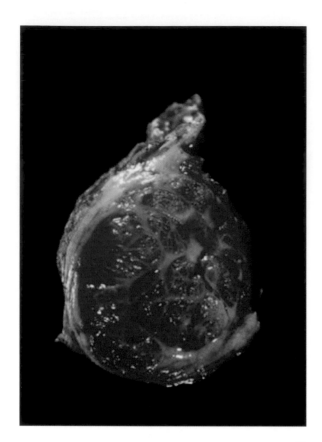
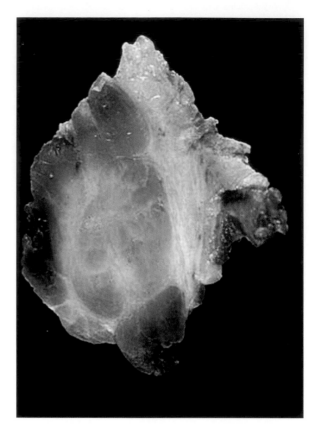

Figure 2-6

PROLIFERATIVE MYOSITIS

Left, Right: The permeative nature of the process is seen, with a tendency to entrap skeletal muscle bundles.

Figure 2-7

PROLIFERATIVE FASCIITIS

This example contains a central, hypovascular, myxedematous zone bordered by granulation tissue-type vasculature. Other examples lack this finding and may have a more infiltrative, stellate configuration at low magnification.

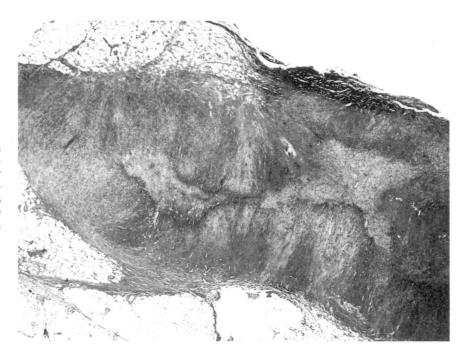

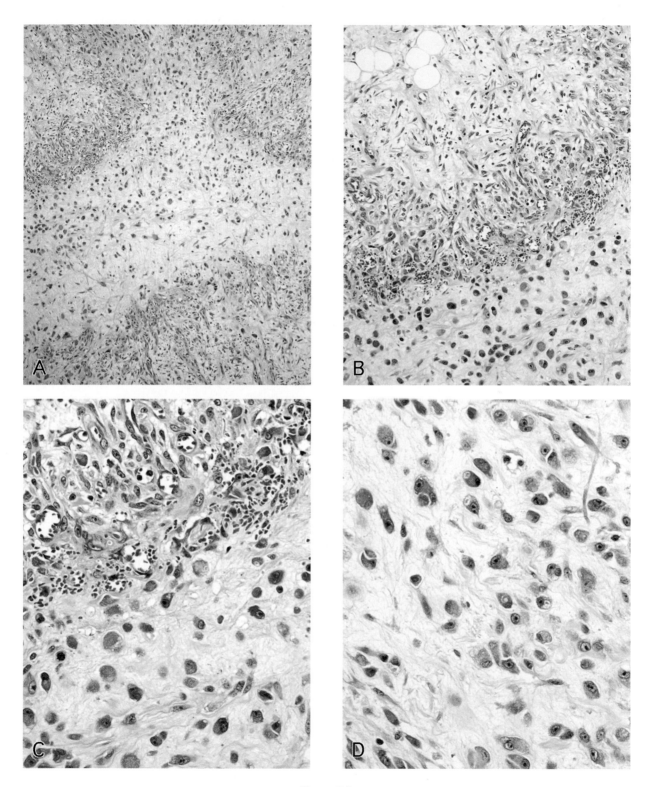

Figure 2-8

PROLIFERATIVE FASCIITIS

Low (A), intermediate (B), and high (C,D) power views show a central, hypovascular, myxedematous zone bordered by granulation tissue-type vasculature. Ganglion cell-like (myo)fibroblasts, spindle cells, and fibrin are present.

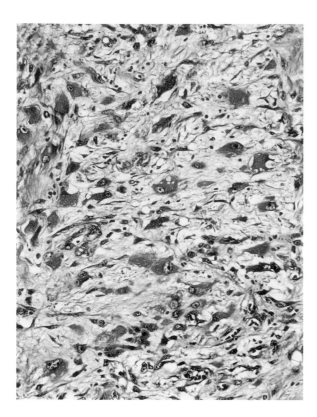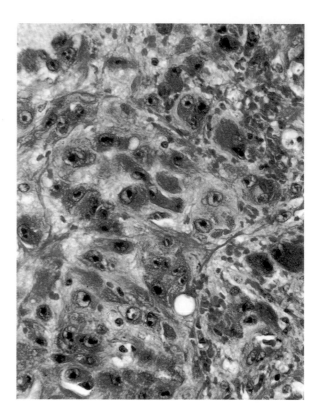

Figure 2-9

PROLIFERATIVE FASCIITIS

Intermediate (left) and high (right) power views of the ganglion cell-like (myo)fibroblasts show abundant amphophilic cytoplasm and large nuclei with a delicate nuclear membrane and prominent central nucleolus. Consistency in nuclear morphology from one cell to the next is a characteristic feature.

stromal mucin (with or without fibrin), bordered by a granulation tissue-type vasculature (figs. 2-7, 2-8). This zonation pattern is more typical of proliferative fasciitis than proliferative myositis. The lesions may, at first glance, appear worrisome for malignancy because of the prominent nucleoli in the ganglion cell-like (myo)fibroblastic component and the presence of scattered mitotic figures. However, the monotony of the population, a vesicular chromatin pattern with a centrally located macronucleolus and delicate nuclear membrane, abundant amphophilic cytoplasm, and lack of atypical mitotic figures help confirm a benign lesion (figs. 2-9, right; 2-10, right). Proliferative fasciitis and myositis have a greater tendency for infiltrative growth than nodular fasciitis, often extending into regional septa and fascia. Permeative growth among skeletal muscle fibers results in a checkerboard-like appearance of proliferative myositis. Up to 9 percent of cases contain small foci of metaplastic bone or cartilage (36,38,39).

When proliferative fasciitis or myositis is encountered in childhood, it often produces a better demarcated, lobular mass with greater cellularity than the adult type (fig. 2-11) (44). Lesions in this setting may have focal necrosis, increased mitotic activity, and a preponderance of ganglion-like cells with exaggerated cytologic features. This constellation of findings can cause confusion with rhabdomyosarcoma.

Special Studies. Spindled lesional cells may be positive for muscle-specific actin and smooth muscle actin, but are usually negative for desmin (41,44,45). The plump cells with ganglion cell-like morphology are generally less reactive for actin, but focal positivity may be noted (41,44). There is a lack of nuclear immunoreactivity for MyoD1 and myogenin.

Genetics. DNA flow cytometric analysis has revealed a diploid pattern for proliferative

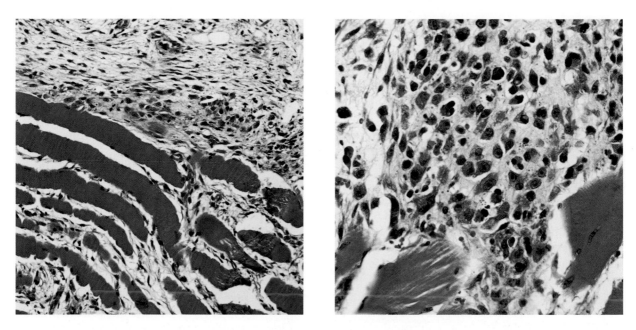

Figure 2-10

PROLIFERATIVE MYOSITIS

This process tends to infiltrate and entrap skeletal muscle fibers (left). The ganglion cell-like (myo)fibroblasts have abundant amphophilic cytoplasm and a large nucleus with an "open" chromatin pattern, a delicate nuclear membrane, and a prominent central nucleolus. The nuclear features are reproducible from one cell to the next (right).

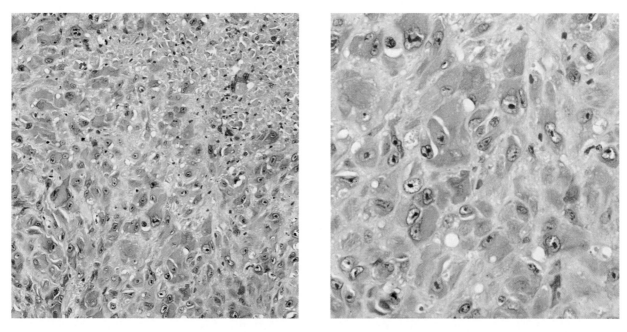

Figure 2-11

PROLIFERATIVE FASCIITIS OF CHILDHOOD

This process often has focal necrosis (left), and there is frequently greater variability in the ganglion cell-like (myo)fibroblastic population (right). The cells, however, maintain abundant amphophilic cytoplasm, and feature an "open" chromatin pattern with a delicate nuclear membrane and prominent central nucleolus. The nuclear features are generally consistent from one cell to the next.

fasciitis and myositis (41,46). There are case reports, however, documenting a trisomy of chromosome 2 by standard cytogenetic analysis for both processes (47,48). There is also a single report of a t(6;14)(q23;q32) in a case of proliferative myositis involving the rectus muscle of a 60-year-old female (49).

Differential Diagnosis. The differential diagnosis for proliferative fasciitis/myositis includes nodular fasciitis, rhabdomyosarcoma, a ganglion cell–rich neural neoplasm, and pleomorphic undifferentiated sarcoma (malignant fibrous histiocytoma). Nodular fasciitis tends to form a better-demarcated mass that displaces rather than incorporates native tissue elements. Also, a ganglion cell–like morphology is not a conspicuous feature of nodular fasciitis. Pleomorphic undifferentiated sarcomas and rhabdomyosarcomas have nuclear pleomorphism and anaplasia, and often contain atypical mitotic figures. Rhabdomyosarcomas have greater immunoreactivity for desmin than smooth muscle actin, and nuclear immunostaining for MyoD1 and/or myogenin. Ganglioneuromas are typically deep-seated, axial lesions with an S-100 protein–positive Schwann cell component.

Treatment and Prognosis. Proliferative fasciitis and proliferative myositis are benign, self-limiting conditions that generally do not recur after simple excision, and special attention to margins is not required (36,38). Recurrence should prompt review of previously sampled material to confirm the accuracy of the initial diagnosis.

ISCHEMIC FASCIITIS

Definition. *Ischemic fasciitis* is a benign proliferation of fibroblasts and myofibroblasts containing large ganglion-like cells and paucicellular zones with fibrinous degeneration. It has a strong predilection for the soft tissues overlying bony prominences. *Atypical decubital fibroplasia* is a synonym.

Clinical Features. Ischemic fasciitis has a peak incidence in the ninth decade of life (50–52). Individuals 70 years of age and older made up more than 70 percent of cases accessioned to the Armed Forces Institute of Pathology (AFIP). We have encountered lesions in two patients in the second decade of life. Occurrence in the third through seventh decades is low, with each decade comprising 3 to 6 percent of cases.

Ischemic fasciitis has a strong predilection for the limb girdles and sacral region, but it also occurs with some frequency on the chest wall and back (50–52). Most patients are debilitated and the lesion may be painful (50–52).

Gross Findings. Examples ranging from 1 to 10 cm in greatest dimension are documented, with a median size in the two largest series ranging from 3.2 to 4.7 cm (50,51). The process is poorly demarcated and features peripheral whitish tan tissue bordering a central area with necrosis, hemorrhage, cystic degeneration, or myxoid change.

Microscopic Findings. Ischemic fasciitis has many features in common with proliferative fasciitis, and it may represent a variant of the latter. It is thought to be an aberrant tissue repair response precipitated by localized tissue ischemia, secondary to chronic trauma or pressure (51,52). At low magnification, ischemic fasciitis generally exhibits a zonal architecture with central fibrinoid degeneration, necrosis, hemorrhage, and/or cystic change, bordered by a granulation tissue–like vascular proliferation (fig. 2-12). Adjacent to the degenerative zone is a proliferation of spindled and large ganglion cell–like (myo)fibroblasts with a prominent central nucleolus and a smudgy "degenerative" chromatin pattern (figs. 2-13, 2-14). These cells morphologically overlap with the cells encountered in proliferative fasciitis. The cells are embedded in myxoid or myxocollagenous matrix, and focal fat necrosis is often present. Regional vessels may exhibit a variety of reactive changes including fibrointimal proliferation, hyalinosis, and thrombosis.

Special Studies. The lesional cells are often focally positive for muscle-specific and smooth muscle actin, and sometimes also for desmin (50,51). CD68 and CD163 highlight accompanying histiocytic cells. Focal keratin immunoreactivity may be present (51). The lesional cells are S-100 protein negative.

Differential Diagnosis. The differential diagnosis is the same as for proliferative fasciitis and myositis. The zonal architecture of ischemic fasciitis, with lesional cells and granulation tissue–type vasculature around a central hypocellular and hypovascular region with fibrinous degeneration, is helpful in establishing the diagnosis. This pattern is rarely encountered in true sarcomas.

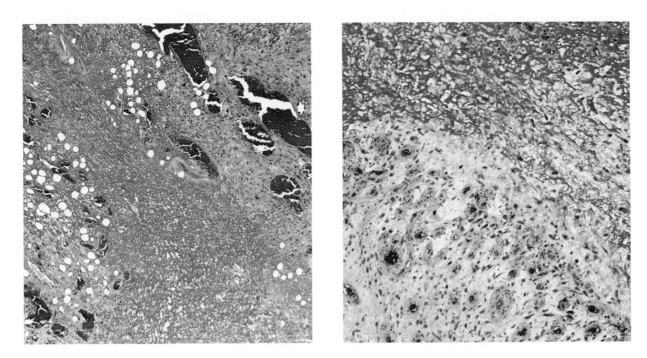

Figure 2-12

ISCHEMIC FASCIITIS

Central fibrinous degeneration and fat necrosis (low power, left) and a zonal granulation tissue-like vascular proliferation (high power, right) are seen.

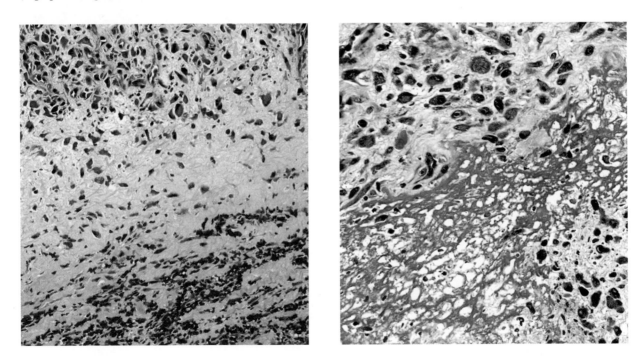

Figure 2-13

ISCHEMIC FASCIITIS

Fibrinous degeneration, a zonal granulation tissue-like vascular pattern (left), and an atypical mesenchymal proliferation (right) that includes plump ganglion cell-like (myo)fibroblasts are present.

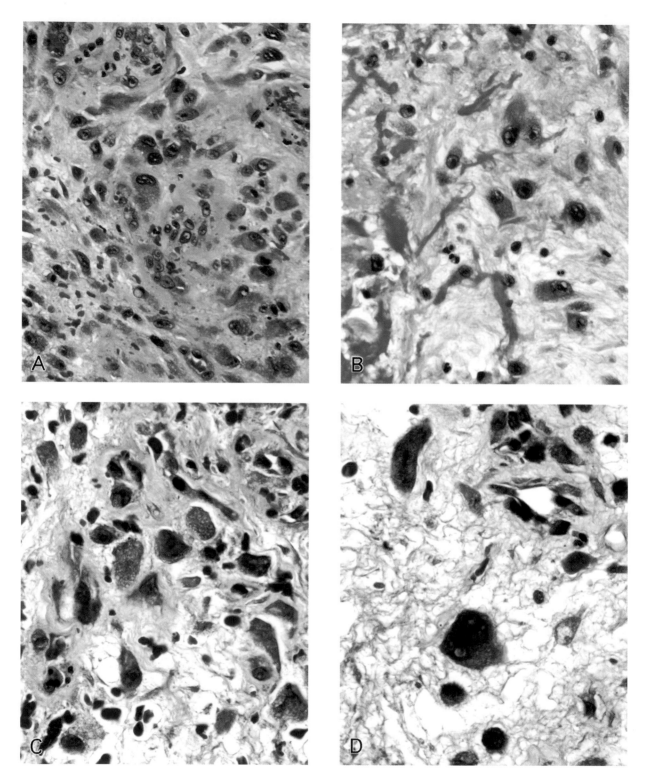

Figure 2-14

ISCHEMIC FASCIITIS

Intermediate (A,B) and high (C,D) power views of the atypical ganglion cell-like (myo)fibroblasts in ischemic fasciitis. The abundant amphophilic cytoplasm contains large pleomorphic nuclei with a smudgy ("degenerative") chromatin pattern.

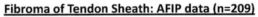
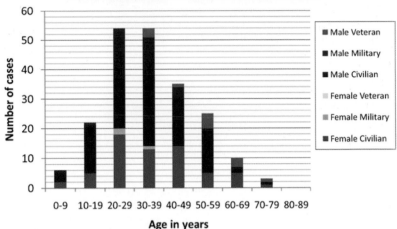
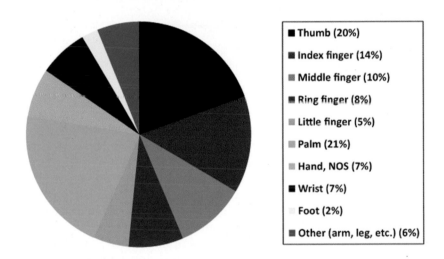

Figure 2-15

FIBROMA OF TENDON SHEATH

Age and sex distribution of 209 cases (top) and anatomic distribution of 215 cases (bottom) of fibroma of tendon sheath reviewed at the Armed Forces Institute of Pathology (AFIP).

Treatment and Prognosis. Simple local excision is sufficient and local recurrences are notably uncommon (50–52).

FIBROMA OF TENDON SHEATH

Definition. *Fibroma of tendon sheath* is a well-demarcated, lobular or multinodular, fibrogenic process that is usually adherent to tenosynovium. It often has paucicellular and moderately cellular foci that may resemble nodular fasciitis or fibrous histiocytoma. *Tenosynovial fibroma* is synonymous.

Clinical Features. Fibromas of tendon sheath affect all age groups, but they occur with greatest frequency in patients in the third and fourth decades of life, with a male predominance (fig. 2-15, top) (53). Most lesions arise in the hand

(especially the thumb, and index and middle fingers), followed in frequency by the wrist, knee, foot, ankle, and elbow (fig. 2-15, bottom). Rare sites of involvement include the forearm, chest wall, and back (53).

A slow-growing mass with no particular clinical symptoms is usually reported, but up to a third of patients note mild tenderness (53). Rarely, there is accompanying carpal tunnel syndrome or local paresthesia. Magnetic resonance imaging (MRI) and computerized tomography (CT) demonstrate a well-demarcated mass intimately associated with a tendon sheath.

Gross Findings. Gross examination generally reveals a small (usually smaller than 2 cm), well-circumscribed, lobulated, rubbery to firm, pearl-white mass that adheres to tendon (53–55).

21

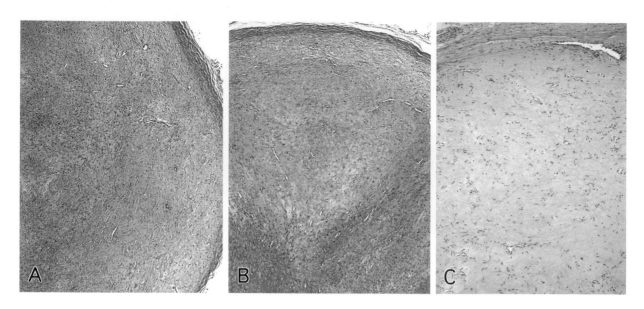

Figure 2-16

FIBROMA OF TENDON SHEATH

The lobular contour (A,B), peripheral slit-like vessels (C), and variable cellularity with focal collagen deposition (B,C) are seen.

Occasional examples are multinodular. Focal myxoid or cystic change may be present.

Microscopic Findings. Histologic examination reveals a lobulated fibrogenic mass with peripherally compressed slit-like vessels, and often, some attached tenosynovium (fig. 2-16). The mass commonly has paucicellular, heavily collagenized areas juxtaposed to moderately cellular foci of bland (myo)fibroblastic cells in haphazard and storiform arrays (fig. 2-17). Focal myxoid matrix may be present, imparting a nodular fasciitis–like appearance, and infrequent giant cells may be evident, resulting in an appearance reminiscent of a fibrous histiocytoma. Rarely, cystic change is present. Xanthoma cells and hemosiderin deposition are usually absent. Exceptional cases with focal pleomorphism have been reported (56).

Special Studies. The lesional cells are often positive for smooth muscle actin (54). Expression of keratin and S-100 protein is absent. One tumor reported as a fibroma of tendon sheath had a t(2;11) involving the 11q12 region (57); however, the accompanying histology leads us to suspect this tumor is actually a desmoplastic fibroblastoma.

Differential Diagnosis. The entities in the differential diagnosis for fibroma of tendon sheath include nodular fasciitis, fibrous histiocytoma, giant cell tumor of tendon sheath, sclerosing perineurioma, desmoplastic fibroblastoma (collagenous fibroma), and palmar/plantar fibromatosis. Differentiation from nodular fasciitis and deep fibrous histiocytoma can sometimes be difficult, but the presence of both cellular and paucicellular collagenous areas is more typical of fibroma of tendon sheath. Fibrous histiocytomas are generally less well marginated and have a heterogeneous cellular makeup. Giant cell tumor of tendon sheath characteristically has a golden brown color on gross examination, and features packeted aggregates of histiocytes, plump histiocytoid cells, and osteoclast-like giant cells, separated by bands of dense collagen. Sclerosing perineurioma closely resembles fibroma of tendon sheath at low magnification, but closer examination reveals corded, branching (basket weave-like) and whorled (onion skin-like) arrays of bland epithelioid and spindled perineurial cells immunoreactive for epithelial membrane antigen (EMA) and GLUT1. Desmoplastic fibroblastoma has a more homogeneous appearance than fibroma of tendon sheath, with uniformly distributed bland stellate-shaped fibroblasts in a hypovascular myxocollagenous matrix.

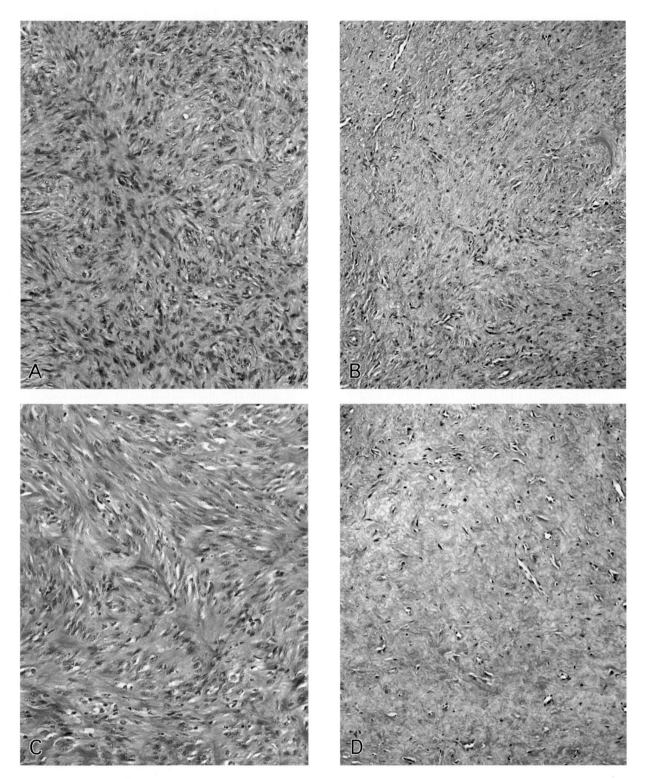

Figure 2-17

FIBROMA OF TENDON SHEATH

High-power magnification demonstrates variable cellularity with some areas exhibiting storiform growth, reminiscent of fibrous histiocytoma (A–C), and other areas having a hypocellular, heavily collagenized appearance (D).

Palmar-plantar fibromatosis arises in the superficial aponeurosis and forms poorly demarcated nodular aggregates of spindle cells.

Treatment and Prognosis. Local excision is the treatment of choice for fibroma of tendon sheath. Postoperative follow-up is recommended because local recurrences, which usually occur within the first 4 months after surgery, are documented in up to 24 percent of patients (53,54). Recurrences are not aggressive and typically respond to local re-excision.

NUCHAL-TYPE FIBROMA

Definition. *Nuchal-type fibroma* is a benign, presumably non-neoplastic, paucicellular, fibrocollagenous, mass-forming lesion that usually involves the dermis and subcutis, with a strong predilection for the posterior neck region. Synonyms include *nuchal fibroma* and *collagenosis nuchae.*

Clinical Features. There is a 4 to 1 male predominance and a peak incidence in the fifth decade of life (58). Most examples present as a firm, slow-growing, painless mass in the posterior neck region, but in one large series, almost 31 percent of cases arose in extranuchal sites (58–62): the back, upper limb girdle, face, and knee. On rare occasion, the process is multifocal. In one series, 11 of 25 patients (44 percent) with follow-up information had diabetes mellitus, and a weak link to Gardner syndrome was noted (58).

Gross Findings. Gross examination reveals a firm, off-white, poorly demarcated superficial mass that extends from the dermis into the underlying soft tissues.

Microscopic Findings. Nuchal-type fibroma is a paucicellular, poorly demarcated process essentially composed of thick collagen bundles, both haphazardly arranged and loosely organized into vaguely lobular aggregates (fig. 2-18). The process typically communicates with the overlying dermis. There is no atypia or notable increase in cellularity. The collagen displaces and entraps regional elements including skin adnexa, fat, and when there is a deep-seated component, skeletal muscle fibers (fig. 2-19A,B). Often, small nerve twigs incorporated within the mass have a splayed, traumatic neuroma–like appearance (fig. 2-19C,D) (58). There is no significant inflammatory component. An elastic stain reveals a delicate network of elastic fibers, but abnormal fibers, as encountered in elastofibroma, are absent.

Special Studies. The sparse mesenchymal cells incorporated within the dense collagen are immunoreactive for CD34 and CD99 (62,63). These cells are typically nonreactive for actin, desmin, and S-100 protein (58,60).

Differential Diagnosis. The differential diagnosis for nuchal-type fibroma includes Gardner-associated fibroma, nuchal fibrocartilaginous pseudotumor, elastofibroma, fibrolipoma, and diabetic scleredema. Some experts regard nuchal-type fibroma and Gardner-associated fibroma as morphologically indistinguishable. Nevertheless, these lesions are separable based on several clinical and subtle histologic differences. Gardner-associated fibromas often develop at a younger age, are more often multifocal, and have a wider anatomic distribution than nuchal-type fibromas. Histologically, they are less likely to be associated with overlying skin, have less patterned collagen with little or no tendency to form lobular aggregates, are not generally associated with small splayed traumatic neuroma-like nerve twigs, and most importantly, typically exhibit mildly increased cellularity whereas nuchal-type fibromas generally appear normocellular.

Nuchal fibrocartilaginous pseudotumor (64–66) is a reactive post-traumatic cartilaginous metaplasia that arises in the posterior nuchal ligament. Fibrolipoma typically presents as a well-demarcated subcutaneous mass that is generally easily "shelled out." Histologically, it contains mature adipocytes, admixed with fibrous connective tissue and a sparse population of spindle cells.

There is morphologic overlap between nuchal-type fibroma and diabetic scleredema, and both processes can occur in the same patient. From a clinical perspective, however, the latter is often either multifocal or diffusely indurative and affects a large anatomic region while nuchal-type fibroma generally manifests as a localized mass.

Treatment and Prognosis. Nuchal fibroma is a benign non-neoplastic process with a low local recurrence rate (58,60). Recurrences are nondestructive and likely reflect persistence of the local or systemic factors that contributed to the lesion's pathogenesis. Simple local re-excision for recurrences is adequate.

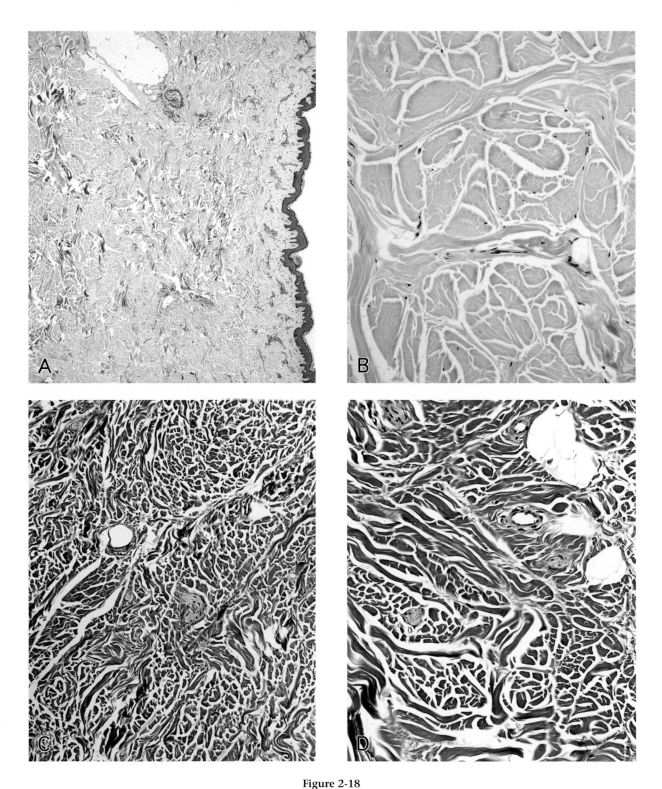

Figure 2-18

NUCHAL-TYPE FIBROMA

A–D: The dermis is expanded by, and the subcutis inflated by thick, haphazardly arranged collagen bundles with low cellularity. The cellularity is typically so low that clinical documentation of a mass lesion is sometimes one of the few clues that this is a pathologic process.

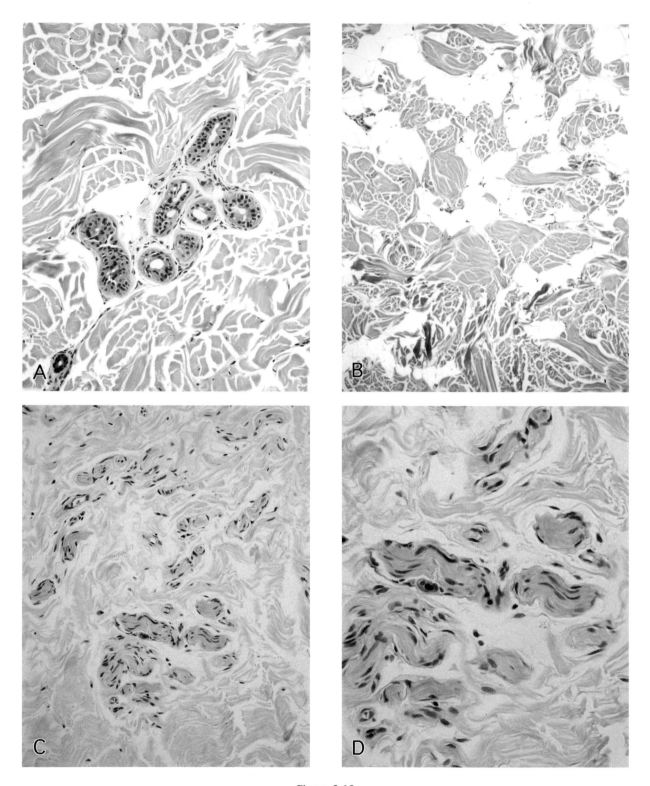

Figure 2-19

NUCHAL-TYPE FIBROMA

Hypocellular, thick collagen bundles infiltrate and entrap skin adnexa (A) and fat (B). Small, splayed nerve twigs with a traumatic neuroma-like appearance are evident within the mass (C,D).

GARDNER-ASSOCIATED FIBROMA

Definition. *Gardner-associated fibroma* is a benign, plaque-like fibrogenic lesion featuring haphazardly arranged collagen bundles and a small number of bland spindle cells. This lesion is associated with familial adenomatous polyposis (Gardner syndrome).

Clinical Features. More than 70 percent of Gardner-associated fibromas are either syndromic or associated with an *APC* mutation, and approximately 38 percent of patients with follow-up have subsequently developed desmoid fibromatosis (67,68). The desmoid tumor can occur in a different anatomic location or arise at the same site as the fibroma, raising the possibility that the latter serves as a precursor lesion.

Gardner-associated fibromas have been reported in individuals from 2 months to 36 years of age, with no gender predilection (67). More than 75 percent of cases are diagnosed in the first decade of life, and only 5 percent occur in those 20 years of age or older. The process typically presents as a slow-growing, plaque-like mass that may be above or below the fascia. The back/paraspinal region is the most common location, with the head and neck, extremities, and chest/abdomen each accounting for 10 to 15 percent of the cases (67,68).

Gross Findings. Gross examination reveals a poorly circumscribed, firm, off-white plaque-like mass, ranging from 0.3 to 12.0 cm (mean, 3.9 cm) in greatest dimension (67). On cut section, yellow streaking secondary to entrapped fat may be noted, but the coarse whorled (uterine leiomyoma–like) appearance characteristic of a desmoid tumor is absent. The lesions are usually subcutaneous masses that do not involve the overlying skin.

Microscopic Findings. Gardner-associated fibroma contains dense, haphazardly arranged, coarse, eosinophilic collagen bundles, separated by clefts and crack-like spaces (figs. 2-20, 2-21, left). The collagen infiltrates and entraps regional structures. While the cellularity is characteristically low, it is generally mildly increased as compared to adjacent normal soft tissue. The lesional cells have bland, somewhat dark-staining nuclei and delicate spindled cytoplasmic processes. The lobular collagen pattern seen in nuchal-type fibroma is typically absent, as are splayed traumatic neuroma-like nerve twigs.

Special Studies. In one large series, 64 percent of cases showed nuclear immunoreactivity for β-catenin (67). The spindle cells within the lesions often express CD34 (fig. 2-21, right), but they typically lack immunoreactivity for actin, desmin, S-100 protein, and estrogen and progesterone receptor proteins (68–70). Gardner-associated fibromas are strongly linked to familial adenomatous polyposis/Gardner syndrome and the patients commonly carry *APC* germline mutations (67).

Differential Diagnosis. The differential diagnosis is similar to that noted above for nuchal-type fibroma.

Treatment and Prognosis. Optimal management for these benign lesions is unresolved, as points for and against surgical excision have been made (67,68). Once diagnosed, however, the patient should be evaluated for familial adenomatous polyposis/Gardner syndrome (67,68). Follow-up is advised to monitor for the subsequent development of a desmoid tumor at the affected site.

DESMOPLASTIC FIBROBLASTOMA

Definition. *Desmoplastic fibroblastoma* is a benign fibroblastic/myofibroblastic tumor characterized by low cellularity, low vascularity, abundant collagenous or myxocollagenous matrix, and bland, uniformly distributed spindle- and stellate-shaped cells. It is synonymous to *collagenous fibroma*

Clinical Features. This process has a strong male predominance, with a ratio of greater than 4 to 1 (71). Patients range in age from the first to ninth decades of life, but the peak incidence is in the sixth decade (fig. 2-22, top) (71). Only 10 percent of cases occur in patients under 30 years of age. Desmoplastic fibroblastoma has a wide anatomic distribution (fig. 2-22, bottom), but is notably uncommon on the head (71–74). Lesions vary from 1 to 20 cm in size, but approximately two thirds of tumors are 2 to 4 cm. Patients typically describe a slow-growing painless mass, often of 6 months' duration or longer.

Imaging studies reveal a well-demarcated ovoid or discoid mass with an MRI signal intensity similar to that of muscle (71). Most examples involve subcutaneous tissue and fascia, but approximately one fourth of cases involve

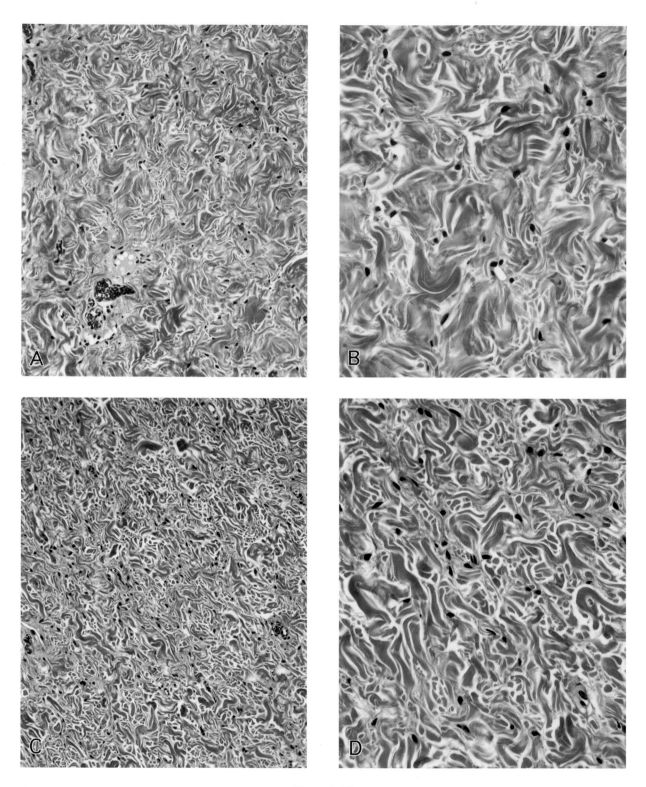

Figure 2-20

GARDNER-ASSOCIATED FIBROMA

A–D: The abundant, thick, wavy collagen is separated by cleft-like spaces. There is a mildly increased number of bland spindle cells.

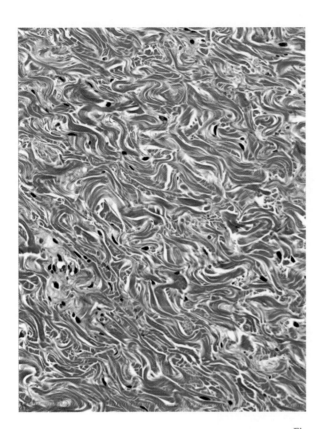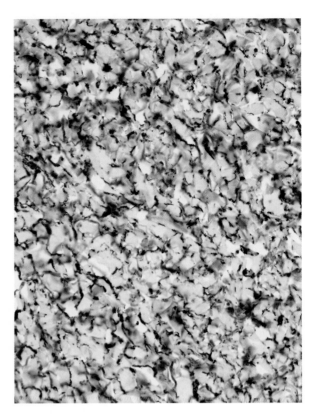

Figure 2-21

GARDNER-ASSOCIATED FIBROMA

Left: Thick, wavy collagen with a mildly increased number of bland spindle cells.
Right: The lesional cells are typically immunoreactive for CD34.

skeletal muscle (71). The preoperative differential diagnosis often includes a lipoma and desmoid tumor, and when acrally located, a fibroma of tendon sheath, tenosynovial giant cell tumor, and ganglion cyst may be considered.

Gross Findings. Desmoplastic fibroblastomas form well-circumscribed fusiform, ovoid, discoid, or multilobulated masses with a rubbery to firm consistency (fig. 2-23). The cut surface may have a homogeneous, pearl-white, fibrous appearance. Occasionally, a mucoid quality, cystic change, calcification, or mottled pinkish areas are evident.

Microscopic Findings. Low magnification usually reveals a lobulated mass with a broad "pushing" border that entraps regional structures at its outer edge (fig. 2-24). The periphery may be moderately cellular, but the central portion of the tumor tends to have low cellularity with a uniformly distributed population of small, bland, spindle- and stellate-shaped cells (figs. 2-25, 2-26). These cells are associated with abundant collagenous or myxocollagenous matrix, and the process has notably low vascularity and no tendency for perivascular hypercellularity. Rare examples have abundant myxoid matrix. Lesional cells have dark-staining, uniform, oval to elongated nuclei with small distinct central nucleoli. Mitotic figures are rare. Vascular invasion is an uncommon finding and has no prognostic significance in this setting (fig. 2-27).

Special Studies. Lesional cells diffusely and variably express actin, often most notable at the tumor periphery (71,74,75). Trace keratin expression is sometimes encountered. No immunoreactivity is reported for CD34, desmin, EMA, S-100 protein, or β-catenin.

Genetics. Clonal chromosomal abnormalities involving 11q12 have been documented in three confirmed cases (76,77). Two of these tumors had a t(2;11)(q31;q12). One additional tumor, reported as a fibroma of tendon sheath

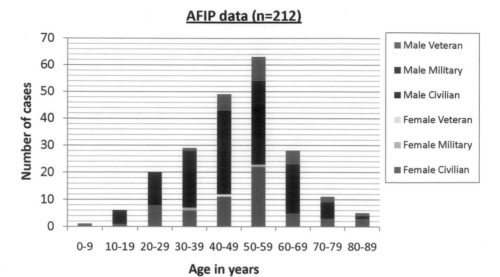

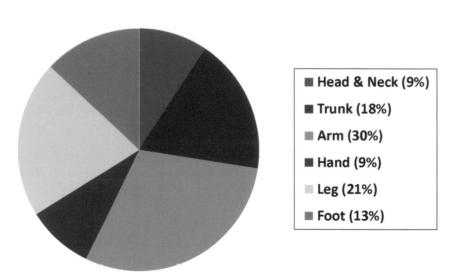

Figure 2-22

DESMOPLASTIC FIBROBLASTOMA

Age and sex distribution of 212 cases (top) and anatomic distribution of 215 cases (bottom) of desmoplastic fibroblastoma (collagenous fibroma) reviewed at the AFIP.

but with the morphology of desmoplastic fibroblastoma, also contained an 11q12 rearrangement with an identical t(2;11) (78).

Differential Diagnosis. The main differential diagnostic considerations are nodular fasciitis, fibroma of tendon sheath, desmoid-type fibromatosis, and low-grade fibromyxoid sarcoma. Nodular fasciitis features greater cellularity, spindled cells, a tissue culture–like growth pattern, and focal mucoid degeneration. The late stages of nodular fasciitis lack the uniform distribution of lesional cells present in desmoplastic fibroblastoma.

In the past, most examples of desmoplastic fibroblastoma involving the hands and feet were considered variants of fibroma of tendon

sheath. However, the latter has greater variability in cellularity and often contains areas reminiscent of fibrous histiocytoma juxtaposed with paucicellular densely collagenized foci.

Desmoid-type fibromatosis is an infiltrative and destructive, fascial-based tumor composed of elongated, mildly atypical spindle cells arranged in loosely organized fascicles and broad storiform arrays. Usually, there is nuclear immunoreactivity for β-catenin. Low-grade fibromyxoid sarcoma may contain paucicellular areas, but foci with increased cellularity (often around vessels), increased vascularity, and mild nuclear atypia and pleomorphism help to differentiate this tumor from desmoplastic fibroblastoma.

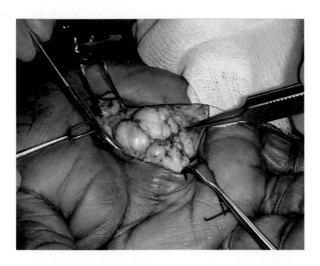
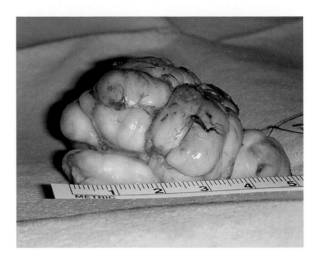

Figure 2-23

DESMOPLASTIC FIBROBLASTOMA

Left, Right: This desmoplastic fibroblastoma, removed from the palm of the hand, has a lobular contour. Examples in this location were often previously misclassified as fibromas of tendon sheath.

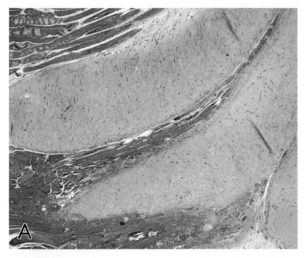
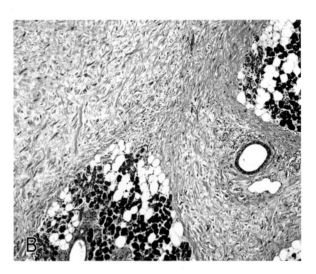

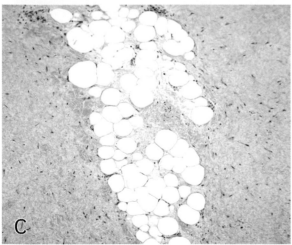

Figure 2-24

DESMOPLASTIC FIBROBLASTOMA

Most examples have a "pushing" border (A), but some lesions are more infiltrative (B,C).

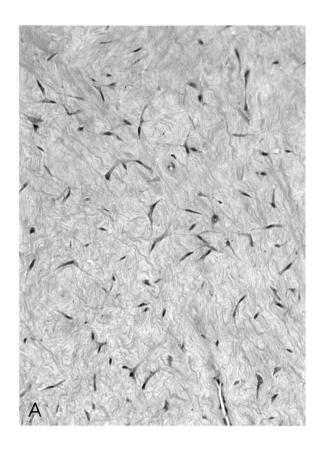

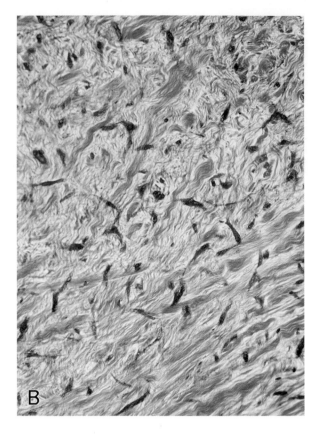

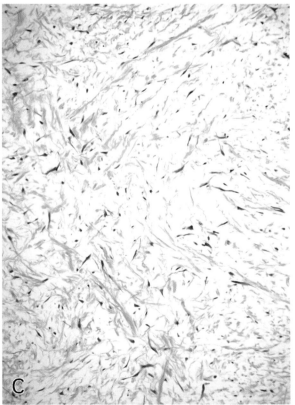

Figure 2-25

DESMOPLASTIC FIBROBLASTOMA

A–C: Minimal vascularity and a fairly uniformly distributed population of relatively bland, stellate- and spindle-shaped cells are seen. The abundant matrix may be heavily collagenized or myxocollagenous. Figure B is a Masson trichrome stain.

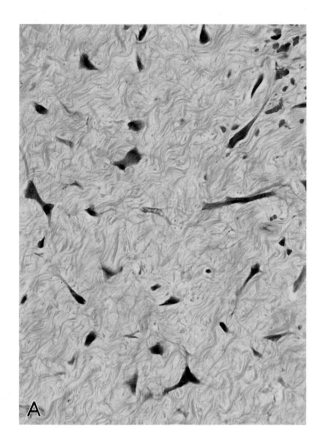

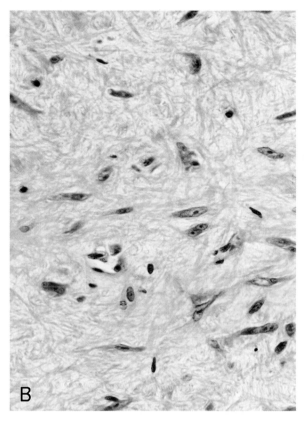

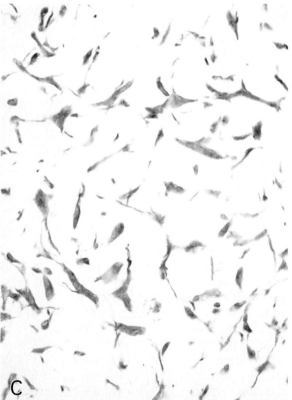

Figure 2-26

DESMOPLASTIC FIBROBLASTOMA

A,B: The mesenchymal cells are fairly evenly distributed, and have uniform morphology. Tumor cell nuclei are mildly hyperchromatic, often with a distinct central nucleolus.

C: An immunostain for vimentin highlights the stellate configuration of the lesional cells.

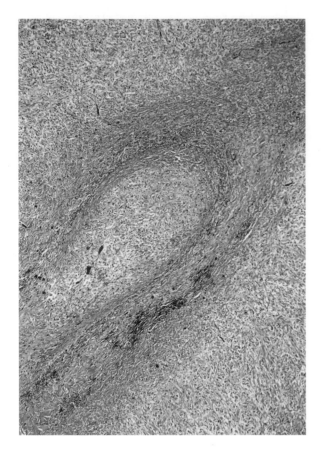 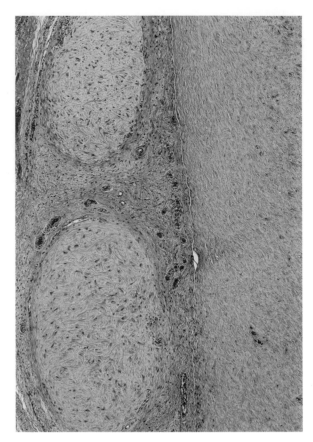

Figure 2-27

DESMOPLASTIC FIBROBLASTOMA

Left, Right: Vascular invasion has no prognostic significance.

ELASTOFIBROMA

Definition. *Elastofibroma* is a fibroblastic tumor-like lesion with numerous abnormal elastic fibers; it almost always occurs between the lower portion of the scapula and chest wall. *Elastofibroma dorsi* is a synonymous term.

Clinical Features. Elastofibroma is a disease of the elderly, with a peak incidence in the seventh decade (fig. 2-28) (79); it is rare before the age of 40. The process has a strong tendency to develop between the inferomedial portion of the scapula and the chest wall at the level of ribs 6 through 8, deep to the latissimus dorsi and rhomboid muscles (79–82). Bilaterality occurs in 10 percent or more of patients (80–82), and some individuals have synchronous lesions or subsequently develop similar lesions in other sites, including the infraolecranon region and overlying the ischial tuberosity (79,82–84).

Slow growth is characteristic, and the process may be asymptomatic, or less often, painful. Most series show a clear female predominance ranging from 2 to 1 to as high as 13 to 1 (79,80,82,85). The process is poorly marginated and typically adherent to fascia and scapular periosteum. In one autopsy study, 24 percent of females and 11 percent of males over the age of 55 had subclinical elastofibroma-like changes documented in the subscapular thoracic fascia (85).

Gross Findings. Gross examination reveals an ill-defined, off-white, rubbery to firm mass with variable amounts of entrapped yellow adipose tissue (fig. 2-29). Lesions range in size from under 2 cm to as large as 20 cm (79).

Microscopic Findings. Elastofibromas form poorly demarcated soft tissue masses that have an admixture of pale eosinophilic collagen bundles, numerous abnormal elastic fibers,

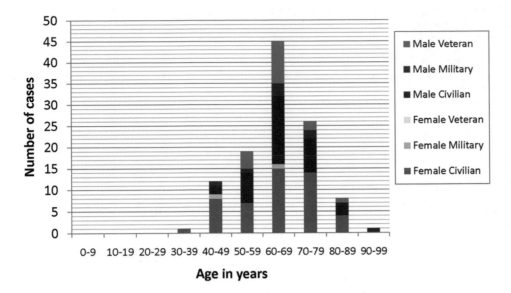

Figure 2-28

ELASTOFIBROMA

Age and sex distribution of 112 patients with elastofibromas reviewed at the AFIP.

scattered bland mononucleated and multinucleated fibroblasts, variable amounts of stromal mucin, and entrapped mature adipocytes (figs. 2-30, 2-31). The elastic tissue exhibits prominent eosinophilia and forms characteristic thick serrated fibers (variously described as resembling a bristled test tube cleaner, beads on a string, and chenille fibers), as well as globules and broken-down irregular grained masses.

Special Studies. Verhoeff elastic stain (fig. 2-32A,B), van Gieson stain, and the elastin immunostain detect large numbers of elastic fibers with varying morphology. Elastic fibers are also usually periodic acid–Schiff (PAS) positive and exhibit autofluorescence (80,82,86,87). Some fibers have an intensely staining central core; others contain several parallel cords associated with a radiating, starburst-like mantle. The fibroblastic cells in elastofibroma often express CD34 (fig. 2-32C) (88).

Genetics. In the small number of examined cases, cytogenetic analysis has revealed significant chromosomal instability, with nonclonal and clonal structural changes predominantly in the form of balanced translocations. Aberrations of 1p (especially 1p32 and 1p13), 3q21, 7q22, and 6p21 are particularly notable (89–92).

Familial occurrence has been reported from Japan and Europe. A third of elastofibromas detected in Okinawa Prefecture, Japan, originated in the same family lines (82). In a Dutch family,

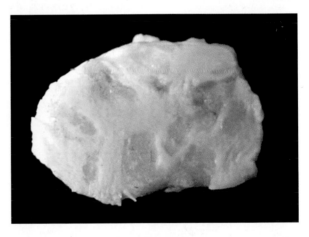

Figure 2-29

ELASTOFIBROMA

The tumor is poorly demarcated. Abundant fibrous connective tissue is admixed with fat.

a mother and her three middle-aged children all had bilateral elastofibromas (91).

Differential Diagnosis. The differential diagnosis for elastofibroma includes atypical lipomatous tumor, fibrolipoma, nuchal-type fibroma, and desmoid-type fibromatosis. Careful review invariably reveals the presence of abnormal elastic fibers and the absence of atypical adipocytic and nonlipogenic elements. Fibrolipomas are typically well-demarcated masses that are usually superficial and easily resected. They lack the abnormal elastic element of elastofibroma.

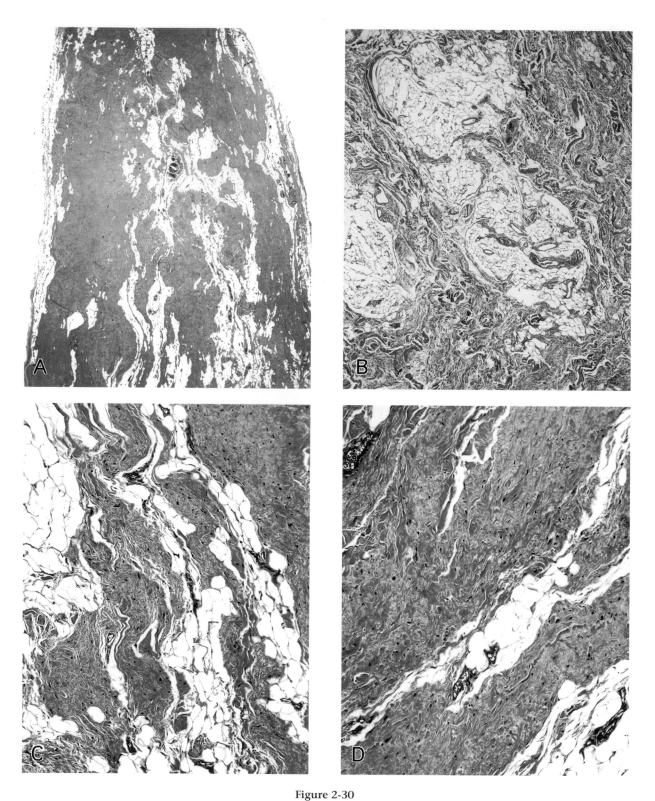

Figure 2-30

ELASTOFIBROMA

A–D: Adipose and fibrous connective tissue are admixed. The latter has mildly increased cellularity and contains numerous abnormal elastic fibers, seen as grayish elements (C,D).

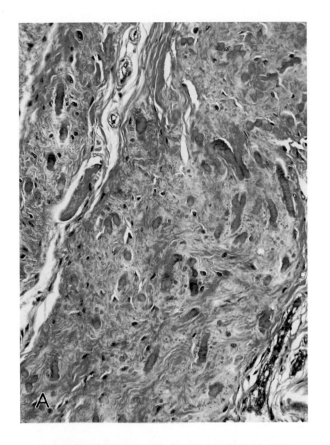

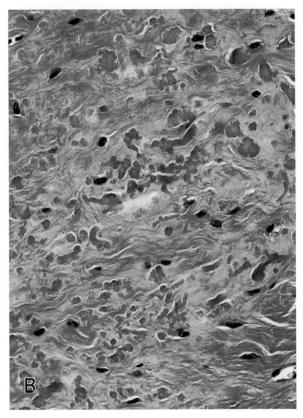

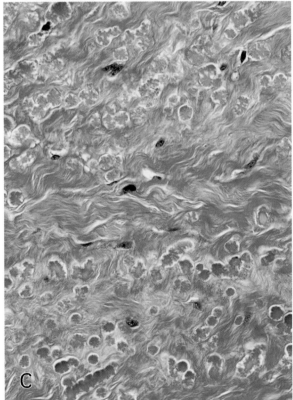

Figure 2-31

ELASTOFIBROMA

A–C: Mesenchymal cells and abnormal elastic fibers are seen within the fibrous connective tissue. The mesenchymal cells may be mononucleated or multinucleated.

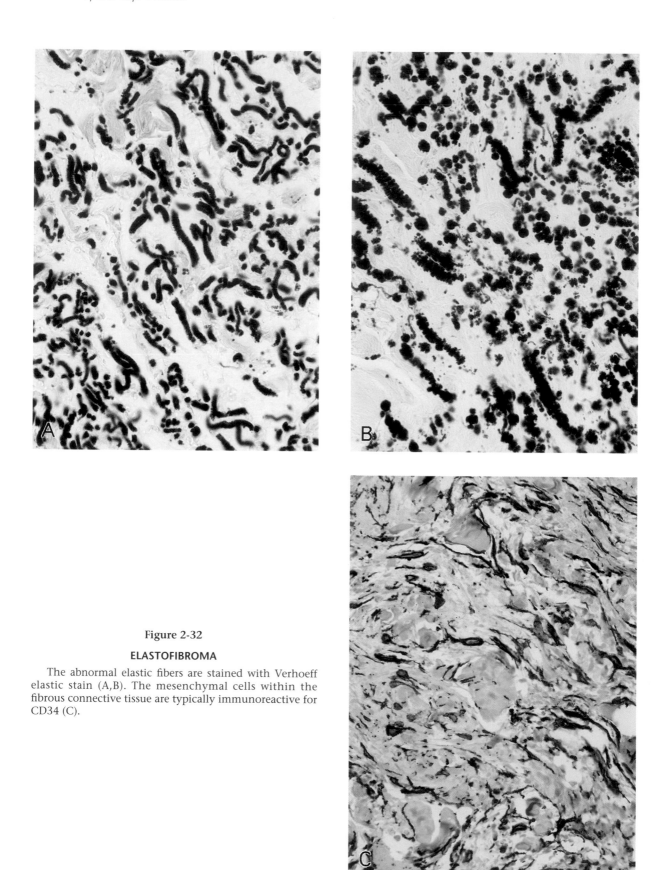

Figure 2-32

ELASTOFIBROMA

The abnormal elastic fibers are stained with Verhoeff elastic stain (A,B). The mesenchymal cells within the fibrous connective tissue are typically immunoreactive for CD34 (C).

Nuchal-type fibromas are collagen-rich, hypocellular, poorly demarcated lesions that contain thin elastic fibers and directly communicate with the dermis. Desmoid-type fibromatosis has greater cellularity and well-developed fascicular and broad storiform growth patterns.

Treatment and Prognosis. Simple local excision is usually curative.

PLEOMORPHIC FIBROMA OF SKIN

Definition. *Pleomorphic fibroma of skin* is a benign cutaneous neoplasm with abundant, haphazardly arranged collagen bundles and sparse spindle- and stellate-shaped and epithelioid mesenchymal cells with pleomorphism and multinucleation and little mitotic activity.

Clinical Features. Based on a small number of reported cases, the patient age ranges from 16 to 67 years, with a peak incidence in middle to late adult life. Females are affected more often than males. The process tends to present as a solitary, flesh-colored, slow-growing, painless, dome-shaped or polypoid mass less than 2 cm in size. Patients often relay a history of the lesion being present for several years prior to removal. The extremities are most often affected, followed by the trunk and head (93–96).

Gross Findings. Pleomorphic fibroma forms a 0.5- to 2.0-cm dome-shaped or polypoid mass with a rubbery to firm consistency and an off-white color.

Microscopic Findings. Histologic examination reveals a fairly well-circumscribed dermal mass with abundant, thick, haphazardly arranged collagen bundles and a sparse population of spindled, stellate-shaped, and epithelioid mesenchymal cells (fig. 2-33). Most cells have large pleomorphic and hyperchromatic nuclei, sometimes with smudgy chromatin and occasionally with small nucleoli. Multinucleation is common, and scattered cells may have a floret-like nuclear arrangement. The atypical cells tend to have scant cytoplasm and indistinct cell borders. Rare mitotic figures may occur, even atypical ones. Sometimes an epidermal collarette is present, and occasional examples have focal myxoid matrix.

Special Studies. The neoplastic cells have variable reactivity for actin and CD34 (93,97,98). S-100 protein, keratins, and desmin are not expressed (97,99).

Differential Diagnosis. The main differential diagnostic considerations are atypical fibroxanthoma, atypical fibrous histiocytoma (fibrous histiocytoma with "monster" giant cells), and pleomorphic lipoma. Atypical fibroxanthoma has greater cellularity and mitotic activity than pleomorphic fibroma. There is more extensive nuclear atypia, with coarsely clumped chromatin and prominent nucleoli. Atypical fibrous histiocytoma has greater cellularity and compositional diversity than pleomorphic fibroma, and it often has a well-developed storiform growth pattern and a stellate interface with adjacent soft tissue. Pleomorphic lipoma generally presents as a well-demarcated subcutaneous mass with mature adipose tissue, ropy collagen, and an admixture of bland spindled cells and pleomorphic multinucleated giant cells with a floret-like nuclear arrangement. We suspect that lesions classified as subungual pleomorphic fibroma (98,100) are more closely linked to superficial acral fibromyxoma.

Treatment. Local excision is generally sufficient.

INTRANODAL (PALISADED) MYOFIBROBLASTOMA

Definition. *Intranodal myofibroblastoma* is a benign intranodal spindle cell proliferation composed of myofibroblastic cells, often with focal nuclear palisading, intralesional hemorrhage, and collagen with stellate or starburst-like extensions. *Intranodal hemorrhagic spindle cell tumor with amianthoid fibers* is synonymous.

Clinical Features. Patients range from 19 to 78 years of age, with a peak incidence in the sixth decade (fig. 2-34) (101–113). The male to female ratio is approximately 3 to 2. The process usually involves a solitary groin lymph node, which may be related to the normal occurrence of immunohistochemically similar intranodal spindle cells in that region (103). Two groin cases have been reported in which more than one lymph node was affected (metachronously) (104,109), and four cases involving a solitary submandibular/neck lymph node have been described (101,106,110). The process is generally slow growing and may be present for many years before resection.

Gross Findings. Gross examination reveals a 0.6- to 6.0-cm (102,113), well-circumscribed,

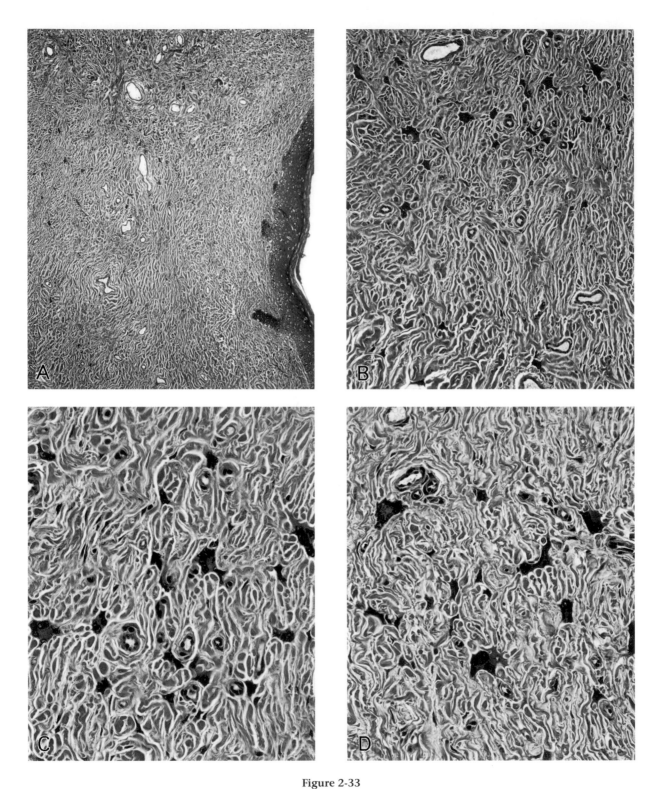

Figure 2-33

PLEOMORPHIC FIBROMA

Low (A), intermediate (B), and high (C,D) power views of pleomorphic fibroma show the abundant collagen, relatively low cellularity, and scattered pleomorphic giant cells. The latter may have a floret-like nuclear arrangement and a morphologic appearance similar to that seen in pleomorphic lipoma.

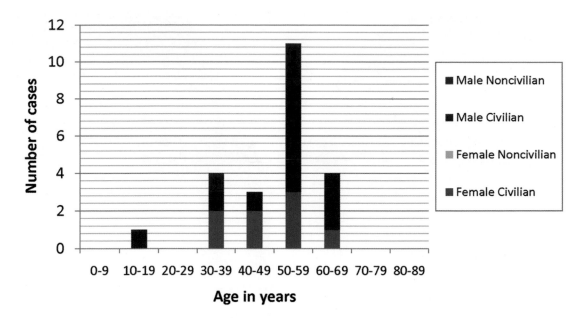

Figure 2-34

INTRANODAL (PALISADED) MYOFIBROBLASTOMA

Age and sex distribution of 23 patients with intranodal (palisaded) myofibroblastoma. This data is derived from histologically confirmed cases identified within the AFIP files and from Suster S, Rosai J. Intranodal hemorrhagic spindle-cell tumor with "amianthoid" fibers. Report of six cases of a distinctive mesenchymal neoplasm of the inguinal region that simulates Kaposi's sarcoma. Am J Surg Pathol 1989;13:347-357.

rubbery to firm mass that on cut section is gray-white with scattered, reddish brown hemorrhagic foci. On close inspection, a rind of residual whitish tan lymphoid tissue may be evident.

Microscopic Findings. Histologic examination demonstrates an intranodal, bland to mildly atypical, spindle cell proliferation arranged in sheets and short intersecting fascicles, often with focal nuclear palisading (figs. 2-35–2-37). Areas of hemorrhage and hemosiderin deposition are usually present, and characteristically, there are scattered islands of collagen with peripheral stellate or starburst-like extensions (resembling amianthoid fibers) (figs. 2-36, 2-37). Mitotic activity is typically low (a few mitotic figures per 50 high-power fields).

The slender elongated spindle cells have tapered nuclei and eosinophilic cytoplasm with poorly defined borders. In some cases, the spindle cells contain lightly eosinophilic intracytoplasmic bodies morphologically similar to those encountered in infantile digital fibroma/fibromatosis (105,106,110,111). These bodies are PAS negative, fuschsinophilic with a Masson trichrome stain, (106,110,111) and at least partially immunoreactive for actin (often with more intense reac-

tivity at the periphery and diminished staining centrally) (105,111). Although the intralesional collagen is often interpreted as forming amianthoid fibers, ultrastructural studies have shown that the giant collagen fibrils characteristic of the latter are absent (105,114).

Special Studies. The spindle cells of intranodal myofibroblastoma are immunoreactive for actin and nonreactive for desmin, S-100 protein, factor VIIIrAg, glial fibrillary acidic protein (GFAP), leu-7, synaptophysin, EMA, and keratin cocktail (101,103,104,108,110). The collagen fibers are predominantly composed of type I collagen, with a lesser amount of peripherally located type III collagen (108,114). Increased actin immunoreactivity is often noted at the periphery of the collagen mats. Examined cases have been negative for human herpesvirus (HHV)-8 or Epstein-Barr virus (EBV) polymerase chain reaction products (104,108).

Differential Diagnosis. The differential diagnosis for intranodal myofibroblastoma includes intranodal schwannoma, Kaposi sarcoma, and metastatic spindle cell sarcoma, not otherwise specified. The cytomorphologic and

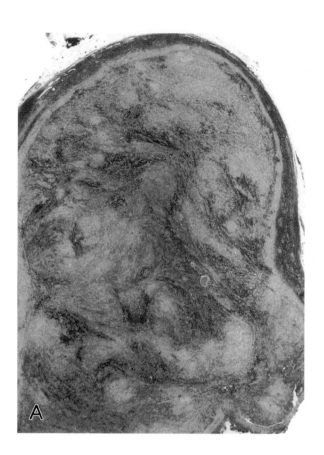

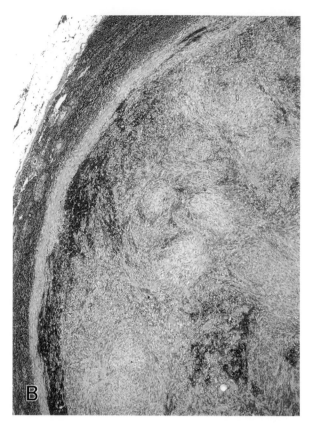

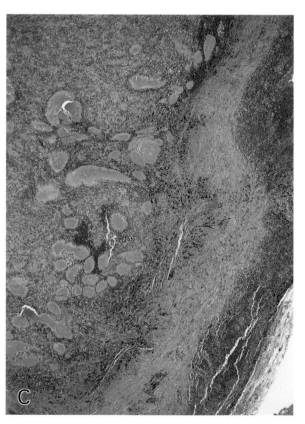

Figure 2-35

INTRANODAL (PALISADED) MYOFIBROBLASTOMA

A–C: Subtotal replacement of a lymph node by a hemorrhagic spindle cell tumor with focal (amianthoid-like) collagen deposition. The latter is best seen in C.

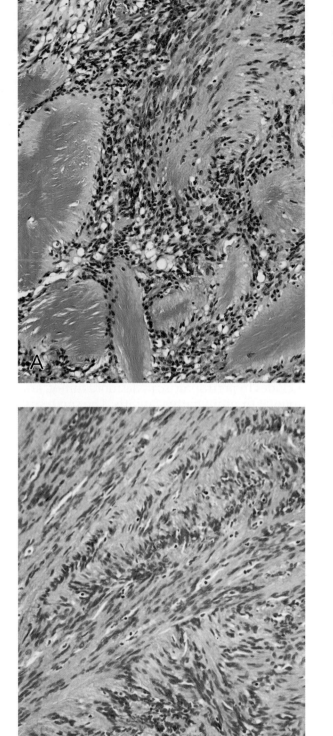

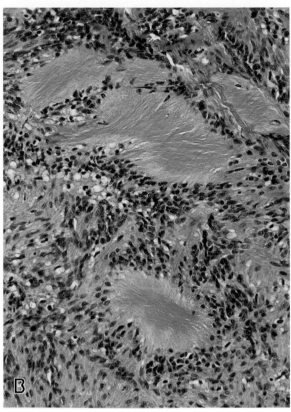

Figure 2-36

INTRANODAL (PALISADED) MYOFIBROBLASTOMA

A–C: Bland spindle cells, focal intralesional hemorrhage, and amianthoid-like collagen (A,B) are seen. The scattered islands of collagen have a starburst-like appearance peripherally.

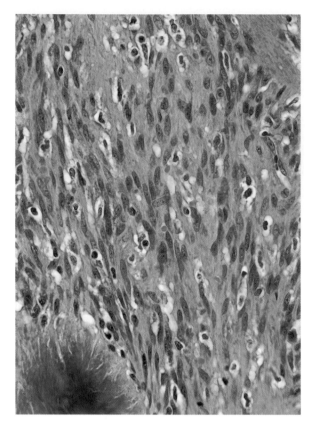

Figure 2-37

INTRANODAL (PALISADED) MYOFIBROBLASTOMA

A high-power view shows the bland, spindled lesional cells.

immunohistochemical features of intranodal myofibroblastoma support myofibroblastic differentiation, and there is no reactivity for S-100 protein or GFAP. Intranodal schwannoma has a predilection for sinusoidal regions of the lymph node and generally exhibits more nuclear atypia and a higher mitotic rate than intranodal myofibroblastoma.

Kaposi sarcoma features numerous slit-like vascular spaces, a lymphoplasmacytic inflammatory infiltrate, grape-like clusters of eosinophilic hyaline bodies, and nuclear immunoreactivity for HHV-8. Nodal sarcoma metastases are uncommon and typically feature much more atypia and mitotic activity than are seen in intranodal myofibroblastoma.

Treatment and Prognosis. Simple local excision is the treatment of choice and typically proves curative (112,113). Two patients had metachronous involvement of multiple regional

groin lymph nodes (104,109). One of the individuals was a renal transplant recipient (104). Both patients had a benign clinical course.

OTHER FIBROMA VARIANTS AND FIBROUS PROLIFERATIONS

Additional fibrogenic lesions that warrant brief mention include fibrous umbilical polyp, sclerotic fibroma, and the cerebriform connective tissue nevus of Proteus syndrome. *Fibrous umbilical polyp* is a distinct fasciitis-like proliferation of early childhood (mean age, 9 months) (115). More than 90 percent of patients are males. The process presents as a dome-shaped or pedunculated mass, 0.4 to 1.2 cm in size. Histologic examination reveals skin with a moderately cellular spindle cell proliferation and variable amounts of collagen (fig. 2-38). The lesional cells have a plump vesicular nucleus with a small nucleolus. Loose storiform and fascicular growth patterns predominate. The spindle cells are focally reactivity for smooth muscle actin, and there may be limited reactivity for desmin. The process is nonreactive for EMA, S-100 protein, CD34, and keratin. The differential diagnosis includes hypertrophic scar, desmoid tumor, and nodular or proliferative fasciitis. The small size, superficial location, patient age, and anatomic site are helpful clues to the correct diagnosis. Simple excision appears adequate.

Sclerotic fibroma (circumscribed storiform collagenoma) is a small, superficial, dome-shaped papule or nodule, usually 1 cm or less in size (116–118). The process has a wide anatomic distribution. Most cases are located on an extremity or the head, but examples are also encountered on the trunk. These lesions are solitary (116–119) or multifocal, the latter often being a manifestation of Cowden disease (multiple hamartoma syndrome) (120–123). Histologic examination reveals a well-circumscribed mass of thick, dense, interwoven collagen bundles separated by cleft-like spaces with "stromal mucin" and arranged in a vaguely storiform pattern (fig. 2-39). The distinctive laminated appearance of the collagen has earned this lesion the nickname "plywood fibroma" (120). The process typically has bland stellate- and spindle-shaped cells, but in some instances, focal multinucleation (fig. 2-39D) or pleomorphism may be encountered (124–126).

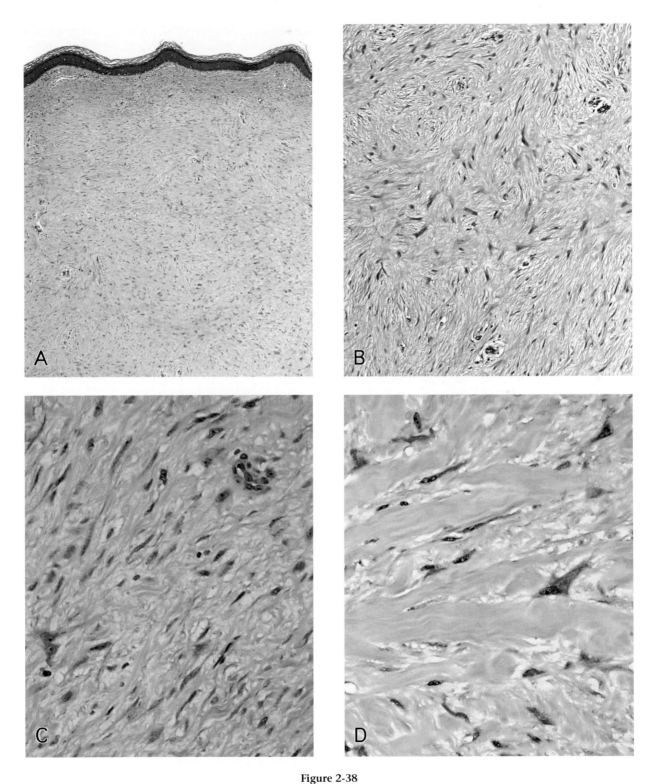

Figure 2-38

FIBROUS UMBILICAL POLYP

Low (A), intermediate (B,C), and high (D) power views of a fibrous umbilical polyp. Moderate cellularity, abundant collagen, and relatively bland "activated" spindle- and stellate-shaped mesenchymal cells are seen. Thick, hyalinized, keloid-like collagen bundles are present (D).

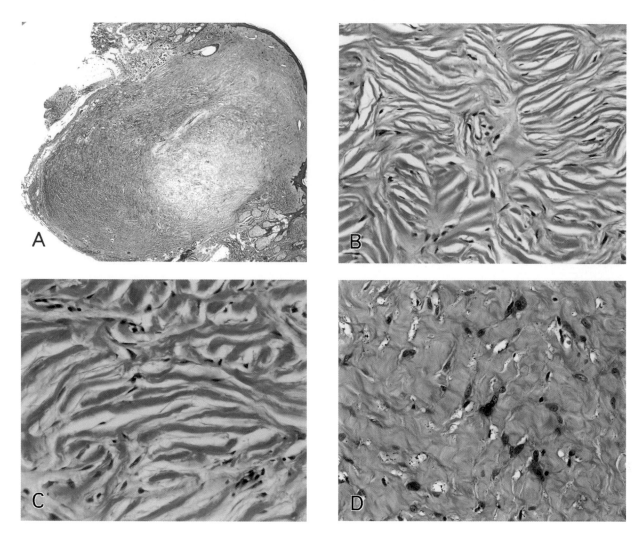

Figure 2-39

SCLEROTIC FIBROMA

Low (A), intermediate (B), and high (C,D) power views of sclerotic fibromas show the small size, superficial location, and well-defined contour of the lesion. The organization and clefted appearance of the collagen bundles are seen (B,C). Infrequent examples contain multinucleated stromal cells (D).

The lesional cells have variable immunoreactivity for CD34 (fig. 2-40) (116,120,127), factor XIIIa (117,124,126–128), and CD99 (116). Focal actin expression may also be present, but S-100 protein is absent (126). Sclerotic fibroma-like changes are sometimes seen in association with other entities, including melanocytic nevi, dermatofibroma/fibrous histiocytoma, neurofibroma, and sclerosing perineurioma (126).

Cerebriform connective tissue nevus (cerebriform fibrous proliferation/fibroplasia) is a highly distinctive manifestation of Proteus syndrome (fig. 2-41) (129–133). This process most commonly involves the plantar surfaces, but the palmar surfaces and other sites, including the neck, abdominal wall, back, eyelids, and nose, may also be affected (134–138). Patients often manifest these lesions within the first 2 years of life, but development may be delayed in some and absent in others (137,138). Biopsy specimens feature abundant dense collagen that expands the dermis and extends into the subcutis. The numerous eccrine glands on the palmar-plantar surfaces tether the skin at regular intervals, producing the characteristic cerebriform or gyriform clinical pattern. Mildly increased cellularity may be present (fig. 2-41C,D), and sometimes, there is a vague nodularity to the deposited collagen (fig. 2-41E,F). Surgical treatment frequently leads to complications, so conservative noninvasive management is generally recommended (136,138).

CALCIFYING FIBROUS (PSEUDO)TUMOR

Definition. *Calcifying fibrous (pseudo)tumor* is a benign, heavily collagenized, mass-forming lesion with a scant population of bland fibroblastic cells, scattered psammomatous and/or dystrophic calcifications, and often, a patchy chronic lymphoplasmacytic inflammatory infiltrate. The process may be solitary or multifocal. Synonyms include *childhood fibrous tumor with psammoma bodies* and *calcifying fibrous tumor*.

General Considerations. There is debate as to whether this is a specific clinicopathologic entity or an endstage morphologic pattern of a variety of different tumors. It has also been questioned whether mesothelial-based (pleural, peritoneal, and scrotal) examples are truly the same process that is encountered in soft tissues. For the time being, we have included all lesions with similar morphology, regardless of anatomic site, under the same designation. Additional study is needed to resolve whether calcifying fibrous (pseudo)tumor is an entirely reactive process or an indolent hypocellular neoplasm.

Clinical Features. Calcifying fibrous (pseudo)tumors are reported in a wide variety of sites, including many soft tissue locations (139–144), visceral organs (heart, small bowel, stomach, and adrenal gland) (145–150), and all of the mesothelial-lined cavities (151–157). Initial studies concentrated on soft tissue examples (158,159), but a current literature review shows the majority of cases actually involve mesothelial-based sites.

Females are affected more often than males. Soft tissue examples have a peak incidence in the first decade of life and a median patient age of 13 years. Pleural and peritoneal examples have a broader age distribution, with median patient ages, at last review, of 35 and 38 years, respectively. Tumors of gastric (144–147,160) or bowel wall (144,148) origin are primarily encountered in adults. These latter examples may form polypoid intraluminal or intramural masses, and may be associated with mucosal

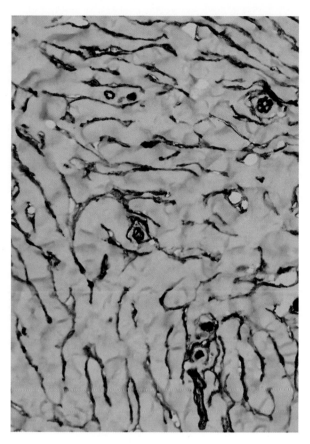

Figure 2-40

SCLEROTIC FIBROMA

Immunoreactivity for CD34 is seen.

ulceration, and on rare occasion, intussusception (148). There are rare reports of calcifying fibrous (pseudo)tumor in the setting of hyaline vascular-type Castleman disease (161), and one report documenting familial susceptibility (162).

Gross Findings. The tumor is a well-circumscribed, solid, rubbery to firm, off-white mass with a gritty cut surface. Soft tissue examples are usually solitary, but mesothelial-based lesions are often multinodular. Tumor nodules range in size from 0.2 to 25.0 cm. More than half of all soft tissue and pleural-based lesions are larger than 5 cm; individual nodules involving the peritoneum are usually 0.5 to 3.0 cm.

Microscopic Findings. Histologic examination reveals a well-demarcated nodular mass that may infiltrate and entrap regional structures at the periphery (fig. 2-42). The mass contains abundant dense collagen in haphazard, vaguely

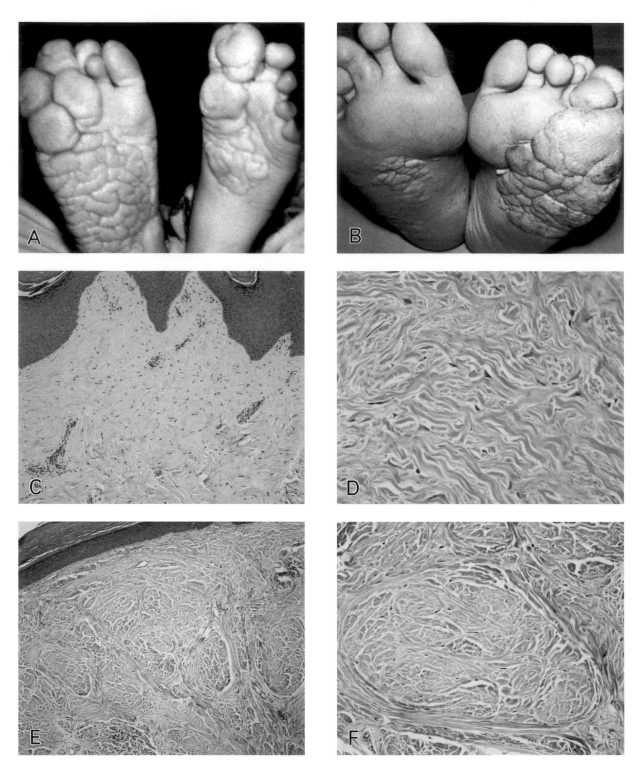

Figure 2-41

CEREBRIFORM CONNECTIVE TISSUE NEVUS OF PROTEUS SYNDROME

Clinical photographs from two patients (A,B) and histologic findings (C–F). Collagen is abundant. Mildly increased cellularity is evident, especially in the superficial dermis (C,D). Sometimes the collagen deposition assumes a vaguely nodular pattern (E,F) (Masson trichrome stain).

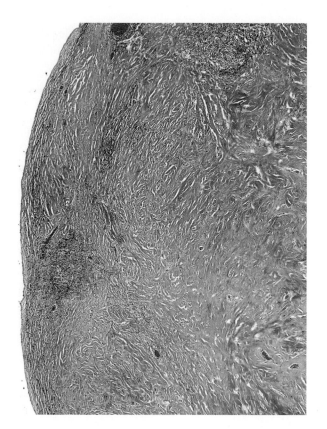 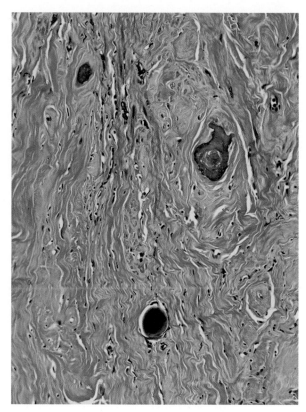

Figure 2-42

CALCIFYING FIBROUS (PSEUDO)TUMOR

The tumor has a lobular contour and lymphoid aggregates (left), abundant dense collagen, and scattered calcifications (right).

storiform and whorled arrangements. There is very low cellularity with infrequent, delicate, bland spindled (fibroblastic) cells, and there is no atypia. Mitotic figures are absent or rare. Scattered psammomatous and dystrophic calcifications are typically present, but these vary considerably in number (fig. 2-43). Infrequent multinucleated giant cells may be seen bordering areas with mineralization (fig. 2-43D). A chronic lymphoplasmacytic inflammatory infiltrate is usually present (fig. 2-44). Germinal centers may be present, and the plasma cell population sometimes contains Russell bodies. Necrosis is absent.

Special Studies. Histochemical stains for amyloid are negative. Immunohistochemical stains reveal variable reactivity for factor XIIIa and CD34 (147,149,154,163,164). Immunostains for keratins, muscle-specific actin, smooth muscle actin, desmin, ALK-1, S-100 protein, CD117, platelet derived growth factor alpha (PDGFRA), and EMA are negative (145,147,149,154,165).

Mesothelial-based examples, however, may contain scattered submesothelial cells with keratin expression.

Differential Diagnosis. Careful sampling to rule out the presence of other clinically relevant findings is mandatory, as there are rare reports of inflammatory myofibroblastic tumors associated with calcifying fibrous (pseudo)tumor-like foci (166–168). Inflammatory myofibroblastic tumors have greater cellularity than calcifying fibrous (pseudo)tumor. They feature plump myofibroblastic cells set in a myxocollagenous stroma with scattered inflammatory cells. Stromal calcifications are uncommon. The myofibroblasts often have an open chromatin pattern, and they may have prominent central nucleoli. Immunoreactivity is typically present for actins, and most tumors express ALK-1. Focal keratin expression may also be present. Clonal cytogenetic aberrations involving the 2p22-24 region with fusion of the *ALK* gene to various partners (e.g.,

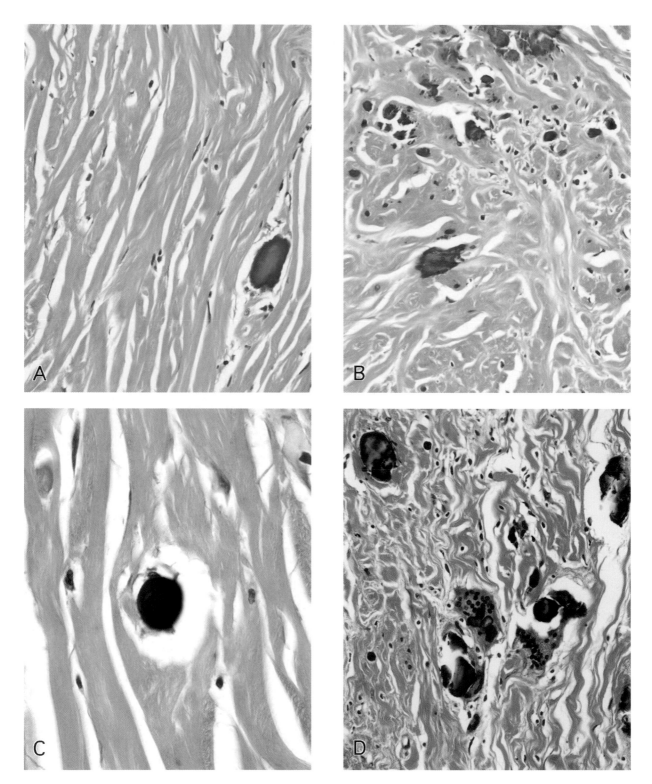

Figure 2-43

CALCIFYING FIBROUS (PSEUDO)TUMOR

A–D: Abundant hypocellular collagen and scattered dystrophic and psammomatous calcifications. The latter may elicit a giant cell reaction (D).

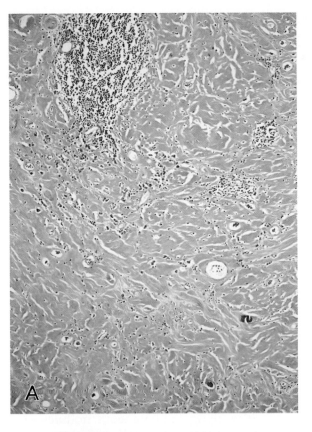

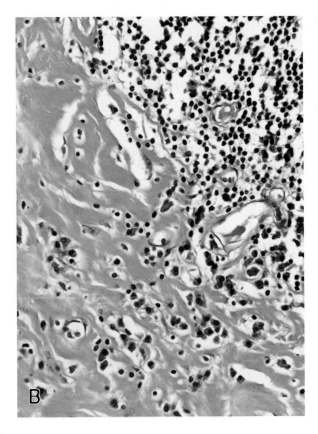

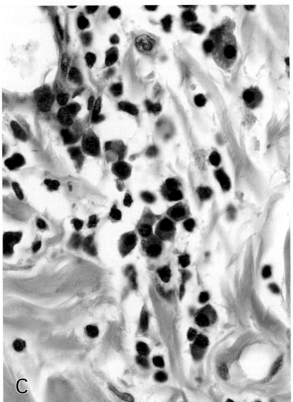

Figure 2-44

CALCIFYING FIBROUS (PSEUDO)TUMOR

Low (A), intermediate (B), and high (C) power views of calcifying fibrous (pseudo)tumor illustrate a patchy lymphoplasmacytic inflammatory infiltrate.

TPM3, TPM4, CLTC) are common in examples diagnosed in children and young adults.

The differential diagnosis also includes an amyloid tumor. Amyloidomas contain abundant amorphous eosinophilic material that may be randomly deposited as well as concentrated around blood vessels. This material is frequently bordered by multinucleated giant cells, and sometimes contains foci with osseous or chondro-osseous metaplasia. A lymphoplasmacytic infiltrate is typically present. Histochemical stains for amyloid (Congo red, Sirius red) are confirmatory.

Reactive nodular fibrous pseudotumor of the gastrointestinal tract and mesentery is generally less well-marginated and has more variable cellularity than calcifying fibrous (pseudo)tumor (169,170). The former typically occurs in adults and is associated with some recognizable insult to the abdominal cavity, such as prior surgical intervention, bowel perforation, or pancreatitis. Cellularity ranges from very low to moderate, but there are characteristically some foci with activated myofibroblasts that have immunoreactivity for actins and sometimes desmin. Hyalinized or keloid-like collagen may be present, but psammomatous calcifications are usually absent. We have seen cases of peritoneal leiomyomatosis, endometriosis, and pelvic inflammatory disease associated with calcifying fibrous (pseudo)tumor-like findings, and these diagnoses also have to be excluded.

Treatment and Prognosis. Calcifying fibrous (pseudo)tumor has a low local recurrence rate (less than 10 percent) when marginally excised. Simple local excision appears to be adequate intervention in most cases. An excision with a margin of normal tissue is justifiable in instances where this can be accomplished without additional morbidity. Recurrent disease is not destructive and carries no risk of metastasis.

JUVENILE HYALINE FIBROMATOSIS

Definition. *Juvenile hyaline fibromatosis* is a non-neoplastic, autosomal recessive disorder that presents in infancy or within the first few years of life and is characterized by the deposition of extracellular, amorphous, eosinophilic hyaline material in the skin, somatic soft tissues, and skeleton. *Infantile systemic hyalinosis* is a closely related allelic condition with similar histology but a rapidly progressive clinical course. Synonyms include *fibromatosis hyalinica multiplex (juvenilis), juvenile systemic hyalinosis, Puretic syndrome*, and *Murray syndrome*.

Clinical Features. Juvenile hyaline fibromatosis affects males and females with equal frequency (171). More than one fourth of the reported patients have consanguineous parents, and sibling cases make up almost 40 percent of the total (171). Approximately one fourth of the documented patients have been Japanese (171).

Juvenile hyaline fibromatosis is always clinically evident by 4 years of age (172–177). The disease often manifests in early infancy and may be evident at birth. The most common presenting feature is flexion contractures (mean onset, about 2 months), followed by gingival hypertrophy (mean onset, about 8 months), and skin and subcutaneous lesions (mean onset, about 22 months) (171). The flexion contractures most often involve the knees and elbows, but other joints may also be affected. The first skin lesions are usually small, pearly white papules, commonly located on the face and neck (178). These may coalesce to form plaques and nodules, particularly on and around the ears, nose, and tips of the digits. Subcutaneous nodules may develop on the scalp, trunk, and extremities. Some lesions ulcerate or develop dystrophic calcification. Occasionally, perianal papules are an early presenting feature (179,180).

Bony abnormalities, including lytic lesions, cortical erosions, and osteoporosis, are also common. The patients characteristically have a normal IQ. Although progressively debilitating, individuals with this disease survive well into adulthood.

Infantile systemic hyalinosis is a much more severe process, with diffusely thickened skin, extensive visceral involvement, intestinal symptoms, recurrent infections, and generally, a rapidly fatal outcome (typically within the first 2 years of life) (181–185).

Gross Findings. Superficial lesions are dome-shaped and attenuate the overlying skin. The cut surface often reveals a circumscribed, solid, off-white to pinkish tan mass that ranges from soft and friable to firm in consistency. Some lesions are translucent.

Microscopic Findings. Individual nodules are often well-demarcated but nonencapsulated. Small early lesions often have high cellularity, whereas larger, more longstanding

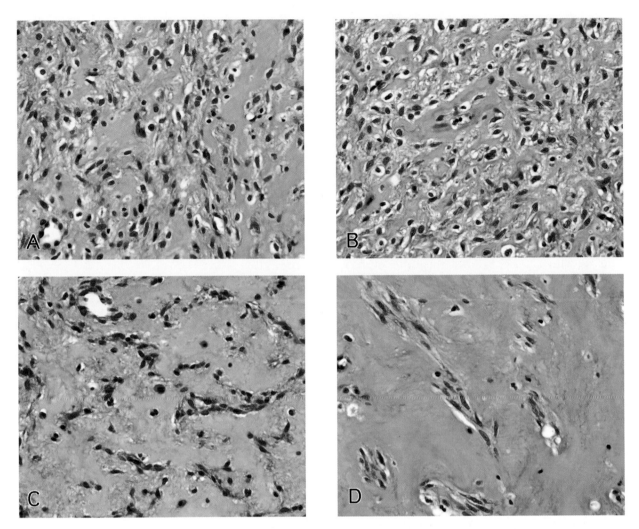

Figure 2-45

JUVENILE HYALINE FIBROMATOSIS

A–D: Bland mesenchymal cells are embedded in a hyaline matrix. Cellularity ranges from moderate to low.

lesions have less cellularity. The process is typified by an abundance of amorphous eosinophilic hyaline extracellular matrix, with some wavy filamentous elements (figs. 2-45, 2-46). Within the matrix are ovoid and spindled (fibroblast-like) mesenchymal cells, present individually and in parallel and interconnecting cords, and sometimes associated with capillary-sized vessels. These mesenchymal cells have bland nuclei and amphophilic to eosinophilic cytoplasm. An accumulation of eosinophilic material within the cytoplasm of some cells resembles extracellular matrix. Mitotic figures are inconspicuous. Also evident are scattered inflammatory cells, including conventional

histiocytes, siderophages, and infrequent lymphocytes. Some of the histiocytic cells have prominent clear cytoplasmic vacuoles that, in the context of abundant extracellular matrix, may lead to a false impression of lacunar spaces and cartilaginous differentiation (186).

Special Studies. The extracellular amorphous hyaline material is PAS positive and diastase resistant. The mesenchymal cells are negative for α-smooth muscle actin, desmin, CD34, and S-100 protein (171,186).

Genetics. This process has been linked to mutations in a gene on chromosome 4q21 that encodes capillary morphogenesis protein 2 (CMG2) (182,187,188). The gene is upregulated

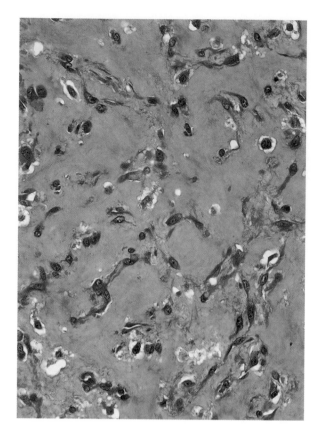
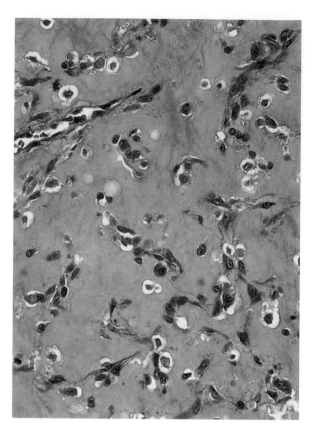

Figure 2-46

JUVENILE HYALINE FIBROMATOSIS

Left, Right: The dense hyalinized matrix, scattered small vessels, spindled mesenchymal cells, and inflammatory cells, including histiocytes, are seen at high power.

in endothelial cells induced to undergo capillary formation. The gene product is a type 1 transmembrane protein with a von Willebrand factor type A extracellular domain that shows strong binding to laminin and collagen IV. These observations suggest CMG2 has an important role in basement membrane matrix assembly and that abnormalities in this protein may lead to leakage of plasma proteins through the capillary basement membrane into the surrounding soft tissue. A variety of different mutations in *CMG2* have been observed, which helps explain the wide phenotypic variability of the disease. While mutation class and position are not fully sufficient to account for all clinical variability, milder forms of juvenile hyaline fibromatosis appear to be linked to in-frame and missense mutations that affect the novel cytoplasmic domain of CMG2, whereas mutations affecting the von Willebrand factor type A extracellular domain

tend to result in more severe disease, analogous to infantile systemic hyalinosis (182).

Differential Diagnosis. The clinical features of juvenile hyaline fibromatosis, coupled with the histopathology, are distinctive. In the absence of a history, myofibroma(tosis) may be considered, but this process features a well-developed, smooth muscle actin-positive spindle cell element, zonated around a well-vascularized, sometimes CD34-positive, pericyte-like component.

Treatment and Prognosis. Juvenile hyaline fibromatosis is a progressive disorder (176,177,179). Treatment is palliative, directed at the relief of local symptoms (176,177,179,180).

FIBROMATOSIS COLLI

Definition. *Fibromatosis colli* is a disease exclusive to infants and children, and characterized by the partial replacement of the sternocleidomastoid muscle by a benign, mass-forming (myo)fibroblastic proliferation. The proliferation regresses spontaneously, but in some instances, is associated with scar formation and muscle shortening, leading to congenital muscular torticollis ("wry neck"). Synonyms include *congenital muscular torticollis* and *pseudotumor of infancy*.

General Considerations. This uncommon process affects 0.4 percent of live births (189, 190). Its etiology is unresolved and may be multifactorial (191–198). The leading theories propose a link to intrauterine crowding and fetal malposition, compromising the vascular supply of the sternocleidomastoid muscle (195) and causing hypoxic tissue injury (more or less a compartment syndrome) (192,193). Less favored theories suggest origin by way of post-traumatic peripartum bleeding with secondary fibrosis, muscle rupture during labor and delivery, or an infectious myopathy. A limited number of familial cases of fibromatosis colli have been reported, but specific genetic information is not currently available (194,197–199). It is important to remember that most cases of fibromatosis colli do not progress to (congenital) muscular torticollis, and that there are a great many causes (more than 80) for muscular torticollis apart from fibromatosis colli (190,193).

Ultrasound is the modality of choice for radiologic evaluation of this disease (193,200). MRI is not recommended for asymptomatic torticollis in an infant, as general anesthesia or sedation would be required, but may have a role in evaluating cases that persist after 12 months of age (200,201).

Clinical Features. Fibromatosis colli affects males and females with approximately equal frequency (189,196,202). Many clinical studies have shown that patients with fibromatosis colli/congenital muscular torticollis are more likely to be first-born children (192,193,199), and the products of a difficult labor and delivery (192,193,199,202,203). Breech presentations have been documented in up to 60 percent of patients (193), and there is an increased incidence of other musculoskeletal positional abnormalities, including developmental dysplasia of the hip (3 to 20 percent of patients), metatarsus adductus, and talipes equinovarus (192,193,196,202–204).

Patients generally appear normal at birth but develop a hard, mobile (often fusiform) mass, with or without tenderness, within the substance of the sternocleidomastoid muscle (usually the lower half), 2 weeks to 2 months later (191,192,195,202,204). Initially, the mass grows fairly rapidly. Then it stabilizes, involutes and disappears over a course of 2 to 8 months (189,191,195,196). Most cases resolve without significant sequelae. Some patients, however, develop torticollis (i.e., a shortened sternocleidomastoid muscle on the affected side with ipsilateral tilting and contralateral rotation of the head), which becomes more apparent with age as the neck lengthens but is tethered on the side with the mass (189,196).

Some patients with congenital muscular torticollis have no history of a transient mass (fibromatosis colli) within the substance of the sternocleidomastoid muscle. For some of these individuals, the mass may have been small and short lived, so that it was overlooked by both parents and pediatrician (189,195).

Gross Findings. It is uncommon to encounter a surgical specimen of fibromatosis colli, because conservative management is widely advocated during the first year of life. Archival specimens typically reveal a 1- to 3-cm, firm, ovoid to fusiform mass within the body of the sternocleidomastoid muscle (195). The cut surface ranges from white to pinkish white, depending on the amount of residual skeletal muscle incorporated within the mass. The interface between lesional tissue and normal muscle is blurred.

Microscopic Findings. The histologic appearance varies with the stage of the process, but examination generally reveals a bland, mildly to moderately cellular, myofibroblastic proliferation with loose myxocollagenous to densely collagenous extracellular matrix (figs. 2-47, 2-48). Varying numbers of degenerating and regenerating skeletal muscle myocytes are incorporated within the mass. The process is confined to the sternocleidomastoid muscle, and often exhibits vague multinodularity due to a tendency to obey normal architectural planes within the muscle. There is no nuclear atypia or pleomorphism, and mitotic figures are usually uncommon and never abnormal. Caution is advised not to overinterpret pyknotic coalesced myocyte nuclei as evidence of atypia. There is usually only a small amount of hemosiderin deposition, and chronic inflammatory cells are uncommon and primarily perivascular in location.

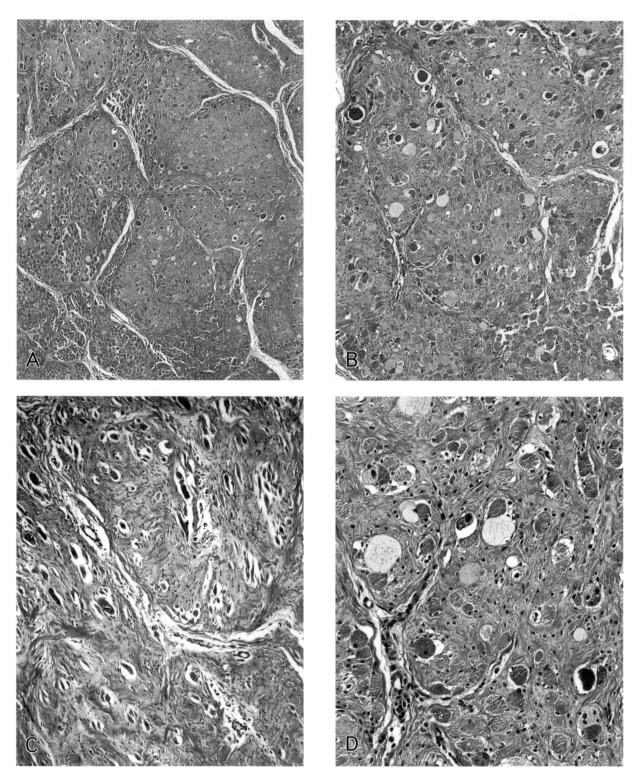

Figure 2-47

FIBROMATOSIS COLLI

Low (A), intermediate (B,C), and high (D) power views show a collagenized spindle cell proliferation with bland cytologic features, a vaguely lobular growth pattern, and entrapment of skeletal muscle fibers.

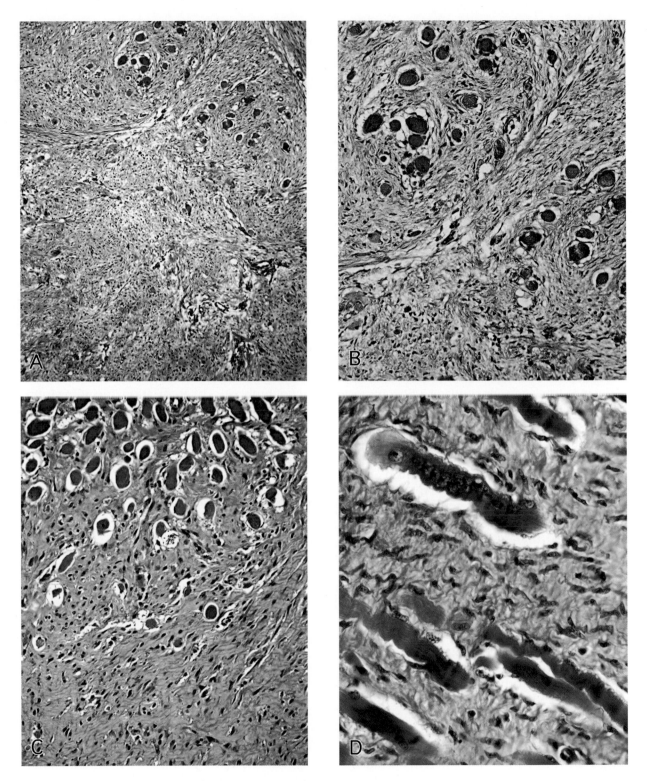

Figure 2-48

FIBROMATOSIS COLLI

Low (A), intermediate (B,C), and high (D) power views illustrate a uniform population of spindle cells with bland cytomorphologic features and entrapment of skeletal muscle fibers. The latter may exhibit degenerative or regenerative features.

Fine needle aspiration cytology, although rarely required for diagnosis, may have some value in selected instances (205,206). Focal immunoreactivity may be present for smooth muscle actin. Nuclear β-catenin expression is absent in the few cases studied to date (207,208).

Differential Diagnosis. The key considerations in the differential diagnosis are desmoid-type fibromatosis, proliferative fasciitis, and fibrosing inflammatory myositis. Desmoid tumors are clinically aggressive neoplasms that tend not to obey normal anatomic boundaries and are almost never confined to the body of the sternocleidomastoid muscle. These tumors contain mildly atypical myofibroblasts with infiltrative and destructive growth. While some myocyte preservation can be present at the periphery of a desmoid tumor, this is not generally encountered centrally. Approximately 80 percent of desmoid-type fibromatoses express nuclear β-catenin.

Proliferative fasciitis preserves skeletal muscle myocytes in a manner similar to fibromatosis colli, but it features an admixture of plump spindled and ganglion cell-like (myo)fibroblasts, set in a loose myxocollagenous matrix. Postinflammatory myositis has more pronounced inflammation than fibromatosis colli.

Treatment and Prognosis. Approximately 70 percent of fibromatosis colli patients, when managed conservatively with observation and physical therapy (possible bracing), have spontaneous resolution of their disease during the first year of life with no significant deficit (192,193,196,202). Conservative intervention is less effective if instituted after the first year of life (192,196,202–204). Surgical intervention (primarily a tenotomy with temporary postoperative bracing) is generally reserved for children over 1 year of age with severe involvement, who have failed a trial of physical therapy (189,192,196,202,204). Botulinum toxin type A has been used with some success as an experimental treatment for recalcitrant disease, but there are associated risks, and long-term results are not currently available (193,209,210). If left uncorrected, muscular torticollis can, in some instances, lead to craniofacial asymmetry, scoliosis, and other problems (189,191,195,202,203).

INFANTILE DIGITAL FIBROMA/FIBROMATOSIS

Definition. *Infantile digital fibroma/fibromatosis* is a benign superficial myofibroblastic tumor with almost exclusive occurrence in the fingers and toes of infants and young children. In most cases, the lesional cells contain eosinophilic intracytoplasmic inclusion bodies. Synonyms are *inclusion body fibromatosis* and *recurring digital fibrous tumor of childhood*.

General Considerations. We support the term infantile digital fibroma over the more recently proposed "inclusion body fibromatosis" (211) because classic examples are largely restricted to the fingers and toes of infants and young children. While cytoplasmic inclusion bodies are a frequent and characteristic feature of this process, they are not absolutely essential for diagnosis (212,213), and outside of the proper clinicopathologic setting, their presence is not specific for this disorder. Similar inclusions occur in toxic oil (epidemic) syndrome, true smooth muscle tumors, and a variety of unrelated soft tissue tumors with myofibroblastic differentiation, including intranodal myofibroblastoma, "fibroepithelial" and phyllodes tumors of the breast, and gynecologic stromal proliferations (214–218).

Clinical Features. This nonfamilial process usually affects infants in the first year of life (fig. 2-49) (212,219–222). One fifth to one third of cases are evident at birth. Less than 20 percent of patients present after 3 years of age. There is no clear sex predilection (213,219,222,223). The process tends to present as a painless, firm, erythematous, dome-shaped mass, usually less than 2 cm in size, on the distal dorsal or dorsolateral aspect of a digit (fig. 2-50). The second through fifth digits are the key sites of involvement, with only rare examples reported elsewhere on the hands and feet (213,221,224,225). The thumb and great toe are almost always spared (212,213,221,222,225). Synchronous or metachronous multifocality is common (213,221–223). Some examples interfere with function and cause bone erosion and joint abnormalities.

Gross and Microscopic Findings. Surgical specimens tend to consist of small, dome-shaped pieces of skin with firm, off-white underlying soft tissue. Histologic examination reveals a poorly demarcated fibrogenic spindle cell proliferation composed of myofibroblasts

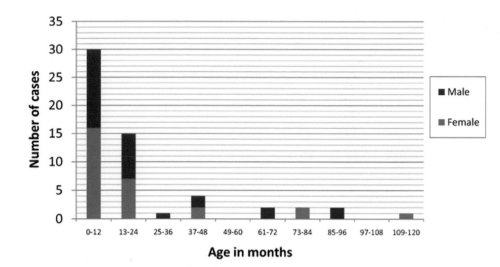

Figure 2-49

INFANTILE DIGITAL FIBROMA/ FIBROMATOSIS

Age and sex distribution at first surgery for 57 patients with infantile digital fibroma/fibromatosis reviewed at the AFIP.

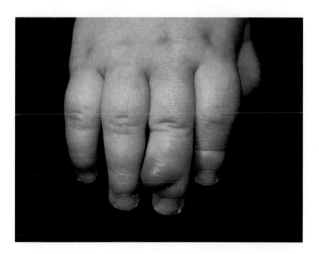

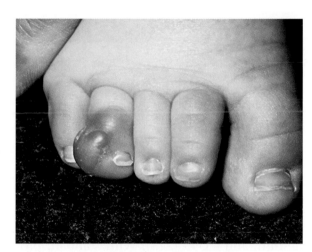

Figure 2-50

INFANTILE DIGITAL FIBROMA/FIBROMATOSIS

A finger (left) and toe (right) are involved.

that form short, randomly intersecting fascicles and cause nodular expansion of the dermis and elevation and attenuation of the overlying epidermis (figs. 2-51, 2-52) (213). The process infiltrates the underlying subcutis and sometimes extends into deeper structures. Lesional cells have elongated nuclei with vesicular chromatin, a small nucleolus, and eosinophilic, vaguely fibrillary, cytoplasm with ill-defined cell borders. In over 80 percent of cases, some spindle cells contain variably sized (usually 3 to 10 μm in diameter; range: 1.5 to 24.0 μm), often juxtanuclear, spherical, intracytoplasmic inclusions with a hyaline pink tinctorial qual-

ity (fig. 2-53) (212, 213). Infrequent cases lack inclusions, or there may be inclusions in one specimen but not others (212,213). Mitotic figures are infrequent.

Special Studies. The characteristic cytoplasmic inclusions in the spindle cell population stain red with the Gomori (fig. 2-53C) and Masson (fig. 2-53D) trichrome stains, deep purple with the phosphotungstic acid-hematoxylin stain, and dark purple to black with an iron hematoxylin stain. The inclusions are PAS and alcian blue negative. The lesional myofibroblasts are immunoreactive for α-smooth muscle actin (often with a "tram-track" pattern), calponin,

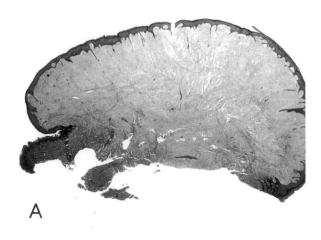

A

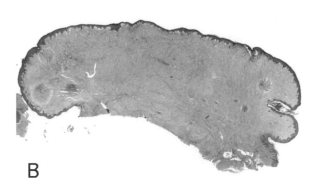

B

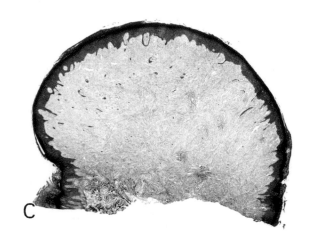

C

Figure 2-51

INFANTILE DIGITAL FIBROMA/FIBROMATOSIS

A–C: Biopsy specimens typically contain a polypoid piece of skin with an expanded dermis (A,B: hematoxylin and eosin [H&E] stain; C: trichrome stain).

desmin, and CD99 (213). With standard processing, the cytoplasmic inclusions are often negative for the aforementioned myoid markers, although a rim of accentuated reactivity may be evident at their periphery (213,226–228). With alcohol-fixed tissue (229,230) or formalin-fixed tissue pretreated with potassium hydroxide (KOH) (in 70 percent alcohol) and trypsin (227), however, the inclusions are actin positive. Nuclear immunoreactivity for β-catenin is usually absent (213).

Ultrastructurally, the inclusions consist of intracytoplasmic, nonmembrane-bound, spherical matted masses of thin filamentous material, admixed with some irregular vesicular and granular structures (228,231–234). Continuity between the inclusion bodies and cytoplasmic actin filaments is often demonstrable.

Differential Diagnosis. Fibrous histiocytomas have a more heterogeneous population of mononucleated and multinucleated cells that characteristically produce stellate-shaped nodules associated with epidermal hyperplasia. Desmoid-type fibromatosis and infantile fibrosarcoma produce more deep-seated masses, and the latter has greater cellularity, mitotic activity, and atypia. Palmar/plantar fibromatosis is characteristically epicentered in an aponeurosis on the ventral or ventrolateral aspect of the hand or foot. True smooth muscle tumors usually contain larger cells with more abundant cytoplasm, and they often have substantial reactivity for h-caldesmon and smooth muscle myosin.

Terminal osseous dysplasia/pigmentary defects syndrome (digitocutaneous dysplasia syndrome/digital fibroma syndrome) (235–237) is an X-linked (male lethal) syndrome that features digital fibromas with a remarkable clinical similarity to those seen in infantile digital fibroma/fibromatosis. However, the digital lesions

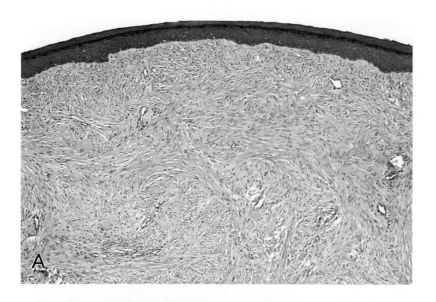

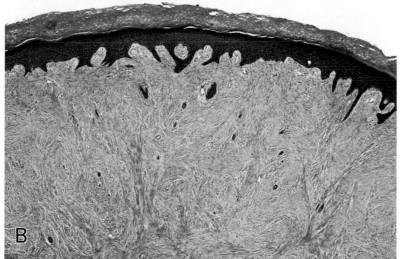

Figure 2-52

INFANTILE DIGITAL FIBROMA/FIBROMATOSIS

Low (A,B) and intermediate (C) power views show an expanded dermis with a bland spindle cell proliferation that exhibits broad storiform and short fascicular growth patterns and contains abundant collagen.

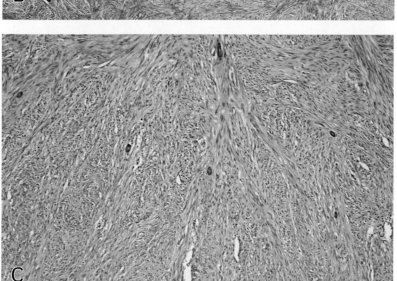

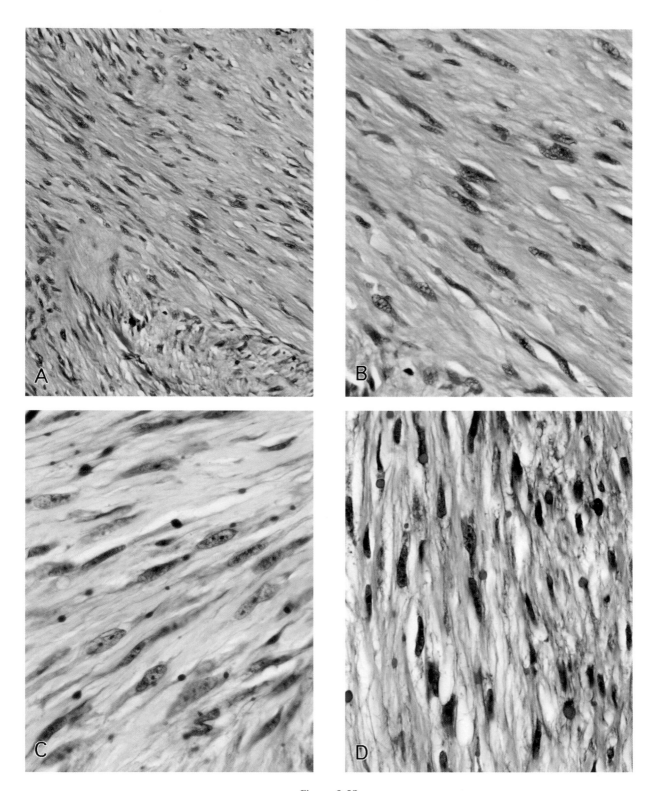

Figure 2-53

INFANTILE DIGITAL FIBROMA/FIBROMATOSIS

Intermediate (A) and high (B–D) power views show bland spindle cells and typical (often juxtanuclear) cytoplasmic inclusions. These inclusions may be highlighted with Gomori (C) and Masson (D) trichrome stains.

have spindle cells that lack inclusions and are apparently nonreactive for actin (236,237). Additionally, all syndromic patients are females who have numerous other clinical manifestations including facial, skeletal, and skin abnormalities. Reported facial abnormalities include iris colobomas, midface hypoplasia, hypertelorism, and eyelid irregularities; skeletal features include distal limb defects such as metacarpal/metatarsal disorganization, brachydactyly/hypodactyly, camptodactyly, and syndactyly; skin changes include punched-out pigmentation defects over the face and scalp, and skin atrophy.

Treatment and Prognosis. Recurrences develop in more than 60 percent of cases, and new lesions may develop in the same or other digits (213,219,220,222). The adequacy of the initial surgical procedure seems to correlate with the rate of recurrence, as lower recurrence rates are reported in some studies where patients have had wider excisions (sometimes with skin grafting and flap placement) (212,213,225). Many experts manage these lesions more conservatively, however, because recurrences are not usually destructive, tumor growth may stabilize over time, some examples spontaneously regress (213,224,238–240), and there are inherent risks associated with more aggressive surgical intervention. More extensive surgery is reserved for lesions that show continued growth and are at risk for causing functional impairment. There are no reports of malignant transformation.

CALCIFYING APONEUROTIC FIBROMA

Definition. *Calcifying aponeurotic fibroma* is a benign soft tissue tumor that occurs predominantly in childhood and has a notable predilection for hands and feet. The tumor features a fibromatosis-like spindle cell component and variable numbers of epithelioid fibroblasts, often associated with scattered distinctive chondrocalcific nodules. *Juvenile aponeurotic fibroma* is synonymous.

General Considerations. This tumor has many features of, and has sometimes been viewed as, a variant of fibromatosis, but the "fibroma" designation is preferred because a predilection for local recurrence, the process generally does not cause tumor-associated deficits, growth often slows over time, and some examples undergo involution.

Clinical Features. Calcifying aponeurotic fibromas have been reported in individuals ranging from under 1 to 67 years of age (241, 242). The peak incidence, however, is in the first decade of life between the ages 6 and 10 years (median age, 12 years), and examples documented after the age of 20 years are rare (fig. 2-54, top) (241). In the AFIP files, the male to female ratio approximates 2 to 1.

The tumor has a strong predilection for the fingers and palm of the hand, but the wrist, plantar surface of the foot, and ankle region are also well-recognized sites of involvement (fig. 2-54, bottom). Less common locations include the lumbosacral area of the back, knee, thigh, forearm, and elbow (241–243). The process is usually less than 3 cm in size and often presents as a nontender mass that involves or encompasses tendon, fascia, aponeurosis, and skeletal muscle. Stippled intralesional calcifications may be evident in radiologic studies (243,244).

Gross Findings. Gross examination reveals a rubbery to firm, off-white mass. Most examples have an irregular contour, but some have a deceptively well-demarcated nodular appearance. The cut surface is often gritty (dependent on the amount of intralesional calcification), and minute granular or chalky areas may be visible to the naked eye (241,243).

Microscopic Findings. This is a spindle cell tumor with randomly intersecting fascicles of (myo)fibroblasts that infiltrate fat, skeletal muscle, and dense regular connective tissue and entrap neurovascular bundles (figs. 2-55, 2-56). Variable numbers of epithelioid or ovoid mesenchymal cells (probably of fibroblastic derivation) are often present and may be loosely grouped into small nests or arranged in parallel cords (figs. 2-56; 2-57A,B). Additionally, most cases contain scattered chondrocalcific nodules, frequently bordered by short radiating columns of plump epithelioid fibroblastic cells and occasional osteoclast-like giant cells (fig. 2-57). Some of these nodules have frank ossification, and rarely, become cystic. In the rare instance where chondrocalcific nodules are absent, the parallel arrays of epithelioid fibroblasts are a helpful clue to the correct diagnosis. Mitotic activity is typically 2 or fewer mitoses per 10 high-power fields.

There are isolated reports of calcifying aponeurotic fibroma undergoing transformation to

63

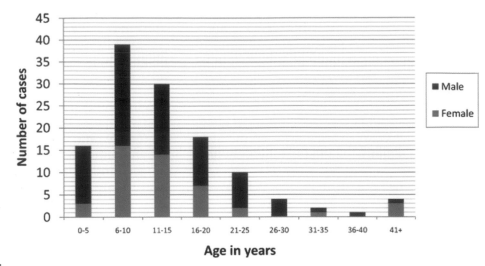

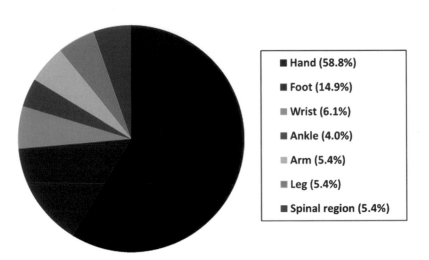

Figure 2-54

CALCIFYING APONEUROTIC FIBROMA

Age and sex (top) and anatomic (bottom) distributions of cases of calcifying aponeurotic fibroma reviewed at the AFIP.

fibrosarcoma (245). We have not been able to identify a single example of this occurrence in the AFIP files and view reported examples with some skepticism.

Special Studies. Immunoreactivity is present, to a varying degree, for actins, CD99, and S-100 protein (241). The last is primarily expressed by chondrocytes within the matrix-producing nodules. Examined tumors have lacked desmin and keratin expression.

Differential Diagnosis. The differential diagnosis includes desmoid-type fibromatosis, palmar/plantar fibromatosis, fibrosarcoma, and synovial sarcoma. Desmoid tumors are rare on palmar and plantar surfaces. Most acral desmoid tumors are dorsally located on the extensor aspect of the hand or foot. These tumors have sheet-like

cell growth with broad fascicular and storiform arrays. They lack parallel cords of plump epithelioid fibroblasts and scattered chondrocalcific nodules. Palmar/plantar fibromatosis is rare in childhood. This process features a multinodular proliferation of myofibroblasts, centered in, and often confined to, the aponeurosis. Fibrosarcoma is an infiltrative, destructive tumor with greater cellularity and mitotic activity than calcifying aponeurotic fibroma. This neoplasm classically exhibits herringbone growth, and may have tumor necrosis. Synovial sarcoma may arise in the same age group and anatomic sites as calcifying aponeurotic fibroma, but this entity usually has focal immunoreactivity for keratin and EMA, and it has a characteristic t(X;18) with *SS18-SSX* fusion transcripts.

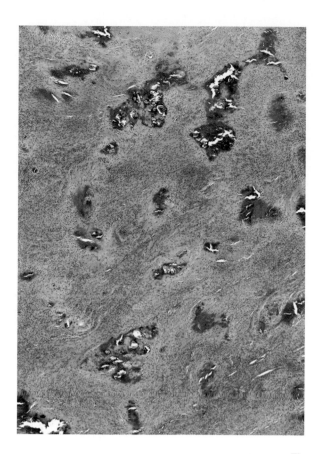 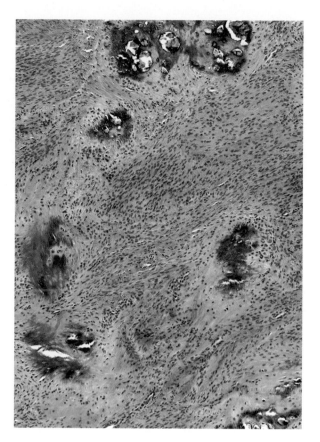

Figure 2-55

CALCIFYING APONEUROTIC FIBROMA

Left, Right: Scattered chondrocalcific nodules are within a fibromatosis-like spindle cell proliferation.

Treatment and Prognosis. Calcifying aponeurotic fibroma is managed with conservative, but as complete as possible, function-preserving intervention, because tumor growth slows over time, there is spontaneous regression, recurrent tumors are not aggressive, and local morbidity is more often an iatrogenic consequence than a direct result of the neoplasm. Conservative excision, however, is associated with a 50 percent local recurrence rate (241,242). The first recurrence usually manifests within 3 years of surgical intervention, but it may take 10 or more years for a recurrence to become clinically apparent. The risk of local recurrence is greatest for patients less than 5 years of age (241).

FIBROUS HAMARTOMA OF INFANCY

Definition. *Fibrous hamartoma of infancy* is a benign pediatric soft tissue tumor (probably neoplasm) that typically forms a superficial mass with three main components: mature fat, a fibromatosis-like spindle cell element with trabecular growth, and scattered small nodules of primitive mesenchymal cells embedded in a myxoid matrix. *Subdermal fibromatous tumor of infancy* is synonymous.

Clinical Features. This nonfamilial process has a male to female ratio of 1.8-2.4 to 1 (fig. 2-58, top) (246). Twenty-three percent of cases are congenital, and approximately 91 percent are evident within the first year of life (246). Only 4 percent of patients present after 2 years of age. Examples are widely distributed (fig. 2-58, bottom), but the most common locations are the axilla, upper arm, upper trunk, inguinal area, and external genitalia (246–250). The head and distal portions of the extremities are uncommon sites, and involvement of a hand or foot is so rare that, in these locations, the diagnosis warrants a healthy dose of skepticism until

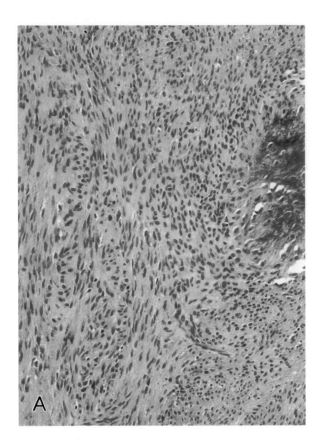

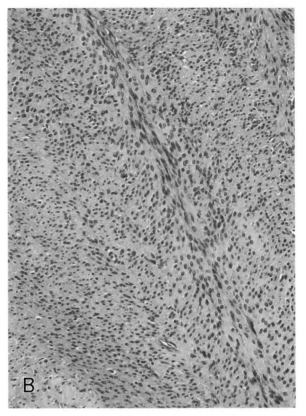

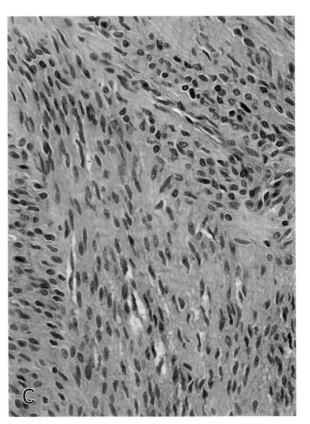

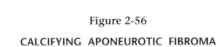

Figure 2-56

CALCIFYING APONEUROTIC FIBROMA

In the fibromatosis-like spindle cell component of calcifying aponeurotic fibroma, the epithelioid fibroblasts are in linear arrays (A–C). The latter cells are an important clue to the diagnosis in early stage lesions in which chondrocalcific nodules may be absent (B,C).

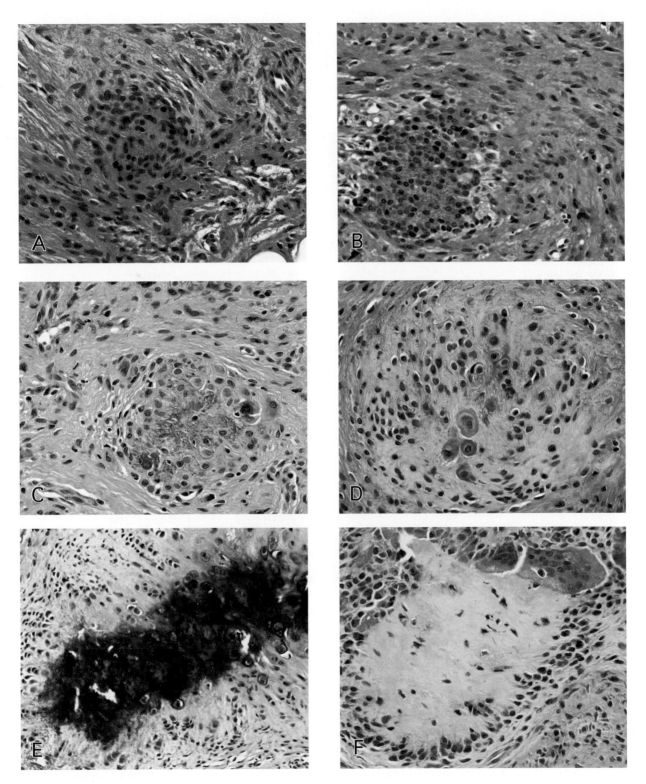

Figure 2-57

CALCIFYING APONEUROTIC FIBROMA

Different stages of the chondrocalcific nodules in calcifying aponeurotic fibroma: early stages (A,B), mature nodules (C,D), and more advanced stages (E,F). A giant cell reaction is seen (F).

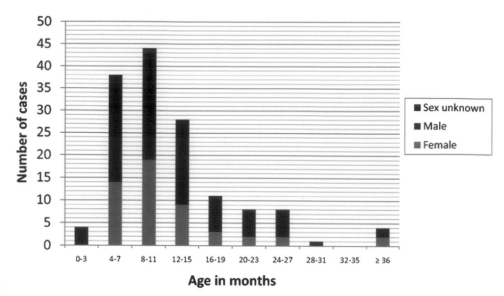

Figure 2-58

FIBROUS HAMARTOMA OF INFANCY

Top: Age and sex distribution of 146 patients with fibrous hamartomas of infancy reviewed at the AFIP.

Bottom: The anatomic distribution of 159 histologically confirmed cases from the same institution.

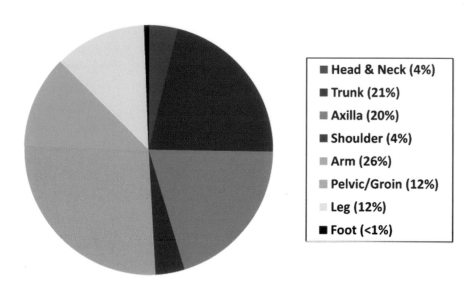

corroborated. There are no examples of fibrous hamartoma of infancy involving a hand and only one involving a foot in the AFIP files.

Most lesions present as a solitary mass centered in the subcutis, sometimes extending into the lower dermis or underlying soft tissue. Rarely, there are changes in the overlying skin, including alterations in pigmentation and increased or coarsened hair (246,250). The tumors are usually painless or only mildly tender to palpation. Initial growth can be rapid, but the rate of growth slows with age. There is no tendency for spontaneous regression (246,251). Four cases have been described as multifocal,

although in some instances, this may have only been a clinical perception (246,251,252).

Gross Findings. Gross examination reveals a poorly marginated mass composed of yellow fat admixed with an irregularly distributed gray-white fibrous element. Examples range in size from 0.5 to 20.0 cm, with an average tumor size of less than 5 cm (246,247,249–251,253).

Microscopic Findings. This poorly demarcated tumor is commonly viewed as having three main components: mature fat; a bland spindle cell element that forms interlacing collagen-rich fascicles; and scattered, small, nodular foci with primitive stellate- and spindle-shaped cells (with or without whorled growth) embedded in a richly vascular myxoid matrix (figs. 2-59–2-61). Zones of dense hyalinized or wiry collagen with admixed spindle cells, referred to in the literature as keloid-like or likened to changes encountered in a neurofibroma ("neurofibroma-like fibrosis"), occur in older children (fig. 2-62) (247,250,253). The proportion of each element varies and one or more of the classic features may be absent, especially in biopsy samples. Nuclear atypia is minimal, and in most cases, mitotic figures are rare.

Special Studies. The spindled fibromatosis-like component is often focally immunoreactive for actin (249,254). Desmin is only rarely expressed (249,253–255). There is no immunoreactivity for myoglobin, cytokeratin, or neurofilament protein (253,254). S-100 protein expression is limited to the adipocytic element. There is question about the diagnosis of cases with published genetic data (256,257), and we view these data with skepticism.

Differential Diagnosis. The differential diagnosis includes lipofibromatosis, desmoid type fibromatosis, calcifying aponeurotic fibroma, and neurofibroma. None of these tumors contain the small myxoid nodules with primitive mesenchymal cells encountered in fibrous hamartoma of infancy. In lipofibromatosis, the fibromatosis-like spindle cell component generally has a more orderly distribution, with a notable tendency to be concentrated within fat septa. Since some fibrous hamartomas of infancy contain areas that closely resemble lipofibromatosis (fig. 2-63), careful sampling is required to identify the distinguishing diagnostic features.

Desmoid-type fibromatosis does not contain an integral fatty component. It is typically intimately associated with fascia and forms a solid, fairly homogeneous, infiltrative mass characterized by sheets of broad, collagen-rich intersecting fascicles. Calcifying aponeurotic fibromas have a notable predilection for acral sites. These tumors feature a fibromatosis-like element with variable numbers of epithelioid fibroblasts and scattered chondrocalcific nodules. Neurofibromas contain S-100 protein–positive neoplastic Schwann cells admixed with CD34-positive fibroblasts and, possibly, residual axons.

Treatment and Prognosis. Local excision, preferably with a small margin of normal tissue if this can be accomplished with minimal morbidity, is optimal. Local recurrences occur in approximately 12 percent of patients, with an average time interval to recurrence of 5.4 months (range, 2 to 11 months) (246). Only 1.3 percent of patients have more than one local recurrence. There are no reports of malignant transformation.

MYOFIBROMA/MYOFIBROMATOSIS

Definition. *Myofibroma,* a solitary, or *myofibromatosis,* a multicentric, process characteristically exhibits biphasic morphology with peripheral nodules of spindled (myoid) cells and centrally located, less differentiated, round to oval cells with a hemangiopericytoma-like vascular pattern. Synonyms for the infantile systemic form are *congenital generalized fibromatosis* and *infantile myofibromatosis.*

General Considerations. This process is solitary (258–262) or multicentric, with or without visceral organ involvement (262–266). The clinicopathologic features overlap with those of infantile hemangiopericytoma (267–270). A derivation from primitive perivascular fibroblast-like cells capable of myofibroblastic or pericytic differentiation has been proposed.

Clinical Features. Myofibromas are seen at any age, from newborn to late adult life, but the peak incidence is in the first decade (fig. 2-64). More than 90 percent of childhood cases are evident by 2 years of age and 60 percent are clinically apparent in the neonate (271). Adult cases are widely distributed through all decades. A male predominance is noted for both solitary and multicentric forms of the disease (272).

The tumors most commonly affect the head and neck region, followed by the trunk and extremities (fig. 2-65). It is estimated that 70 to 80 percent of patients present with solitary lesions and the remainder have multicentric disease (271). Patients with multicentric disease usually have lesions clinically apparent at birth, and just over one third of infants with multiple lesions have visceral involvement (272).

Approximately half of all solitary lesions present as superficial masses involving the skin or subcutis (271,272). Most of the remaining cases involve deep soft tissue sites such as skeletal muscle. Approximately 9 percent of solitary lesions involve bone, and rarely, visceral sites (e.g., the larynx or gastrointestinal tract) (272).

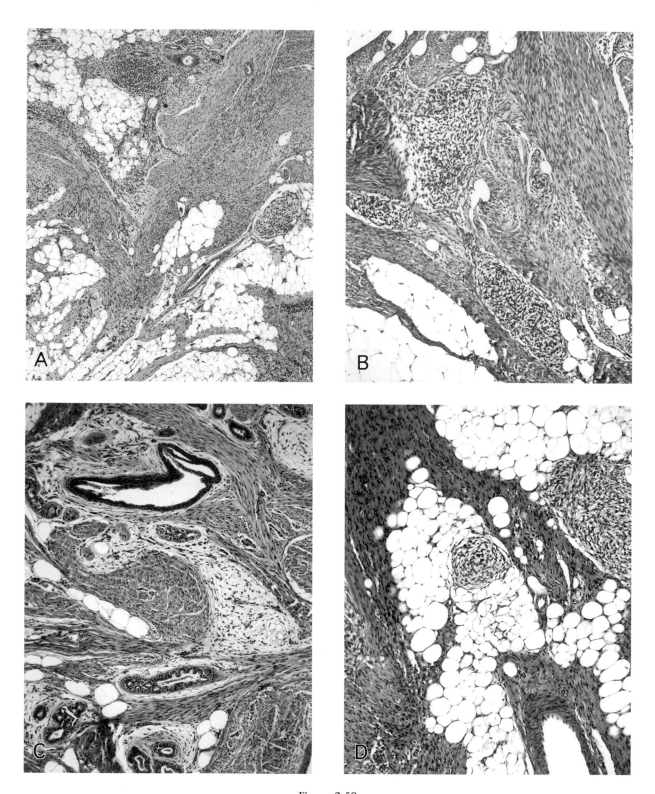

Figure 2-59

FIBROUS HAMARTOMA OF INFANCY

A–D: Several fibrous hamartomas of infancy illustrate mature fat, a fibromatosis-like spindle cell component, and bluish myxoid mesenchymal nodules with primitive stellate- and spindle-shaped cells.

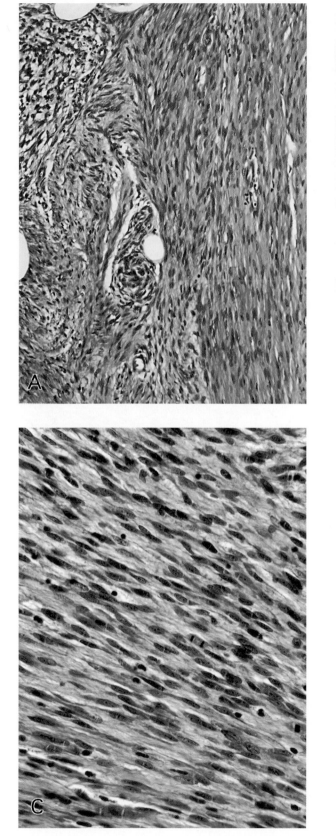

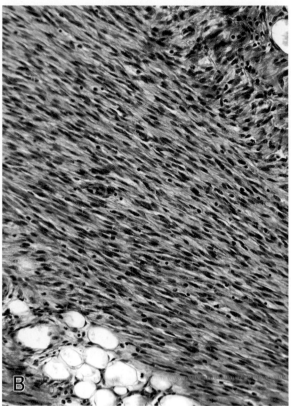

Figure 2-60

FIBROUS HAMARTOMA OF INFANCY

The fibromatosis-like element of the tumor is seen here. This component usually has low to moderate cellularity and a low mitotic rate (A,B). Infrequent examples, however, contain areas with increased cellularity and notable mitotic activity (C).

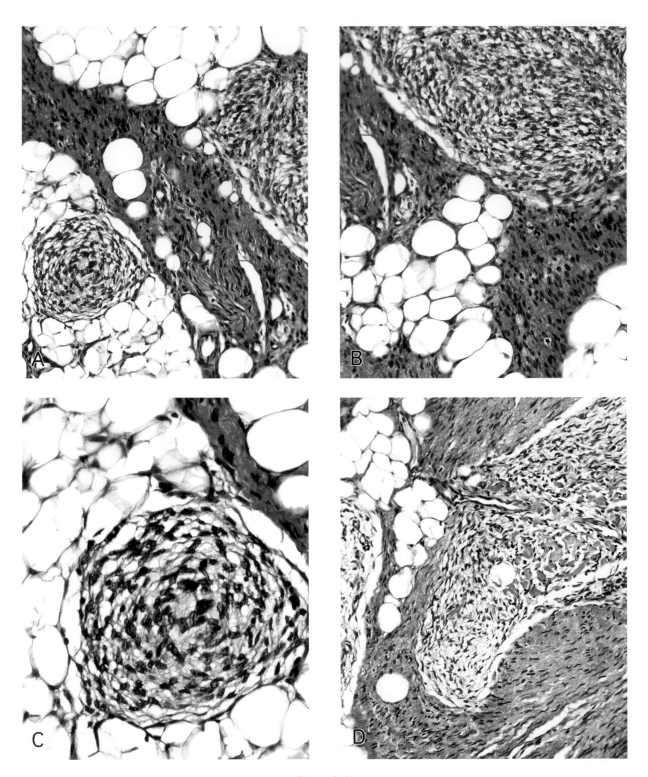

Figure 2-61

FIBROUS HAMARTOMA OF INFANCY

The primitive myxoid mesenchymal nodules frequently exhibit a whorled growth pattern (A–C). These nodules vary in cellularity. Sometimes they contain collagenized stroma (D), suggesting they may give rise to the fibrosing foci illustrated in figure 2-62.

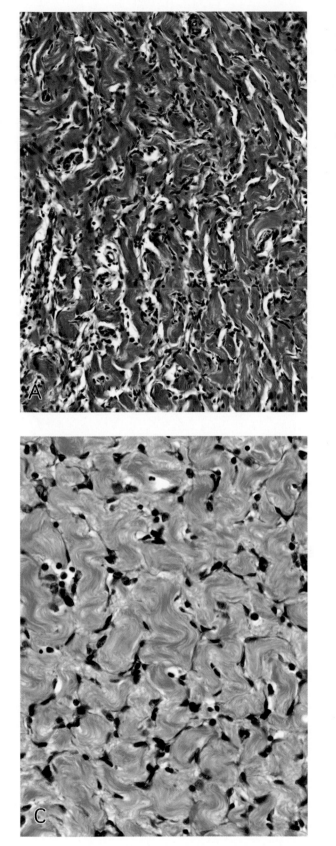

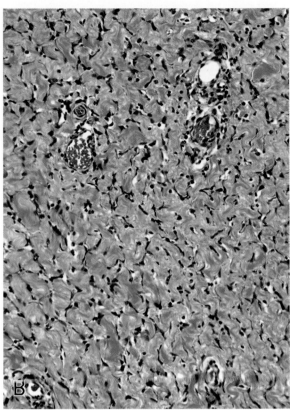

Figure 2-62

FIBROUS HAMARTOMA OF INFANCY

A–C: The collagenized (so-called neurofibroma-like fibrosing) element is often present and is a very helpful feature for diagnosis.

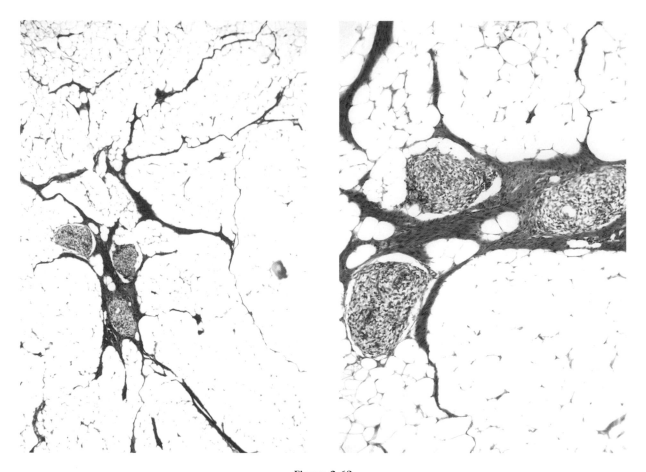

Figure 2-63

FIBROUS HAMARTOMA OF INFANCY

Left, Right: The abundant fat and a fibrogenic element closely resembling that seen in lipofibromatosis are seen here. The primitive myxoid mesenchymal nodules are a defining feature of fibrous hamartoma of infancy and are absent in lipofibromatosis.

Figure 2-64

MYOFIBROMA/ MYOFIBROMATOSIS

Age and sex distribution of 295 patients with either a solitary myofibroma or multifocal myofibromatosis reviewed at the AFIP.

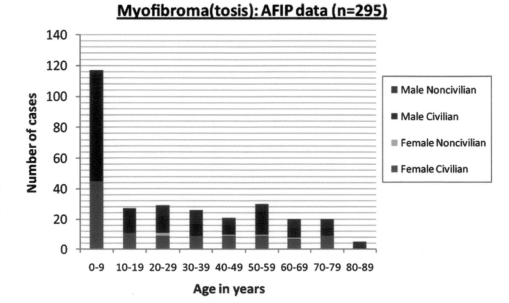

Anatomic distribution for 113 patients ≤ 12 years old presenting with a solitary myofibroma

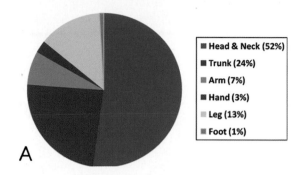

- Head & Neck (52%)
- Trunk (24%)
- Arm (7%)
- Hand (3%)
- Leg (13%)
- Foot (1%)

A

Anatomic distribution for 113 patients ≤ 12 years old presenting with a solitary myofibroma

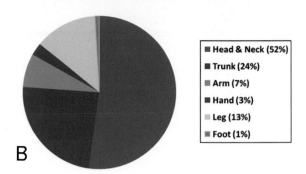

- Head & Neck (52%)
- Trunk (24%)
- Arm (7%)
- Hand (3%)
- Leg (13%)
- Foot (1%)

B

Solitary myofibroma: anatomic distribution for 77 patients ≥ 50 years old

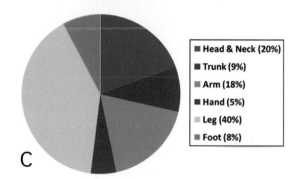

- Head & Neck (20%)
- Trunk (9%)
- Arm (18%)
- Hand (5%)
- Leg (40%)
- Foot (8%)

C

Figure 2-65

MYOFIBROMA/MYOFIBROMATOSIS

Anatomic distribution of solitary myofibromas from patients 12 years old and younger (A), 13 to 49 years old (B), and 50 years old and older (C) reviewed at the AFIP. The anatomic distribution shifts with increasing age.

Patients with multicentric disease have 2 to over 100 lesions (272,273). The skin, subcutis, or skeletal muscle is involved in 98 percent of patients. Bone is involved in 57 percent, lung in 23 percent, heart in 16 percent, and the gastrointestinal tract in 14 percent of patients (272). A variety of other sites may also be affected.

Bone involvement is primarily present in infancy and early childhood. Solitary bone lesions usually involve the skull or mandible (274). Bone lesions are more widely distributed in multicentric disease, often affecting the metaphyseal region of long bones, as well as the ribs, vertebrae, and pelvis. The typical radiologic appearance is a well-demarcated, lucent mass with a sclerotic rim (273,275). Some examples have central mineralization (258)

Superficial lesions typically present as rubbery to firm, mobile masses that are usually painless. When skin is involved, the process may have a macular appearance with a purplish hue, reminiscent of a hemangioma. Rare examples ulcerate the overlying skin. Deep-seated tumors may be fixed to fascia or other adjacent anatomic structures.

Gross Findings. Myofibromas range in size from 0.5 to 7.0 cm in greatest dimension, but most are under 2 cm (273). The process forms a firm, well-demarcated, nodular or multinodular mass, often with a grayish white cut surface. The center of the tumor may have a purple tinge due to increased vascularity or yellow discoloration due to necrosis.

Microscopic Findings. The prototypic myofibroma is a well-defined, nodular, biphasic tumor with peripherally located spindled cells zonated around more primitive, small, round to oval cells associated with a prominent hemangiopericytoma-like capillary network (figs. 2-66, 2-67). The spindled cells have elongated, rounded, or blunt-ended nuclei and abundant eosinophilic to clear cytoplasm. Occasionally, juxtanuclear vacuoles are noted (fig. 2-68, left).

The spindle cells form short, loosely organized fascicles or have a whorled arrangement, and they are often embedded in a

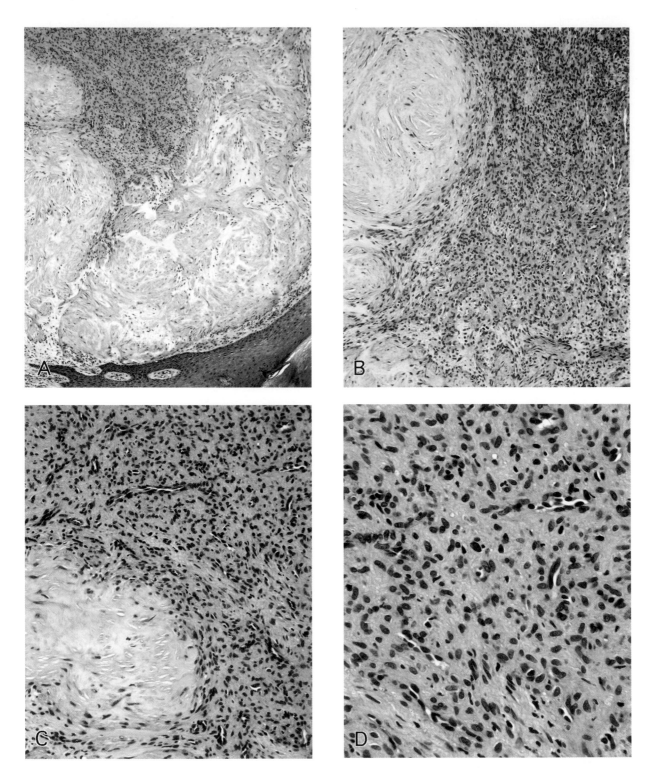

Figure 2-66

MYOFIBROMA

Low (A), intermediate (B,C), and high (D) power views of a myofibroma illustrate the biphasic morphology. The peripherally located myoid element is embedded in a myxocollagenous matrix. The centrally located component is composed of small ovoid and spindled cells with a pericyte-like appearance.

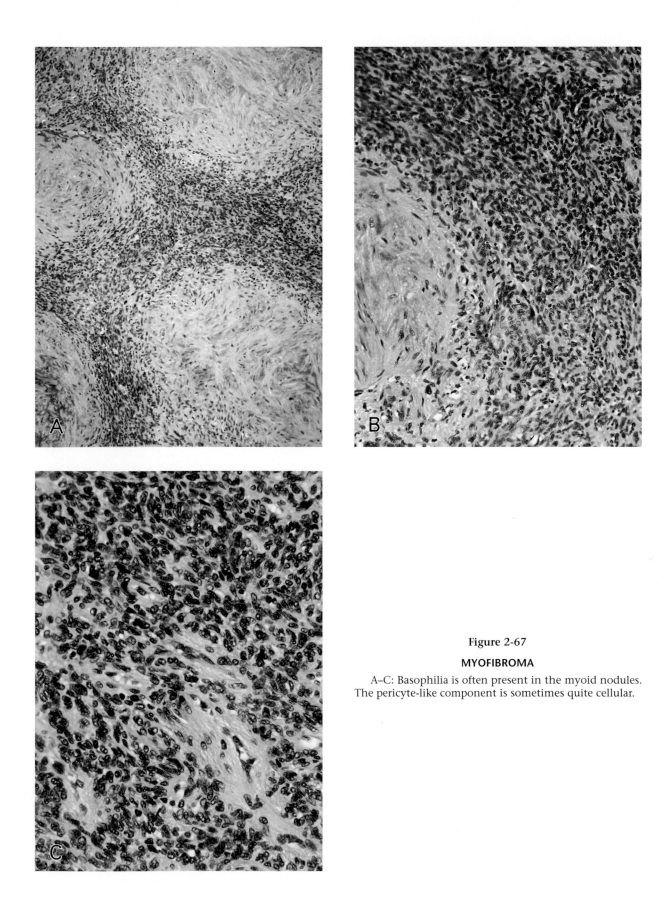

Figure 2-67

MYOFIBROMA

A–C: Basophilia is often present in the myoid nodules. The pericyte-like component is sometimes quite cellular.

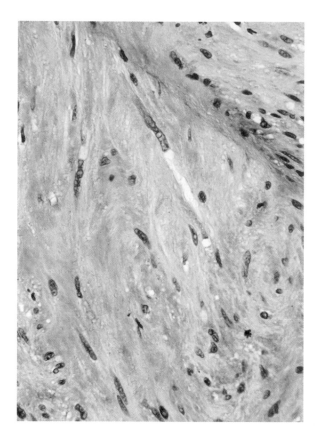 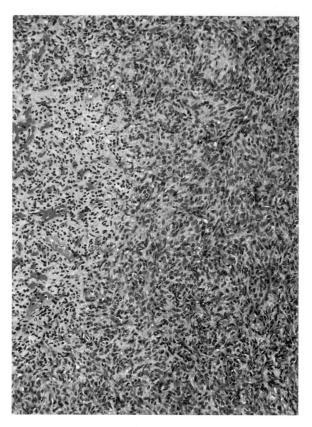

Figure 2-68

MYOFIBROMA

The spindled myoid cells contain juxtanuclear vacuoles and are typically embedded in abundant, basophilic, myxocollagenous matrix (left). The cellular pericyte-like component has foci with zonal necrosis (right).

myxocollagenous or densely hyalinized matrix. In contrast, the centrally located, more primitive cells have scant cytoplasm with poorly defined cell borders and round to oval, dark-staining and slightly pleomorphic nuclei. This latter element is often associated with a prominent branching microvascular network, and it may contain areas of necrosis (fig. 2-68, right) (271,276), hemorrhage, or calcification. Mitotic figures are usually sparse and never atypical, but infrequently, there are more than 5 mitotic figures per 10 high-powered fields. Focal intravascular growth is a well-described phenomenon in this setting. Neither the level of mitotic activity nor the presence of intravascular growth influence behavior.

Variations in composition and growth pattern are well documented (fig. 2-69) (260,267, 277,278). In some examples, there is a reversal in the zonation pattern. In others, the spindled (myoid) or the hemangiopericytoma-like element is largely absent. The small round cell component may predominate in newly formed lesions, whereas the spindled component is more prevalent in later stages of the process. Visceral and osseous examples tend to have greater compositional variance than superficial lesions (259,271,274). Mucosal-based examples may assume a polypoid configuration with surface ulceration (259,271).

Special Studies. The spindled (myoid) lesional cells typically express α-smooth muscle actin, but desmin is usually absent (259,260, 268,277,279,280). The more primitive, small, round to oval cells associated with accentuated vascularity may also have limited α-smooth muscle actin expression, but most cells are negative for this marker. Tumor cells are nonreactive for S-100 protein, EMA, and keratins (259,260,268,277,278).

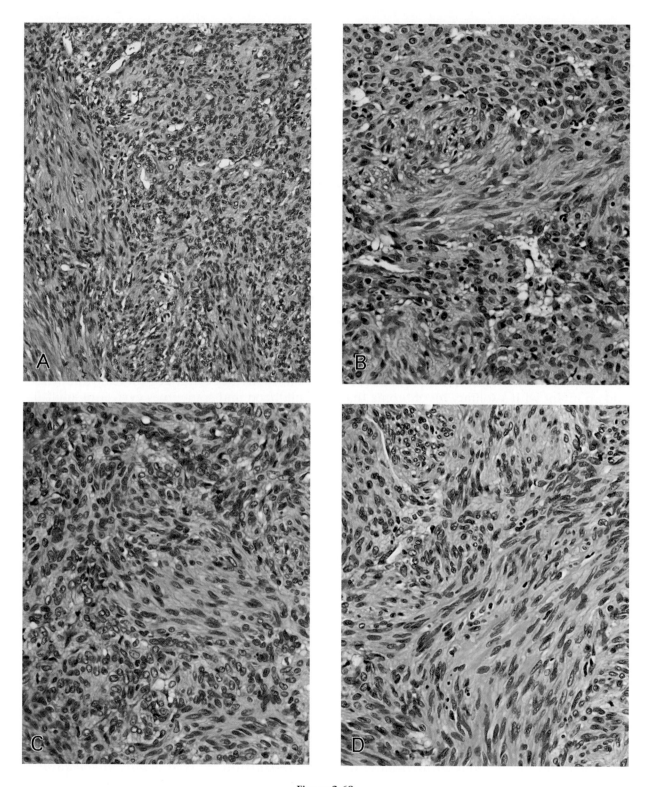

Figure 2-69

MYOFIBROMA/MYOFIBROMATOSIS

A–D: Myofibroma from a pediatric patient with myofibromatosis. Some examples, as illustrated here, have a more disorganized admixture of myoid and pericytic-like components.

Genetics. A small number of familial cases of myofibroma(tosis) have been reported (259,263, 266,281,282). No ethnic or sex predilection has been demonstrated for familial tumors. The documentation of individuals in the same kindred with multicentric myofibromatosis (with or without visceral involvement) and solitary myofibromas supports the view that these are forms of the same disease process (273). There is speculation that this disease may have more than one genetic pathway (263,273,282): while most kindreds follow a vertical pattern of inheritance consistent with an autosomal dominant trait with variable penetrance and expressivity (266,278,282,283), a smaller number of kindreds exhibit a horizontal pattern of inheritance, occasionally associated with parental consanguinity, that suggests an autosomal recessive disorder (263,281). One patient with Turner syndrome and generalized myofibromatosis has been reported (284). There are also reports of a newborn with a solitary myofibroma that had a tumor karyotype of 46,XX,der(9;16)(q10;q10),+16 and an infant with a solitary myofibroma that had a del(6)(q12;q15) as the sole cytogenetic abnormality (261,285).

Differential Diagnosis. The differential diagnosis includes a smooth muscle tumor, fibrous histiocytoma, infantile hemangiopericytoma, congenital fibrosarcoma, and the recently described myopericytoma. Smooth muscle tumors tend to have well-developed fascicular growth and extensive desmin expression. Fibrous histiocytomas generally form superficial masses with a stellate configuration, and they feature epithelioid and spindled cells with a well-developed storiform growth pattern. Congenital fibrosarcomas may contain areas with immature fibroblastic cells arranged around a prominent hemangiopericytoma-like vascular network, bearing some resemblance to the immature component encountered in myofibroma. However, as a general rule, congenital fibrosarcoma is a more cellular, infiltrative, and mitotically active process, often dominated by a population of uniform spindled cells with well-developed fascicular and herringbone growth patterns. Also, most congenital fibrosarcomas are believed to harbor *ETV6-NTRK3* gene fusions.

Myopericytoma (286,287) is primarily encountered in adults and has features that overlap with angioleiomyoma. It typically forms a well-demarcated mass with numerous blood vessels surrounded by spindled cells with well-developed smooth muscle morphology and smaller ovoid cells with a pericytic appearance.

Treatment and Prognosis. Behavior and outcome are strongly linked to the age of the patient, number of lesions, and anatomic distribution. Solitary myofibromas are invariably benign. In children, they tend to spontaneously regress, regardless of location (272). In adults, however, spontaneous regression is thought to be uncommon (260). The risk of recurrence after local excision of a myofibroma is reportedly about 10 percent, with re-excision almost invariably curative (271,272). The risk of recurrence after marginal excision of an osseous myofibroma appears negligible (274).

Patients with multicentric disease without visceral involvement also frequently have an excellent prognosis (271,272). There is spontaneous regression of the lesions over time, although new lesions may continue to develop throughout childhood and sometimes even into adult life (267,271). On rare occasion, some lesions are associated with a protracted destructive course.

Of patients with multicentric disease with visceral involvement, 73 percent die (272). The risk of fatality is greatest in the first few weeks of life and is generally attributable to cardiopulmonary and gastrointestinal complications related to mass effect or obstruction (266,272,288). Limited visceral disease, especially when critical sites are spared, is compatible with a good prognosis (288).

There is no consensus on optimal treatment for patients with severe multicentric disease (282,289). Reportedly, some patients have benefitted from low-dose chemotherapy or interferon alpha, but it is difficult to judge the efficacy of these treatments given the very limited number of "successfully treated" patients and the natural tendency for pediatric lesions to regress spontaneously (264,290–292).

PALMAR/PLANTAR FIBROMATOSIS

Definition. *Palmar/plantar fibromatosis* is a benign (myo)fibroblastic proliferation that arises within aponeurosis on the palmar and plantar surfaces of the hands and feet. The process is commonly multinodular and frequently

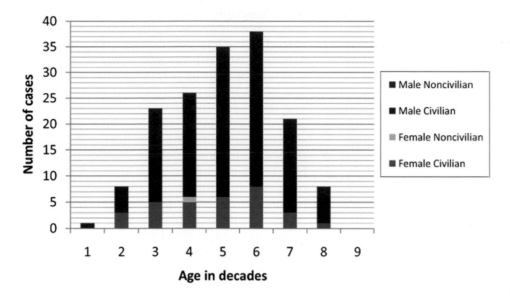

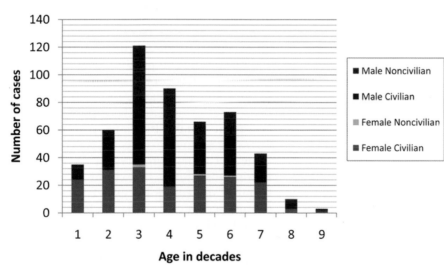

Figure 2-70

PALMAR/PLANTAR FIBROMATOSIS

Age and sex distribution of 160 patients with palmar fibromatosis (top) and 501 patients with plantar fibromatosis (bottom) reviewed at the AFIP.

multicentric. Synonyms include *superficial fibromatosis, Dupuytren disease* (palmar), and *Ledderhose disease* (plantar).

General Considerations. We regard "superficial fibromatosis" as a too generic designation to be used for diagnostic purposes and prefer the older entrenched terminology for this site-specific process. Palmar/plantar fibromatosis is the most common type of fibromatosis.

Clinical Features. There is a well-documented genetic predisposition for palmar/plantar fibromatosis among individuals of northern European ancestry (293–295). Most pedigrees appear to follow an autosomal dominant

pattern of inheritance, with age-related and incomplete penetrance (294–298). A variety of factors, including trauma, chronic alcohol abuse (295,299–302), smoking (299,303,304), and diabetes (295,305), act as disease promoters. Disease prevalence increases with advancing age (295,304,306–308). Plantar fibromatosis often manifests earlier in life than palmar fibromatosis (309–312) and has a peak surgical incidence in the third decade (fig. 2-70, bottom) (310). In contrast, the peak surgical incidence for palmar fibromatosis is in the sixth decade (fig. 2-70, top) (310). Bilaterality is common for both plantar and palmar fibromatoses (298,310,312–314).

Palmar fibromatosis affects males with much greater frequency than females up through mid adult life, but, with advancing age, decreases to less than 2 to 1 (295,306,307,315). Palmar lesions arise in any location containing an aponeurosis, but they most commonly affect the ulnar aspect of the palm, with the greatest effect on the 4th and 5th fingers (293,312,316–318). Lesions close to digits have the greatest risk for causing permanent contractures (316,319,320).

Knuckle pads (302,310,318,321,322), Peyronie disease of the penis (294,323–326), and epilepsy (295,302,310,327,328) occur with a higher frequency in patients with palmar fibromatosis, and there may be an increased propensity for keloids (309,310,326,329,330) and other less well-characterized fibrogenic lesions (309,310, 312,331,332). The rate of disease progression is highly variable (293,316–318).

Plantar fibromatosis is less studied than palmar fibromatosis. Females appear to be affected more often than males through adolescence (310), but the gender ratio in adulthood is even (331,333,334). Lesions on the foot typically involve the medial plantar arch region, and in the absence of close proximity to a digit, have little risk for contracture (309,310,312,331,332).

The initial clinical manifestation of the disease is usually a small, firm, superficial nodule situated within an aponeurosis on the palm or sole. Over time, additional nodules develop and others may regress. The affected areas become associated with cords of fibrous tissue that tend to progressively shorten, and when the process overlies a joint, this leads to a permanent and increasingly severe flexion contracture. The nodules are often asymptomatic, but they may become painful with prolonged pressure.

Gross Findings. Gross examination reveals dense fibrous connective tissue with adherent subcutaneous fat. One or more gray-white nodular masses (typically 0.5 to 2.5 cm) may be apparent within the fibrous connective tissue. When the lesions are small, they may escape visual detection, but they can usually be found with careful palpation because they have a firmer consistency than the surrounding normal soft tissue. Careful gross examination and tissue processing greatly enhance accurate early diagnosis of this disease.

Microscopic Findings. Low-power examination reveals dense, regular connective tissue with the characteristic features of aponeurosis. Arising within this layer is a nodular or multinodular spindle cell proliferation composed of fibroblasts and myofibroblasts (figs. 2-71, 2-72). The ratio of fibroblasts to myofibroblasts, the degree of cellularity, and the level of mitotic activity vary with the duration and stage of the lesion. Early proliferative lesions have both high cellularity and frequent mitotic figures, but neither is an indication of malignant potential in this setting. Older lesions often have lower cellularity, fewer mitoses, and more abundant collagen. The spindle cells have uniform, normochromatic or slightly dark-staining nuclei with small nucleoli, and pleomorphism is absent. Infrequent multinucleated stromal cells with nuclei in clumped, linear, or wreath-like arrangements may be present (fig. 2-72D,E) (309,310,335,336). Necrosis is rarely observed, and atypical mitotic figures are not present.

The spindle cell proliferation generally does not extend beyond the adipose tissue adjacent to the aponeurotic layer, and involvement of the overlying dermis or underlying skeletal muscle is rare and usually associated with a postsurgical recurrence. On rare occasion, foci of metaplastic bone or cartilage are present. Whereas palmar fibromatosis tends to exhibit a randomly distributed multinodular growth pattern within the aponeurotic layer, plantar lesions often form discrete wreath-like multinodular masses with a centrally spared aponeurosis (310).

Special Studies. The spindle cell population is variably immunoreactive for muscle-specific and smooth muscle actins, reflecting myofibroblastic differentiation. Focal nuclear positivity for β-catenin may be present (337). Immunostains for keratins, EMA, and S-100 protein are negative.

Genetics. Most karyotypic studies have yielded normal results or single chromosome trisomies (338–340). One study of palmar fibromatosis demonstrated heterogeneous clonal or sporadic chromosomal changes in 69 percent of cases (341). Palmar/plantar fibromatosis lacks *CTNNB1*/β-*catenin* and *APC* gene mutations and appears genetically unrelated to desmoid fibromatosis (337).

Differential Diagnosis. The differential diagnosis includes scar tissue, fibrous histiocytoma,

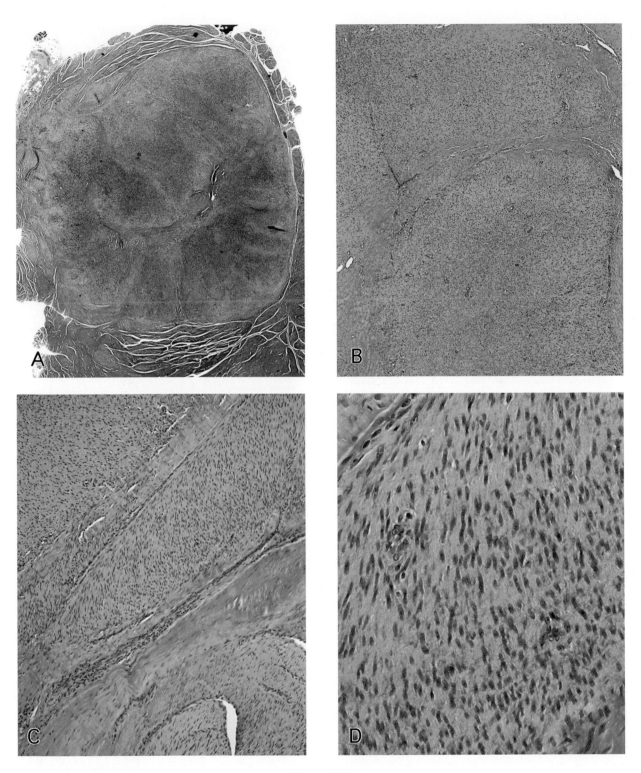

Figure 2-71

PALMAR/PLANTAR FIBROMATOSIS

Low (A), intermediate (B,C), and high (D) power views show localization within dense regular connective tissue (aponeurosis). The garland-like growth pattern (A) is typical for plantar fibromatosis, whereas palmar fibromatosis generally exhibits a less organized multinodular growth pattern.

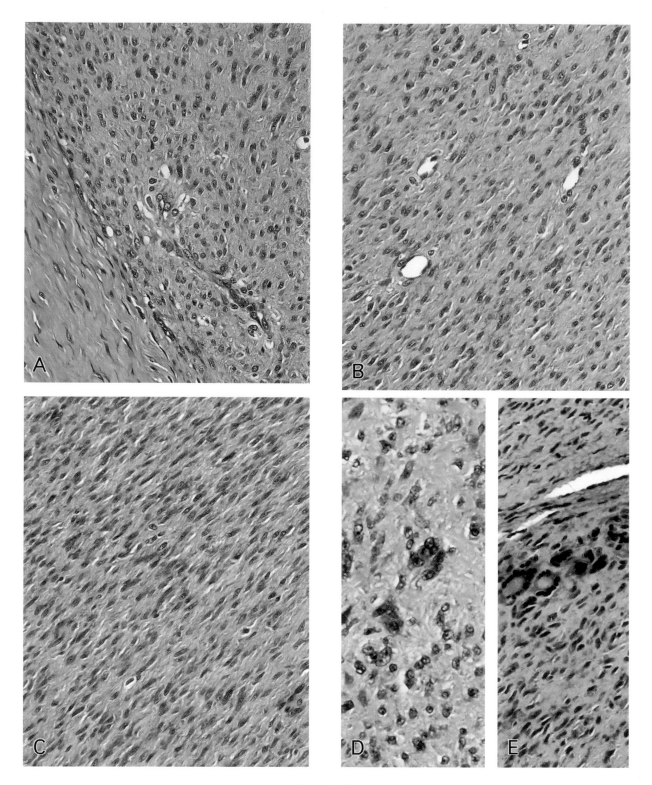

Figure 2-72

PALMAR/PLANTAR FIBROMATOSIS

A fairly uniform population of mildly atypical spindle cells is arranged in a loosely fascicular growth pattern (A–C). Some multinucleated lesional cells are present (D,E).

calcifying aponeurotic fibroma, desmoid-type fibromatosis, fibrosarcoma, and monophasic fibrous-type synovial sarcoma. Palmar/plantar fibromatosis is usually easily distinguished from these entities by correlation with preoperative clinical findings and recognition of the characteristic localization within the aponeurotic layer. Scar tissue is usually less cellular than palmar/plantar fibromatosis, and it generally lacks localization to an aponeurosis. Fibrous histiocytomas tend to be epicentered in the dermis, and they typically have a stellate configuration and greater cellular heterogeneity. Calcifying aponeurotic fibromas feature a spindled fibromatosis-like element admixed with scattered distinctive chondrocalcific nodules and/or plump epithelioid fibroblasts in corded arrays. Desmoid-type fibromatosis, fibrosarcoma, and synovial sarcoma all arise deep to the aponeurosis. The last two entities typically exhibit the cytomorphologic hallmarks of a malignant process, and in the case of synovial sarcoma, there is typically focal keratin and EMA immunoreactivity.

Treatment and Prognosis. It is difficult to predict behavior in an individual case for palmar/plantar fibromatosis. Factors reported to correlate with more aggressive behavior include early disease onset (322,328,342–344), a strong family history (300,322,345), bilateral involvement or coexisting palmar and plantar disease (322,345), the presence of knuckle pads (300,322), and a history of epilepsy or alcoholism (300,322,328). Some authors also add the male sex to this list (328,344).

Optimal treatment is controversial (310,314, 315,346,347). Plantar disease rarely causes contractures, so surgical intervention is often unnecessary. The management of palmar disease is more complicated and influenced by symptomatology, location of the tumor nodules, and risk of contracture formation. In palmar fibromatosis, surgery is often reserved for early contractures overlying the proximal interphalangeal joints of the hand, especially when the little finger is involved (293,319,320). A wide or radical fasciectomy or dermofasciectomy with skin graft reduces the risk of local recurrence (314,331,333,345,348), but the more aggressive the intervention, the longer the post-surgical recovery interval. Local recurrences are usually evident within 12 to 24 months of follow-up.

LIPOFIBROMATOSIS

Definition. *Lipofibromatosis* is a benign tumor of childhood characterized by the presence of abundant, usually mature, adipose tissue admixed with a spindle cell (fibromatosis-like) component that tends to be concentrated in septal and perimysial locations.

General Considerations. In the past, tumors of this type were usually classified as infantile/juvenile fibromatosis, fibrous hamartoma of infancy, or a cellular variant of lipoblastoma. It is our opinion that this entity warrants separate classification.

Clinical Features. Lipofibromatosis is a pediatric tumor (fig. 2-73, top) (349–353). Patients range from newborn (350–352,354) to 14 years of age (349), with congenital cases representing approximately 20 percent of the total. There is a greater than 2 to 1 male predominance. The process typically presents as a painless mass in the extremities. Approximately 34 percent of cases involve the hand and 15 percent involve the foot (fig. 2-73, bottom). Less common locations include the head and neck region, chest wall, abdominal wall, back, and pelvis. The tumors are either subcutaneous or deep-seated, and usually poorly demarcated.

MRI shows high signal intensity on both T1- and T2-weighted images, consistent with fat, and in some instances, multiple internal septations are evident (352,355,356). The radiologic appearance often leads to a differential diagnosis that includes lipoma, lipoblastoma, fibrous hamartoma of infancy, and hemangioma or lymphangioma with so-called fatty overgrowth.

Gross Findings. The tumors usually range from 1 to 5 cm (median, 2 cm), but a few have measured 7 cm or more, and rare examples have involved an entire extremity (352,354). The process consists of an irregular, poorly marginated, yellowish or yellow-tan mass of fatty or fibrofatty tissue. Fibrous streaks are occasionally grossly visible within the fat. Depending on the depth of the process, fascia or skeletal muscle may be present.

Microscopic Findings. Abundant adipose tissue typically comprises more than 50 percent of the tumor volume (figs. 2-74, 2-75). The adipocytes are usually mature and lack atypia. In newborn patients, however, the fat lobules may have an immature appearance with a myxoid matrix, as is sometimes encountered in early-stage lipoblastoma (fig. 2-76).

85

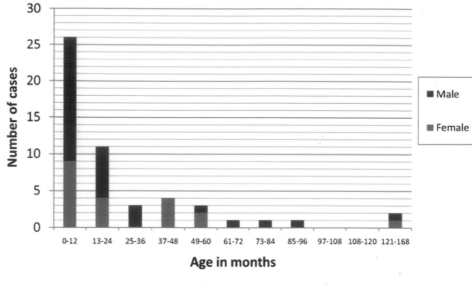

Figure 2-73

LIPOFIBROMATOSIS

Age and sex (top) and anatomic (bottom) distributions of patients with lipofibromatosis. These data are derived from 45 cases reviewed at the AFIP and 8 adequately documented cases retrieved from the medical literature. The gender was not provided for one AFIP patient.

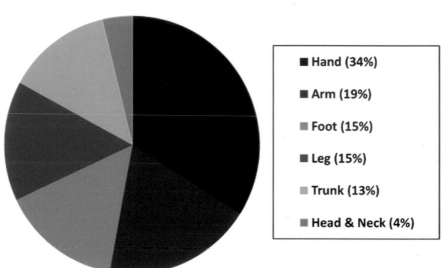

In addition to the fatty element, the tumors have a fibroblastic component that characteristically forms fascicles concentrated in septal regions and along the perimysium of accompanying skeletal muscle (figs. 2-74, 2-75). The fibroblastic cells show only mild atypia (fig. 2-77), and mitotic figures are uncommon (rarely exceeding 5 mitoses per 50 high-power fields). The spindle cells may spill over into the fat lobules and focally replace skeletal muscle, but there is no sheet-like growth pattern of fibroblasts. Small collections of univacuolated cells may be noted between the spindled fibroblasts and the mature adipocytes. In rare instances, melanin-laden pigmented cells are seen among the fibroblastic population (349,351). The tumors lack organoid nodules of primitive mesenchymal cells, foci with a hyalinized, wavy (neurofibroma-like) collagen pattern, and chondrocalcific nodules bordered by plump epithelioid mesenchymal cells.

Special Studies. The fibroblastic component has variable immunoreactivity for CD99, CD34, smooth muscle actin, and bcl-2 (351,355). Some examples have focal reactivity for S-100 protein, muscle-specific actin, and rarely, EMA (351). No reactivity is present for desmin or keratins. The few cases thus far tested have lacked nuclear reactivity for β-catenin (357,358). The exceptionally uncommon pigmented cells described

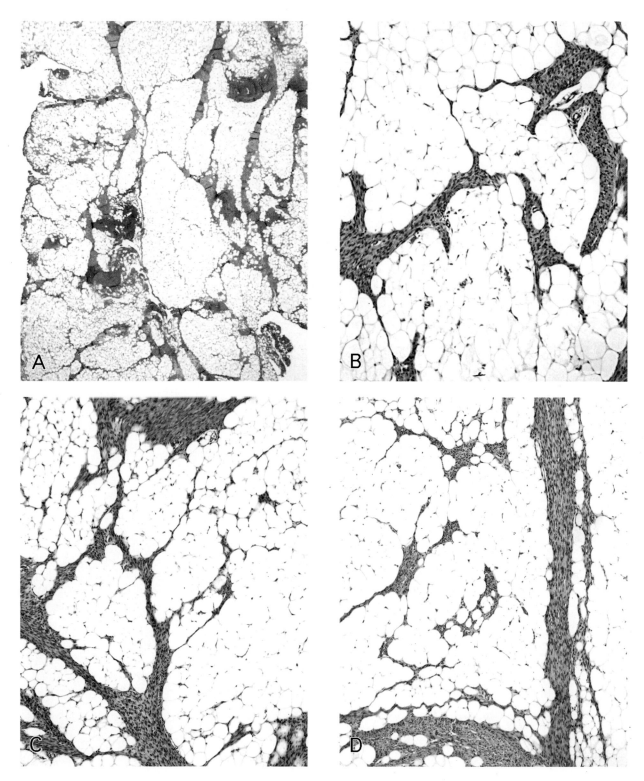

Figure 2-74

LIPOFIBROMATOSIS

A–D: Abundant mature adipose tissue and a moderately cellular spindle cell proliferation with fascicular growth are seen. The spindle cells have a notable tendency to reside within fat septa.

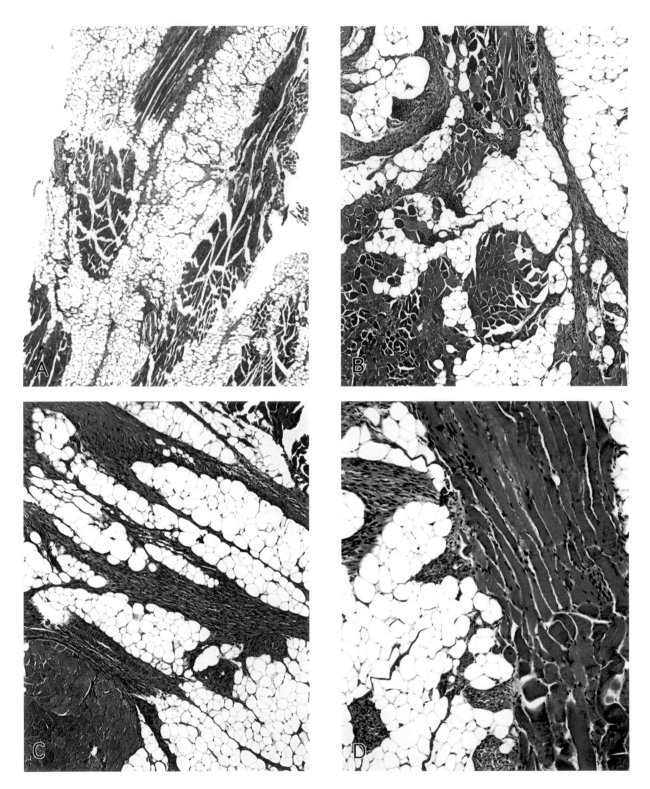

Figure 2-75

LIPOFIBROMATOSIS

A–D: Lipofibromatosis involving skeletal muscle is displaced by abundant mature adipose tissue and a spindle cell proliferation that tends to involve fat septa and perimysium.

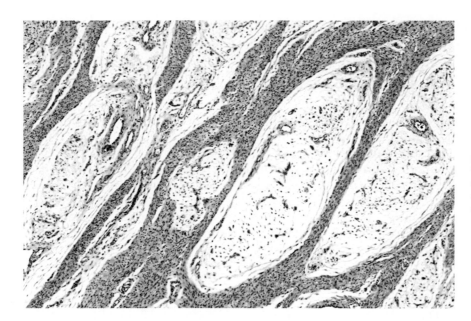

Figure 2-76

LIPOFIBROMATOSIS

In this neonate, abundant myxoid matrix is present within the immature fat lobules. This change is analogous to that encountered within fat in very early stages of lipoblastoma.

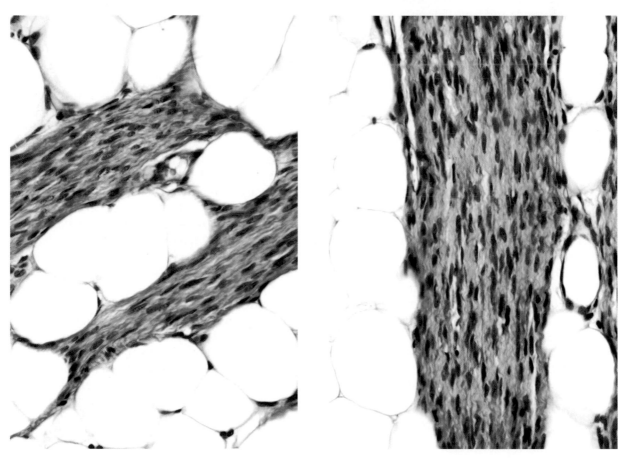

Figure 2-77

LIPOFIBROMATOSIS

Left, Right: Mildly atypical spindle cells with fascicular growth.

above express melan-A, HMB-45, and tyrosinase (349,351). One example of lipofibromatosis, removed from a 5-year-old boy, contained a balanced three-way t(4;9;6)(q21;q22;q2?4) translocation (359).

Differential Diagnosis. The prominent adipocytic component and the growth pattern of the fibroblastic element distinguish lipofibromatosis from infantile diffuse fibromatosis and juvenile desmoid tumor. A predilection for the distal portions of the extremities and the absence of both organoid islands of primitive mesenchymal cells in a myxoid matrix and a neurofibroma-like pattern of fibrosis set it apart from fibrous hamartoma of infancy. While lipoblastomas may have mildly increased septal cellularity, this is never present to the extent seen in lipofibromatosis.

Calcifying aponeurotic fibroma is a fibroblast- and collagen-rich tumor with a notable predilection for the hands and feet. This entity has broad fascicles of spindled cells with sheet-like growth, commonly punctuated with scattered chondrocalcific nodules bordered by plump epithelioid fibroblasts. In its earliest stages, the distinctive chondrocalcific nodules may be absent, and recognition hinges on the identification of small clusters of epithelioid fibroblasts in corded arrays.

Infantile diffuse fibromatosis features ovoid to spindled fibroblasts with a permeative, diffuse, sheet-like growth pattern. Infantile fibrosarcoma also has a diffuse sheet-like growth pattern, often with better developed fascicular growth, more mitotic activity, and somewhat greater nuclear atypia. Fat is not an integral component of calcifying aponeurotic fibroma, infantile diffuse fibromatosis, or infantile fibrosarcoma.

The designation "lipofibromatosis" has also been used in the orthopedic literature for an unrelated congenital process associated with macrodactyly (also termed macrodactylia fibrolipomatosis, macrodystrophia lipomatosa, megalodactyly, dactylomegaly, and local gigantism) (360). This process is said to contain abundant fibrofatty tissue that is increased in amount but otherwise normal.

Treatment and Prognosis. Lipofibromatosis has a notable tendency for local recurrence when incompletely excised, but there are no reports of metastasis (351). In this AFIP series, over 70 percent of patients at last follow-up had either regrowth of their tumor or persistent disease. As a result, complete excision is preferable if this can be accomplished with minimal morbidity. Factors potentially linked to recurrence include congenital onset of disease, male sex, acral location, mitotic activity in the fibroblastic component, and incomplete excision (351).

DIFFUSE INFANTILE FIBROMATOSIS

Definition. *Diffuse infantile fibromatosis* is a rare benign mesenchymal tumor of infancy and early childhood, characterized by a diffuse proliferation of oval to spindled fibroblasts that infiltrate and entrap skeletal muscle, fat, and other regional structures. Synonyms include *congenital/infantile/juvenile fibromatosis variant.*

General Considerations. This term was introduced by Enzinger in 1965 (361). Over the years, we have encountered a small number of tumors that match the description presented here, but this remains a poorly characterized process that conceptually is still in a state of evolution. This is one of the rarest recognized variants of infantile/juvenile fibromatosis.

Clinical Features. Diffuse infantile fibromatosis has a male predominance and is almost always discovered within the first 3 years of life (361). Approximately 12 percent of cases are congenital. The process generally presents as an asymptomatic, poorly demarcated, deep-seated mass that is not fixed to the overlying skin. A wide variety of sites may be involved, but the majority of cases affect the upper extremity and head and neck region (361,362). The hands and feet are typically spared.

Gross Findings. Grossly, the tumor forms a nondescript, poorly delineated, whitish to yellow-tan mass that chiefly involves skeletal muscle. It may extend along the fascial plain, entrap tendons, and infiltrate into subcutaneous fat.

Microscopic Findings. Histologically, there is a diffuse proliferation of small oval to spindled fibroblasts with only mild atypia (fig. 2-78). The cells are loosely and somewhat haphazardly arranged in a myxocollagenous matrix, and they infiltrate and entrap skeletal muscle and other regional structures. There is no pleomorphism, extreme cellularity with herringbone growth, high mitotic activity, or necrosis, in contrast with fibrosarcoma. Fat is not an integral component of this process. This tumor does not have a well-

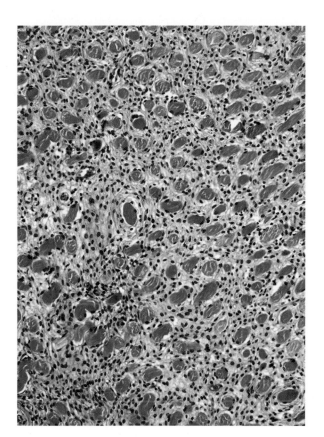 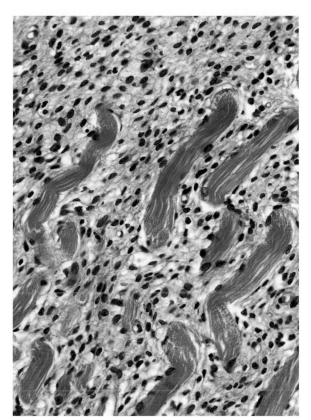

Figure 2-78

DIFFUSE INFANTILE FIBROMATOSIS

Left, Right: A uniform population of small, oval to spindled fibroblastic cells entrap skeletal muscle fibers.

documented immunohistochemical profile. No genetic data are available.

Differential Diagnosis. Key considerations in the differential diagnosis include lipofibromatosis, desmoid-type fibromatosis, and infantile fibrosarcoma. Lipofibromatosis typically has a dominant fatty component that is considered integral to the process and is visible both grossly and by imaging analysis. While its fibroblastic component may have small areas with a permeative/diffuse growth pattern, there is a notable tendency for this element to be concentrated within fat septa and along the perimysial surface of muscle bundles.

There is no evidence that diffuse infantile fibromatosis or lipofibromatosis undergoes "maturation" to a desmoid tumor. Desmoid tumors are infiltrative and destructive, and have a greater tendency to replace muscle and other regional structures than diffuse infantile fibromatosis. Desmoids also have larger spindled cells with a well-developed myofibroblastic phenotype and

more abundant collagen, and they tend to feature broad storiform and loose fascicular growth patterns with evenly spaced vessels.

Infantile fibrosarcoma has greater cellularity and more mitotic activity than diffuse infantile fibromatosis. It often contains areas with solid sheet-like or classic herringbone growth; foci with necrosis and hemorrhage are frequent. In addition, most infantile fibrosarcomas contain *ETV6/NTRK3* fusion transcripts.

Treatment and Prognosis. Diffuse infantile fibromatosis has a strong predilection (over 35 percent) for local recurrence if incompletely excised, and recurrences may be multiple (361). There are no reports of metastasis. Complete excision with documented margins is advisable if this can be accomplished without undue morbidity. Aggressive surgical intervention that may impair function is not generally advocated except in extreme instances were tumor size and extent make this absolutely necessary.

DESMOID-TYPE FIBROMATOSIS

Definition. *Desmoid-type fibromatosis* is a benign, usually fascia-associated (myo)fibroblastic neoplasm that characteristically involves deep soft tissue, exhibits infiltrative growth, and has a strong tendency for local recurrence but does not metastasize. Synonyms include *aggressive fibromatosis, musculoaponeurotic fibromatosis, deep fibromatosis,* and *desmoid tumor.*

General Considerations. This tumor is separate and distinct from palmar/plantar fibromatosis. Desmoid tumors are commonly subclassified by location: abdominal wall, extra-abdominal, and intra-abdominal/mesenteric because the various subgroups have different clinical demographics and recurrence rates. All desmoid tumors share similar morphologic features. True desmoid tumors in the pediatric population are no different from desmoid tumors in adults (363–366), and we believe they should be classified as such and not as infantile fibromatosis. We restrict use of the term infantile fibromatosis to more primitive pediatric fibroblastic tumors, such as diffuse infantile fibromatosis.

Genetic, hormonal, and physical factors are all implicated in the pathogenesis of desmoid-type fibromatosis. Familial adenomatous polyposis (FAP) is an autosomal dominant disorder caused by a germline mutation in the *APC* tumor-suppressor gene on chromosome 5q21 (367–370). The incidence of desmoid tumors in this setting is reported to range from 4 to 38 percent, with cumulative life-time risk estimates ranging from 10 to 21 percent (371–375). The relative risk of developing a desmoid tumor in an FAP patient is estimated to be 852 to 1,240 times that of the general population (368,371,373,374,376). The designation Gardner syndrome has also been used for FAP, including desmoid tumors as a manifestation, especially in the past.

Hormonal factors (especially high endogenous estrogen levels) influence the development and growth of desmoid tumors, particularly those arising in the abdominal wall and pelvic region (377–380). Accelerated tumor growth has been documented in women using oral contraceptives (374,378), and antiestrogenic and progestational agents have proven beneficial in the treatment of some tumors (378,381–384).

Trauma (either spontaneous or iatrogenic) is linked to the development of an estimated 12 to 33 percent (with studies reporting an association as high as 63 percent) of abdominal wall and extra-abdominal fibromatoses (364,385–388). Surgical trauma, usually related to colectomy, precedes the development of 68 to 83 percent of intra-abdominal desmoids in FAP patients (372–374,389).

Clinical Features. Based on a Finnish study, it is estimated that 2.4 to 4.3 new cases of desmoid-type fibromatosis are diagnosed per 10^6 population/year (379,390). These tumors occur in all age groups, but are least common in the first decade. There is a nearly equal sex distribution (or a mild male predominance in some series) in pediatric cases and these tumors primarily are extra-abdominal (363,365,366,386,391).

Apart from pediatric cases, extra-abdominal desmoid tumors have a female predominance of 1.8-3.1 to 1.0 and a peak incidence in the third to fourth decades of life (392–396). They are widely distributed but most commonly affect the chest wall/back (397,398), shoulder/upper arm (399), and buttock/thigh regions (396). Abdominal (wall) tumors, which represent the single largest subgroup of desmoid tumors, have a very strong female predominance, about 9 to 1 in AFIP files) (392–394,400,401) and are usually encountered between the ages of 18 and 40 years (peak incidence, third decade) (377,390). They originate primarily from the rectus and internal oblique musculature and fascia and often present during or within the first year after a pregnancy (especially after the second pregnancy) (377,380).

Intra-abdominal desmoids are subcategorized as pelvic, mesenteric (401–403), or retroperitoneal. Pelvic examples have a strong female predominance and are usually located in the iliac fossa or lower pelvic region (404–406). They occur over the same age range as, but are more than 20 times rarer than, abdominal wall tumors. Although no clear link between pelvic desmoids and pregnancy or childbirth has been reported, a recent review of AFIP material, showed a possible association with gestation in up to 40 percent of cases. Mesenteric desmoids have a female to male ratio of approximately 1.0 to 1.2 and a peak incidence in the fourth decade (average age, 41 years) (389). Most examples involve the small bowel mesentery, but the ileocolic mesentery, gastrocolic ligament, omentum, and ligamentum teres are also affected.

The anatomic distribution of desmoid tumors in FAP patients is as follows: 50 to 72 percent intra-abdominal (372,373,376), 27 to 48 percent abdominal wall (373), and 2 to 14 percent extra-abdominal (368,373,407,408). In contrast, the distribution for sporadic desmoid tumors is 49 percent abdominal wall, 43 percent extra-abdominal, and only 8 to 11 percent intra-abdominal (374,376).

Desmoid tumors typically present as firm, fixed, deep-seated masses that grow insidiously and are often painless. When the tumors have reached sufficient size to compromise regional structures, decreased joint mobility and neurologic symptoms may ensue. Intra-abdominal tumors may cause abdominal pain, gastrointestinal bleeding, bowel obstruction, and perforation.

A small percentage of desmoid tumors appear to be multifocal within one general area (e.g., a limb or the abdominal cavity) (365,389, 407,409,410). Careful inspection sometimes reveals communication between these tumors due to insidious growth along fascial planes. An even rarer occurrence is true multicentric disease, where patients develop multiple widely separated tumors, often in different body sites (364,407,411–413). Both events are substantially more common in FAP patients than individuals with sporadic disease. In one large FAP series, female patients more frequently manifested multifocal disease than male patients (407).

Gross Findings. Desmoid tumors are usually (with the exception of mesenteric fibromatosis) adherent to and intimately associated with fascia and skeletal muscle (fig. 2-79). These tumors often have a deceptively well-demarcated gross appearance, but careful inspection usually reveals signs of infiltration. Tumors arising outside the abdominal cavity may extend up into the subcutis, but when this occurs, the process still tends to be associated with fascia. It is our opinion, based on extensive case review, that most true desmoid-type fibromatoses of the breast have a fascial association/derivation (371,411,414). Desmoid tumors have a firm gritty consistency, and on cut section, have an off-white color and a coarsely trabeculated surface, reminiscent of a uterine leiomyoma (fig. 2-79A). Abdominal wall tumors average 3 to 7 cm (377,400,408), extra-abdominal tumors average 5 to 10 cm (398,408,415), and intra-abdominal tumors tend to be the largest, with an average size of 13 to 15 cm (389,403,405).

Microscopic Findings. Desmoid-type fibromatoses are morphologically similar, regardless of patient age or anatomic site (figs. 2-80, 2-81). With the exception of mesenteric fibromatosis, most examples involve fascia and skeletal muscle. The tumors are moderately cellular, infiltrative, and composed of spindled cells with only mild nuclear atypia (fig. 2-81B,C) and no significant pleomorphism. The neoplastic cells have somewhat hyperchromatic nuclei, and often, small but distinct central nucleoli. Mitotic activity is variable but usually low, rarely exceeding 5 mitoses per 10 high-power fields. Abundant collagenous or myxocollagenous matrix is present, and the lesional cells are generally arranged in loose, sweeping fascicular and broad storiform arrays. Keloid-like collagen bundles may be evident (fig. 2-81A).

The vasculature tends to be evenly spaced and consists primarily of small arteries and compressed thin-walled veins. Perivascular edema and microhemorrhages may be noted. Peripherally entrapped multinucleated myocytes may give a false impression of pleomorphism and should be discounted. Exceptional cases contain small foci with metaplastic cartilage or bone. Mesenteric tumors often contain more abundant myxoid matrix than other examples, and when this is prominent, fascicular growth is only vaguely represented (389).

Special Studies. Focal immunoreactivity is often present for α-smooth muscle actin, muscle-specific actin, and sometimes for desmin (416,417). Over 80 percent of desmoid tumors have at least focal nuclear staining for β-catenin (fig. 2-81D) (371,418–421). Desmoid tumors are typically negative for KIT/CD117, and lack reactivity for CD34, DOG-1, S-100 protein, and keratins.

Genetics. These tumors are clonal neoplasms, as evidenced by karyotypic analyses and X chromosome inactivation patterns (422–428). Most have somatic activating mutations of the β-*catenin* (*CTNNB1*) gene (39 to 87 percent) or biallelic loss of function mutations of the *APC* gene, including a heterozygous germline mutation in hereditary cases (370,429–433). Both scenarios lead to an intranuclear accumulation of β-catenin protein, which leads to constitutive activation of the Wnt signaling pathway

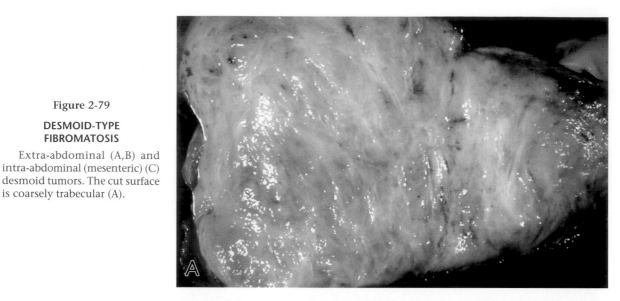

Figure 2-79

DESMOID-TYPE FIBROMATOSIS

Extra-abdominal (A,B) and intra-abdominal (mesenteric) (C) desmoid tumors. The cut surface is coarsely trabecular (A).

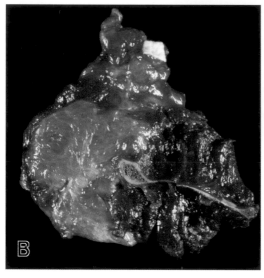

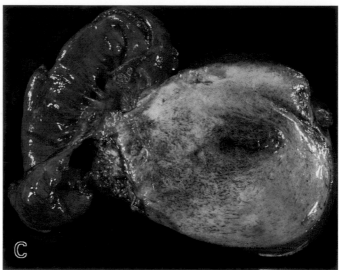

promoting cell proliferation (420,421,434–436). The location of the *APC* mutations (over 700 *APC* mutations have been reported, to date) influences the phenotypic expression pattern and disease severity (367,369,437–439). Desmoid tumors occur with greater frequency in patients who have truncating *APC* mutations involving codons 1445 to 1580, than in patients with mutations before codon 1387 (367,433,438,440,441). Some patients with *APC* mutations have an attenuated phenotype with a diminished number or absence of colonic polyps (367,439).

Additional genetic events in desmoid tumors include trisomies of chromosomes 8 and 20 (424,425,442–444). These changes are more read-

ily detected with fluorescence in situ hybridization (FISH) than conventional cytogenetics, presumably because the trisomic population has a growth disadvantage and is overgrown by diploid cells in culture (424,445,446). These trisomies are thought to most likely be secondary events and are not considered key to the pathogenesis of the tumors. Gains in chromosomal regions 1q21 and 9p12; losses in 6q16-q21, 5q14-q15, and 13q21-q31; and other aberrant genetic events have been documented in a small percentage of cases (425,442,444,447,448).

Differential Diagnosis. The differential diagnosis for desmoid-type fibromatosis includes scar tissue, palmar/plantar (so-called superficial)

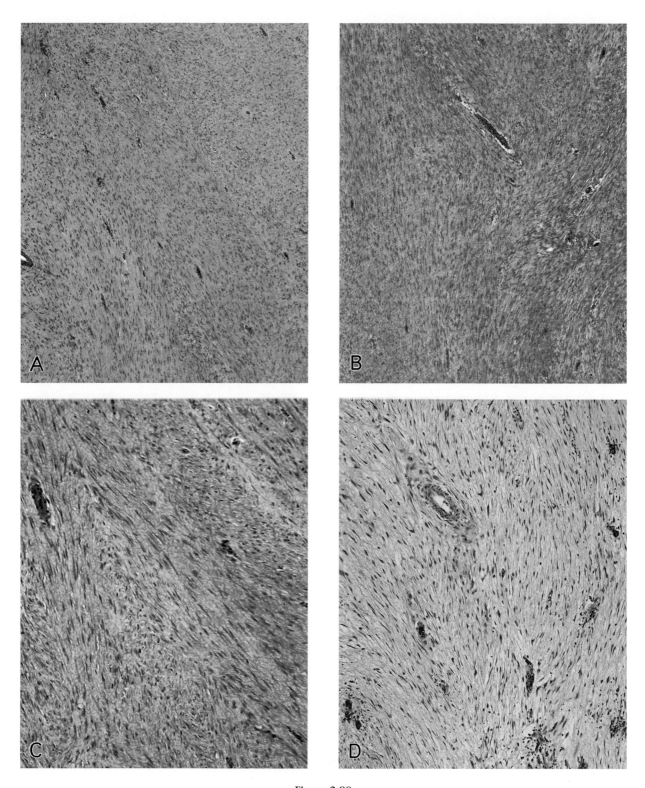

Figure 2-80

DESMOID-TYPE FIBROMATOSIS

A–D: A uniform population of spindled cells with a loose fascicular growth pattern, abundant extracellular matrix, and a fairly evenly distributed vasculature is seen. The extracellular matrix ranges from collagenous to myxocollagenous.

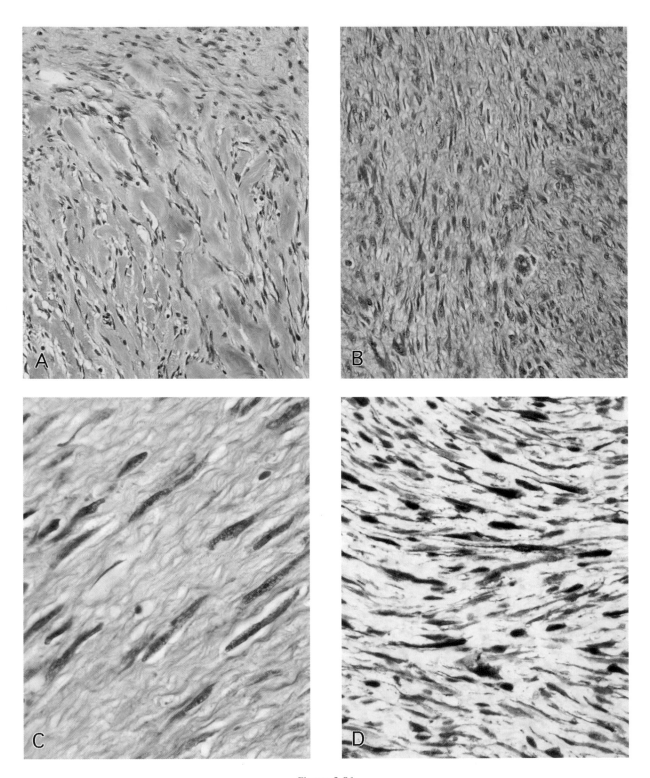

Figure 2-81

DESMOID-TYPE FIBROMATOSIS

Keloid-like collagen bundles (A) and tumor cells with characteristic mild nuclear atypia (B,C) are seen. There is coarsening of the nuclear chromatin with small but distinct central nucleoli. Both nuclear and cytoplasmic β-catenin expression is often detectable with immunohistochemistry (D).

fibromatosis, fibromatosis colli, Gardner-associated fibroma, desmoplastic fibroblastoma (collagenous fibroma), low-grade fibromyxoid sarcoma, and low-grade fibrosarcoma. For intra-abdominal fibromatosis, idiopathic retroperitoneal fibrosis and gastrointestinal stromal tumor (GIST) also warrant some consideration.

Scar tissue generally presents as a smaller mass, accompanied by some past history of trauma. Scar tissue has more variable cellularity than a desmoid tumor, and it often has granulation tissue–type vasculature, areas of hemorrhage or hemosiderin deposition, and a number of secondary inflammatory elements. Nuclear β-catenin expression is absent (418).

Palmar/plantar fibromatosis is a multinodular myofibroblastic proliferation, typically confined to the aponeurosis of the palm or sole. Muscle invasion is uncommon. Fibromatosis colli presents as a soft tissue mass within the sternocleidomastoid muscle (especially the lower half of the muscle) of an infant. This process typically has vaguely lobular growth and characteristically entraps residual degenerating and regenerating skeletal muscle fibers.

Gardner-associated fibromas are strongly associated with FAP/Gardner syndrome and present at a young age. These lesions are considerably less cellular and more collagenous than a desmoid tumor and are CD34 positive, with focal nuclear β-catenin expression in some cases. Desmoplastic fibroblastoma (collagenous fibroma) has less cellularity and less vascularity than a desmoid tumor. Low-grade fibromyxoid sarcomas contain areas that closely resemble a desmoid tumor, but helpful features that aid in recognition include foci with myxoid change and microvasculature accentuation, zones with perivascular hypercellularity, and hyalinizing nodules bordered by epithelioid cells (so-called giant rosettes). These tumors typically contain a t(7;16) with *FUS/CREB3L2* fusion transcripts.

Fibrosarcoma has greater cellularity than a desmoid tumor, with herringbone patterns, and usually greater atypia and mitotic activity. Idiopathic retroperitoneal fibrosis is an inflammatory fibrosclerotic process that often causes compression or obstruction of the ureters and other regional structures (including major vessels). Histologically, this process commonly contains abundant hyalinized collagen, strongly actin-positive but sparse myofibroblasts, and a mixed chronic inflammatory infiltrate. GISTs usually arise within the alimentary canal wall. In general, these tumors are more cellular and have less collagenous matrix than a desmoid tumor. In contrast to desmoid tumor, the neoplastic cells in GISTs characteristically express CD117, DOG1, and CD34; have variable reactivity for smooth muscle actin and desmin; and lack nuclear β-catenin expression (416).

Treatment and Prognosis. Desmoid tumors have a propensity for local recurrence when incompletely excised, but they do not metastasize. Recurrence rates vary by subgroup (388,389,393,400,403), with generally accepted ranges of 35 to 68 percent for extra-abdominal tumors and 10 to 30 percent for abdominal wall tumors. Intra-abdominal tumors have an overall recurrence rate of approximately 20 percent, but the risk of recurrence is markedly higher in FAP/Gardner patients (about 90 percent of these individuals experience a recurrence versus a reported low of 11 percent for patients with sporadic intra-abdominal tumors) (403). Approximately 3 to 6 percent of desmoids resolve spontaneously (373,374,395,449,450).

Optimal management is influenced by a number of factors including the following: anatomic site, tumor size, patient age, FAP status, and risk for involvement of vital structures (374,401,431,451,452). Extra-abdominal fibromatoses are only rarely fatal, and when they are, it is usually because of involvement of vital structures (453,454). In contrast, unresectable mesenteric fibromatosis has a mortality rate as high as 30 percent, and intra-abdominal desmoid tumors are the most frequent extracolonic cause of death (usually secondary to bowel obstruction, ischemic necrosis, and septicemia) in FAP patients (374).

For intra-abdominal tumors, many experts consider first-line management to be sulindac, often in combination with a selective estrogen receptor modulator (e.g., tamoxifen, toremifene, or raloxifene) (368,375,383,452,455). If this treatment fails and the desmoid is resectable without sacrificing small bowel function, surgical intervention (primarily for non-FAP patients) is often recommended (374,402). Radiation is not generally advisable in this setting, and cytotoxic chemotherapy is often reserved for patients with either unresectable or unresponsive tumors that threaten vital structures (368,375,402,455,456).

Extra-abdominal and abdominal wall desmoid tumors are generally managed with wide local excision (368,394,397,400,452,457). When resection cannot be achieved without undue morbidity, alternate intervention is often advocated because of a lack of metastatic potential (397,431,452,458–460). In cases where tumor-free margins are not achievable, postoperative radiation therapy (primarily reserved for adult patients) (386,413,461–463) may be beneficial (431,452,456,459,464,465) or pharmacologic therapy (including nonsteroidal anti-inflammatory drugs, antiestrogenic agents [378,383,466], sunitinib [412], and cytotoxic chemotherapy) (374,381,382,386,458) may be tried. Radical surgery is generally reserved for cases in which all other reasonable treatment options have been exhausted.

BENIGN FIBROUS HISTIOCYTOMA (DERMATOFIBROMA)

Definition. *Benign fibrous histiocytoma* (BFH), or *dermatofibroma*, is a fibroblastic-myofibroblastic neoplasm almost always based in skin or subcutis and often extensively infiltrated by histiocytes. Previous terminology includes *sclerosing hemangioma*, *histiocytoma*, and *subepidermal nodular fibrosis*.

General Comments. The most common form of BFH is a small cutaneous papule or nodule. These tumors have a predilection for young adults, although some variants occur in older populations (467,468). Discussed here are histologic variants (fewer than 10 percent of all cases) that form soft tissue tumors and even simulate a sarcoma. Common to most of them is a fibroblastic-myofibroblastic neoplastic cell population, which is accompanied by variable numbers of infiltrating non-neoplastic histiocytes (hence the old term "fibrohistiocytic"). The presence of clonal genetic changes and proliferative activity in the fibroblasts, but not in the histiocytes, seems to support the concept of a fibroblastic-myofibroblastic neoplasm, as opposed to a reactive process.

Although most benign fibrous histiocytomas are skin based, many also involve the subcutis, sometimes exclusively. Those lesions that are located in areas with superficially located skel-etal muscle, such as face and neck, may extend into muscle and have a higher rate of recurrence because of commonly applied tissue-sparing surgery in sensitive facial sites (469). Most intramuscular tumors historically designated as "deep fibrous histiocytoma" belong to other entities, especially solitary fibrous tumor and low-grade fibromyxoid sarcoma.

Immunohistochemistry often shows focal to extensive smooth muscle actin expression, reflecting myofibroblastic differentiation, and some variants are focally positive for CD34 and desmin. CD10 expression is a typical feature, as is common to many other fibroblastic lesions, benign and malignant. Consistent negativity for S-100 protein helps to separate BFH from nerve sheath and melanocytic tumors (467,468).

Management generally includes simple excision, but complete excision whenever possible without undue morbidity is necessary for those variants that have a significant potential to recur (aneurysmal, cellular, and atypical variants). The fibrous histiocytoma variants of greater importance to soft tissue pathology are discussed here: 1) aneurysmal, 2) cellular, 3) lipidized, and 4) atypical fibrous histiocytoma.

Aneurysmal Fibrous Histiocytoma. This rare variant (2 percent of all BFHs) occurs in a wide age range, but especially in young adults, with a mild female predominance and a predilection for proximal parts of the extremities. The tumor size ranges from less than 0.5 to 4.0 cm. Grossly, there is a blue or dark surface and cystic consistency, with some examples potentially clinically simulating Kaposi sarcoma or melanoma. Intratumoral hematoma formation may result in worrisome lesional enlargement, prompting medical attention. This variant can also form a large, exophytic sessile polypoid cutaneous mass. Reported recurrence rates vary from 0 to 19 percent, and there are at least three reports of regional lymph node metastasis without evidence of progressive disease (470–475).

Histologically, aneurysmal fibrous histiocytoma is characterized by cysts and hemorrhagic spaces without endothelial lining and containing extravasated erythrocytes and xanthoma cells. There is often a vague storiform architecture, and a hemangiopericytoma-like vascular pattern may be present. Focal stromal sclerosis and hemosiderin deposition are common.

Mitotic activity of up to 5 mitoses per 10 high-power fields is common. Plump, slightly epithelioid or polygonal cells admixed with histiocytes comprise the main cellular component (fig. 2-82). Some cases contain inclusions of entrapped skin adnexal epithelia, which can be slightly proliferative.

This variant should not be confused with angiomatoid fibrous histiocytoma, a childhood tumor composed of densely cellular sheets of round to spindled cells. Aneurysmal fibrous histiocytoma is separated from Kaposi sarcoma by a more heterogeneous cellular composition and immunohistochemical differences (negative for CD34 and HHV-8). A t(12;19)(p12;q13) chromosomal translocation was reported in one case (476).

Cellular Fibrous Histiocytoma. This variant has a predilection for the proximal lower and upper extremities; approximately 20 percent of cases occur in the head and neck region. There is a moderate male predilection (468,477). Recurrence is more frequent than in other variants and occurs in up to 25 percent of patients. A small number of cases with pulmonary metastases have been reported at 1.5 to 23.0 years after the primary tumor, sometimes preceded by multiple recurrences. These metastases have formed cystic, often multiple, pulmonary lesions, and the clinical course has been indolent during limited follow-up (474,478–480).

Cellular fibrous histiocytoma often involves the dermis and subcutis, and usually measures 0.5 to 2.5 cm in maximum diameter. Histologically, it is composed of cellular fascicles of spindle cells without significant nuclear atypia or variability. The mitotic rate is higher than for common benign fibrous histiocytomas (up to 10 mitoses per 10 high-power fields). The tumor often extends into subcutaneous fat with a wide pushing border, and central necrosis may be present (fig. 2-83). Immunohistochemical features include nearly consistent expression of smooth muscle actin, focal desmin expression in a third of cases, and CD34 expression in rare cases (481).

Lipidized Fibrous Histiocytoma. The lipidized variant occurs more often in older adults, and has some predilection for the distal lower extremity. It sometimes forms larger masses larger than other BFHs (5 cm or more). This variant is histologically characterized by abundant lipid-laden xanthoma cell-like histiocytes with variably clear cytoplasm and a prominent capillary pattern with hyalinized vessel walls (fig. 2-84) (468,482). There is no significant association with hyperlipidemia. This lesion should be distinguished from xanthomas that tend to contain cholesterol crystals and are composed of a nearly purely histiocytic population (483).

Atypical Fibrous Histiocytoma. Atypical fibrous histiocytoma, also designated as *pseudosarcomatous fibrous histiocytoma* or *dermatofibroma with monster cells*, occurs in a wide age range with a predilection to young adults, among which males predominate. The anatomic distribution is wide, and some examples are larger than usual fibrous histiocytomas (up to 8 cm). Atypical fibrous histiocytomas have a greater potential to recur than usual BFH, and rare metastases thought to be comparable with aneurysmal and cellular BFH have been reported to other sites of skin, colon, and lung. Complete excision and follow-up are advisable.

Histologically, the tumor shows features of conventional BFH, but in addition, contains focal cytologic atypia (fig. 2-85). The scattered atypical cells have large nuclei, often with prominent nucleoli, and some also have abundant cytoplasm. Mitotic activity is minimal, but atypical mitoses may be present. Some examples are CD34 positive, but based on the cytology (heterogeneous cellular composition), they are not likely confused with dermatofibrosarcoma protuberans (with a greater cellular homogeneity). The small number of atypical cells distinguishes this tumor from atypical fibroxanthoma, where the atypia is pervasive and atypical mitoses often numerous (468,484–488).

Immunohistochemical Findings. The tumor cells are almost always negative for CD34, and a peripheral rim of positive innate dermal fibroblasts should not be confused with tumor cell positivity. Focal to extensive positivity for α-smooth muscle actin is common. The tumor cells are generally negative for desmin, keratins, and S-100 protein. Variable numbers of tumor-infiltrating histiocytes are positive for the histiocytic markers factor XIIIa, CD68, and CD163, but the fibroblastic tumor cells are negative.

Differential Diagnosis. Dermatofibrosarcoma protuberans is a cytologically homogeneous, less histiocyte-rich, CD34-positive neoplasm typically showing a storiform or

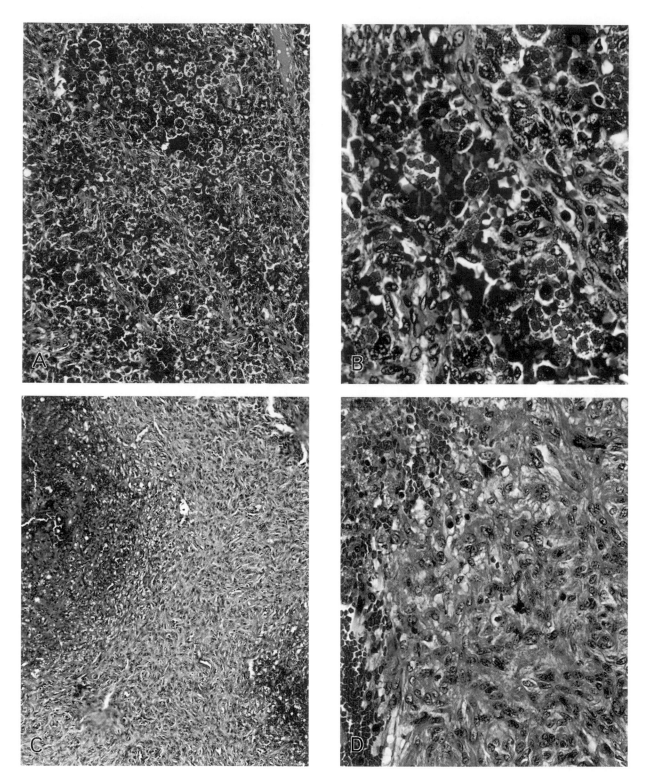

Figure 2-82

ANEURYSMAL FIBROUS HISTIOCYTOMA

A–D: An aneurysmal fibrous histiocytoma contains blood-filled spaces with hemosiderin-laden macrophages. The lesional cells are oval to spindled, and fairly uniform in size.

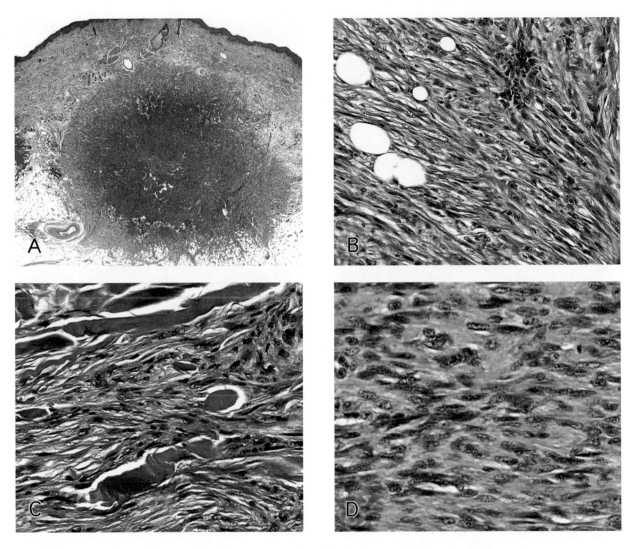

Figure 2-83

CELLULAR FIBROUS HISTIOCYTOMA

A: At low magnification, this cellular fibrous histiocytoma forms a deep dermal mass that also involves the subcutis and infiltrates the fat at the irregular deep border.

B: Uniform spindled tumor cells have a tendency to fascicular organization.

C: The collagen trapping typical of fibrous histiocytoma is evident.

D: At high magnification, the spindled cells have elongated nuclei with delicate nucleoli.

cartwheel pattern and extensively infiltrating the subcutaneous fat. Some BFH variants infiltrate focally in the subcutaneous fat, usually with a pushing border. Juvenile xanthogranuloma is a true histiocytic lesion positive for CD163 and often containing Touton giant cells with a ring-like nuclear arrangement.

Treatment and Prognosis. BFH is generally treated by simple excision. The variants with an increased risk of recurrence (cellular and atypical variants) should be completely excised, however,

whenever possible. The frequency of recurrence of usual variants is probably less than 10 percent, whereas the cellular variant has a recurrence rate of 25 percent. On rare occasion, regional lymph node metastases have been reported in the cellular variant. There are isolated cases of pulmonary metastases of BFH (especially aneurysmal, cellular, and atypical types). Such metastases are often multiple and occur years after the primary tumor; however, limited follow-up shows the disease course seems to be indolent.

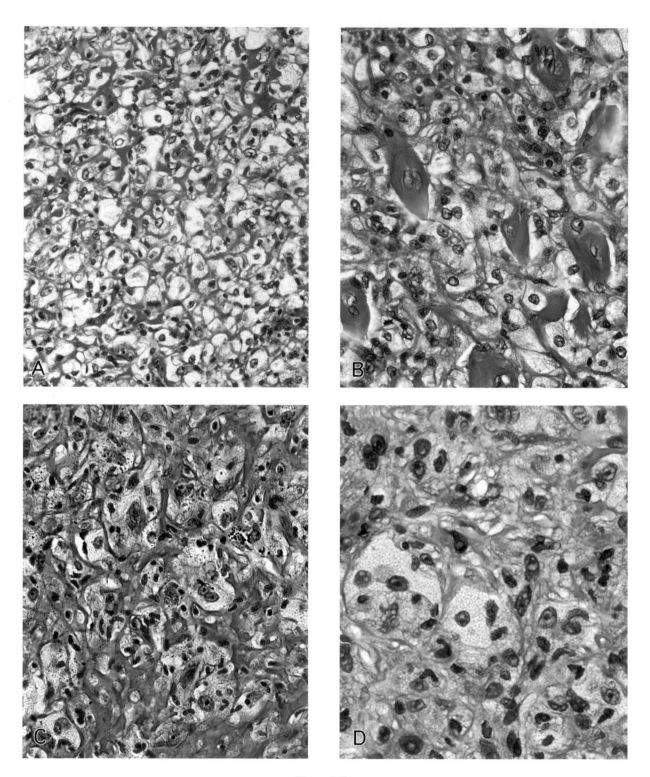

Figure 2-84

LIPIDIZED FIBROUS HISTIOCYTOMA

A,B: Lipidized fibrous histiocytoma contains pale cytoplasmic lipidized cells. Focal or more extensive sclerosis is often present.
C: Focal hemosiderin deposition is often present.
D: At high magnification, the lipidized cells have a pale, multivacuolated cytoplasm.

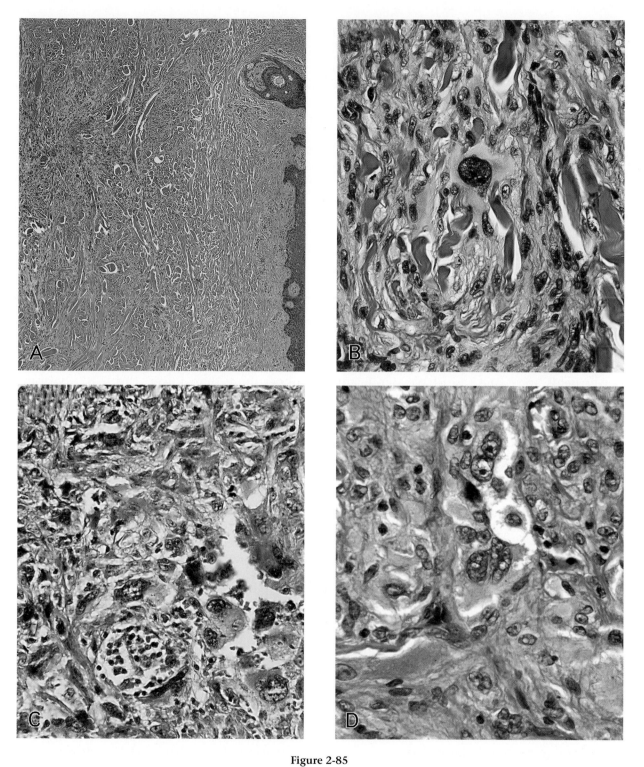

Figure 2-85

ATYPICAL FIBROUS HISTIOCYTOMA

A: At low magnification, larger atypical nuclei stand out in the lower middle portion of this dermal atypical fibrous histiocytoma.

B: Moderately atypical cells in the same case.

C,D: Nuclear atypia in two other atypical fibrous histiocytomas.

NON-NEURAL GRANULAR CELL TUMOR

Definition. *Non-neural granular cell tumor* is a mesenchymal, fibroblastic-myofibroblastic, S-100 protein–negative neoplasm with a prominent content of cells with granular cytoplasm. This tumor is also called *granular cell dermatofibroma* and *primitive non-neural granular cell tumor of skin* (489–493).

Clinical Features. The reported rare cases have occurred in young adults with a male predominance. The lesions have a predilection to shoulder, neck, and back. The tumors may involve skin and subcutis and vary from small papules to nodules of 2 to 3 cm or more (489–493).

Microscopic Findings. The tumor is composed of cells with abundant granular cytoplasm, similar to ordinary S-100 protein–positive granular cell tumors, but the tumor cells are negative for S-100 protein. Some examples also contain spindle cells or areas resembling conventional BFH (fig. 2-86). Mitotic activity consists of 2 to 12 mitotic figures per 10 high-power fields and some cases have significant nuclear atypia including pleomorphism. Non-neural granular cell tumor differs conceptually from atypical fibroxanthoma by the presence of widespread, often malignant fibrous histiocytoma-like cytologic atypia in the latter.

Treatment and Prognosis. Although most examples are benign, regional lymph node metastasis has been reported in at least one case. This was associated with a benign clinical course after local excision. Atypical examples should be managed with complete excision and follow-up.

NEUROTHEKEOMA

Definition. *Neurothekeoma* is a mesenchymal neoplasm of the skin and subcutis that characteristically forms a small, multinodular mass composed of spindled and epithelioid cells with a notable tendency for whorled and focal fascicular growth. S-100 protein expression is characteristically absent. Examples are subclassified as cellular, mixed type, or myxoid, based on the amount extracellular matrix.

General Considerations. Over the years, many authors have use the terms "neurothekeoma" and "nerve sheath myxoma" as synonyms (494,495). More recently, some authors have selectively used the designation "myxoid neurothekeoma" as a synonym for "nerve sheath myxoma" (496,497). We do not support either approach, because there is ample evidence that neurothekeomas (whether cellular, mixed type, or myxoid) are unrelated to true nerve sheath myxomas (495,498–501)

There is no substantive evidence that neurothekeomas, whether cellular, mixed type, or myxoid, have a neural derivation (495,499,500). Recent observations suggest that neurothekeoma is a special type of fibroblastic/myofibroblastic (or "fibrohistiocytic") tumor, and that existing nomenclature is inaccurate (495,499–502). Some morphologic overlap with plexiform fibrohistiocytic tumor has been noted (497,499,502–504).

Clinical Features. There is a 2 to 1 female predominance, and a strong predilection for the first three decades of life, with a peak incidence in the second decade (fig. 2-87, top) (495,499,500). There is a well-recognized tendency for lesions to affect the head and neck, trunk, and proximal portions of the extremities (upper more than lower) (fig. 2-87, bottom) (499,500,505). Patients generally present with a small, superficial, painless mass of several weeks' to many years' duration.

Gross Findings. This process forms a dermal and/or subcutaneous mass that is usually 1 cm or smaller (499,500,505). Fewer than 10 percent of cases are 2 cm or larger. On cut section, the lesional boundaries are often poorly defined. Some tumors are solid and have a firm consistency, whereas others are soft and highly myxoid.

Microscopic Findings. Histologic examination reveals a multinodular dermal and/or subcutaneous neoplasm composed of spindled and epithelioid cells with abundant granular eosinophilic cytoplasm (fig. 2-88). Most examples have no more than mild atypia, but occasional tumors have focal, or even more generalized, moderate atypia and pleomorphism (499,500,505,506). The degree of mitotic activity is variable (499,500,505,506). In one study (499), 69 percent of cases had 0 to 5 mitotic figures per 25 wide high-power fields, but 14 percent of cases had over 10 mitotic figures per 25 wide high-power fields. Rarely, atypical mitotic figures are seen (499,500).

There is a notable tendency for tumor cells within individual nodules to exhibit whorled and focal fascicular growth. The cells may be

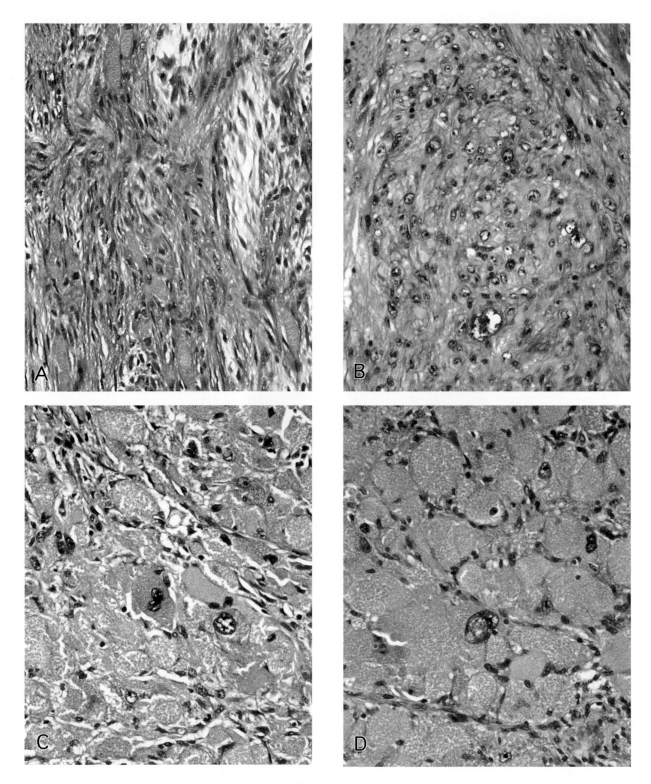

Figure 2-86

NON-NEURAL GRANULAR CELL TUMOR

A non-neural, S-100 protein–negative granular cell tumor contains a spindle cell element (A) and a prominent epithelioid granular cell component with significant focal nuclear pleomorphism (B–D).

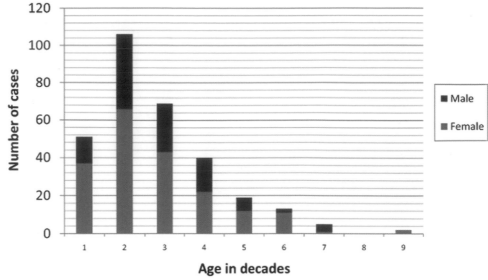

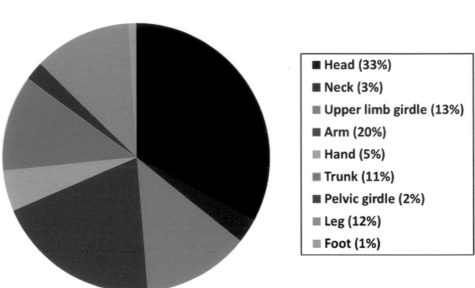

Figure 2-87

NEUROTHEKEOMA

Age and sex (top) and anatomic (bottom) distributions for patients with neurothekeomas. These data are derived from series published by Fetsch et al. (499) and Hornick and Fletcher (500).

closely apposed with indistinct borders, or they can be widely separated by abundant extracellular myxoid matrix (fig. 2-89). We subclassify tumors with 10 percent or less myxoid matrix as *cellular neurothekeomas*, with more than 10 but 50 percent or less myxoid matrix as *mixed-type neurothekeomas*, and with more than 50 percent myxoid matrix as *myxoid neurothekeomas* (499). Individual tumor nodules are often bordered by fibrous connective tissue. Occasional osteoclast-like giant cells are admixed with tumor cells in approximately 40 percent of neurothekeomas (fig. 2-88C,D) (499). Some inflammatory cells, including lymphocytes, plasma cells, conven-

tional histiocytes, eosinophils, and polymorphonuclear leukocytes, may also be present.

Special Studies. The neoplastic cells of neurothekeoma are typically immunoreactive for CD10, CD63, and microphthalmia transcription factor (MITF) (fig. 2-90) (499,500,506,507). Immunoreactivity is also commonly present for CD99. Approximately 60 percent of cases are positive for PGP9.5, and 38 to 57 percent of cases have at least focal reactivity for smooth muscle actin (499–502,508). In the two largest series, with a combined total of 311 cases (499, 500), no tumor was immunoreactive for S-100 protein. Barring the unforeseen exception, S-100

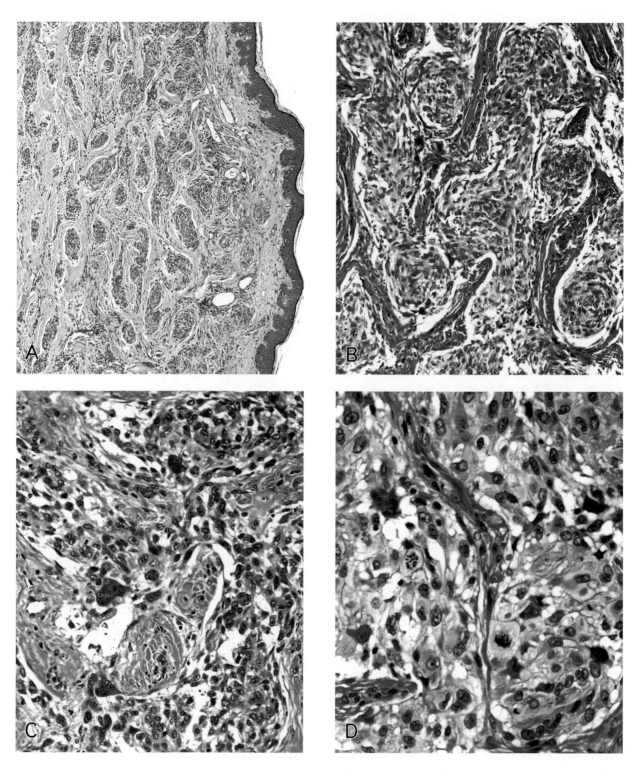

Figure 2-88

NEUROTHEKEOMA

Low (A), intermediate (B,C), and high (D) power views of neurothekeoma, cellular type. The superficial location, multinodular growth pattern, and tendency for whorled growth are seen. The neoplastic cells have abundant cytoplasm and focal nuclear atypia. Scattered osteoclast-like giant cells are present in many examples (C,D). Mitotic activity is variable (D).

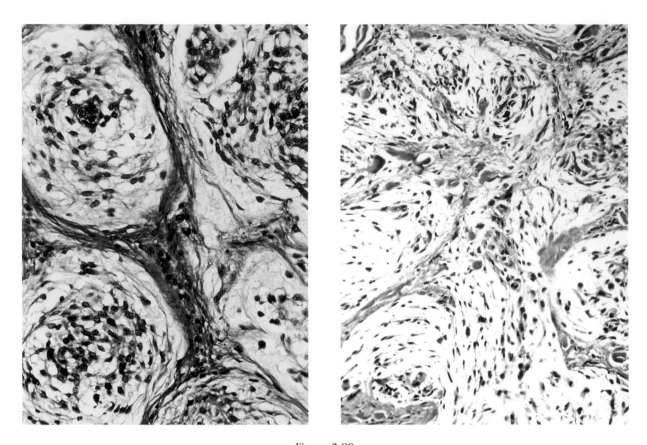

Figure 2-89

MYXOID NEUROTHEKEOMA

There is a tendency for whorled growth (left). The latter example has areas with increased nuclear atypia and pleomorphism, features that are occasionally present in neurothekeomas but are absent in true nerve sheath myxomas (right).

protein immunoreactivity in a tumor that has been classified as a neurothekeoma is generally explainable in one of two ways: 1) S-100 protein-positive, nonlesional "antigen-presenting," dendritic cells have been misinterpreted as tumor cells. In this setting, the S-100 protein-positive cells are typically sparsely distributed in a "pepper and salt" fashion, or 2) the tumor is actually a peripheral nerve sheath tumor (e.g., nerve sheath myxoma, schwannoma, or neurofibroma) or melanocytic neoplasm and not a neurothekeoma. In this setting, the S-100 protein-positive cells are present in great abundance, because both benign neoplastic Schwann cells and melanocytes tend to be diffusely and strongly reactive for this marker. This pattern is never encountered in a true neurothekeoma.

Differential Diagnosis. Two key considerations in the differential diagnosis of neurothek-

eoma are nerve sheath myxoma and plexiform fibrohistiocytic tumor. Nerve sheath myxomas (498,509–512) have often been confused with the myxoid variant of neurothekeoma, because both processes are matrix rich and form superficial, multinodular masses in dermal and subcutaneous tissue. There are a number of clinical and histopathologic differences, however, that allow clear separation of these entities. Nerve sheath myxomas have a strong predilection for the distal portions of the extremities, and there is a tendency to involve the fingers and knee region (498,509–511). Second, from a histopathologic perspective, nerve sheath myxomas are true peripheral nerve sheath tumors. They contain bland neoplastic Schwann cells, present singly, in corded arrays, and syncytial-like aggregates (fig. 2-91). Some of the Schwann cells have spindled morphology, some are epithelioid, and

108

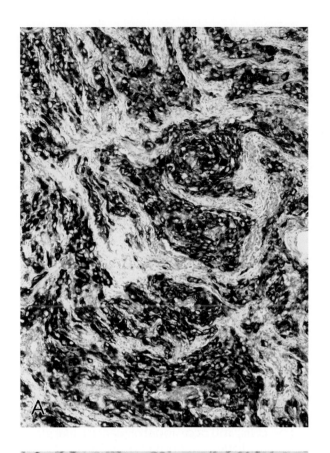

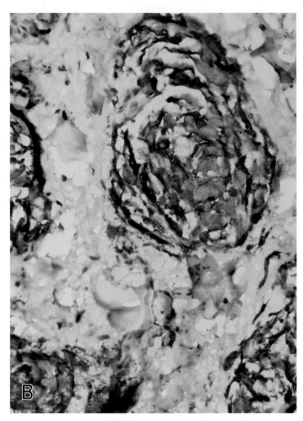

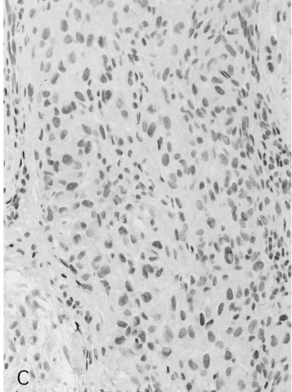

Figure 2-90

NEUROTHEKEOMA

Immunoreactivity is present for CD63 (A), CD10 (B), and microphthalmia transcription factor (MITF) (C).

others have spider-like cytoplasmic processes or a vacuolated appearance; cytoplasmic-nuclear invaginations are common (fig. 2-91D). The neoplastic Schwann cells are diffusely immunoreactive for S-100 protein (495,508–510,512) and GFAP (fig. 2-92), and they are nonreactive for CD10 (498,499,501). In contrast, neurothekeomas express CD10, are nonreactive for S-100 protein and GFAP, and lack a peripheral cuff of EMA-positive perineurial cells. From a management perspective, nerve sheath myxomas have a much greater propensity for local recurrence when incompletely excised than do neurothekeomas. In a recent AFIP study (498), 47 percent of patients with a nerve sheath myxoma developed a recurrence, and in 15 percent of these individuals, the recurrences were multiple.

Plexiform fibrohistiocytic tumor has a number of clinicopathologic features that overlap with neurothekeoma (497,499,503,504). Both entities have a similar age range, female predominance, and anatomic distribution. Both also form multinodular masses with spindle cells, have areas with fascicular growth, and can have osteoclast-like giant cells. Overlapping immunohistochemical features have also been reported. These similarities raise the possibility that the two processes are closely related, and it is only fair to point out that there are cases where a clear distinction between the two cannot be made. At present, we believe the following features favor a diagnosis of plexiform fibrohistiocytic tumor: predominantly subcutaneous localization with sparing of the upper dermis, well-developed fascicular growth dominated by spindle cells with myofibroblastic features, and lack of whorled architecture. Plexiform fibrohistiocytic tumors also typically lack the nuclear variability and pleomorphism that are sometimes seen in neurothekeomas.

Other entities that enter into the differential diagnosis of neurothekeoma include melanocytic tumors, superficial angiomyxoma, and reticulohistiocytoma.

Treatment and Prognosis. Surgical specimens of neurothekeoma commonly show tumor extending to the tissue margin. In spite of this, the local recurrence rate for this process, based on the two largest series published to date (499,500), is only approximately 15 percent, and this figure may well be an overestimation

of the "true" recurrence rate, because the data are derived from consultative services. The following factors may correlate with increased potential for local recurrence: highly myxoid tumors, facial location, incomplete excision with the absence of subcutaneous tissue in the surgical specimen, and female sex (499).

While the presence of atypical cytologic features (i.e., at least moderate nuclear atypia and pleomorphism, increased mitotic activity, or atypical mitotic figures) and large tumor size (most neurothekeoma are smaller than 2 cm) have not been shown to adversely affect outcome (499,500,506), we view this as a gray area that warrants further study and advocate complete excision and follow-up for tumors with these findings as a precautionary measure.

PLEXIFORM FIBROHISTIOCYTIC TUMOR

Definition. *Plexiform fibrohistiocytic tumor* is a borderline/very low malignant potential neoplasm characterized by multinodular/plexiform growth within dermal and subcutaneous tissue. The process features spindled (myo)fibroblastic cells (often with fascicular growth), ovoid histiocytoid cells, and occasional osteoclast-like giant cells with little cellular pleomorphism.

General Considerations. This process is sometimes difficult to distinguish from neurothekeoma (513,514). Histomorphologic features that aid in the distinction are provided in the differential diagnosis section of neurothekeoma. In cases where precise classification is problematic, complete excision with follow-up should be encouraged.

Clinical Features. This neoplastic process occurs over a wide age range (2 months to 77 years), but over 50 percent of the patients are under 20 years of age (median, 13 to 20 years in various reports) (515–518). A striking female predominance has been noted in some series (515,518). The most common site of involvement is the upper extremity (ranging from shoulder to hand), followed in descending frequency by the lower extremity (especially the thigh region), trunk, and head and neck area (515,517,518). Patients typically present with a slow-growing, painless mass that may elevate the overlying skin. Occasional examples display central dimpling.

Gross Findings. Plexiform fibrohistiocytic tumors typically form poorly demarcated, gray-white

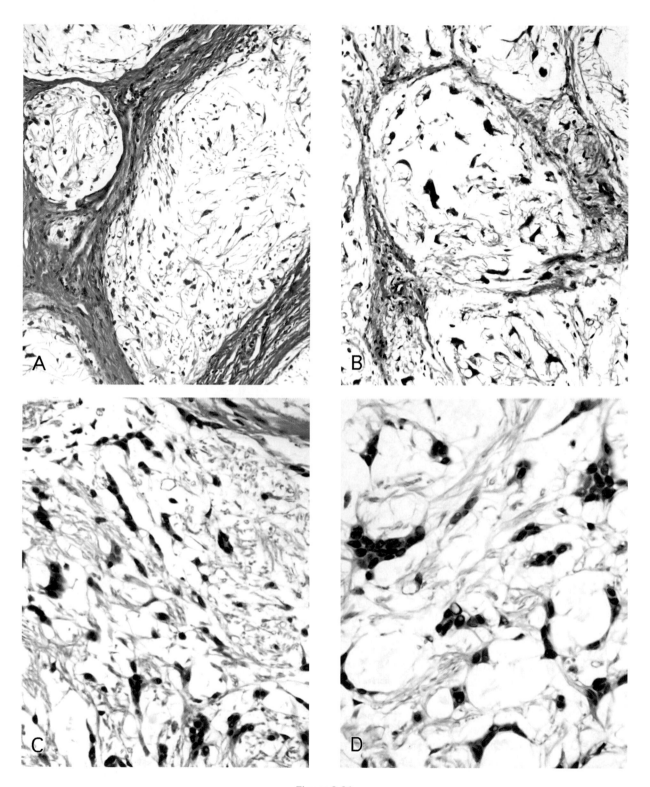

Figure 2-91

NERVE SHEATH MYXOMA

Multinodularity, abundant myxoid matrix, and scattered, bland, neoplastic (Schwann) cells often arranged in cords and syncytial-like clusters (A–D). Some tumor cells have cytoplasmic-nuclear invaginations (D).

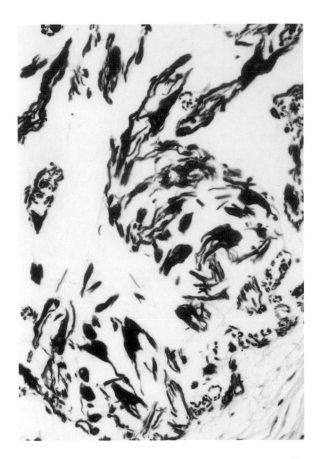
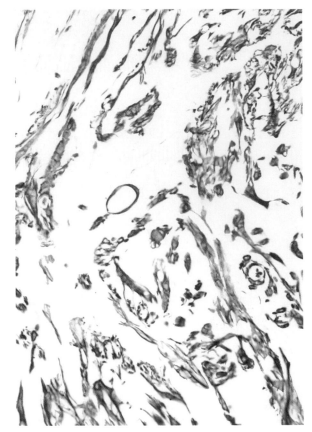

Figure 2-92

NERVE SHEATH MYXOMA

Strong and diffuse immunoreactivity for S-100 protein (left) and glial fibrillary acidic protein (GFAP) (right) in nerve sheath myxoma. All variants of neurothekeoma (cellular, mixed-type, and myxoid) are nonreactive for both markers.

to tan masses, epicentered in the lower dermis and subcutis. Close inspection of the cut surface may reveal a coarsely trabecular growth pattern. Reported examples have ranged in size from 0.3 to 8.5 cm in greatest dimension, but most examples are in the 1- to 3-cm range (515,518,519).

Microscopic Findings. Low-power microscopic examination demonstrates a multinodular or plexiform proliferation concentrated in the deep dermis and subcutis (fig. 2-93), occasionally extending into underlying skeletal muscle. The composition of individual tumor nodules varies from case to case and even from one area to the next in a given tumor, but characteristically, there are spindled (myo)fibroblasts and/or round to oval pale-staining histiocytoid cells with somewhat granular cytoplasm, admixed with varying numbers of osteoclast-like giant cells (fig. 2-94) (515–518). In cases with an abundance of spindled cells, fascicular growth tends to be well developed. Cellular pleomorphism is minimal (with rare exception), and necrosis is characteristically absent.

Mitotic activity can range from 0 to more than 10 mitoses per 10 high-power fields, but most examples have 3 or fewer mitoses (515,518). Only rarely have atypical mitotic figures been reported (517,518). Focal intravascular growth (presently of uncertain prognostic significance) is present in a few instances (515,517,518,529). Additional findings include dense perinodular fibrosis, patchy chronic inflammation, intralesional microhemorrhage, focal myxoid change, and rarely, osseous metaplasia.

Special Studies. Focal immunoreactivity for α-smooth muscle actin and muscle-specific actin is often demonstrable in the spindled tumor cells (516,517,519). CD68 highlights the osteoclast-like

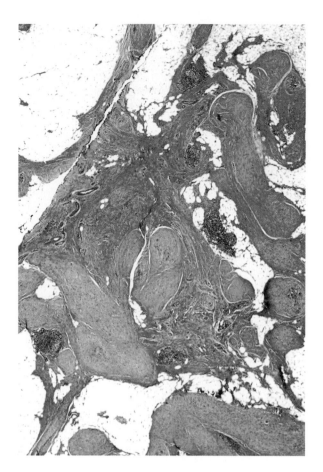

Figure 2-93

PLEXIFORM FIBROHISTIOCYTIC TUMOR

A plexiform fibrohistiocytic tumor involving subcutaneous fat has the distinctive growth pattern and accompanying inflammatory reaction.

giant cells and is more weakly expressed in other lesional cells (fig. 2-94F). We have noted CD10 expression. Immunostains for calponin, desmin, keratin, and S-100 protein are negative (516–518). CD34 expression is usually absent (517).

Genetics. There are two case reports describing genetic alterations in neoplasms that have been classified as plexiform fibrohistiocytic tumors. One tumor had a karyotype of 46, XY, -6,-8, del(4)(q25q31), del(20)(q11.2), +der (8)t(8;?)(p22;?), +mar (521). The other tumor had a simpler karyotype of 46, XY, t(4;15)(q21;q15) (522). The histologic illustration accompanying the second case does not seem fully convincing for a plexiform fibrohistiocytic tumor, but the brief text description is supportive.

Differential Diagnosis. The key consideration in the differential diagnosis is cellular neurothekeoma. This has been discussed in the section on neurothekeoma.

Additional considerations in the differential diagnosis include giant cell tumor of soft parts and plexiform xanthomatous tumor. The former tends to grow as a discrete nodular mass and has histologic features reminiscent of giant cell tumor of bone. The latter characteristically occurs in older patients, exhibits multinodular/plexiform growth within the dermis and subcutis, and features spindled fibroblasts and xanthomatous histiocytes, admixed with scattered cholesterol clefts, and lacks osteoclast-like giant cells (523).

Treatment and Prognosis. Most patients with plexiform fibrohistiocytic tumor have a benign clinical course. Approximately two thirds of patients are cured by local excision. An estimated one third experience local recurrence (actual recurrence rates in published series range from 12.5 to 50.0 percent) and require re-excision (515,516,518). Regional lymph node and distant metastases are rare, and typically are preceded by a local recurrence (515,518,520). Histomorphologic features are not predictive of outcome (515,518). A wide local excision and long-term follow-up with appropriate chest imaging studies are generally considered optimal management techniques.

SUPERFICIAL ACRAL FIBROMYXOMA

Definition. *Superficial acral fibromyxoma* is a benign dermal fibroblastic tumor of acral sites, with a predilection for periungual locations in digits. Most examples have bland cytomorphology, loose fascicular or broad storiform growth, abundant myxoid to collagenous matrix, mildly accentuated vasculature, and immunoreactivity for CD34.

General Considerations. It is the authors' experience that this benign process is not as rare as the literature currently suggests. Most examples in the past have been classified as a fibrous histiocytoma variant, (periungual) fibroma, fibromyxoma, or neurofibroma. Tumors recently described as *cellular digital fibroma* and *digital fibromyxoma* are considered part of this histologic spectrum.

Clinical Features. Superficial acral fibromyxomas have been documented in individuals

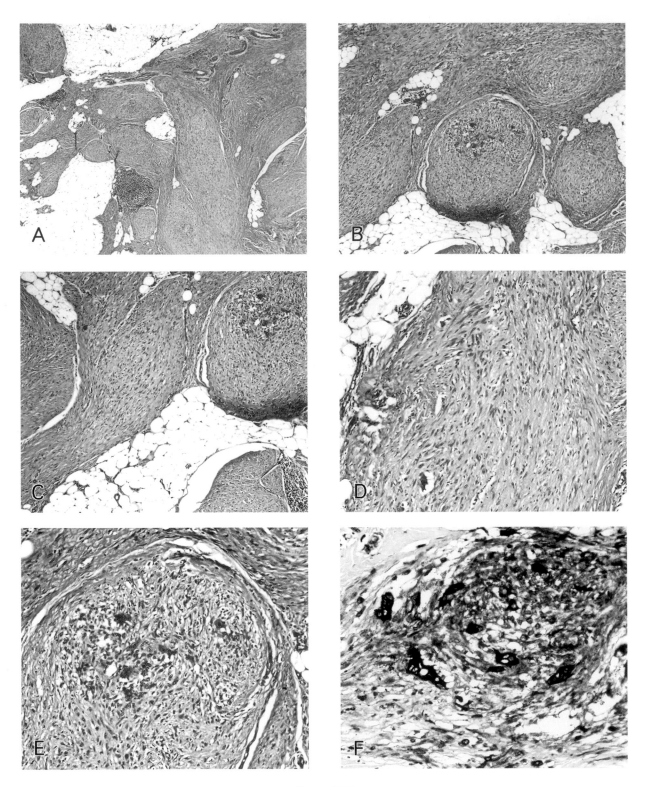

Figure 2-94

PLEXIFORM FIBROHISTIOCYTIC TUMOR

The spindled tumor cells have a fairly uniform morphology and broad fascicular growth pattern (A–E). The osteoclast-like giant cells (E) are strongly reactive for CD68 (F).

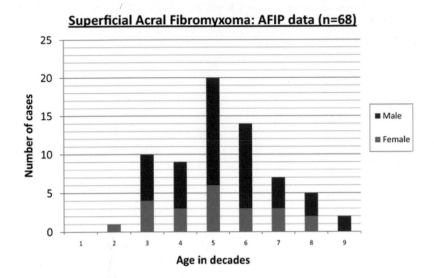

Figure 2-95

SUPERFICIAL ACRAL FIBROMYXOMA

Age and sex distribution of 68 patients with a superficial acral fibromyxoma reviewed at the AFIP.

ranging in age from 14 to 82 years, but approximately 70 percent of patients are 40 years of age or older (fig. 2-95) (524–531). Male patients have outnumbered female patients by a 2 to 1 margin (524,525,529). The typical example presents as a solitary, slow-growing, painless mass on a finger or toe. The most frequently affected site is the great toe (524,525,529). Up to two thirds of cases are reported to be periungual, but other acral sites, including the palms and soles, may also be affected (524,525,529). Some examples cause nail deformities, and rare examples cause scalloping of the underlying bone (525,531).

Gross Findings. Gross examination reveals a superficial, dome-shaped, polypoid or verrucoid mass (0.6 to 5.0 cm; median, 1.5 cm) just beneath the epidermis (525). In many resection specimens, portions of the nail and nail bed are present. The process has a soft to firm consistency and an off-white color, and the cut surface ranges from myxoid to solid and fibrous.

Microscopic Findings. Histologic examination reveals a moderately cellular, dermal-based proliferation of spindle- and stellate-shaped fibroblasts embedded in a myxoid to collagenous matrix (figs. 2-96, 2-97). The cells have random, loose fascicular and broad storiform growth patterns, and there is often accentuated microvasculature with many mast cells. In most instances, mitotic figures are uncommon (typically less than 1 mitotic figure per 10 high-power fields). Most tumor cells are mononuclear, but sparsely distributed multinucleated cells are seen in approximately half of the cases. Only rare examples have focally moderate or more pronounced atypia (524,525,527,529). These latter cases retain a low mitotic count, and atypical mitotic figures are absent. Extension into the superficial subcutis is common, and rarely, the process involves underlying fascia or abuts bone. Up to two thirds of cases are closely associated with the nail bed (524,525,525a).

Special Studies. The tumor cells are typically immunoreactive for CD34 (fig. 2-97D), and there is often reactivity for CD99 (524–527,529). Some investigators have reported a high percentage of cases with focal EMA expression, whereas others report this marker to be negative (524,525,527,529,530). This discordance is likely due to differing EMA antibodies and antigen retrieval techniques. More recently, CD10 expression has been noted in some cases (528,530). S-100 protein, HMB-45, GFAP, actin, desmin, and keratin are, for practical purposes, not expressed. No genetic information is currently available for this tumor.

Differential Diagnosis. The differential diagnosis for superficial acral fibromyxoma includes fibrous histiocytoma, acquired digital/periungual fibrokeratoma, superficial angiomyxoma (cutaneous myxoma), and neurofibroma. Fibrous histiocytomas tend to have more compact growth with well-developed storiform architecture and greater cellular diversity. These

115

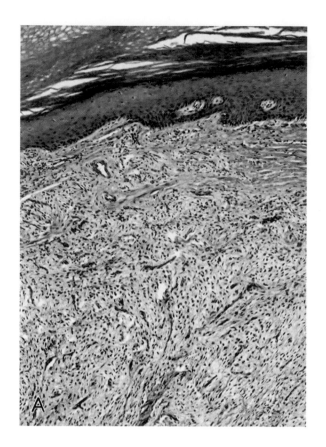

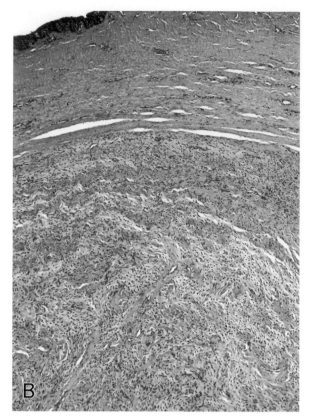

Figure 2-96

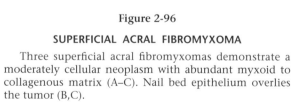

SUPERFICIAL ACRAL FIBROMYXOMA

Three superficial acral fibromyxomas demonstrate a moderately cellular neoplasm with abundant myxoid to collagenous matrix (A–C). Nail bed epithelium overlies the tumor (B,C).

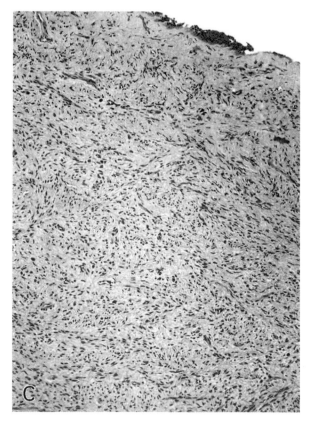

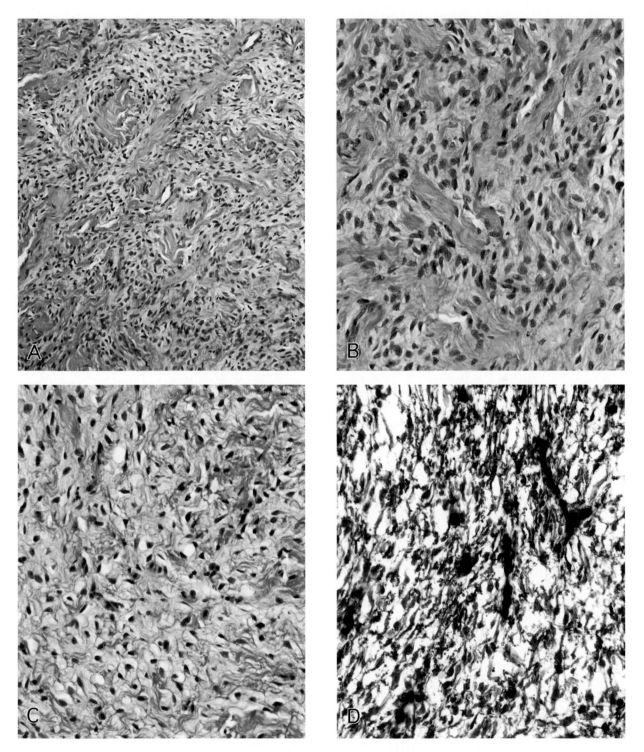

Figure 2-97

SUPERFICIAL ACRAL FIBROMYXOMA

Three prototypic superficial acral fibromyxomas show moderate cellularity, both random and loose storiform growth patterns, and abundant matrix that ranges from myxoid to collagenous. Tumors of this type usually feature a fairly uniform population of stellate- and spindle-shaped cells (as illustrated), but rare examples may have increased atypia and pleomorphism (A–C). Immunoreactivity is typically present for CD34 (D).

lesions are typically CD34 negative, and often have a stellate interface with adjacent soft tissue. Acquired digital/periungual fibrokeratomas are generally smaller, more exophytic, more heavily collagenized (with collagen bundles classically oriented in the vertical axis of the lesion), less cellular, and less vascularized than superficial acral fibromyxomas. The periungual fibromas (Koenen tumors) of tuberous sclerosis are histologically similar to fibrokeratomas, but they are often multifocal. Superficial angiomyxomas typically present as multinodular/multilobular masses with pleomorphic, mononucleated and multinucleated mesenchymal cells embedded in an abundant myxoid matrix; 30 percent of cases have cystic epithelial inclusions. Neurofibromas contain S-100 protein–positive Schwann cells with elongated cytoplasmic processes and undulating tapered nuclei but they also contain a subpopulation of CD34-positive fibroblastic cells.

Treatment and Prognosis. Most superficial acral fibromyxomas are treated by local excision. The overall recurrence rate when managed accordingly is low, probably in the 15 to 20 percent range (524,525). Because the full potential of lesions with more pronounced cytologic atypia is unknown, we generally advise complete local excision and follow-up.

SUPERFICIAL ANGIOMYXOMA (CUTANEOUS MYXOMA)

Definition. *Superficial angiomyxoma* (SAM), also termed *cutaneous myxoma*, is a benign, often multinodular soft tissue tumor that arises in the skin or subcutis and contains pools of myxoid matrix, a variable number of vessels, and scattered mildly atypical and somewhat pleomorphic, mononucleated and multinucleated, stellate- and spindle-shaped cells. Epithelial inclusions of skin adnexa are present in approximately 25 percent of cases.

General Considerations. Most SAMs occur as sporadic, solitary lesions, unassociated with a syndrome (532–534). They are also recognized as one of the major diagnostic criteria for Carney complex (535–539), a disorder characterized by skin pigmentary abnormalities, myxomas (involving the heart, skin, subcutis, breasts, oropharynx, and genital tract), endocrine overactivity (Cushing syndrome), and schwannomas

and other tumors. SAMs in Carney complex patients often manifest earlier in life than sporadic examples (usually between birth and the fourth decade), and they are frequently multifocal (537,540). A summary of the major diagnostic criteria and supplementary criteria for Carney complex is found in the provided references (535,537–539). Most patients previously diagnosed with the NAME (nevi, atrial myxomas, ephelides) (541) and LAMB (lentigines, atrial myxoma, blue nevi) (542) syndromes are now included under the Carney complex umbrella (532,539,543).

Clinical Features. SAMs occur in all decades of life (fig. 2-98, top) (532,533,540). Sporadic, nonsyndromic cases are usually solitary, and have a peak incidence in the fourth decade, with a male predominance (532). Cases associated with Carney complex are multifocal in over 70 percent of patients, and tend to present at an earlier age (mean, 18 years), with no clear sex predilection (540). SAMs have a very wide anatomic distribution (532–534,540), and are seen with similar frequency in the trunk, pelvic region, leg, upper extremity, and head and neck area (fig. 2-98, bottom). In the setting of Carney complex, notable sites of involvement include the eyelids, external ear canals (544), and nipples (539,540,543).

Patients often present with a history of a slow-growing lesion of less than 6 months' duration. Most are asymptomatic, but some lesions are painful with pressure. The process forms a superficial, mobile mass that often causes dome-shaped elevation of the overlying skin. More advanced lesions may be pedunculated. The various clinical appearances can be confused with an epidermal inclusion cyst, neurofibroma, and fibroepithelial polyp (skin tag, acrocodon).

Gross findings. Gross examination reveals a superficial lesion, usually 2 cm or smaller but occasionally as large as 10 cm, involving the dermis and/or subcutis (532–534,540,544). The skin surface may be flat or mildly to moderately elevated, papillary or polypoid. On cut section, the process is typically described as gelatinous (or mucoid) and translucent. Some examples may be hemorrhagic and others may contain golden-brown foci secondary to hemosiderin deposition. The tumors form multiple, small nodules separated by thin fibrous septa, or less often, single

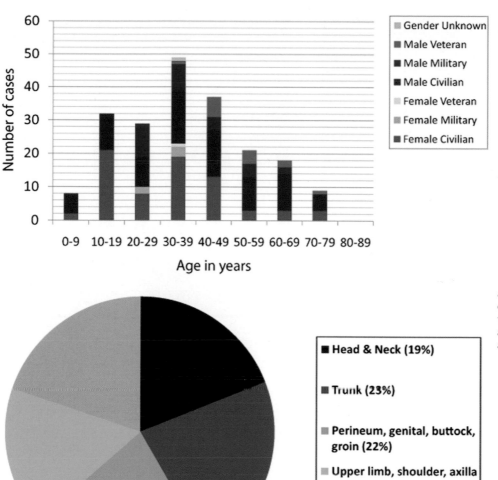

Figure 2-98

SUPERFICIAL ANGIOMYXOMA

Age and sex (top) and anatomic (bottom) distributions of patients with superficial angiomyxoma reviewed at the AFIP.

well-demarcated myxoid masses. Some contain small, firm, off-white, cystic adnexal inclusions that may have keratinous debris.

Microscopic Findings. SAMs usually form multinodular masses within the dermis and subcutis (figs. 2-99–2-102). Infrequently, they extend into underlying skeletal muscle, although this usually occurs with large or recurrent lesions at sites where the muscle is loosely organized and not associated with a well-developed fascial layer. The tumors always have an abundant, hyaluronic acid-rich, myxoid matrix that often forms paucicellular pools and peripherally located clefts (fig. 2-99).

The cellularity ranges from low to moderate and consists of loosely organized, stellate- and spindle-shaped neoplastic cells with indistinct cell borders and smudgy nuclear chromatin, sometimes with cytoplasmic-nuclear invaginations (figs. 2-100, 2-101). The tumor cells are mononucleated or multinucleated; mild atypia and pleomorphism are common. Hyperchromatic nuclei with coarse chromatin and prominent nucleoli are not present, and mitoses are uncommon. A variably accentuated capillary network is often present, and this is occasionally associated with degenerative changes such as perivascular hyalinization and fibrosis, thrombus

119

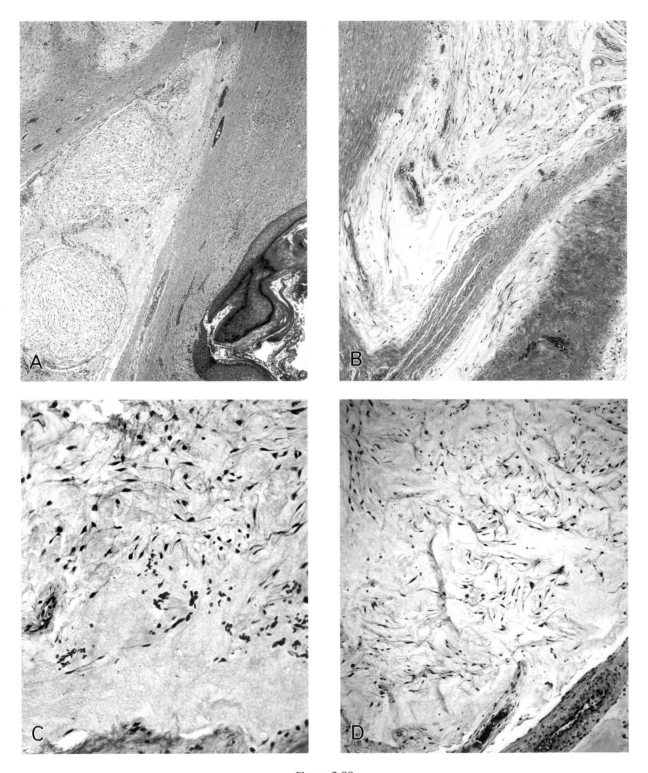

Figure 2-99

SUPERFICIAL ANGIOMYXOMA

In this superficial angiomyxoma involving the skin and subcutis, the abundant myxoid matrix has a tendency to form acellular pools and peripheral clefts (A,B). A mildly pleomorphic population of stellate- and spindle-shaped mesenchymal cells and generally low vascularity are seen (C,D).

formation, and hemosiderin deposition. Perivascular hypercellularity, as seen in association with myxoid sarcomas, is absent.

Commonly, the myxoid matrix contains small numbers of inflammatory cells, including lymphocytes, polymorphonuclear leukocytes, and eosinophils (figs. 2-100, 2-101). Approximately 25 percent of cases contain skin adnexal inclusions (fig. 2-101D) (532–534,540). These may be cystic or filled with keratin, and may contain peripheral basaloid buds or epithelial strands.

Special Studies. SAMs are usually immunoreactive for CD34 (fig. 2-100D) (534). Some also stain (generally weak) for S-100 protein, and occasionally, small numbers of actin-positive cells are present. The process is nonreactive for GFAP, desmin, estrogen and progesterone receptor proteins, and AE1/AE3 keratin cocktail.

Genetics. There is no genetic information available for sporadic SAMs. Carney complex has been reported in all ethnic groups and is inherited in an autosomal dominant manner (538,539,545,546). Approximately 70 percent of patients have an affected parent, and the remainder presumably have a de novo mutation (536,539,543,545,547).

Loss of function mutations in the *PRKAR1A* gene on chromosome 17q23-q24 have been identified in approximately 60 percent of affected individuals overall and 80 percent or more of patients when primary pigmented nodular adrenocortical disease is present (539,548–550). At least 117 different *PRKAR1A* mutations have been identified over the entire open reading frame of the gene (539,545,550). Documented molecular changes include single base substitutions, small (15 bp or less) and relatively large deletions (547), insertions, and combined rearrangements. *PRKAR1A* functions as a classic tumor suppressor gene, and most mutations lead to premature stop codon and protein abrogation (536,539,548,550,551). Approximately 20 percent of Carney complex patients have a 2p16 chromosomal locus (CNC2) and one or more additional loci may also exist (539,543,546,547,550). Disease penetrance in patients with a documented *PRKAR1A* mutation is greater than 95 percent by 50 years of age (550). Most patients with Carney complex have a normal lifespan, but because some individuals die at an early age, the average life expectancy is approximately 50 years (539).

Differential Diagnosis. The differential diagnosis for SAM includes various mesenchymal processes with abundant myxoid matrix, including focal mucinosis, digital mucous cyst, myxoid spindle cell lipoma, intramuscular myxoma, juxta-articular myxoma, and low-grade myxofibrosarcoma (low-grade myxoid malignant fibrous histiocytoma). Focal mucinosis is a cutaneous deposition of stromal mucin (hyaluronic acid) with minimal if any vascular accentuation and very low cellularity (552,553). Digital mucous cyst is a mucoid cystic process related to ganglion cyst that occurs on the fingers and toes (554,555). The mucin in this setting is extravasated from the underlying synovium. Myxoid spindle cell lipomas form well-demarcated subcutaneous masses that primarily occur on the head, neck, and upper back of adults. These lesions contain CD34-positive spindle cells with bland nuclear features (with or without longitudinal nuclear grooves), variable amounts of ropy collagen, and mature adipocytes. The last is sometimes sparsely distributed. Intramuscular and juxta-articular myxomas are associated with deep soft tissue and have little vascularity and cellularity. Myxofibrosarcoma (myxoid malignant fibrous histiocytoma) tends to form a fascial-based mass that generally has greater atypia and more mitotic activity than SAM. It may also contain areas with malignant fibrous histiocytoma/pleomorphic undifferentiated sarcoma-like morphology.

Nerve sheath myxoma (556) and neurothekeoma (557,558), two separate and distinct clinicopathologic entities, also warrant special consideration in the differential diagnosis. Nerve sheath myxomas have a peak incidence in the fourth decade, a predilection for the extremities (especially the distal portions), and a high local recurrence rate. These lesions contain small epithelioid Schwann cells in corded, nested, and syncytial aggregates, as well as Schwann cells with ring-like, stellate, and conventional spindled morphology. There is always abundant myxoid matrix, and the neoplastic cells strongly and diffusely express S-100 protein and GFAP, and lack reactivity for CD34 and CD10. Neurothekeoma has a peak incidence in the second decade, a predilection for the head and proximal

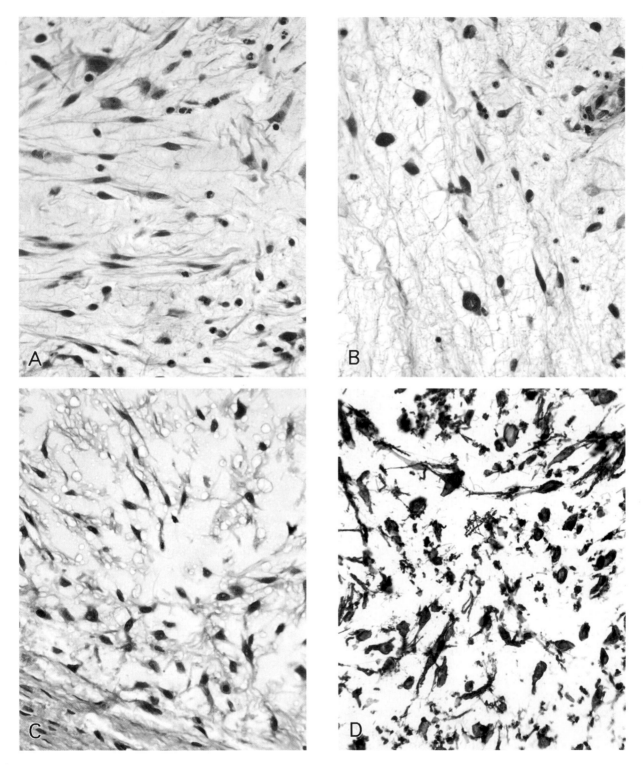

Figure 2-100

SUPERFICIAL ANGIOMYXOMA

At high power, the mesenchymal cells of superficial angiomyxoma show mild atypia, focal pleomorphism, and multinucleation, as well as the presence of some cytoplasmic-nuclear invaginations. Occasional inflammatory cells are within the myxoid matrix (A–C). The tumor is immunoreactive for CD34 (D).

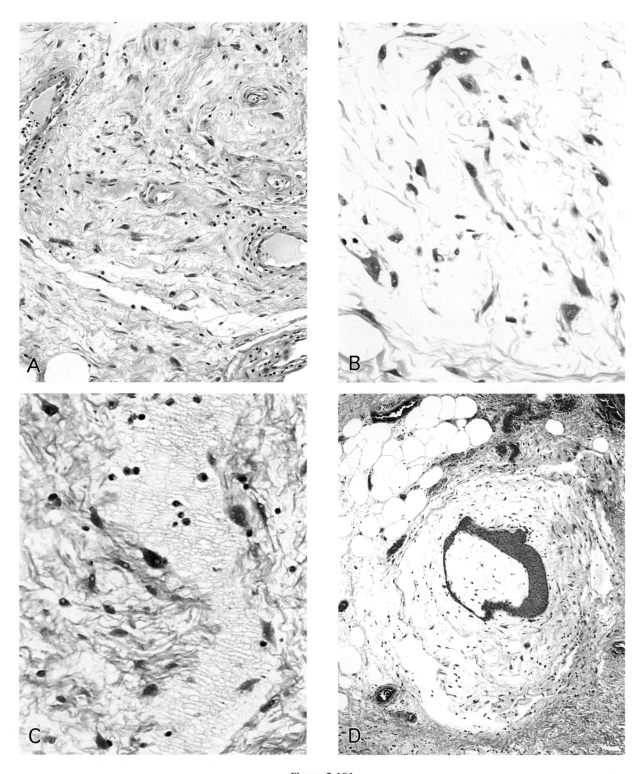

Figure 2-101

SUPERFICIAL ANGIOMYXOMA

Mild hyperchromasia, some pleomorphism, focal multinucleation, and scattered cytoplasmic-nuclear invaginations are seen in the neoplastic cells (A–C). This process often zonates around skin adnexa (D), and may contain a variety of epithelial inclusions.

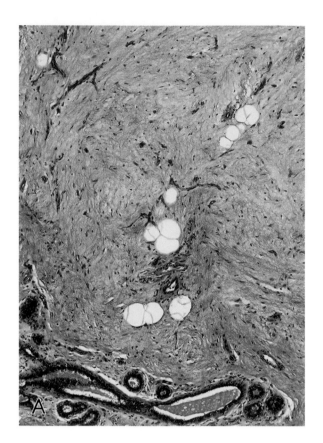

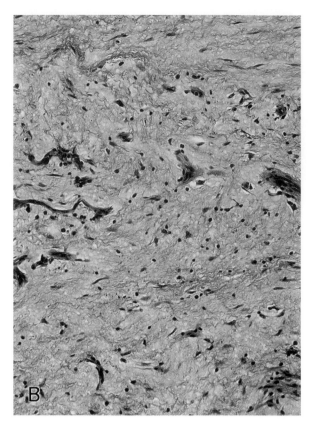

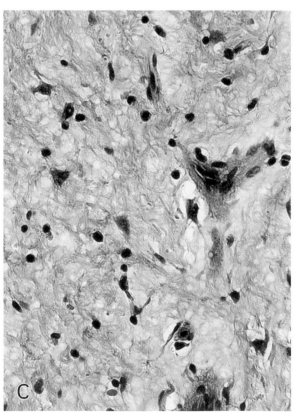

Figure 2-102

SUPERFICIAL ANGIOMYXOMA

Superficial angiomyxomas involving the female breast are morphologically similar to examples encountered in other cutaneous/subcutaneous sites.

A: Lesion involving breast lobule.

B: Prominent myxoid matrix, blood vessels, and focal lymphocytes.

C: Mild nuclear pleomorphism is present.

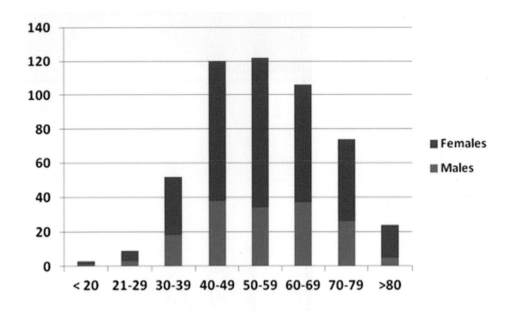

Figure 2-103

INTRAMUSCULAR MYXOMA

Age and sex distribution and anatomic location of 650 intramuscular myxomas.

portions of the extremities, and a low recurrence rate. This tumor features epithelioid and spindled cells with varying degrees of nuclear atypia and generally abundant eosinophilic cytoplasm. The neoplastic cells have a tendency for whorled growth. A myxoid matrix may be present or absent, and approximately one third of cases contain osteoclast-like giant cells. The neoplastic cells express CD10, CD63, and MITF, and there can be some reactivity for α-smooth muscle actin and CD68. The tumor cells are nonreactive for S-100 protein, GFAP, and CD34.

Treatment and Prognosis. SAMs are best managed by complete local excision, since approximately one third of cases recur when marginally excised (532–534). There are no reports of malignant behavior. When SAMs manifest at an unusually young age, are multiple, or are associated with other clinical findings such as abundant lentigines, endocrine abnormalities, or various uncommon tumors, evaluation for Carney complex is advisable (537,539,540).

INTRAMUSCULAR MYXOMA

Definition. *Intramuscular myxoma* is a benign fibromyxoid neoplasm, usually paucicellular and poorly vascularized, with an abundant myxoid matrix that involves fascial planes and skeletal muscle.

Clinical Features. Intramuscular myxoma is a rare tumor. Older studies estimated its annual incidence as 1 per million people, but judging from the more recently radiologically detected small tumors it may be twice as common. The tumor typically occurs in middle-aged adults between 40 and 70 years, with a 2 to 1 female predominance (fig. 2-103). The most common sites are thigh, buttock, proximal arm, and chest wall (fig. 2-104). The tumor is slow growing and the size varies from a small nodule of less than 1 cm to a sizable mass exceeding 20 cm. The latter is especially true with tumors located in the thigh or buttock.

Rare patients (less than 5 percent) have multiple intramuscular myxomas together with polyostotic fibrous dysplasia of bone, which can involve adjacent or distant bones (559–562). This combination occurs in Mazabraud and McCune-Albright syndromes. The latter syndrome also includes cutaneous hyperpigmentation and endocrine abnormalities.

Gross Findings. Grossly typical is a round to ovoid circumscribed mass, which often infiltrates skeletal muscle at the periphery. The cut surface is gelatinous, pale gray-white, and glistening (fig. 2-105). Macroscopic cysts are present in larger tumors. Gross necrosis is seen.

Microscopic Findings. Intramuscular myxoma typically infiltrates between edematous skeletal muscle fibers at its periphery. The tumor is paucicellular and hypovascular, but contains a number of small capillaries with narrow lumens (fig. 106A–C). The cellular main elements are fibroblasts and myofibroblasts, which are embedded in a myxoid, focally collagenous matrix

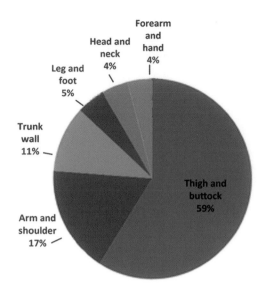

Figure 2-104

INTRAMUSCULAR MYXOMA

Anatomic locations of 650 intramuscular myxomas.

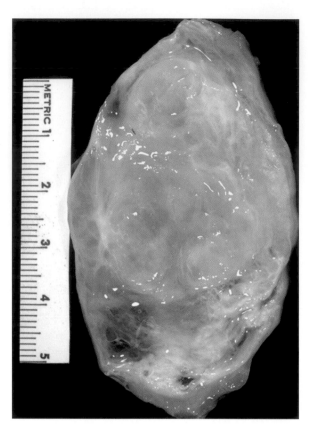

Figure 2-105

INTRAMUSCULAR MYXOMA

Intramuscular myxoma has a glistening cut surface.

containing hyaluronic acid–rich mucopolysaccharides. The stroma may have a vacuolar appearance. The tumor cells contain small nuclei with dense chromatin and elongated, but often weakly staining cytoplasm. Variants with a higher cellularity also occur; these may have some potential for recurrence, but none for metastasis (fig. 2-106D). Mitotic activity is inconspicuous. In addition, numerous histiocytes are present and often constitute a significance percentage of the overall cellularity. A more cellular variant has been reported, and such tumors may have an increased risk for recurrence (563,564).

Special Studies. The tumor cells are immunohistochemically positive for vimentin and often focally positive for smooth muscle actin and CD34, but are negative for S-100 protein and desmin. Large numbers of histiocytes are CD163 positive (565,566). The myxoid matrix is alcian blue positive.

Genetics. Both Mazabraud and McCune-Albright syndromes are associated with somatic or mosaic germline *GNAS* gene mutations encoding a protein regulating cellular cyclic AMP levels. Mutations R261C or R261H (*GNAS* exon 8) are typical of both intramuscular myxoma and fibrous dysplasia lesions (567–569).

Differential Diagnosis. Myxofibrosarcoma/myxoid malignant fibrous histiocytoma generally shows a higher cellularity and more prominent vascularity, along with at least focal nuclear atypia. Mitotic activity, including atypical mitoses, is generally evident. Myxoid liposarcoma is also hypervascular with a network of delicate capillaries, surrounded by evenly spaced oval cells in a greater density than cells in myxoma, with varying numbers of fat cells. If the tumor were not muscle associated, then the generic designation "myxoma" would be appropriate. Distinction from juxta-articular myxoma requires clinicoradiologic correlation.

Treatment and Prognosis. Specific preoperative diagnosis by radiologic studies (MRI) or biopsy allows for more conservative surgery. The typical radiologic features include a peritumoral fat-like zone consisting of atrophic muscle and a water-like character (high signal in T2-weighted images), gadolinium enhancement in 50 percent of cases, and often cyst-like low attenuation in the CT (570,571).

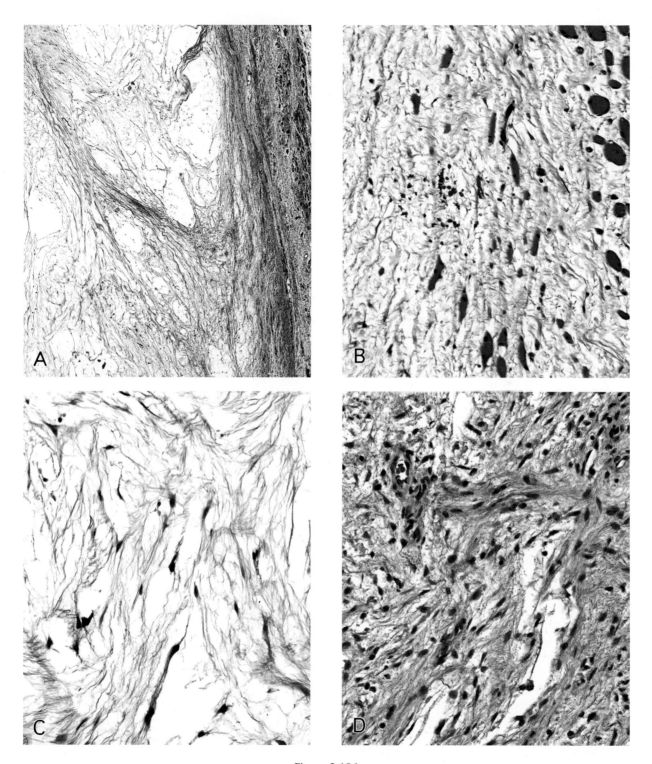

Figure 2-106

INTRAMUSCULAR MYXOMA

Cellular intramuscular myxoma has dense cellularity but no nuclear atypia.

A–C: A paucicellular mass contains areas of microcystic degeneration. At the periphery, the tumor often infiltrates skeletal muscle.

D: A more cellular example of intramuscular myxoma.

Intramuscular myxoma is benign and simple excision is sufficient. Recurrences are rare (less than 5 percent), but the cellular variant may have a higher risk for recurrence; no metastases have been reported (565,566,572,573).

JUXTA-ARTICULAR MYXOMA

Definition. *Juxta-articular myxoma* is a periarticular myxoma often associated with internal joint derangement, such as meniscal tear and cysts.

General Considerations. The nature of this joint-associated myxoma is unclear. Although coexistence with internal knee derangements, such as meniscal tear, and histologic resemblance to ganglion cyst have been found in a number of cases, the greater than 30 percent potential for recurrence may suggest a neoplasm.

Clinical Features. Juxta-articular myxoma occurs predominantly in adults, and 60 percent of cases are seen between the ages of 20 and 50 years. There is a 3 to 1 male predominance. The most common sites of occurrence are around large joints, such as the lateral or medial side of the knee (80 to 90 percent), and less commonly, the shoulder, elbow, hip, or ankle (see fig. 11-8). The lesion can involve the subcutis, joint capsule, synovium, and rarely, skeletal muscle. Most lesions are smaller than 5 cm but rare lesions are larger than 10 cm (574,575).

The clinical manifestations include swelling and pain, and some examples are incidentally detected. Recurrence was reported in 34 percent of cases in the original series (574). Most recurrences occur within 2 years, but some occur 10 to 15 years after the first surgery (576). Radiologic studies commonly show joint pathology such as meniscal tear, suggesting that some examples of this tumor are reactive lesions related to joint pathology and extrusion of mucinous synovial fluid into surrounding soft tissue.

Gross and Microscopic Findings. Juxta-articular myxoma greatly resembles intramuscular myxoma. Grossly, the lesion is gelatinous and gray-white to pale tan. Microscopically, it is paucicellular, with fine alternating streaks of collagen and myxoid areas (fig. 2-107). Often there are ganglion-like cysts with a collagenous, acellular lining. Juxta-articular myxoma may have a richer vascular pattern and show a greater cellularity than intramuscular myxoma.

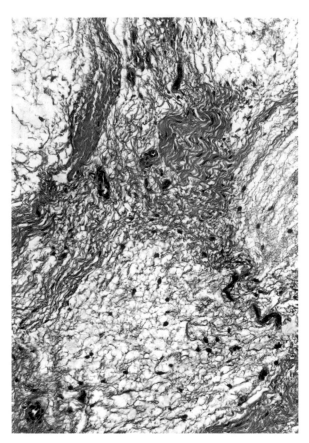

Figure 2-107

JUXTA-ARTICULAR MYXOMA

Uniform spindled cells in a myxoid matrix.

Genetics. The *GNAS* mutations typically seen in intramuscular myxoma do not seem to occur in juxta-articular myxoma, based on the examination of five cases in one study (576). Clonal chromosomal changes have been reported in one case (577).

Treatment. Local excision is sufficient, although recurrence is possible.

AGGRESSIVE ANGIOMYXOMA

Definition. *Aggressive angiomyxoma* is a benign, hormonally-influenced, mesenchymal neoplasm that typically arises in the deep soft tissue of the pelvicoperineal region in women. The tumor has infiltrative growth, an abundant myxedematous matrix, and a dominant population of small stellate- and spindle-shaped cells that exhibit some myoid differentiation. *Deep angiomyxoma* is a synonym.

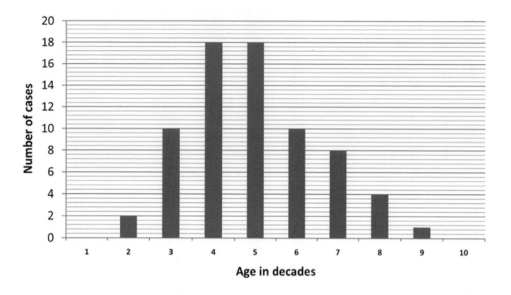

Figure 2-108

AGGRESSIVE ANGIOMYXOMA

Age distribution of 71 female patients with an aggressive angiomyxoma reviewed at the AFIP.

General Considerations. Caution is advised when considering this diagnosis in the male population. While we cannot totally exclude the occurrence of aggressive angiomyxoma in males, many tumors classified as such in the literature are unrelated neoplasms, often either a well-differentiated liposarcoma (atypical lipomatous tumor) variant or cellular angiofibroma (male angiomyofibroblastoma-like tumor) (578–581).

Clinical Features. Aggressive angiomyxoma usually affects adult females in the third to seventh decades, with a peak incidence in the fourth and fifth decades (fig. 2-108) (582–584). Prepubertal girls are almost never affected (585).

Patients generally present with a slow-growing mass in the pelvicoperineal region that is either asymptomatic, or associated with dull pain, vague discomfort, a pressure-like sensation, or dyspareunia (583). On physical examination, the tumor size is often significantly underestimated, because the bulk of the process tends to be concealed within the deep soft tissues (583). This commonly leads to false preoperative clinical impressions of a Bartholin gland cyst, vaginal cyst, hernia, or lipoma (582–584,586). When the full tumor size becomes apparent through imaging, more than half of the lesions are 10 cm or larger (583).

CT imaging reveals a hypoattenuated or isoattenuated mass that typically grows around pelvic floor structures without causing significant disruption of the vaginal or rectal musculature (587,588). In T1-weighted MRIs, a hypointense

to isointense mass is present, whereas T2-weighted MRIs reveal a mass with high signal intensity (587–589). Both T2-weighted MRI and enhanced CT images demonstrate a distinctive swirled or layered internal architecture (588). These imaging techniques provide critical information about tumor extent and whether the pelvic diaphragm has been traversed, factors important for selecting an optimal surgical approach (588,589).

Gross Findings. Resected tumors are commonly larger than 10 cm and not infrequently larger than 20 cm (583,586). Tumors under 5 cm make up less than 10 percent of examples in the AFIP files. The neoplasms often have a lobular contour and adhere to fat, muscle, and other regional structures. The tumor consistency ranges from soft to moderately firm or rubbery, and the cut surface is commonly glistening or myxedematous with a pink or reddish tan color. Hemorrhagic foci and areas with cystic change may be present.

Microscopic Findings. Aggressive angiomyxomas generally have low to moderate cellularity. They feature small, stellate- and spindle-shaped cells embedded in a loosely collagenized, myxedematous matrix, with scattered vessels of varying caliber and a variety of entrapped regional structures (figs. 2-109, 2-110). The dominant neoplastic population has scant eosinophilic cytoplasm, and there is no significant atypia, pleomorphism, or mitotic activity (fig. 2-111). Multinucleation is also uncommon (fig. 2-111, right).

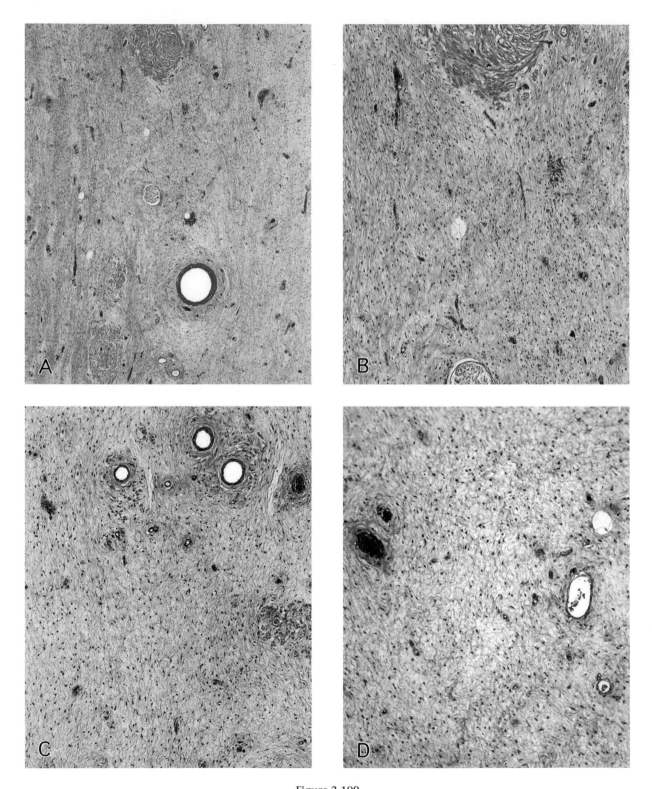

Figure 2-109

AGGRESSIVE ANGIOMYXOMA

A–D: Uniform cellularity, abundant myxedematous extracellular matrix, mild vascular accentuation, entrapment of regional structures, and a proliferation of plump myoid cells around some nerves and vessels are seen.

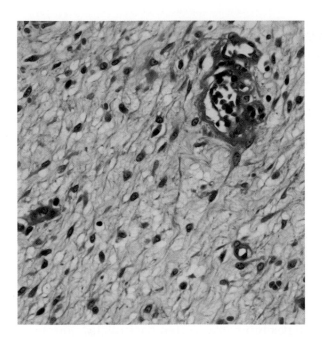 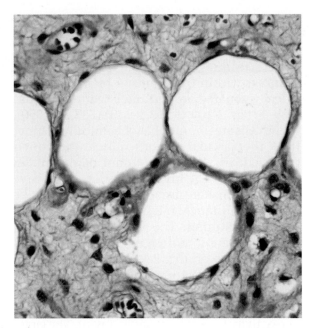

Figure 2-110

AGGRESSIVE ANGIOMYXOMA

Left, Right: The uniform appearance of the neoplastic cells and their scant eosinophilic cytoplasm are seen. This process has abundant myxedematous matrix and infiltrative growth. Biopsies taken from the tumor periphery may be confused with a fatty neoplasm (right).

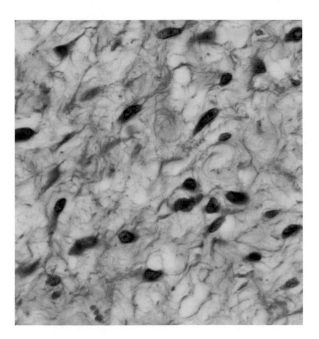 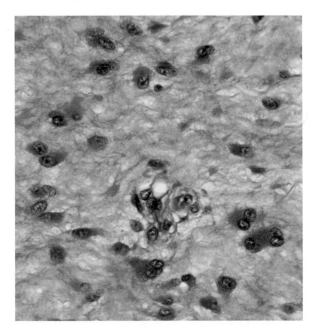

Figure 2-111

AGGRESSIVE ANGIOMYXOMA

At high power, the nuclei are often mildly hyperchromatic, with slightly coarsened chromatin; they contain small distinct central nucleoli (left). Infrequent tumor cells may be multinucleated (right).

A helpful feature is the common presence of scattered larger spindled cells with well-developed myoid (myofibroblastic versus true smooth muscle) features, randomly distributed in small numbers within the tumor or more characteristically zonated around the larger nerves and vessels (figs. 2-109, 2-112, 2-113) (583,584,590). These cells are immunohistochemically distinct from the vascular smooth muscle they often encircle (583). While the tumor name implies an abundance of myxoid matrix, aggressive angiomyxomas are usually only weakly positive for mucosubstances (583).

Special Studies. The neoplastic cells often have moderate to diffuse nuclear immunoreactivity for estrogen (fig. 2-113) and progesterone (580,583,591) receptor proteins, and variable levels of reactivity for desmin and actins (583, 584). CD34 expression, if present, is only focal. Immunoreactivity for S-100 protein is absent. The larger well-developed myoid cells that are a focal finding, often detected around nerves and vessels, have stronger and more uniform actin (fig. 2-113) and desmin expression than the smaller tumor cells with less abundant cytoplasm (583).

In some but not all tumors, there is aberrant nuclear HMGA2 (HMGIC) protein expression. (592). While this finding is not unique to aggressive angiomyxoma (it has also been noted in other soft tissue entities including uterine leiomyomas), it is reportedly absent in normal vulvovaginal soft tissue and several soft tissue tumors that are important considerations in the differential diagnosis (e.g., angiomyofibroblastoma) (592).

Genetics. Cytogenetic analyses of aggressive angiomyxoma have often demonstrated aberrations involving chromosome 12, with the *HMGA2 (HMGIC)* gene implicated in several studies (593–596). The simplest karyotypic abnormalities reported for aggressive angiomyxoma include: 46,XX, t(12;21)(q15;q21.1); 46,XX,t(1;12)(p32;q15); 46,XX, t(11;12)(q23;q15); 46,XX,t(8;12) (p12;q15); 46,XX,t(7;12)(q22~31;q13~14); and 46,XX,t(5;8)(p15;q22) (596,597).

Differential Diagnosis. The differential diagnosis of aggressive angiomyxoma includes angiomyofibroblastoma, cellular angiofibroma, true myxoid and edematous smooth muscle tumors, pelvic fibromatosis, and various sarcoma types that may have a myxoid matrix. Detailed discussions of angiomyofibroblastoma and cellular angiofibroma are found elsewhere in this chapter. True myxoid and edematous smooth muscle tumors feature an abundance of large spindled cells that often have longitudinal cytoplasmic striations (highlighted with the Masson trichrome stain) and may have juxtanuclear vacuoles. These tumors generally have more extensive immunoreactivity for smooth muscle actin and desmin than aggressive angiomyxoma. Myxoid smooth muscle tumors also have more abundant hyaluronic acid than is typically encountered in aggressive angiomyxoma.

Pelvic fibromatosis has the classic features of a desmoid tumor, with abundant collagen, mildly atypical spindled cells in loose fascicular and broad storiform arrangements, and fairly uniformly distributed small to medium-sized vessels with slit-like or patent lumens. Desmoid-type fibromatoses often have nuclear immunoreactivity for β-catenin.

Sarcomas that enter into the differential diagnosis include myxofibrosarcoma or variants of liposarcoma. These tumors have a peak incidence in late adulthood, and even when low grade, have more obvious atypia and pleomorphism than is acceptable in aggressive angiomyxoma.

In the absence of relevant clinical information, certain physiologic conditions, such as childhood asymmetric labium majus enlargement (also termed prepubertal vulvar fibroma) (598–600) and vulvar hypertrophy with lymphedema (601), have the potential in biopsy samples of being confused with aggressive angiomyxoma. Recognition that the specimen contains a superficial, poorly demarcated, bland process that lacks the characteristic histologic features described above for aggressive angiomyxoma is important to proper diagnosis. An elucidated history often resolves the diagnosis, but the presence of dilated tortuous lymphatics aids in recognition of vulvar hypertrophy with lymphedema, and the presence of CD34-positive, desmin-negative fibroblastic stromal cells that tend to grow within widened septa between preserved fat lobules is a helpful clue to the diagnosis of childhood asymmetric labium majus enlargement.

Treatment and Prognosis. Aggressive angiomyxoma has a local recurrence rate that exceeds 35 percent (582–584,586). Complete excision is the preferred management when it can be

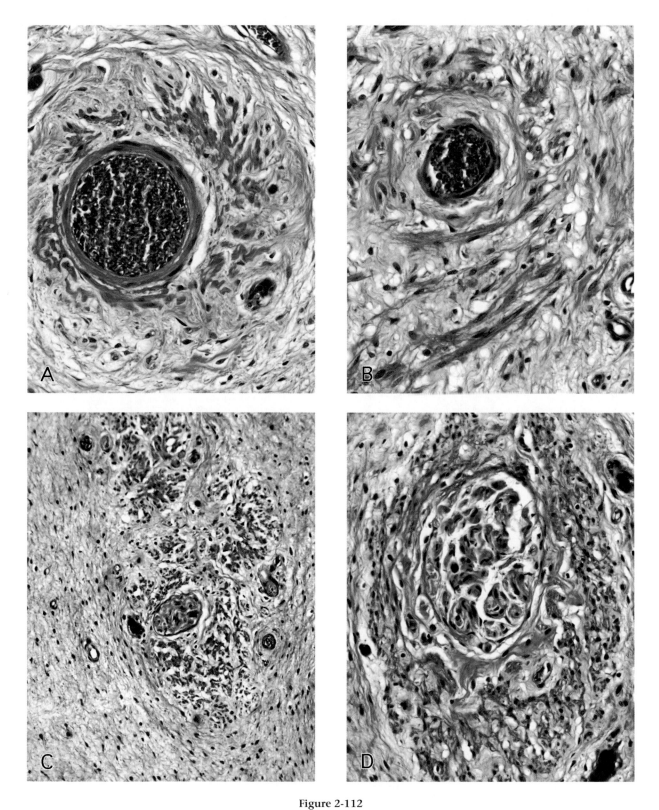

Figure 2-112

AGGRESSIVE ANGIOMYXOMA

Myoid proliferation is often encountered around vessels (A,B) and nerves (C,D) in aggressive angiomyxoma.

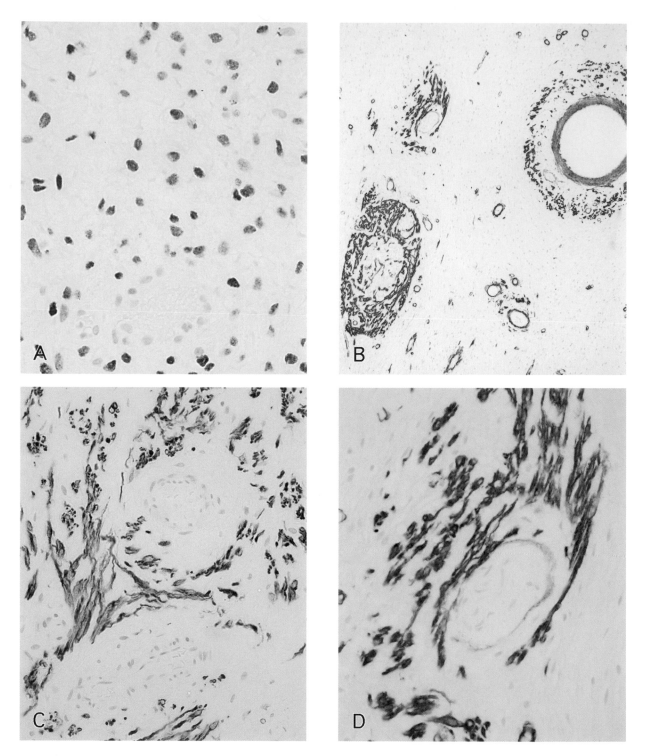

Figure 2-113

AGGRESSIVE ANGIOMYXOMA

Estrogen receptor protein (A), smooth muscle actin (B,D), and D33 desmin (C) immunostains in aggressive angiomyxoma. Estrogen receptor protein is usually strongly expressed in tumor cell nuclei. Smooth muscle actin highlights the perivascular and perineurial myoid populations. The perivascular myoid cells express D33 desmin, but the vessel walls are desmin negative. Although not illustrated, the small conventional tumor cells in aggressive angiomyxoma are also often desmin positive.

accomplished without undue morbidity. When the risk of morbidity is high or when there is a desire to preserve fertility, lesser intervention is acceptable, assuming the risk of recurrence and the potential need for additional surgical intervention are understood (582). All patients require long-term follow-up with periodic imaging analysis because tumor growth tends to be slow and recurrences late in onset, and physical examination has low sensitivity for detecting a recurrence (582,583). There is no proven role for adjuvant radiotherapy or chemotherapy. There are some reports describing a dramatic response to hormonal therapy (gonadotropin-releasing hormone [GnRH] agonist), and this may be a valuable therapeutic tool in selected instances, but additional study is required (591,602).

There are two published reports purporting a metastasizing aggressive angiomyxoma (603,604). The initial case report (604) is not convincing, as the patient's primary pelvic tumor appears by illustration to be an unrelated myxoid sarcoma. The most recent case report (603) is more difficult to dismiss, but additional studies are needed to ascertain the true significance of this observation. Certainly, metastatic behavior of aggressive angiomyxoma is exceptional, if it occurs.

ANGIOMYOFIBROBLASTOMA

Definition. *Angiomyofibroblastoma* is a benign, well-demarcated neoplasm that typically arises in the subcutis of the vulvoperineal region. It contains a hormonally influenced population of polymorphic epithelioid and spindled cells that have a notable tendency to aggregate around vessels and are often admixed with a variable amount of intralesional fat.

General Considerations. This process somewhat overlaps morphologically with cellular angiofibroma. Many tumors previously reported as angiomyofibroblastomas involving the uterine cervix or vagina proper (not in continuity with the introitus) (605) are more appropriately classified as superficial (cervicovaginal) myofibroblastomas.

Clinical Features. Angiomyofibroblastoma is primarily a tumor of adult females (fig. 2-114) (606–610). The process has infrequently been described in males in the inguinoscrotal region, but most of these cases are not fully convincing, and some seem more compatible with the more recently described cellular angiofibroma (angiomyofibroblastoma-like tumor of the male genital tract). Female patients typically present with a painless, well-demarcated, subcutaneous mass in the vulvoperineal region. Infrequent examples involve the vagina, but these are usually located near the introitus.

Gross Findings. The resected lesions typically form well-circumscribed masses with a soft to rubbery consistency. Most are smaller than 5 cm, but rare examples larger than 10 cm have been reported (605,607). The cut surface is pinkish tan to yellow, and often has a mucoid or myxedematous quality. Intralesional fat may be grossly apparent.

Microscopic Findings. This process forms a well-demarcated mass of low to moderate cellularity. A polymorphic population of epithelioid and spindled cells is embedded in a myxedematous, loosely collagenized stroma with numerous, fairly uniformly distributed, capillary-sized vessels and small venous segments (fig. 2-115). The polymorphic cells are mononucleated or multinucleated, and some epithelioid cells with abundant eosinophilic cytoplasm have a plasmacytoid appearance. The neoplastic cells tend to form corded, nested, and trabecular arrangements, and to aggregate around the vasculature. Atypia is usually mild, although foci with more pronounced "degenerative" changes have been observed. Mitotic activity is characteristically minimal. Occasional cases show perivascular hyalinization, similar to that seen in cellular angiofibroma.

Although some authors report intralesional fat to be an uncommon element (607), this is present in over 50 percent of examples accessioned to the AFIP (609). In a small percentage of cases, fat is a dominant feature, as documented in the lipomatous variant of angiomyofibroblastoma (fig. 2-116) (606,609).

Special Studies. Immunoreactivity for desmin and estrogen and progesterone receptors is typical (605,607–610). Reactivity for actins is variable, but generally, there is little or no expression (607–611). CD34 is uncommon in conventional cases, but it is detected with some frequency in the lipomatous variant of angiomyofibroblastoma (606,609,611). S-100 protein reactivity and nuclear reactivity for HMGA2 (HMGIC) are absent (612). Some vaginal tumors reported as angiomyofibroblastomas

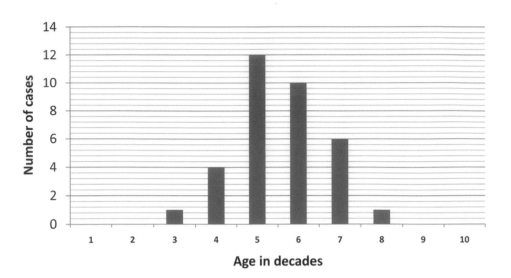

Figure 2-114

ANGIOMYO-FIBROBLASTOMA

Age distribution of 34 female patients with angiomyofibroblastoma reviewed at the AFIP.

with co-expression of desmin and CD34 (605) are, in our opinion, better classified as superficial (cervicovaginal) myofibroblastomas.

Genetics. Genetic data are limited, but recent observations suggest that this tumor lacks the *HMGA2* rearrangements encountered in a small but significant percent of aggressive angiomyxomas (613). Flow cytometric analyses yield DNA indices consistent with both diploidy (610,611) and aneuploidy (611).

Differential Diagnosis. The differential diagnosis includes aggressive angiomyxoma, cellular angiofibroma, and superficial (cervicovaginal) myofibroblastoma. Aggressive angiomyxoma generally presents as a large deep-seated mass that infiltrates and entraps regional structures. The process is dominated by a more uniformly distributed population of small, monomorphic, stellate- and spindle-shaped cells; scattered well-developed smooth muscle-like cells are often present.

Cellular angiofibroma shares a number of features with angiomyofibroblastoma, including superficial location, circumscription, numerous vessels, a spindle cell component, and the occasional presence of intralesional fat. However, the former tends to lack the polymorphism encountered in the latter, and the lesional cells do not aggregate around the vasculature.

Superficial (cervicovaginal) myofibroblastoma (614,615) preferentially involves the uterine cervix and vagina, whereas angiomyofibroblastoma primarily affects the vulva. The former arises just beneath the mucosal surface, and often co-expresses desmin and CD34 (614,615).

Treatment and Prognosis. Angiomyofibroblastomas with conventional morphology are typically cured by simple local excision (605,607,609,611). There is one unique case report of an angiomyofibroblastoma with sarcomatous transformation (containing foci resembling a myxofibrosarcoma/myxoid malignant fibrous histiocytoma) that occurred in an elderly female (616).

CELLULAR ANGIOFIBROMA

Definition. *Cellular angiofibroma (angiomyofibroblastoma-like tumor)* is a benign, typically well-demarcated, spindle cell tumor that usually arises in the subcutis of the inguinoscrotal and vulvoperineal regions. The process characteristically has many fairly uniformly distributed thick-walled vessels, a loose myxocollagenous matrix, and variable amounts of intralesional fat.

General Considerations. This recently described tumor has some morphologic overlap with angiomyofibroblastoma and spindle cell lipoma (617–621). Features that aid in differentiating these entities are provided in the differential diagnosis section.

Clinical Features. This tumor primarily arises in the vulvoperineal region in women (size range, 0.6 to 25.0 cm; median size, 2.8 cm) and the inguinoscrotal region in men (size range, 2.5 to 25.0 cm; median size, 6 cm) (619,620,622). The median age at resection is 52 years for women and 60 years for men. The process usually presents as a well-demarcated, painless mass situated within the subcutis. Rare primary sites

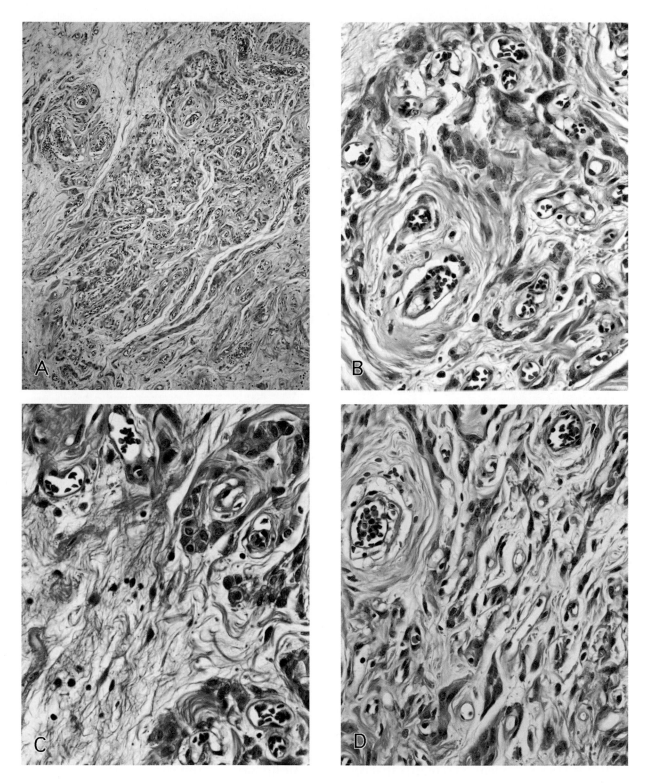

Figure 2-115

ANGIOMYOFIBROBLASTOMA

A–D: The loosely collagenized extracellular matrix, vascular accentuation, and tendency for tumor cells to zonate around the vessels are seen. The tumor cells may be epithelioid or spindled and mononucleated or multinucleated.

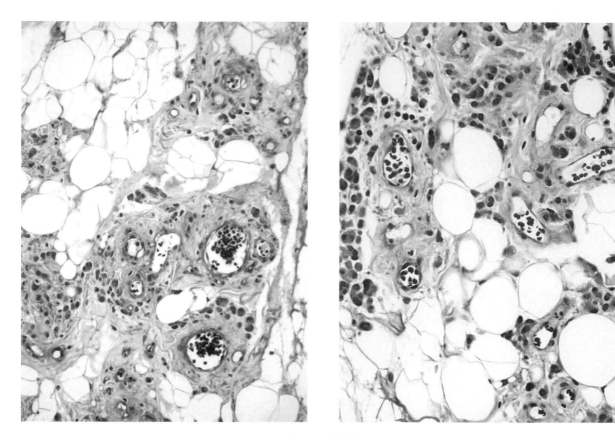

Figure 2-116

ANGIOMYFIBROBLASTOMA: LIPOMATOUS VARIANT

Left, Right: Mature fat is abundant. The epithelioid, mononucleated, and multinucleated tumor cells have a tendency to zonate around vessels.

include the retroperitoneum, lumbar region, and trunk (619).

Gross Findings. Gross examination generally reveals a well-delineated off-white to yellowish mass (usually 3 cm or smaller in women and 8 cm or smaller in men), with a soft to firm consistency. The cut surface may be mucoid or myxedematous. Some examples have gross evidence of intralesional fat.

Microscopic Findings. This process is typically well-marginated, and contains a moderately cellular population of spindle cells that usually have only mild atypia, although rare examples have focally more pronounced atypia (figs. 2-117, 2-118). The spindle cells are embedded in a myxedematous matrix that contains wispy collagen bundles. Some hyalinized collagen and variable amounts of fat may be present. A variety of degenerative changes are noted, including hemorrhage, cystic change,

and localized accumulations of myxoid matrix resulting in a pseudoangiomatous pattern.

The lesions commonly have uniformly distributed, small to medium-sized vessels, frequently with perivascular hyalinization or fibrosis. There is no predilection for lesional cells to assume an epithelioid morphology and zonate around the vasculature. Mitotic activity is generally sparse, but in exceptional instances, is more pronounced. Atypical mitotic figures and tumor necrosis are absent in conventional cases.

Recently, a case report (623) and a small series (624) of cellular angiofibromas with "sarcomatous transformation" have been reported. The sarcomatous component resembled pleomorphic liposarcoma in two cases, an atypical lipomatous tumor in three cases, and a pleomorphic spindle cell sarcoma, not otherwise specified, in five cases. The significance of these observations is, at present, unclear. We would classify

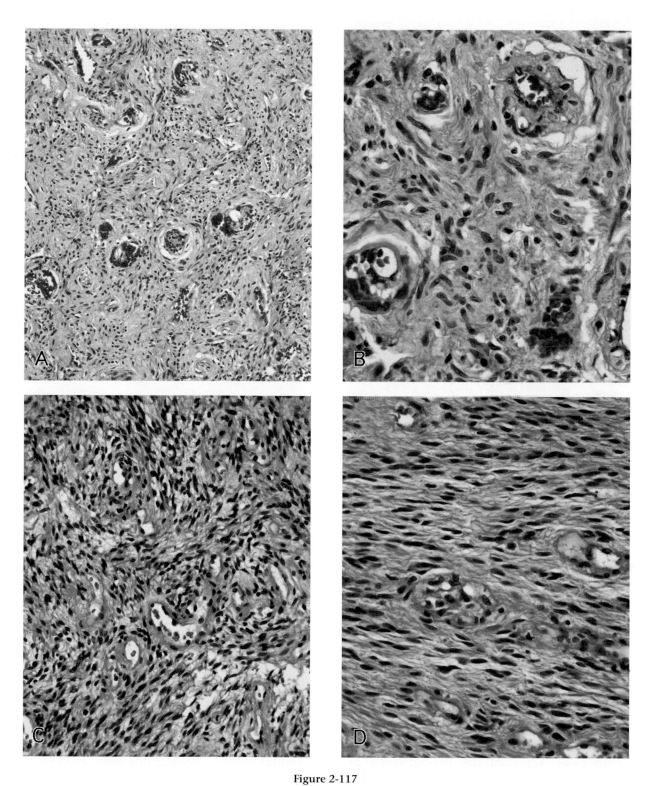

Figure 2-117

CELLULAR ANGIOFIBROMA

A–D: The uniform population of spindled cells has only mild atypia and increased vascularity. Some vessels have a hyalinized wall with focal hemosiderin deposition. There is no appreciable tendency for the neoplastic cells to tightly zonate around the vessels.

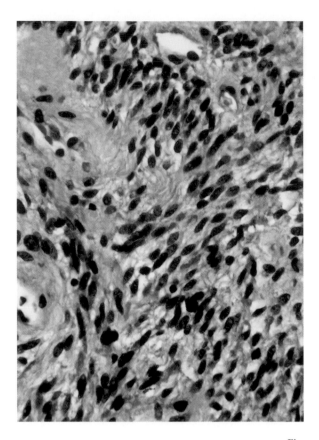 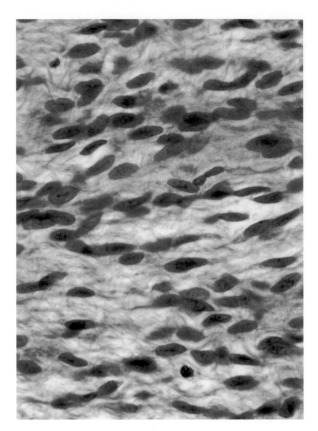

Figure 2-118

CELLULAR ANGIOFIBROMA

Left: High power shows the uniformity of the neoplastic cells

Right: Some longitudinal nuclear grooves, similar to those encountered in spindle cell lipoma and mammary myofibroblastoma, are evident.

the tumors with a lipoblastic component as liposarcoma variants rather than cellular angiofibromas with sarcomatous transformation. The other five cases lacked sufficient illustration to formulate a clear opinion. These observations support the need for thorough sampling and careful histopathologic review.

Special Studies. There are discrepancies in the reported immunohistochemical profile for this tumor, so additional study is required for clarification (619,620,622,625). CD34, estrogen receptor protein, and progesterone receptor protein have been documented in about half of the cases. Actin and desmin expression are reported in less than 20 percent and less than 10 percent of cases, respectively.

Genetics. Genetic information is available for only a small number of cases. DNA imaging analysis in one case revealed a diploid DNA pattern (626). One karyotyped tumor from a 60-year-old man had complex findings with monosomy 16, loss of one chromosome 13, and unbalanced rearrangements involving the remaining chromosome 13 (618). Another tumor from a 52-year-old man was shown by interphase FISH analysis to have deletion of the region on chromosome 13q14 spanning the RB1 and FOX1A1 loci (621). A third tumor from a 55-year-old woman had monoallelic FOX1A1/13q14 loss (621), and FISH analysis of seven cases (617) revealed monoallelic deletion of RB1 from chromosome 13q14.2. These findings suggest a genetic link between cellular angiofibroma, spindle cell lipoma, and mammary-type myofibroblastoma (617,618,621). In another study, *HMGA2* and *HMGA1* rearrangements were not identified in six tumors examined with FISH (627).

Differential Diagnosis. Cellular angiofibroma has some morphologic overlap with angiomyofibroblastoma (618,620) and spindle cell lipoma (619–622). Angiomyofibroblastoma generally exhibits more cellular heterogeneity, with an admixture of spindled and epithelioid cells that are often both mononucleated and multinucleated, and there is a strong tendency for these cells to aggregate around the vasculature. There are some tumors, however, where a clear morphologic distinction between angiomyofibroblastoma and cellular angiofibroma cannot be made. Fortunately, this doesn't appear to have clinical significance.

Spindle cell lipomas are uncommon in the genital area. They usually feature a greater adipocytic component, more ropy collagen, and a less pronounced vasculature than cellular angiofibroma. The spindle cells in spindle cell lipoma are more consistently immunoreactivity for CD34 than the spindle cells in cellular angiofibroma.

Treatment and Prognosis. Complete local excision is considered optimal management for conventional cases (629,620,622). Local recurrences are uncommon (620,625). For the rare examples with increased mitotic activity or foci with significant atypia, special attention to margins is advisable. There are no documented instances of metastasis. To date, none of the purported examples with sarcomatous transformation behaved aggressively (623,624).

REFERENCES

Introduction

1. Schürch W, Seemayer TA, Gabbiani G. The myofibroblast: a quarter century after its discovery. Am J Surg Pathol 1998;22:141-147.

Nodular Fasciitis

2. Hutter RV, Foote FW, Francis KC, Higinbotham NL. Parosteal fasciitis. A self-limiting benign process that simulates a malignant neoplasm. Am J Surg 1962;104:800-807.
3. Allen PW. Nodular fasciitis. Pathology 1972;4:9-26.
4. Bernstein KE, Lattes R. Nodular (pseudosarcomatous) fasciitis, a nonrecurrent lesion: clinicopathologic study of 134 cases. Cancer 1982;49:1668-1678.
5. Konwaler BE, Keasbey L, Kaplan L. Subcutaneous pseudosarcomatous fibromatosis (fasciitis). Am J Clin Pathol 1955;25:241-252.
6. Dahl I, Jarlstedt J. Nodular fasciitis in the head and neck. A clinicopathological study on 18 cases. Acta Otolaryngol 1980;90:152-159.
7. Meister P, Bückmann FW, Konrad E. Nodular fasciitis (analysis of 100 cases and review of the literature). Pathol Res Pract 1978;162:133-165.
8. Montgomery EA, Meis JM. Nodular fasciitis. Its morphologic spectrum and immunohistochemical profile. Am J Surg Pathol 1991;15:942-948.
9. Price EB Jr, Silliphant WM, Shuman R. Nodular fasciitis: a clinicopathologic analysis of 65 cases. Am J Clin Pathol 1961;35:122-136.
10. Goodlad JR, Fletcher CD. Intradermal variant of nodular 'fasciitis'. Histopathology 1990;17:569-571.
11. Patchefsky AS, Enzinger FM. Intravascular fasciitis: a report of 17 cases. Am J Surg Pathol 1981;5:29-36.
12. Lauer DH, Enzinger FM. Cranial fasciitis of childhood. Cancer 1980;45:401-406.
13. Patterson JW, Moran SL, Konerding H. Cranial fasciitis. Arch Dermatol 1989;125:674-678.
14. Rapanà A, Iaccarino C, Bellotti A, Marsicano C, Donnianni T, Tedeschi E. Exclusively intracranial and cranial fasciitis of the adult age. Clin Neurol Neurosurg 2002;105:35-38.
15. Sarangarajan R, Dehner LP. Cranial and extracranial fasciitis of childhood: a clinicopathologic and immunohistochemical study. Hum Pathol 1999;30:87-92.
16. Sayama T, Morioka T, Baba T, Tkezaki K, Fukin M. Cranial fasciitis with massive intracranial extension. Child Nerv Syst 1995;11:242-245.
17. O'Connell JX, Young RH, Nielsen GP, Rosenberg AE, Bainbridge TC, Clement PB. Nodular fasciitis of the vulva: a study of six cases and literature review. Int J Gynecol Pathol 1997;16:117-123.
18. Shimizu S, Hashimoto H, Enjoji M. Nodular fasciitis: an analysis of 250 patients. Pathology 1984;16:161-166.
19. Wirman JA. Nodular fasciitis, a lesion of myofibroblasts: an ultrastructural study. Cancer 1976;38:2378-2389.

20. Perez-Montiel MD, Plaza JA, Dominguez-Malagon H, Suster S. Differential expression of smooth muscle myosin, smooth muscle actin, h-caldesmon, and calponin in the diagnosis of myofibroblastic and smooth muscle lesions of skin and soft tissue. Am J Dermatopathol 2006;28:105-111.

21. Carlson JW, Fletcher CD. Imunohistochemistry for beta-catenin in the differential diagnosis of spindle cell lesions: analysis of a series and review of the literature. Histopathology 2007;51:509-514.

22. Koizumi H, Mikami M, Doi M, Tadokoro M. Clonality analysis of nodular fasciitis by HU-MARA-methylation-specific PCR. Histopathology 2005;47:320-321.

23. Donner LR, Silva T, Dobin SM. Clonal rearrangement of 15p11.2, 16p11.2, 16p13.3 in a case of nodular fasctiitis: additional evidence favoring nodular fasciitis as a benign neoplasm and not a reactive tumefaction. Cancer Genet Cytogenet 2002;139:138-140.

24. Sawyer JR, Sammartino G, Baker GF, Bell JM. Clonal chromosome aberrations in a case of nodular fasciitis. Cancer Genet Cytogenet 1994;76:154-156.

25. Velagaleti GV, Tapper JK, Panova NE, Miettinen M, Gatalica Z. Cytogenetic findings in a case of nodular fasciitis of subclavicular region. Cancer Genet Cytogenet 2003;141:160-163.

26. Weibolt VM, Buresh CJ, Roberts CA, et al. Involvement of 3q21 in nodular fasciitis. Cancer Genet Gytogenet 1998;106:177-179.

26a. Erickson-Johnson MR, Chou MM, Evers BR, et al. Nodular fasciitis: a novel model of transient neoplasia induced by MYH9-USP6 gene fusion. Lab Invest 2011;91:1427-1433.

27. Dahl I, Angervall L. Pseudosarcomatous proliferative lesions of soft tissue with or without bone formation. Acta Pathol Microbiol Scand A 1977;85:577-589.

28. Daroca PJ Jr, Pulitzer DR, LoCicero J 3rd. Ossifying fasciitis. Arch Pathol Lab Med 1982;106:682-685.

29. Kwittken J, Branche M. Fasciitis ossificans. Am J Clin Pathol 1969;51:251-255.

30. Bacac M, Migliavacca E, Stehle JC, et al. A gene expression signature that distinguishes desmoid tumors from nodular fasciitis. J Pathol 2006;208:543-553.

31. Fetsch JF, Brinsko RW, Davis CJ Jr, Mostofi FK, Sesterhenn IA. A distinctive myointimal proliferation ("myointimoma") involving the corpus spongiosum of the glans penis: a clinicopathologic and immunohistochemical analysis of 10 cases. Am J Surg Pathol 2000;24:1524-1530.

32. McKenney JK, Collins MH, Carretero AP, Boyd TK, Redman JF, Parham DM. Penile myointimoma in children and adolescents: a clinicopathologic study of 5 cases supporting a distinct entity. Am J Surg Pathol 2007;31:1622-1626.

33. Robbins JB, Kohler S. Penile nodule in a 54-year-old man: a case of a myointimoma. J Am Acad Dermatol 2005;53:1084-1086.

34. Schwartz SL, Perkins PL, Ritchey ML. Angiocentric myofibroblastic tumor of the penis in a child: case report and literature review. J Urol 1993;149:1114-1115.

35. Vardar E, Gunlusoy B, Arslan M, Kececi S. Myoinitimoma of the glans penis. Pathol Int 2007;57:158-161.

Proliferative Fasciitis and Proliferative Myositis

36. Chung EB, Enzinger FM. Proliferative fasciitis. Cancer 1975;36:1450-1458.

37. Dent CD, DeBoom GW, Hamlin ML. Proliferative myositis of the head and neck. Report of a case and review of the literature. Oral Surg Oral Med Oral Pathol 1994;78:354-358.

38. Enzinger FM, Dulcey F. Proliferative myositis: report of thirty-three cases. Cancer 1967;20:2213-2223.

39. Kern WH. Proliferative myositis: a pseudosarcomatous reaction to injury: a report of seven cases. Arch Pathol 1960;69:209-216.

40. Kitano M, Iwasaki H, Enjoji M. Proliferative fasciitis. A variant of nodular fasciitis. Acta Pathol Jpn 1977;27:485-493.

41. Lundgren L, Kindblom LG, Willems J, Falkmer U, Angervall L. Proliferative myositis and fasciitis. A light and electron microscopic, cytologic, DNA-cytometric and immunohistochemical study. APMIS 1992;100:437-448.

42. Diaz-Flores L, Martin Herrera AI, Garcia Montelongo R, Gutiérrez García R. Proliferative fasciitis: ultrastructure and histogenesis. J Cutan Pathol 1989;16:85-92.

43. Rose AG. An electron microscopic study of the giant cells in proliferative myositis. Cancer 1974;33:1543-1547.

44. Meis JM, Enzinger FM. Proliferative fasciitis and myositis in childhood. Am J Surg Pathol 1992;16:364-372.

45. El-Jabbour JN, Bennett MH, Burke MM, Lessells A, O'Halloran A. Proliferative myositis. An immunohistochemical and ultrastructural study. Am J Surg Pathol 1991;15:654-659.

46. El-Jabbour JN, Wilson GD, Bennett MH, Burke MM, Davey AT, Eames K. Flow cytometric study of nodular fasciitis, proliferative fasciitis, and proliferative myositis. Hum Pathol 1991;22:1146-1149.

47. Dembinski A, Bridge JA, Neff JR, Berger C, Sandberg AA. Trisomy 2 in proliferative fasciitis. Cancer Genet Cytogenet 1992;60:27-30.

48. Ohjimi Y, Iwasaki H, Ishiguro M, Tsayama T, Kaneko Y. Trisomy 2 found in proliferative myositis cultured cell. Cancer Genet Cytogenet 1994;76:157.

49. McComb EN, Neff JR, Johansson SL, Nelson M, Bridge JA. Chromosomal anomalies in a case of proliferative myositis. Cancer Genet Cytogenet 1997;98:142-144.

Ischemic Fasciitis

50. Liegl B, Fletcher CD. Ischemic fasciitis: analysis of 44 cases indicating an inconsistent association with immobility or debilitation. Am J Surg Pathol 2008;32:1546-1552.

51. Montgomery EA, Meis JM, Mitchell MS, Enzinger FM. Atypical decubital fibroplasia. A distinctive fibroblastic pseudotumor occurring in debilitated patients. Am J Surg Pathol 1992;16:708-715.

52. Perosio PM, Weiss SW. Ischemic fasciitis: a juxta-skeletal fibroblastic proliferation with a predilection for elderly patients. Mod Pathol 1993;6:69-72.

Fibroma of Tendon Sheath

53. Chung EB, Enzinger FM. Fibroma of tendon sheath. Cancer 1979;44:1945-1954.

54. Hashimoto H, Tsuneyoshi M, Daimaru Y, Daimaru Y, Ushijima M, Enjoji M. Fibroma of tendon sheath: a tumor of myofibroblasts. A clinocopathologic study of 18 cases. Acta Pathol Jpn 1985;35:1099-1107.

55. Millon SJ, Bush DC, Garbes AD. Fibroma of tendon sheath in the hand. J Hand Surg Am 1994;19:788-793.

56. Lamovec J, Bracko M, Voncina D. Pleomorphic fibroma of tendon sheath. Am J Surg Pathol 1991;15:1202-1205.

57. Dal Cin P, Sciot R, De Smet L, Van Den Berghe H. Translocation 2;11 in a fibroma of tendon sheath. Histopathology 1998;32:433-435.

Nuchal-Type Fibroma

58. Michal M, Fetsch JF, Hes O, Miettinen M. Nuchal-type fibroma. A clinicopathologic study of 52 cases. Cancer 1999;85:156-163.

59. Abraham Z, Rozenbaum M, Rosner I, Naschitz Y, Boss Y, Rosenmann E. Nuchal fibroma. J Dermatol 1997;24:262-265.

60. Balachandran K, Allen PW, MacCormac LB. Nuchal fibroma. A clinicopathologic study of nine cases. Am J Surg Pathol 1995;19:313-317.

61. Banney LA, Weedon D, Muir JB. Nuchal fibroma associated with scleredema, diabetes mellitus and organic solvent exposure. Australas J Dermatol 2000;41:39-41.

62. Diwan AH, Graves ED, King JA, Horenstein MG. Nuchal-type fibroma in two related patients with Gardner's syndrome. Am J Surg Pathol 2000;24:1563-1567.

63. Zamecnik M, Michal M. Nuchal-type fibroma is positive for CD34 and CD99. Am J Surg Pathol 2001;25:970.

64. Laskin WB, Fetsch JF, Miettinen M. Nuchal fibrocartilaginous pseudotumor: a clinicopathologic study of five cases and review of the literature. Mod Pathol 1999;12:663-668.

65. O'Connell JX, Janzen DL, Hughes TR. Nuchal fibrocartilaginous pseudotumor: a distinctive soft tissue lesion associated with prior neck injury. Am J Surg Pathol 1997;21:836-840.

66. Zamecnik M, Michal M. Nuchal fibrocartilaginous pseudotumor: immunohistochemical and ultrastructural study of two cases. Pathol Int 2001;51:723-728.

Gardner-Associated Fibroma

67. Coffin CM, Hornick JL, Zhou H, Fletcher CD. Gardner fibroma: a clinicopathologic and immunohistochemical analysis of 45 patients with 57 fibromas. Am J Surg Pathol 2007;31:410-416.

68. Wehrli BM, Weiss SW, Yandow S, Coffin CM. Gardner-associated fibromas (GAF) in young patients. A distinct fibrous lesion that identifies unsuspected Gardner syndrome and risk for fibromatosis. Am J Surg Pathol 2001;25:645-651.

69. Michal M. Non-nuchal-type fibroma associated with Gardner's syndrome. A hitherto-unreported mesenchymal tumor different from fibromatosis and nuchal-type fibroma. Pathol Res Pract 2000;196:857-860.

70. Michal M, Boudova L, Mukensnabl P. Gardner's syndrome associated fibromas. Pathol Int 2004;54:523-526.

Desmoplastic Fibroblastoma

71. Miettinen M, Fetsch JF. Collagenous fibroma (desmoplastic fibroblastoma): a clincopathological analysis of 63 cases of a distinctive soft tissue lesion with stellate-shaped fibroblasts. Hum Pathol 1998;29:676-682.

72. Evans HL. Desmoplastic fibroblastoma. A report of seven cases. Am J Surg Pathol 1995;19:1077-1081.

73. Hasegawa T, Shimoda T, Hirohashi S, Hizawa K, Sano T. Collagenous fibroma (desmoplastic fibroblastoma). Report of four cases and review of the literature. Arch Pathol Lab Med 1998;122:455-460.

74. Nielsen GP, O'Connell JX, Dickersin GR, Rosenberg AE. Collagenous fibroma (desmoplastic fibroblastoma): a report of seven cases. Mod Pathol 1996;9:781-785.

75. Takahara M, Ichikawa R, Oda Y, et al. Desmoplastic fibroblastoma: a case presenting as a protruding nodule in the dermis. J Cutan Pathol 2008;35(Suppl 1):70-73.

76. Bernal K, Nelson M, Neff JR, Nielsen SM, Bridge JA. Translocation (2;11)(q31;q12) is recurrent in collagenous fibroma (desmoplastic fibroblastoma). Cancer Genet Cytogenet 2004;149:161-163.

77. Sciot R, Samson I, van den Berghe H, Van Damme B, Dal Cin P. Collagenous fibroma (desmoplastic fibroblastoma): genetic link with fibroma of tendon sheath? Mod Pathol 1999;12:565-568.

78. Dal Cin P, Sciot R, De Smet L, Van den Berghe H. Translocation 2;11 in a fibroma of tendon sheath. Histopathology 1998;32:433-435.

Elastofibroma

79. Kransdorf MJ, Meis JM, Montgomery E. Elastofibroma: MR and CT appearance with radiologic-pathologic correlation. AJR Am J Roentgenol 1992;159:575-579.

80. Järvi OH, Saxén AE, Hopsu-Havu VK, Wartiovarra JJ, Vaissalo VT. Elastofibroma—a degenerative pseudotumor. Cancer 1969;23:42-63.

81. Machens HG, Mechtersheimer R, Göhring U, Schlag PN. Bilateral elastofibroma dorsi. Ann Thorac Surg 1992;54:774-776.

82. Nagamine N, Nohara Y, Ito E. Elastofibromas in Okinawa. A clinicopathologic study of 170 cases. Cancer 1982;50:1794-1805.

83. Cross DL, Mills SE, Kulund DN. Elastofibroma arising in the foot. South Med J 1984;77:1194-1196.

84. Enjoji M, Sumiyoshi K, Sueyoshi K. Elastofibromatous lesion of the stomach in a patient with elastofibroma dorsi. Am J Surg Pathol 1985;9:233-237.

85. Järvi OH, Länsimies PH. Subclinical elastofibromas in the scapular region in an autopsy series. Acta Pathol Microbiol Scand A 1975;83:87-108.

86. Benisch B, Peison B, Marquet E, Sobel HJ. Pre elastofibroma and elastofibroma (the continuum of elastic-producing fibrous tumors). A light and ultrastructural study. Am J Clin Pathol 1983;80:88-92.

87. Fukuda Y, Miyake H, Masuda Y, Masugi Y. Histogenesis of unique elastinophilic fibers of elastofibroma: ultrastructural and immunohistochemical studies. Hum Pathol 1987;18:424-429.

88. Hisaoka M, Hashimoto H. Elastofibroma: clonal fibrous proliferation with predominant CD34-positive cells. Virchows Arch 2006;448:195-199.

89. Batstone P, Forsyth L, Goodlad J. Clonal chromosome aberrations secondary to chromosome instability in an elastofibroma. Cancer Genet Cytogenet 2001;128:46-47.

90. McComb EN, Feely MG, Neff JR, Johansson SL, Nelson M, Bridge JA. Cytogenetic instability, predominantly involving chromosome 1, is characteristic of elastofibroma. Cancer Genet Cytogenet 2001;126:68-72.

91. Schepel JA, Wille J, Seldenrijk CA, vam Ramshorst B. Elastofibroma: a familial occurrence. Eur J Surg 1998;164:557-558.

92. Vanni R, Marras S, Faa G, et al. Chromosome instability in elastofibroma. Cancer Genet Cytogenet 1999;111:182-183.

Pleomorphic Fibroma of Skin

93. Ahn SK, Won JH, Lee SH, Lee WS, Choi SJ. Pleomorphic fibroma on the scalp. Dermatology 1995;191:245-248.

94. Chen TM, Purohit SK, Wang AR. Pleomorphic sclerotic fibroma: a case report and literature review. Am J Dermatopathol 2002;24:54-58.

95. García-Doval I, Casas L, Toribio J. Pleomorphic fibroma of the skin, a form of sclerotic fibroma: an immunohistochemical study. Clin Exp Dermatol 1998;23:22-24.

96. Kamino H, Lee JY, Berke A. Pleomorphic fibroma of the skin: a benign neoplasm with cytologic atypia. A clinicopathologic study of eight cases. Am J Surg Pathol. 1989;13:107-113.

97. Layfield LJ, Fain JS. Pleomorphic fibroma of skin. A case report and immunohistochemical study. Arch Pathol Lab Med 1991;115:1046-1049.

98. Hassanein A, Telang G, Benedetto E, Spielvogel K. Subungual myxoid pleomorphic fibroma. Am J Dermatopathol 1998;20:502-505.

99. Rudolph P, Schubert C, Zelger BG, Zelger B, Parwanesch K. Differential expression of CD34 and Ki-M1p in pleomorphic fibroma and dermatofibroma with monster cells. Am J Dermatopathol 1999;21:414-419.

100. Hsieh YJ, Lin YC, Wu YH, Su HY, Billings SD, Hood AF. Subungual pleomorphic fibroma. J Cutan Pathol 2003;30:569-571.

Intranodal (Palisaded) Myofibroblastoma

101. Alguacil-Garcia A. Intranodal myofibroblastoma in a submandibular lymph node. A case report. Am J Clin Pathol 1992;97:69-72.

102. Basu A, Harvey DR. Palisaded myofibroblastoma—an uncommon tumour of lymph nodes. Eur J Surg Oncol 1998;24:609.

103. Bigotti G, Coli A, Mottolese M, De Filippo F. Selective localization of palisaded myofibroblastoma with amianthoid fibers. J Clin Pathol 1991;44;761-764.

104. Creager AJ, Garwacki CP. Recurrent intranodal palisaded myofibroblastoma with metaplastic bone formation. Arch Pathol Lab Med 1999;123:433-436.

105. Eyden BP, Harris M, Greywoode GI, Christensen L, Bauergee SS. Intranodal myofibroblastoma: report of a case. Ultrastruct Pathol 1996;20:79-88.

106. Fletcher CD, Stirling RW. Intranodal myofibroblastoma presenting in the submandibular region: evidence of a broader clinical and histological spectrum. Histopathology 1990;16:287-293.

107. Hisaoka M, Hashimoto H, Daimaru Y. Intranodal palisaded myofibroblastoma with so-called amianthoid fibers: a report of two cases with a review of the literature. Pathol Int 1998;48:307-312.

108. Kleist B, Poetsch M, Schmoll J. Intranodal palisaded myofibroblastoma with overexpression of cyclin D1. Arch Pathol Lab Med 2003;127:1040-1043.

109. Lioe TF, Allen DC, Bell JC. A case of multicentric intranodal palisaded myofibroblastoma. Histopathology 1994;24:173-175.

110. Michal M, Chlumská A, Povýšilová V. Intranodal "amianthoid" myofibroblastoma. Report of six cases immunohistochemical and electron microscopical study. Pathol Res Pract 1992;188:199-204.

111. Rossi A, Bulgarini A, Rondanelli E, Incensati R. Intranodal palisaded myofibroblastoma: report of three new cases. Tumori 1995;81:464-468.

112. Suster S, Rosai J. Intranodal hemorrhagic spindle-cell tumor with "amianthoid" fibers. Report of six cases of a distinctive mesenchymal neoplasm of the inguinal region that simulates Kaposi's sarcoma. Am J Surg Pathol 1989;13:347-357.

113. Weiss SW, Gnepp DR, Bratthauer GL. Palisaded myofibroblastoma. A benign mesenchymal tumor of lymph node. Am J Surg Pathol 1989;13:341-346.

114. Skálová A, Michal M, Chlumská A, Leivo J. Collagen composition and ultrastructure of the so-called amianthoid fibres in palisaded myofibroblastoma. Ultrastructural and immunohistochemical study. J Pathol 1992;167:335-340.

Other Fibroma Variants and Fibrous Proliferations

115. Vargas SO. Fibrous umbilical polyp: a distinct fasciitis-like proliferation of early childhood with a marked male predominance. Am J Surg Pathol 2001;25:1438-1442.

116. Mahmood MN, Salama ME, Chaffins M, et al. Solitary sclerotic fibroma of skin: a possible link with pleomorphic fibroma with immunophenotypic expression for O13 (CD99) and CD34. J Cutan Pathol 2003;30:631-636.

117. Metcalf JS, Maize JC, LeBoit PW. Circumscribed storiform collagenoma (sclerosing fibroma). Am J Dermatopathol 1991;13:122-129.

118. Rapini RP, Golitz LE. Sclerotic fibromas of the skin. J Am Acad Dermatol 1989;20:266-271.

119. Lo WL, Wong CK. Solitary sclerotic fibroma. J Cutan Pathol 1990;17:269-273.

120. Hanft VN, Shea CR, McNutt NS, Pullitzer D, Horenstein MG, Prieto VO. Expression of CD34 in sclerotic ("plywood") fibromas. Am J Dermatopathol 2000;22:17-21.

121. Requena L, Gutiérrez J, Yus ES. Multiple sclerotic fibromas of the skin. A cutaneous marker of Cowden's disease. J Cutan Pathol 1992;19:346-351.

122. Starink TM, Meijer CJ, Brownstein MH. The cutaneous pathology of Cowden's disease: new findings. J Cutan Pathol 1985;12:83-93.

123. Weary PE, Gorlin RJ, Gentry WC Jr, Comer JE, Greer KE. Multiple hamartoma syndroma (Cowden's disease). Arch Dermatol 1972;106:682-690.

124. Chen TM, Purohit SK, Wang AR. Pleomorphic sclerotic fibroma: a case report and literature review. Am J Dermatopathol 2002;24:54-58.

125. García-Doval I, Casas L, Toribio. Pleomorphic fibroma of the skin, a form of sclerotic fibroma: an immunohistochemical study. Clin Exp Dermatol 1998;23:22-24.

126. Martin-López R, Feal-Cortizas C, Fraga J. Pleomorphic sclerotic fibroma. Dermatology 1999;198:69-72.

127. Shitabata PK, Crouch EC, Fitzgibbon JF, Swanson PE, Adesokan PN, Wick MR. Cutaneous sclerotic fibroma. Immunohistochemical evidence of a fibroblastic neoplasm with ongoing type I collagen synthesis. Am J Dermatopathol 1995;17:339-343.

128. High WA, Stewart D, Essary LR, Kageyama NP, Hoang MP, Cockerell CJ. Sclerotic fibroma-like change in various neoplastic and inflammatory skin lesions: is sclerotic fibroma a distinct entity? J Cutan Pathol 2004;31:373-378.

129. Cohen MM Jr. Proteus syndrome: clinical evidence for somatic mosaicism and selective review. Am J Med Genet 1993;47:645-652.

130. Cohen MM Jr. Proteus syndrome: an update. Am J Med Genet C Semin Med Genet 2005;137C:38-52.

131. Gordon PL, Wilroy RS, Lasater OE, Cohen MM Jr. Neoplasms in Proteus syndrome. Am J Med Genet 1995;57:74-78.

132. Happle R. The manifold faces of Proteus syndrome. Arch Dermatol 2004;140:1001-1002.

133. Wiedemann HR, Burgio GR, Aldenhoff P, Kunze J, Kaufmann HJ, Schirg E. The proteus syndrome. Partial gigantism of the hands and/or feet, nevi, hemihypertrophy, subcutaneous tumors, macroceophaly, or other skull anomalies and possible accelerated growth and visceral affections. Eur J Pediatr 1983;140:5-12.

134. Biesecker LG, Happle R, Mulliken JB, et al. Proteus syndrome: diagnostic criteria, differential diagnosis, and patient evaluation. Am J Med Genet 1999;84:389-395.

135. Cohen MM Jr. Putting a foot in one's mouth or putting a foot down: nonspecificity v. specificity of the connective tissue nevus in Proteus syndrome. Proc Greenwood Genet Center 1995;14:11-13.

136. Nguyen D, Turner JT, Olsen C, Biesecker LG, Darling TN. Cutaneous manifestations of proteus syndrome: correlations with general clinical severity. Arch Dermatol 2004;140:947-953.

137. Turner JT, Cohen MM Jr, Biesecker LG. Reassessment of the Proteus syndrome literature: application of diagnostic criteria to published cases. Am J Med Genet A 2004;130A:111-122.

138. Twede JV, Turner JT, Biesecker LG, Darling TN. Evolution of skin lesions in Proteus syndrome. J Am Acad Dermatol 2005;52:834-838.

Calcifying Fibrous (Pseudo)tumor

139. Chon SH, Lee CB, Oh YH. Calcifying fibrous pseudotumor causing thoracic outlet syndrome. Eur J Cardiothorac Surg 2005;27:353-355.

140. Hill KA, Gonzalez-Crussi F, Chou PM. Calcifying fibrous pseudotumor versus inflammatory myofibroblastic tumor: a histological and immunohistochemical comparison. Mod Pathol 2001;14:784-790.

141. Hoffmann H, Beaver ME, Maillard AA. Calcifying fibrous pseudotumor of the neck. Arch Pathol Lab Med 2000;124:435-437.

142. Maeda A, Kawabata K, Kusuzaki K. Rapid recurrence of calcifying fibrous pseudotumor (a case report). Anticancer Res 2002;22:1795-1797.

143. Mangat A, Schiller C, Mengoni P, Reynolds C, Jeruss JS. Calcifying fibrous pseudotumor of the breast. Breast J 2009;3:299-301.

144. Nascimento AF, Ruiz R, Hornick JL, Fletcher CD. Calcifying fibrous 'pseudotumor': clinicopathologic study of 15 cases and analysis of its relationship to inflammatory myofibroblastic tumor. Int J Surg Pathol 2002;10:189-196.

145. Agaimy A, Bihl MP, Tornillo L, Wünsch PH, Hartmann A, Michal M. Calcifying fibrous tumor of the stomach: clinicopathologic and molecular study of seven cases with literature review and reappraisal of histogenesis. Am J Surg Pathol 2010;34:271-278.

146. Attila T, Chen D, Gardiner GW, Ptak TW, Marcon NE. Gastric calcifying fibrous tumour. Can J Gastroenterol 2006;20:487-489.

147. Elpek GÖ, Küpesiz GY, Ögüs M. Incidental calcifying fibrous tumor of the stomach presenting as a polyp. Pathol Int 2006;56:227-231.

148. Emanuel P, Qin L, Harpaz N. Calcifying fibrous tumor of small intestine. Ann Diagn Pathol 2008;12:138-141.

149. Lau SK, Weiss LM. Calcifying fibrous tumor of the adrenal gland. Hum Pathol 2007;38:656-659.

150. Shigematsu H, Sano Y, Kasahara S, Yanai H, Date H. Calcifying fibrous tumor arising from the heart. J Thorac Cardiovasc Surg 2006;132:e21-22.

151. Ammar A, El Hammami S, Horchani H, Sellami N, Kilani T. Calcifying fibrous pseudotumor of the pleura: a rare location. Ann Thorac Surg 2003;76:2081-2082.

152. Kirby PA, Sato Y, Tannous R, Dehner LP. Calcifying fibrous pseudotumor of the myocardium. Pediatr Dev Pathol 2006;9:384-387.

153. Lee HY, Chuah KL, Tan PH. Test and teach. Number fifty-three. Diagnosis: calcifying fibrous pseudotumor. Pathology 2003;35:166-169.

154. Lee JC, Lien HC, Hsiao CH. Coexisting sclerosing angiomatoid nodular transformation of the spleen with multiple calcifying fibrous pseudotumors in a patient. J Formos Med Assoc 2007;106:234-239.

155. Medina AM, Alexis JB. A 27-year-old woman with incidental omental nodules. Arch Pathol Lab Med 2006;130:563-564.

156. Shibata K, Yuki D, Sakata K. Multiple calcifying fibrous pseudotumors disseminated in the pleura. Ann Thorac Surg 2008;85:e3-5.

157. Suh JH, Shin OR, Kim YH. Multiple calcifying fibrous pseudotumor of the pleura. J Thorac Oncol 2008;3:1356-1358.

158. Fetsch JF, Montgomery EA, Meis JM. Calcifying fibrous pseudotumor. Am J Surg Pathol 1993;17:502-508.

159. Rosenthal NS, Abdul-Karim FW. Childhood fibrous tumor with psammoma bodies. Clinicopathologic features in two cases. Arch Pathol Lab Med 1988;112:798-800.

160. Delbecque K, Legrand M, Boniver J, Lauwers GY, de Leval L. Calcifying fibrous tumour of the gastric wall. Histopathology 2004;44:399-400.

161. Dargent JL, Delplace J, Roufosse C, Laget JP, Lespagnard L. Development of a calcifying fibrous pseudotumour within a lesion of Castleman disease, hyaline-vascular subtype. J Clin Pathol 1999;52:547-549.

162. Chen KT. Familial peritoneal multifocal calcifying fibrous tumor. Am J Clin Pathol 2003;119:811-815.

163. Kawahara K, Yasukawa M, Nakagawa K, Katsura H, Nagano T, Iwasaki T. Multiple calcifying fibrous tumor of the pleura. Virchows Arch 2005;447:1007-1008.

164. Mourra N, Bell S, Parc R, Flejou JF. Calcifying fibrous pseudotumour: first case report in the gallbladder. Histopathology 2004;44:84-86.

165. Kocova L, Michal M, Sulc M, et al. Calcifying fibrous pseudotumour of visceral peritoneum. Histopathology 1997;31:182-184.

166. Lee D, Suh YL, Lee SK. Calcifying fibrous pseudotumour arising in a gastric inflammatory myofibroblastic tumour. Pathology 2006;38:588-591.

167. Pomplun S, Goldstraw P, Davies SE, Burke MM, Nicholson AG. Calcifying fibrous pseudotumour arising within an inflammatory pseudotumour: evidence of progression from one lesion to the other? Histopathology 2000;37:380-382.

168. Van Dorpe J, Ectors N, Geboes K, D'Hoore A, Sciot R. Is calcifying fibrous pseudotumor a late sclerosing stage of inflammatory myofibroblastic tumor? Am J Surg Pathol 1999;23:329-335.

169. Chatelain D, Manaouil D, Levy P, Joly JP, Sevestre H, Regimbeau JM. Reactive nodular fibrous pseudotumor of the gastrointestinal tract and mesentery. Am J Surg Pathol 2004;28:416.

170. Yantiss RK, Nielsen GP, Lauwers GY, Rosenberg AE. Reactive nodular fibrous pseudotumor of the gastrointestinal tract and mesentery; a clinicopathologic study of five cases. Am J Surg Pathol 2003;27:532-540.

Juvenile Hyaline Fibromatosis

171. Senzaki H, Kiyozuka Y, Uemura Y, Shikata N, Ueda S, Tsibira A. Juvenile hyaline fibromatosis: a report of two unrelated adult sibling cases and a literature review. Pathol Int 1998;48:230-236.

172. Fayad MN, Yacoub A, Salman S, Khudr A, Der Kaloustian VM. Juvenile hyaline fibromatosis: two new patients and review of the literature. Am J Med Genet 1987;26:123-131.

173. Kitano Y, Horiki M, Aoki T, Sagami S. Two cases of juvenile hyalin fibromatosis. Some histological, electron microscopic, and tissue culture observations. Arch Dermatol 1972;106:877-883.

174. Kitano Y. Juvenile hyalin fibromatosis. Arch Dermatol 1976;112:86-88.

175. O'Neill DB, Kasser JR. Juvenile hyaline fibromatosis. A case report and review of musculoskeletal manifestations. J Bone Joint Surg Am 1989;71:941-944.

176. Quintal D, Jackson R. Juvenile hyaline fibromatosis. A 15 year follow-up. Arch Dermatol 1985;121:1062-1063.

177. Remberger K, Krieg T, Kunze D, Weinmann HM, Hübner G. Fibromatosis hyalinica multiplex (juvenile hyalin fibromatosis). Light microscopic, electron microscopic, immunohisto-chemical, and biochemical findings. Cancer 1985;56:614-624.

178. Finlay AY, Ferguson SD, Holt PJ. Juvenile hyaline fibromatosis. Br J Dermatol 1983;108:609-616.

179. Kan AE, Rogers M. Juvenile hyaline fibromatosis: an expanded clinicopathologic spectrum. Pediatr Dermatol 1989;6:68-75.

180. Urbina F, Sazunic I, Murray G. Infantile systemic hyalinosis or juvenile hyaline fibromatosis? Pediatr Dermatol 2004;21:154-159.

181. Glover MT, Lake BD, Atherton DJ. Clinical, histologic, and ultrastructural findings in two cases of infantile systemic hyalinosis. Pediatr Dermatol 1992;9:255-258.

182. Hanks S, Adams S, Douglas J, et al. Mutations in the gene encoding capillary morphogenesis protein 2 cause juvenile hyaline fibromatosis and infantile systemic hyalinosis. Am J Hum Genet 2003;73:791-800.

183. Landing BH, Nadorra R. Infantile systemic hyalinosis: report of four cases of a disease, fatal in infancy, apparently different from juvenile systemic hyalinosis. Pediatr Pathol 1986;6:55-79.

184. Mancini GM, Stojanov L, Willemsen R, et al. Juvenile hyaline fibromatosis: clinical heterogeneity in three patients. Dermatology 1999;198:18-25.

185. Sahn EE, Salinas CF, Sens MA, Key J, Swiger FK Jr, Holbrook KA. Infantile systemic hyalinosis in a black infant. Pediatr Dermatol 1994;11:52-60.

186. Haleem A, Al-Hindi HN, Juboury MA, Husseini HA, Ajlan AA. Juvenile hyaline fibromatosis: morphologic, immunohisto- chemical, and ultrastructural study of three siblings. Am J Dermatopathol 2002;24:218-224.

187. Dowling O, Difeo A, Ramirez MC, et al. Mutations in capillary morphogenesis gene-2 result in the allelic disorders juvenile hyaline fibromatosis and infantile systemic hyalinosis. Am J Hum Genet 2003;73:957-966.

188. Rahman N, Dunstan M, Teare MD, et al. The gene for juvenile hyaline fibromatosis maps to chromosome 4q21. Am J Hum Genet 2002;71:975-980.

Fibromatosis Colli

189. Coventry MB, Harris LE, Bianco AJ Jr, Bulbulian AH. Congenital muscular torticollis (wry neck). Postgrad Med 1960;28:383-392.

190. Kiwak KJ. Establishing an etiology for torticollis. Postgrad Med 1984;75:126-134.

191. Armstrong D, Pickrell K, Fetter B, Pitts W. Torticollis: an analysis of 271 cases. Plast Recon Surg 1965;35:14-25.

192. Davids JR, Wenger DR, Mubarak SJ. Congenital muscular torticollis: sequela of intrauterine or perinatal compartment syndrome. J Pediatr Orthop 1993;13:141-147.

193. Do TT. Congenital muscular torticollis: current concepts and review of treatment. Curr Opin Pediatr 2006;18:26-29.

194. Engin C, Yavuz SS, Sahin FI. Congenital muscular torticollis: is heredity a possible factor in a family with five torticollis patients in three generations? Plast Reconstr Surg 1997;99:1147-1150.

195. Kiesewetter WB, Nelson PK, Palladino VS, Koop CE. Neonatal torticollis. J Am Med Assoc 1955;157:1281-1285.

196. Lawrence WT, Azizkhan RG. Congenital muscular torticollis: a spectrum of pathology. Ann Plast Surg 1989;23:523-530.

197. Suzuki S, Yamamuro T, Fujita A. The aetiological relationship between congenital torticollis and obstetrical paralysis. Int Orthop 1984;8:175-181.

198. Thompson F, McManus S, Colville J. Familial congenital muscular torticollis: case report and review of the literature. Clin Orthop Relat Res 1986;202:193-196.

199. Macdonald D. Sternomastoid tumor and muscular torticollis. J Bone Joint Surg Br 1969;51:432-443.

200. Parikh SN, Crawford AH, Choudhury S. Magnetic resonance imaging in the evaluation of infantile torticollis. Orthopedics 2004;27:509-515.

201. Whyte AM, Lufkin RB, Bredenkamp J, Hoover L. Sternocleidomastoid fibrosis in congenital muscular torticollis: MR appearance. J Comput Assist Tomogr 1989;13:163-164.

202. Binder H, Eng GD, Gaiser JF, et al. Congenital muscular torticollis: results of conservative management with long-term follow-up in 85 cases. Arch Phys Med Rehabil 1987;68:222-225.

203. Canale ST, Griffin DW, Hubbard CN. Congenital muscular torticollis. A long-term follow-up. J Bone Joint Surg Am 1982;64:810-816.

204. Bredenkamp JK, Hoover LA, Berke GS, Shaw A. Congenital muscular torticollis. A spectrum of disease. Arch Otolaryngol Head Neck Surg 1990;116:212-216.

205. Sauer T, Selmer L, Freng A. Cytologic features of fibromatosis colli of infancy. Acta Cytol 1997;41:633-635.

206. Wakely PE Jr, Price WG, Frable WJ. Sternomastoid tumor of infancy (fibromatosis colli): diagnosis by aspiration cytology. Mod Pathol 1989;2:378-381.

207. Carlson JW, Fletcher CD. Immunohistochemistry for beta-catenin in the differential diagnosis of spindle cell lesions: analysis of a series and review of the literature. Histopathology 2007;51:509-514.

208. Thway K, Gibson S, Ramsay A, Sebire NJ. Beta-catenin expression in pediatric fibroblastic and myofibroblastic lesions: a study of 100 cases. Pediatr Dev Pathol 2009;12:292-296.

209. Joyce MB, de Chalain TM. Treatment of recalcitrant idiopathic muscular torticollis in infants with botulinum toxin type a. J Craniofac Surg 2005;16:321-327.

210. Oleszek JL, Chang N, Apkon SD, Wilson PE. Botulinum toxin type a in the treatment of children with congenital muscular torticollis. Am J Phys Med Rehabil 2005;84:813-816.

Infantile Digital Fibroma/Fibromatosis

211. Zardawi IM, Earley MJ. Inclusion body fibromatosis. J Pathol 1982;137:99-107.

212. Allen PW. Recurring digital fibrous tumours of childhood. Pathology 1972;4:215-223.

213. Laskin WB, Miettinen M, Fetsch JF. Infantile digital fibroma/fibromatosis: a clinicopathologic and immunohistochemical study of 69 tumors from 57 patients with long-term follow-up. Am J Surg Pathol 2009;33:1-13.

214. Dundr P, Povysil C, Tvrdik D. Leiomyoma of the gastrointestinal tract with intracytoplasmic inclusion bodies. Report of three cases. Cesk Patol 2006;42:139-144.

215. Hayashi T, Tsuda N, Chowdhury PR, Takahashi Y, Nakajima H. Infantile digital fibromatosis: a study of the development and regression of cytoplasmic inclusion bodies. Mod Pathol 1995;8:548-552.

216. Ortega E, Aranda FI, Chuliá MT, Niveiro M, Paya A, Segui J. Phyllodes tumor of the breast with actin inclusions in stromal cells: diagnosis by fine-needle aspiration cytology. Diagn Cytopathol 2001;25:115-117.

217. Pettinato G, Manivel JC, Gould EW, Albores-Saavedra J. Inclusion body fibromatosis of the breast. Two cases with immunohistochemical and ultrastructural findings. Am J Clin Pathol 1994;101:714-718.

218. Yusoff KL, Spagnolo DV, Digwood KI. Atypical cervical polyp with intracytoplasmic inclusions. Pathology 1998;30:215-217.

219. Beckett JH, Jacobs AH. Recurring digital fibrous tumors of childhood: a review. Pediatrics 1977;59:401-406.

220. Dabney KW, MacEwen GD, Davis NE. Recurring digital fibrous tumor of childhood: case report with long-term follow-up and review of the literature. J Pediatr Orthop 1986;6:612-617.

221. Ryman W, Bale P. Recurring digital fibromas of infancy. Australas J Dermatol 1985;26:113-117.

222. Santa Cruz DJ, Reiner CB. Recurrent digital fibroma of childhood. J Cutan Pathol 1978;5:339-346.

223. Shapiro L. Infantile digital fibromatosis and aponeurotic fibroma. Case reports of two rare pseudosarcomas and review of the literature. Arch Dermatol 1969;99:37-42.

224. Ishii N, Matsui K, Ichiyama S, Takahashi Y, Nakajima H. A case of infantile digital fibromatosis showing spontaneous regression. Br J Dermatol 1989;121:129-133.

225. Rimareix F, Bardot J, Andrac L, Vasse D, Galinier P, Magalon G. Infantile digital fibroma. Report on eleven cases. Eur J Pediatr Surg 1997;7:345-348.

226. Hiraoka N, Mukai M, Hosoda Y, Hata J. Phyllodes tumor of the breast containing the intracytoplasmic inclusion bodies identical with infantile digital fibromatosis. Am J Surg Pathol 1994;18:506-511.

227. Mukai M, Torikata C, Iri H, Hata J, Naito M, Shimoda T. Immunohistochemical identification of aggregated actin filaments in formalin-fixed, paraffin-embedded sections. I. A study of infantile digital fibromatosis by a new pretreatment. Am J Surg Pathol 1992;16:110-115.

228. Yun K. Infantile digital fibromatosis. Immunohistochemical and ultrastructural observations of cytoplasmic inclusions. Cancer 1988;61:500-507.

229. Choi KC, Hashimoto K, Setoyama M, Kagetsu N, Ironnier M, Sturman S. Infantile digital fibromatosis. Immunohistochemical and immunoelectron microscopic studies. J Cutan Pathol 1990;17:225-232.

230. Fringes B, Thais H, Böhm N, Altmannsberger M, Osborn N. Identification of actin microfilaments in the intracytoplasmic inclusions present in recurring infantile digital fibromatosis (Reye tumor). Pediatr Pathol 1986;6:311-324.

231. Battifora H, Hines JR. Recurrent digital fibromas of childhood. An electron microscope study. Cancer 1971;27:1530-1536.

232. Bhawan J, Bacchetta C, Joris I, Majno G. A myofibroblastic tumor. Infantile digital fibroma (recurrent digital fibrous tumor of childhood). Am J Pathol 1979;94:19-36.

233. Iwasaki H, Kikuchi M, Ohtsuki I, Enjoji M, Suenaga N, Mori R. Infantile digital fibromatosis. Identification of actin filaments in cytoplasmic inclusions by heavy meromyosin binding. Cancer 1983;52:1653-1661.

234. McKenzie AW, Innes FL, Rack JM, Breathnack AS, Gross M. Digital fibrous swellings in children. Br J Dermatol 1970;83:446-458.

235. Bacino CA, Stockton DW, Sierra RA, Heilstedt HA, Lewandrwski R, Van den Veyver JB. Terminal osseous dysplasia and pigmentary defects: clinical characterization of a novel male lethal X-linked syndrome. Am J Med Genet 2000;94:102-112.

236. Breuning MH, Oranje AP, Langemeijer RA, et al. Recurrent digital fibroma, focal dermal hypoplasia, and limb malformations. Am J Med Genet 2000;94:91-101.

237. Drut R, Pedemonte L, Rositto A. Noninclusion-body infantile digital fibromatosis; a lesion heralding terminal osseous dysplasia and pigmentary defects syndrome. Int J Surg Pathol 2005;13:181-184.

238. Azam SH, Nicholas JL. Recurring infantile digital fibromatosis: report of two cases. J Pediatr Surg 1995;30:89-90.

239. Bean SF. Infantile digital fibroma. Arch Dermatol 1969;100:124.

240. Bittesini L, DeiTos AP, Doglioni C, Della Libera D, Laurino L, Fletcher CD. Fibroepithelial tumor of the breast with digital fibroma-like inclusions in the stromal component. Case report with immunocytochemical and ultrastructural analysis. Am J Surg Pathol 1994;18:296-301.

Calcifying Aponeurotic Fibroma

241. Fetsch JF, Miettinen M. Calcifying aponeurotic fibroma: a clinicopathologic study on 22 cases arising in uncommon sites. Hum Pathol 1998;29:1504-1510.

242. Goldman RL. The cartilage analogue of fibromatosis (aponeurotic fibroma). Further observations based on 7 new cases. Cancer 1970;26:1325-1331.

243. Allen PW, Enzinger FM. Juvenile aponeurotic fibroma. Cancer 1970;26:857-867.

244. Keasbey LE. Juvenile aponeurotic fibroma (calcifying fibroma): a distinctive tumor arising in the palms and soles of young children. Cancer 1953;6:338-346.

245. Lafferty KA, Nelson EL, Demuth RJ, Miller SH, Harrison MW. Juvenile aponeurotic fibroma with disseminated fibrosarcoma. J Hand Surg Am 1986;11:737-740.

Fibrous Hamartoma of Infancy

246. Dickey GE, Sotelo-Avila C. Fibrous hamartoma of infancy: current review. Pediatr Dev Pathol 1999;2:236-243.

247. Enzinger FM. Fibrous hamartoma of infancy. Cancer 1965;18:241-248.

248. Paller AS, Gonzalez-Crussi F, Sherman JO. Fibrous hamartoma of infancy. Eight additional cases and a review of the literature. Arch Dermatol 1989;125:88-91.

249. Popek EJ, Montgomery EA, Fourcroy JL. Fibrous hamartoma of infancy in the genital region: findings in 15 cases. J Urol 1994;152:990-993.

250. Sotelo-Avila C, Bale PM. Subdermal fibrous hamartoma of infancy: pathology of 40 cases and differential diagnosis. Pediatr Pathol 1994;14:39-52.

251. Efem SE, Ekpo MD. Clinicopathological features of untreated fibrous hamartoma of infancy. J Clin Pathol 1993;46:522-524.

252. Jung PM, Hong EK. Fibrous hamartoma of infancy manifested as multiple nodules—a case report. J Korean Med Sci 1990;5:243-247.

253. Fletcher CD, Powell G, van Noorden S, McKee PH. Fibrous hamartoma of infancy: a histochemical and immunohistochemical study. Histopathology 1988;12:65-74.

254. Michal M, Mukenšnábl P, Chlumská A, Kodet R. Fibrous hamartoma of infancy. A study of eight cases with immunohistochemical and electron microscopical findings. Pathol Res Pract 1992;188:1049-1053.

255. Groisman G, Lichtig C. Fibrous hamartoma of infancy: an immunohistochemical and ultrastructural study. Hum Pathol 1991:22:914-918.

256. Rougemont AL, Fetni R, Murthy S, Fournet JC. A complex translocation (6;12;8)(q25;q24.3;q13) in a fibrous hamartoma of infancy. Cancer Genet Cytogenet 2006;171:115-118.

257. Tassano E, Nozza P, Tavella E, Garaventa A, Panarello C, Morerio C. Cytogenetic characterization of a fibrous hamartoma of infancy with complex translocations. Cancer Genet Cytogenet 2010;201:66-69.

Myofibroma/Myofibromatosis

258. Chateil JF, Brun M, Lebail B, Perel Y, Castell JF, Diard F. Infantile myofibromatosis. Skeletal Radiol 1995; 24:629-632.

259. Foss RD, Ellis GL. Myofibromas and myofibromatosis of the oral region: A clinicopathologic analysis of 79 cases. Oral Surg Oral Med Oral Pathol Oral Radiol Endod 2000;89:57-65.

260. Requena L, Kutzner H, Hügel H, Rütten A, Furio V. Cutaneous adult myofibroma: a vascular neoplasm. J Cutan Pathol 1996;23:445-457.

261. Sirvent N, Perrin C, Lacour JP, Maire G, Attias R, Pedeutour F. Monosomy 9q and trisomy 16q in a case of congenital solitary infantile myofibromatosis. Virchows Arch 2004;445:537-540.

262. Vered M, Allon I, Buchner A, Dayan D. Clinico-pathologic correlations of myofibroblastic tumors of the oral cavity. II. Myofibroma and myofibromatosis of the oral soft tissues. J Oral Pathol Med 2007;36:304-314.

263. Arcangeli F, Calista D. Congenital myofibromatosis in two siblings. Eur J Dermatol 2006;16:181-183.

264. Auriti C, Kieran MW, Deb G, Devito R, Pasquini L, Danhaive O. Remission of infantile generalized myofibromatosis after interferon alpha therapy. J Pediatr Hematol Oncol 2008;30:179-181.

265. Gopal M, Chahal G, Al-Rifai Z, Eradi B, Nnan G, Nour S. Infantile myofibromatosis. Pediatr Surg Int 2008;24:287-291.

266. Ikediobi NI, Iyengar V, Hwang L, Collins WE, Metry DW. Infantile myofibromatosis: support for autosomal dominant inheritance. J Am Acad Dermatol 2003;49:S148-150.

267. Briselli MF, Soule EH, Gilchrist GS. Congenital fibromatosis: report of 18 cases of solitary and 4 cases of multiple tumors. Mayo Clin Proc 1980;55:554-562.

268. Coffin CM, Neilson KA, Ingels S, Fran-Gerszberg K, Dehner LP. Congenital generalized fibromatosis: a disseminated angiocentric myofibromatosis. Pediatr Pathol Lab Med 1995;15:571-587.

269. Mentzel T, Calonje E, Nascimento AG, et al. Infantile hemangiopericytoma versus infantile myofibromatosis. Study of a series suggesting a continuous spectrum of infantile myofibroblastic lesions. Am J Surg Pathol 1994;18:922-930.

270. Variend S, Bax NM, Van Gorp J. Are infantile myofibromatosis, congenital fibrosarcoma and congenital haemangiopericytoma histogenetically related? Histopathology 1995;26:57-62.

271. Chung EB, Enzinger FM. Infantile myofibromatosis. Cancer 1981;48:1807-1818.

272. Wiswell TE, Davis J, Cunningham BE, Solenberger R, Thomas PJ.. Infantile myofibromatosis: the most common fibrous tumor of infancy. J Pediatr Surg 1988;23:314-318.

273. Bracko M, Cindro L, Golouh R. Familial occurrence of infantile myofibromatosis. Cancer 1992;69:1294-1299.

274. Inwards CY, Unni KK, Beabout JW, Shives TC. Solitary congenital fibromatosis (infantile myofibromatosis) of bone. Am J Surg Pathol 1991;15:935-941.

275. Vigneswaran N, Boyd DL, Waldron CA. Solitary infantile myofibromatosis of the mandible. Report of three cases. Oral Surg Oral Med Oral Pathol 1992;73:84-88.

276. Fukasawa Y, Ishikura H, Takada A, et al. Massive apoptosis in infantile myofibromatosis. A putative mechanism of tumor regression. Am J Pathol 1994;144:480-485.

277. Beham A, Badve S, Suster S, Fletcher CD. Solitary myofibroma in adults: clinicopathological analysis of a series. Histopathology 1993;22:335-341.

278. Zelger BW, Calonje E, Sepp N, Fink FM, Zelger BG, Schmid KW. Monophasic cellular variant of infantile myofibromatosis. An unusual histopathologic pattern in two siblings. Am J Dermatopathol 1995;17:131-138.

279. Daimaru Y, Hashimoto H, Enjoji M. Myofibromatosis in adults (adult counterpart of infantile myofibromatosis). Am J Surg Pathol 1989;13:859-865.
280. Smith KJ, Skelton HG, Barrett TL, Lupton GP, Graham JH. Cutaneous myofibroma. Mod Pathol 1989;2:603-609.
281. Narchi H. Four half-siblings with infantile myofibromatosis: a case for autosomal-recessive inheritance. Clin Genet 2001;59:134-135.
282. Zand DJ, Huff D, Everman D, et al. Autosomal dominant inheritance of infantile myofibromatosis. Am J Med Genet 2004;126A:261-266.
283. Jennings TA, Duray PH, Collins FS, Sabetta J, Enzinger FM. Infantile myofibromatosis. Evidence for an autosomal-dominant disorder. Am J Surg Pathol 1984;8:529-538.
284. Savasan S, Fulgenzi LA, Rabah R, Mohamed AN, Ravindranath Y. Generalized infantile myofibromatosis in a patient with Turner's syndrome: a trial of interferon-alpha. J Pediatr 1998;133:694-696.
285. Stenman G, Nadal N, Persson S, Gunterberg B, Angervall L. del(6)(q12q15) as the sole cytogenetic abnormality in a case of solitary infantile myofibromatosis. Oncol Rep 1999;6:1101-1104.
286. Granter SR, Badizadegan K, Fletcher CD. Myofibromatosis in adults, glomangiopericytoma, and myopericytoma. A spectrum of tumors showing perivascular myoid differentiation. Am J Surg Pathol 1998;22:513-525.
287. Mentzel T, Dei Tos AP, Sapi Z, Kutzner H. Myopericytoma of skin and soft tissues: clinicopathologic and immunohistochemical study of 54 cases. Am J Surg Pathol 2006;30:104-113.
288. Hatzidaki E, Korakaki E, Voloudaki A, Daskaloyannaki M, Manoura A, Giannakopoulou C. Infantile myofibromatosis with visceral involvement and complete spontaneous regression. J Dermatol 2001;28:379-382.
289. Zeller B, Storm-Mathisen I, Smevik B, Sund S, Danielsen K, Lie SO. Cure of infantile myofibromatosis with severe respiratory complications without antitumour therapy. Eur J Pediatr 1997;156:841-844.
290. Day M, Edwards AO, Weinberg A, Leavey PJ. Brief report: successful treatment of a patient with infantile generalized myofibromatosis. Med Pediatr Oncol 2002;38:371-373.
291. Gandhi MM, Nathan PC, Weitzman S, Levitt GA. Successful treatment of life-threatening generalized infantile myofibromatosis using low-dose chemotherapy. J Pediatr Hematol Oncol 2003;25:750-754.
292. Williams W, Craver RD, Correa H, Velez M, Gardner RV. Use of 2-chlorodeoxyadenosine to treat infantile myofibromatosis. J Pediatr Hematol Oncol 2002;24:59-63.

Palmar/Plantar Fibromatosis

293. Benson LS, Williams CS, Kahle M. Dupuytren's contracture. J Am Acad Orthop Surg 1998;6:24-35.
294. Burge P. Genetics of Dupuytren's disease. Hand Clin 1999;15:63-71.
295. Ross DC. Epidemiology of Dupuytren's disease. Hand Clin 1999;15:53-62.
296. Chen KT, Van Dyne DA. Familial plantar fibromatosis. J Surg Oncol 1985;29:240-241.
297. Ling RS. The genetic factor in Dupuytren's disease. J Bone Joint Surg Br 1963;45:709-718.
298. Nyberg LM Jr, Bias WB, Hochberg MC, Walsh PC. Identification of an inherited form of Peyronie's disease with autosomal dominant inheritance and association with Dupuytren's contracture and histocompatibility B7 cross-reacting antigens. J Urol 1982;128:48-51.
299. Burge P, Hoy G, Regan P, Milne R. Smoking, alcohol and the risk of Dupuytren's contracture. J Bone Joint Surg Br 1997;79B:206-210.
300. Hueston JT. Dermofasciectomy for Dupuytren's disease. Bull Hosp Jt Dis Orthop Inst 1984;44:224-232.
301. Noble J, Arafa M, Royle SG, McGeorge G, Crank S. The association between alcohol, hepatic pathology and Dupuyten's disease. J Hand Surg Br 1992;17B:71-74.
302. Paletta FX. Dupuytren's contracture. Am Fam Physician 1981;23:85-90.
303. An HS, Southworth SR, Jackson WT, Russ B. Cigarette smoking and Dupuytren's contracture of the hand. J Hand Surg Am 1988;13A:872-874.
304. Gudmundsson KG, Arngrímsson R, Sigfússon N, Björnsson A, Jónsson T. Epidemiology of Dupuytren's disease: clinical, serological, and social assessment. The Reykjavik study. J Clin Epidemiol 2000;53:291-296.
305. Arkkila PE, Kantola IM, Viikari JS, Ronnemaa T, Vahatalo MA. Dupuytren's disease in type 1 diabetic patients: a five-year prospective study. Clin Exp Rheumatol 1996;14:59-65.
306. Early PF. Population studies in Dupuytren's contracture. J Bone Joint Surg Br 1962;44B:602-613.
307. Hueston JT. The incidence of Dupuytren's contracture. Med J Aust 1960;6:999-1002.
308. Yost J, Winters T, Fett HC Sr. Dupuytren's contracture; a statistical study. Am J Surg 1955;90:568-571.

309. Allen RA, Woolner LB, Ghormley RK. Soft-tissue tumors of the sole; with special reference to plantar fibromatosis. J Bone Joint Surg Am 1955;37A:14-26.

310. Fetsch JF, Laskin WB, Miettinen M. Palmarplantar fibromatosis in children and preadoleascents: a clinicopathological study of 56 cases with newly recognized demographics and extended follow-up information. Am J Surg Pathol 2005;29:1095-1105.

311. Pickren JW, Smith AG, Stevenson TW Jr, Stout AP. Fibromatosis of the plantar fascia. Cancer 1951;4:846-856.

312. Ushijima M, Tsuneyoshi M, Enjoji M. Dupuytren type fibromatoses. A clinicopathologic study of 62 cases. Acta Pathol Jpn 1984;34:991-1001.

313. Godette GA, O'Sullivan M, Menelaus MB. Plantar fibromatosis of the heel in children: a report of 14 cases. J Pediatr Orthop 1997;17:16-17.

314. Sammarco GJ, Mangone PG. Classification and treatment of plantar fibromatosis. Foot Ankle Int 2000;21:563-569.

315. Rayan GM. Dupuytren disease: anatomy, pathology, presentation, and treatment. J Bone Joint Surg Am 2007;89:189-198.

316. Luck JV. Dupuytren's contracture; a new concept of the pathogenesis correlated with surgical management. J Bone Joint Surg Am 1959;41-A:635-664.

317. Mikkelsen OA. Dupuytren's disease—initial symptoms, age of onset and spontaneous course. Hand 1977;9:11-15.

318. Rayan GM. Clinical presentation and types of Dupuytren's disease. Hand Clin 1999;15:87-96.

319. Honner R, Lamb DW, James JI. Dupuytren's contracture. Long term results after fasciectomy. J Bone Joint Surg Br 1971;53:240-246.

320. McFarlane RM, Jamieson WG. Dupuytren's contracture. The management of one hundred patients. J Bone Joint Surg Am 1966;48:1095-1105.

321. Hueston JT. Some observations on knuckle pads. J Hand Surg Br 1984;9:75-78.

322. Hueston JT. Dupuytren diathesis. In: Dupuytren's disease. McFarlane RM, McGrouther DA, Flint MH, eds. New York: Churchill Livingstone 1990; 246-252.

323. Bivalacqua TJ, Purohit SK, Hellstrom WJ. Peyronie's disease: advances in basic science and pathophysiology. Curr Urol Rep 2000;1:297-301.

324. Davis CJ Jr. The microscopic pathology of Peyronie's disease. J Urol 1997;157:282-284.

325. Hellstrom WJ, Bivalacqua TJ. Peyronie's disease: etiology, medical and surgical therapy. J Androl 2000;21:347-354.

326. Lee YC, Chan HH, Black MM. Aggressive polyfibromatosis: a 10 year follow-up. Australas J Dermatol 1996;37:205-207.

327. Arafa M, Noble J, Royle SG, Trail JA, Allen J. Dupuytren's and epilepsy revisited. J Hand Surg Br 1992;17B:221-224.

328. McFarlane RM, Botz JS, Cheung H. Epidemiology of surgical patients. In: Dupuytren's disease. McFarlane RM, McGrouther DA, Flint MH, eds. New York: Churchill Livingstone 1990; 201-238.

329. González-Martínez R, Marín-Bertolín S, Amorrortu-Velayos J. Association between keloids and Dupuytren's disease: case report. Br J Plast Surg 1995;48:47-48.

330. Tsekouras AA, McGeorge DD. Palmar fascietomy and keloid formation. Br J Plast Surg 1999;52:593-594.

331. Lund M. Dupuytren's contracture and epilepsy. Acta Psych Neurol Scand 1941;16:465-492.

332. Aviles E, Arlen M, Miller T. Plantar fibromatosis. Surgery 1971;69:117-120.

333. Landers PA, Yu GV, White JM, Farrer AK. Recurrent plantar fibromatosis. J Foot Ankle Surg 1993;32:85-93.

334. Meyerding HW, Shellito JG. Dupuytren's contracture of the foot. J Int Coll Surg 1948;11:595-603.

335. Allen PW. The fibromatoses: a clinicopathologic classification based on 140 cases. Am J Surg Pathol 1977;1:255-270.

336. Evans HL. Multinucleated giant cells in plantar fibromatosis. Am J Surg Pathol 2002;26:244-248.

337. Montgomery E, Lee JH, Abraham SC, Wu TT. Superficial fibromatoses are genetically distinct from deep fibromatoses. Mod Pathol 2001;14:695-701.

338. Breiner JA, Nelson M, Bredthaucr BD, Neff JR, Bridge JA. Trisomy 8 and trisomy 14 in plantar fibromatosis. Cancer Genet Cytogenet 1999;108:176-177.

339. Dal Cin P, De Smet L, Sciot R, Van Damme B, Van den Berghe H. Trisomy 7 and trisomy 8 in dividing and non-dividing tumor cells in Dupuytren's disease. Cancer Genet Cytogenet 1999;108:137-140.

340. De Wever I, dal Cin P, Fletcher CD, Mandahl N, Mertens F. Cytogenetic, clinical, and morphologic correlations in 78 cases of fibromatosis: a report from the CHAMP study group. Mod Pathol 2000;13:1080-1085.

341. Casalone R, Mazzola D, Meroni E, et al. Cytogenetic and interphase cytogenetic analyses reveal chromosome instability but no clonal trisomy 8 in Dupuytren contracture. Cancer Genet Cytogenet 1997;99:73-76.

342. Gudmundsson KG, Arngrimsson R, Jónsson T. Eighteen years follow-up study of the clinical manifestations and progression of Dupuytren's disease. Scand J Rheumatol 2001;30:31-34.

343. Rombouts JJ, Noël H, Legrain Y, Munting E. Prediction of recurrence in the treatment of Dupuytren's disease: evaluation of a histologic classification. J Hand Surg Am 1989;14:644-652.

344. Wilbrand S, Ekbom A, Gerdin B. The sex ratio and rate of reoperation for Dupuytren's contracture in men and women. J Hand Surg Br 1999;24:456-459.

345. Aluisio FV, Mair SD, Hall RL. Plantar fibromatosis: treatment of primary and recurrent lesions and factors associated with recurrence. Foot Ankle Int 1996;17:672-678.

346. de Bree E, Zoetmulder FA, Keus RB, Peterse HL, van Coevorden F. Incidence and treatment of recurrent plantar fibromatosis by surgery and postoperative radiotherapy. Am J Surg 2004;187:33-38.

347. Skoff HD. The surgical treatment of Dupuytren's contracture: a synthesis of techniques. Plast Reconstr Surg 2004;113:540-544.

348. Wapner KL, Ververeli PA, Moore JH Jr, Hecht PJ, Becker CE, Lackman RD. Plantar fibromatosis: a review of primary and recurrent surgical treatment. Foot Ankle Int 1995;16:548-551.

Lipofibromatosis

349. Ayadi L, Charfi S, Hamed YB, et al. Pigmented lipofibromatosis in unusual location: case report and review of the literature. Virchows Arch 2008;452:115-117.

350. Deepti AN, Madhuri V, Walter NM, Cherian RA. Lipofibromatosis: report of a rare paediatric soft tissue tumour. Skeletal Radiol 2008;37:555-558.

351. Fetsch JF, Miettinen M, Laskin WB, Michal M, Enzinger FM. A clinicopathologic study of 45 pediatric soft tissue tumors with an admixture of adipose tissue and fibroblastic elements, and a proposal for classification as lipofibromatosis. Am J Surg Pathol 2000;24:1491-1500.

352. Greene AK, Karnes J, Padua HM, Schmidt BA, Kasser JR, Labow BI. Diffuse lipofibromatosis of the lower extremity masquerading as a vascular abnormality. Ann Plast Surg 2009;62:703-706.

353. Sari A, Tunakan M, Bolat B, Cakmakçi H, Ozer E. Lipofibromatosis in a two-year-old girl: a case report. Turk J Pediatr 2007;49:319-321.

354. Teo HE, Peh WC, Chan MY, Walford N. Infantile lipofibromatosis of the upper limb. Skeletal Radiol 2005;34:799-802.

355. Kabasawa Y, Katsube K, Harada H, et al. A male infant case of lipofibromatosis in the submental region exhibited the expression of the connective tissue growth factor. Oral Surg Oral Med Oral Pathol Oral Radiol Endod 2007;103:677-682.

356. Sasaki D, Hatori M, Hosaka M, Watanabe M, Kokubun S. Lipofibromatosis arising in a pediatric forearm—a case report. Ups J Med Sci 2005;110:259-266.

357. Carlson JW, Fletcher CD. Immunohistochemistry for beta-catenin in the differential diagnosis of spindle cell lesions: analysis of a series and review of the literature. Histopathology 2007;51:509-514.

358. Thway K, Gibson S, Ramsay A, Sebire NJ. Beta-catenin expression in pediatric fibroblastic and myofibroblastic lesions: a study of 100 cases. Pediatr Dev Pathol 2009;12:292-296.

359. Kenney B, Richkind KE, Friedlaender G, Zambrano E. Chromosomal rearrangements in lipofibromatosis. Cancer Genet Cytogenet 2007;179:136-139.

360. Grogan DP, Bernstein RM, Habal MB, Zambrano E. Congenital lipofibromatosis associated with macrodactyly of the foot. Foot Ankle Int 1991;12:40-46.

Diffuse Infantile Fibromatosis

361. Enzinger FM. Fibrous tumors of infancy. In: Cumley RW, McCay J, Beane DA, et al, eds. Tumors of bone and soft tissue. Chicago, IL: Year Book Medical Publishers; 1965:375-396.

362. Chung EB. Pitfalls in diagnosing benign soft tissue tumors in infancy and childhood. Pathol Annu 1985;20(Pt 2):323-346.

Desmoid-Type Fibromatosis

363. Ayala AG, Ro JY, Goepfert H, Cangir A, Khorsand J, Flake G. Desmoid fibromatosis: a clinicopathologic study of 25 children. Semin Diagn Pathol 1986;3:138-150.

364. Bonvalot S, Eldweny H, Haddad V, et al. Extra-abdominal primary fibromatosis: aggressive management could be avoided in a subgroup of patients. Eur J Surg Oncol 2008;34:462-468.

365. Faulkner LB, Hajdu SI, Kher U, et al. Pediatric desmoid tumor: retrospective analysis of 63 cases. J Clin Oncol 1995;13:2813-2818.

366. Taylor LJ. Musculoaponeurotic fibromatosis. A report of 28 cases and review of the literature. Clin Orthop Relat Res 1987;224:294-302.

367. Galiatsatos P, Foulkes WD. Familial adenomatous polyposis. Am J Gastroenterol 2006;101:385-398.

368. Groen EJ, Roos A, Muntinghe FL, et al. Extra-intestinal manifestations of familial adenomatous polyposis. Ann Surg Oncol 2008;15:2439-2450.

369. Gryfe R, Swallow C, Bapat B, Redston M, Gallinger S, Couture J. Molecular biology of colorectal cancer. Curr Probl Cancer 1997;21:235-299.

370. Latchford A, Volikos E, Johnson V, et al. APC mutations in FAP-associated desmoid tumours are non-random but not 'just right'. Hum Mol Genet 2007;16:78-82.

371. Abraham SC, Reynolds C, Lee JH, et al. Fibromatosis of the breast and mutations involving the APC/beta-catenin pathway. Hum Pathol 2002;33:39-46.

372. Gurbuz AK, Giardiello FM, Petersen GM, et al. Desmoid tumours in familial adenomatous polyposis. Gut 1994;35:377-381.

373. Heiskanen I, Järvinen HJ. Occurrence of desmoid tumours in familial adenomatous polyposis and results of treatment. Int J Colorectal Dis 1996;11:157-162.

374. Knudsen AL, Bülow S. Desmoid tumour in familial adenomatous polyposis. A review of literature. Fam Cancer 2001;1:111-119.

375. Seow-Choen F. The management of desmoids in patients with familial adenomatous polyposis (FAP). Acta Chir Iugosl 2008;55:83-87.

376. Fallen T, Wilson M, Morlan B, Lindor NM. Desmoid tumors—a characterization of patients seen at Mayo Clinic 1976-1999. Fam Cancer 2006;5:191-194.

377. Brasfield RD, Das Gupta TK. Desmoid tumors of the anterior abdominal wall. Surgery 1969;65:241-246.

378. Deyrup AT, Tretiakova M, Montag AG. Estrogen receptor-beta expression in extraabdominal fibromatosis: an analysis of 40 cases. Cancer 2006;106:208-213.

379. Häyry P, Reitamo JJ, Tötterman S, Hopfner-Hallikainen D, Sivula A. The desmoid tumor. II. Analysis of factors possibly contributing to the etiology and growth behavior. Am J Clin Pathol 1982;77:674-680.

380. Reitamo JJ, Scheinin TM, Häyry P. The desmoid syndrome. New aspects in the cause, pathogenesis and treatment of the desmoid tumor. Am J Surg 1986;151:230-237.

381. Hansmann A, Adolph C, Vogel T, Unger A, Moeslein G. High-dose tamoxifen and sulindac as first-line treatment for desmoid tumors. Cancer 2004;100:612-620.

382. Janinis J, Patriki M, Vini L, Aravantinos G, Whelan JS. The pharmacological treatment of aggressive fibromatosis: a systematic review. Ann Oncol 2003;14:181-190.

383. Picariello L, Tonelli F, Brandi ML. Selective oestrogen receptor modulators in desmoid tumours. Expert Opin Investig Drugs 2004;13:1457-1468.

384. Wilcken N, Tattersall MH. Endocrine therapy for desmoid tumors. Cancer 1991;68:1384-1388.

385. Aaron AD, O'Mara JW, Legendre KE, Evans SR, Attinger CE, Montgomery EA. Chest wall fibromatosis associated with silicone implants. Surg Oncol 1996;5:93-99.

386. Buitendijk S, van de Ven CP, Dumans TG, et al. Pediatric aggressive fibromatosis: a retrospective analysis of 13 patients and review of the literature. Cancer 2005;104:1090-1099.

387. Kumar V, Khanna S, Khanna AK, Khanna R. Desmoid tumors: experience of 32 cases and review of the literature. Indian J Cancer 2009; 46:34-39.

388. Pignatti G, Barbanti-Bròdano G, Ferrari D, et al. Extraabdominal desmoid tumor. A study of 83 cases. Clin Orthop Relat Res 2000;375:207-213.

389. Burke AP, Sobin LH, Shekitka KM, Federspiel BH, Helwig EB. Intra-abdominal fibromatosis. A pathologic analysis of 130 tumors with comparison of clinical subgroups. Am J Surg Pathol 1990;14:335-341.

390. Reitamo JJ, Häyry P, Nykyri E, Saxén E. The desmoid tumor. I. Incidence, sex-, age- and anatomical distribution in the Finnish population. Am J Clin Pathol 1982;77:665-673.

391. Ramirez RN, Otsuka NY, Apel DM, Bowen RE. Desmoid tumor in the pediatric population: a report of two cases. J Pediatr Orthop B 2009; 18:141-144.

392. Gronchi A, Casali PG, Mariani L, et al. Quality of surgery and outcome in extra-abdominal aggressive fibromatosis: a series of patients surgically treated at a single institution. J Clin Oncol 2003;21:1390-1397.

393. Merchant NB, Lewis JJ, Woodruff JM, Leung DH, Brennan MF. Extremity and trunk desmoid tumors: a multifactorial analysis of outcome. Cancer 1999;86:2045-2052.

394. Phillips SR, A'Hern R, Thomas JM. Aggressive fibromatosis of the abdominal wall, limbs and limb girdles. Br J Surg 2004;91:1624-1629.

395. Reitamo JJ. The desmoid tumor. IV. Choice of treatment, results, and complications. Arch Surg 1983;118:1318-1322.

396. Rock MG, Pritchard DJ, Reiman HM, Soule EH, Brewster RC. Extra-abdominal desmoid tumors. J Bone Joint Surg Am 1984;66:1369-1374.

397. Abbas AE, Deschamps C, Cassivi SD, et al. Chest wall desmoid tumors: results of surgical intervention. Ann Thorac Surg 2004;78:1219-1223.

398. Dashiell TG, Payne WS, Hepper NG, Soule EH. Desmoid tumors of the chest wall. Chest 1978;74:157-162.

399. Enzinger FM, Shiraki M. Musculo-aponeurotic fibromatosis of the shoulder girdle (extra-abdominal desmoid). Analysis of thirty cases followed up for ten or more years. Cancer 1967;20:1131-1140.

400. Bertani E, Chiappa A, Testori A, et al. Desmoid tumors of the anterior abdominal wall: results from a monocentric surgical experience and review of the literature. Ann Surg Oncol 2009;16:1642-1649.

401. Stoeckle E, Coindre JM, Longy M, et al. A critical analysis of treatment strategies in desmoid tumours: a review of a series of 106 cases. Eur J Surg Oncol 2009;35:129-134.

402. Bertagnolli MM, Morgan JA, Fletcher CD, et al. Multimodality treatment of mesenteric desmoid tumours. Eur J Cancer 2008;44:2404-2410.

403. Burke AP, Sobin LH, Shekitka KM. Mesenteric fibromatosis. A follow-up study. Arch Pathol Lab Med 1990;114:832-835.

404. Manetta A, Abt AB, Mamourian AC, et al. Pelvic fibromatosis: case report and review of literature. Gynecol Oncol 1989;32:91-94.

405. Mariani A, Nascimento AG, Webb MJ, Sim FH, Podratz KC. Surgical management of desmoid tumors of the female pelvis. J Am Coll Surg 2000;191:175-183.

406. Simon NL, Mazur MT, Shingleton HM. Pelvic fibromatosis: an unusual gynecologic tumor. Obstet Gynecol 1985;65:767-769.

407. Clark SK, Neale KF, Landgrebe JC, Phillips RK Desmoid tumours complicating familial adenomatous polyposis. Br J Surg 1999;86:1185-1189.

408. Ferenc T, Sygut J, Kopczynski J, et al. Aggressive fibromatosis (desmoid tumors): Definition, occurrence, pathology, diagnostic problems, clinical behavior, genetic background. Pol J Pathol 2006;57:5-15.

409. Lopez R, Kemalyan N, Moseley HS, Dennis D, Vetto RM. Problems in diagnosis and management of desmoid tumors. Am J Surg 1990;159:450-453.

410. Sundaram M, Duffrin H, McGuire MH, Vas W. Synchronous multicentric desmoid tumors (aggressive fibromatosis) of the extremities. Skeletal Radiol 1988;17:16-19.

411. Reis-Filho JS, Milanezi F, Pope LZ, Fillus-Neto J, Schmitt FC. Primary fibromatosis of the breast in a patient with multiple desmoid tumors—report of a case with evaluation of estrogen and progesterone receptors. Path Res Pract 2001;197:775-779.

412. Skubitz KM, Manivel JC, Clohisy DR, Frolich JW. Response of imatinib-resistant extra-abdominal aggressive fibromatosis to sunitinib: case report and review of the literature on response to tyrosine kinase inhibitors. Cancer Chemother Pharmacol 2009;64:635-640.

413. Spiegel DA, Dormans JP, Meyer JS, et al. Aggressive fibromatosis from infancy to adolescence. J Pediatr Orthop 1999;19:776-784.

414. Wargotz ES, Norris HJ, Austin RM, Enzinger FM. Fibromatosis of the breast. A clinical and pathological study of 28 cases. Am J Surg Pathol 1987;11:38-45.

415. Ballo MT, Zagars GK, Pollack A, Pisters PW, Pollack RA. Desmoid tumor: prognostic factors and outcome after surgery, radiation therapy, or combined surgery and radiation therapy. J Clin Oncol 1999;17:158-167.

416. Montgomery E, Torbenson MS, Kaushal M, Fisher C, Abraham SC. Beta-catenin immunohistochemistry separates mesenteric fibromatosis from gastrointestinal stromal tumor and sclerosing mesenteritis. Am J Surg Pathol 2002;26:1296-1301.

417. Schmidt D, Klinge P, Leuschner I, Harms D. Infantile desmoid-type fibromatosis. Morphological features correlate with biological behavior. J Pathol 1991;164:315-319.

418. Bhattacharya B, Dilworth HP, Iacobuzio Donahue C, et al. Nuclear beta-catenin expression distinguishes deep fibromatosis from other benign and malignant fibroblastic and myofibroblastic lesions. Am J Surg Pathol 2005;29:653-659.

419. Carlson JW, Fletcher CD. Immunohistochemistry for beta-catenin in the differential diagnosis of spindle cell lesions: analysis of a series and review of the literature. Histopathology 2007;51:509-514.

420. Ng TL, Gown AM, Barry TS, et al. Nuclear beta-catenin in mesenchymal tumors. Mod Pathol 2005;18:68-74.

421. Saito T, Oda Y, Kawaguchi K, et al. Possible association between higher beta-catenin mRNA expression and mutated beta-catenin in sporadic desmoid tumors: real-time semiquantitative assay by TaqMan polymerase chain reaction. Lab Invest 2002;82:97-103.

422. Alman BA, Pajerski ME, Diaz-Cano S, Corboy K, Wolfe HJ. Aggressive fibromatosis (desmoid tumor) is a monoclonal disorder. Diagn Mol Pathol 1997;6:98-101.

423. Bridge JA, Meloni AM, Neff JR, et al. Deletion 5q in desmoid tumor and fluorescence in situ hybridization for chromosome 8 and/or 20 copy number. Cancer Genet Cytogenet 1996;92:150-151.

424. Bridge JA, Swarts SJ, Buresh C, et al. Trisomies 8 and 20 characterize a subgroup of benign fibrous lesions arising in both soft tissue and bone. Am J Pathol 1999;154:729-733.

425. De Wever I, Dal Cin P, Fletcher CD, et al. Cytogenetic, clinical, and morphologic correlations in 78 cases of fibromatosis: a report from the CHAMP study group. Mod Pathol 2000;13:1080-1085.

426. Li M, Cordon-Cardo C, Gerald WL, Rosai J. Desmoid fibromatosis is a clonal process. Hum Pathol 1996;27:939-943.

427. Lucas DR, Shroyer KR, McCarthy PJ, Markham NE, Fujita M, Enomoto TE. Desmoid tumor is a clonal cellular proliferation: PCR amplification of HUMARA for analysis of patterns of X-chromosome inactivation. Am J Surg Pathol 1997;21:306-311.

428. Middleton SB, Frayling IM, Phillips RK. Desmoids in familial adenomatous polyposis are monoclonal proliferations. Br J Cancer 2000;82:827-832.

429. Alman BA, Li C, Pajerski ME, Diaz-Cano S, Wolfe HJ. Increased beta-catenin protein and somatic APC mutations in sporadic aggressive fibromatoses (desmoid tumors). Am J Pathol 1997;151:329-334.

430. Heinrich MC, McArthur GA, Demetri GD, et al. Clinical and molecular studies of the effect of imatinib on advanced aggressive fibrmatosis (desmoid tumor). J Clin Oncol 2006;24:1195-1203.

431. Lazar AJ, Hajibashi S, Lev D. Desmoid tumor: from surgical extripation to molecular dissection. Curr Opin Oncol 2009;21:352-359.

432. Miyoshi Y, Iwao K, Nawa G, Yoshikawa H, Ochi T, Nakamura Y. Frequent mutations in the beta-catenin gene in desmoid tumors from patients without familial adenomatous polyposis. Oncol Res 1998;10:591-594.

433. Tejpar S, Michils G, Denys H, et al. Analysis of Wnt/Beta catenin signaling in desmoid tumors. Acta Gastroenterol Belg 2005;68:5-9.

434. Li C, Bapat B, Alman BA. Adenomatous polyposis coli gene mutation alters proliferation through its beta-catenin-regulatory function in aggressive fibromatosis (desmoid tumor). Am J Pathol 1998;153:709-714.

435. Saito T, Oda Y, Tanaka K, et al. Beta-catenin nuclear expression correlates with cyclin D1 overexpression in sporadic desmoid tumours. J Pathol 2001;195:222-228.

436. Tejpar S, Nollet F, Li C, et al. Predominance of beta-catenin mutations and beta-catenin dysregulation in sporadic aggressive fibromatosis (desmoid tumor). Oncogene 1999;18:6615-6620.

437. Caspari R, Friedl W, Mandl M, et al. Familial adenomatous polyposis: mutation at codon 1309 and early onset of colon cancer. Lancet 1994;343:629-632.

438. Caspari R, Olschwang S, Friedl W, et al. Familial adenomatous polyposis: desmoid tumours and lack of ophthalmic lesions (CHRPE) associated with APC mutations beyond codon 1444. Hum Mol Genet 1995;4:337-340.

439. Couture J, Mitri A, Lagace R, et al. A germline mutation at the extreme 3' end of the APC gene results in a severe desmoid phenotype and is associated with overexpression of beta-catenin in the desmoid tumor. Clin Genet 2000;57:205-212.

440. Giarola M, Wells D, Mondini P, et al. Mutations of adenomatous polyposis coli (APC) gene are uncommon in sporadic desmoid tumours. Br J Cancer 1998;78:582-587

441. Palmirotta R, Curia MC, Esposito DL, et al. Novel mutations and inactivation of both alleles of the APC gene in desmoid tumors. Hum Mol Genet 1995;4:1979-1981.

442. Brandal P, Micci F, Bjerkehagen B, et al. Molecular cytogenetic characterization of desmoid tumors. Cancer Genet Cytogenet 2003;146:1-7.

443. Kouho H, Aoki T, Hisaoka M, Hashimoto H. Clinicopathological and interphase cytogenetic analysis of desmoid tumors. Histopathology 1997;31:336-341.

444. Larramendy ML, Virolainen M, Tukiainen E, Elomaa I, Knuutila S. Chromosome band 1q21 is recurrently gained in desmoid tumors. Genes Chromosomes Cancer 1998;23:183-186.

445. Dal Cin P, Sciot R, Aly MS, et al. Some desmoid tumors are characterized by trisomy 8. Genes Chromosomes Cancer 1994;10:131-135.

446. Fletcher JA, Naeem R, Xiao S, Corson JM. Chromosome aberrations in desmoid tumors. Trisomy 8 may be a predictor of recurrence. Cancer Genet Cytogenet 1995;79:139-143.

447. Dangel A, Meloni AM, Lynch HT, Sandberg AA. Deletion (5q) in a desmoid tumor of a patient with Gardner's syndrome. Cancer Genet Cytogenet 1994;78:94-98.

448. Mertens F, Willén H, Rydholm A, et al. Trisomy 20 is a primary chromosome aberration in desmoid tumors. Int J Cancer 1995;63:527-529.

449. Dalén BP, Bergh PM, Gunterberg BU. Desmoid tumors: a clinical review of 30 patients with more than 20 years' follow-up. Acta Orthop Scand 2003;74:455-459.

450. Dalén BP, Geijer M, Kvist H, Bergh PM, Gunterberg BU. Clinical and imaging observations of desmoid tumors left without treatment. Acta Orthop Scand 2006;77:932-937.

451. Hosalkar HS, Fox EJ, Delaney T, Torbert JT, Ogilvie CM, Lackman RD. Desmoid tumors and current status of management. Orthop Clin North Am 2006;37:53-63.

452. Melis M, Zager JS, Sondak VK. Multimodality management of desmoid tumors: how important is a negative surgical margin? J Surg Oncol 2008;98:594-602.

453. Masson JK, Soule EH. Desmoid tumors of the head and neck. Am J Surg 1966;112:615-622.

454. Posner MC, Shiu MH, Newsome JL, Hajdu SI, Gaynor JJ, Brennan MF. The desmoid tumor. Not a benign disease. Arch Surg 1989;124:191-196.

455. Sturt NJ, Clark SK. Current ideas in desmoid tumours. Fam Cancer 2006;5:275-285.

456. Schlemmer M. Desmoid tumors and deep fibromatoses. Hematol Oncol Clin North Am 2005;19:565-571.

457. Leithner A, Gapp M, Leithner K, et al. Margins in extra-abdominal desmoid tumors: a comparative analysis. J Surg Oncol 2004;86:152-156.

458. Lackner H, Urban C, Benesch M, et al. Multi-modal treatment of children with unresectable or recurrent desmoid tumors: an 11-year longitudinal observational study. J Pediatr Hematol Oncol 2004;26:518-522.

459. Lev D, Kotilingam D, Wei C, et al. Optimizing treatment of desmoid tumors. J Clin Oncol 2007;25:1785-1791.

460. Lewis JJ, Boland PJ, Leung DH, Woodruff JM, Brennan MF. The enigma of desmoid tumors. Ann Surg 1999;229:866-873.

461. Biermann JS. Desmoid tumors. Curr Treat Options Oncol 2000;1:262-266.

462. Merchant TE, Nguyen D, Walter AW, Pappo AS, Kun LE, Rao BN. Long-term results with radiation therapy for pediatric desmoid tumors. Int J Radiat Oncol Biol Phys 2000;47:1267-1271.

463. Sharma A, Ngan BY, Sándor GK, Campisi P, Forte V. Pediatric aggressive fibromatosis of the head and neck: a 20-year retrospective experience. J Pediatr Surg 2008;43:1596-1604.

464. Jelinek JA, Stelzer KJ, Conrad E, et al. The efficacy of radiotherapy as postoperative treatment for desmoid tumors. Int J Radiation Oncology Biol Phys 2001;50:121-125.

465. Nuyttens JJ, Rust PF, Thomas CR Jr, Turrisi AT 3rd. Surgery versus radiation therapy for patients with aggressive fibromatosis or desmoid tumors: A comparative review of 22 articles. Cancer 2000;88:1517-1523.

466. Kinzbrunner B, Ritter S, Domingo J, Rosenthal CJ. Remission of rapidly growing desmoid tumors after tamoxifen therapy. Cancer 1983;52:2201-2204.

Benign Fibrous Histiocytoma

467. Zelger B, Zelger BG, Burgdorf WH. Dermatofibroma—a critical evaluation. Int J Surg Pathol 2004;12:333-344.

468. Luzar B, Calonje E. Cutaneous fibrohistiocytic tumors—an update. Histopathology 2010;56:148-165.

469. Mentzel T, Kutzner H, Rütten A, Hügel H. Benign fibrous histiocytoma (dermatofibroma) of the face. Clinicopathological and immunohistochemical study of 34 cases associated with an aggressive clinical course. Am J Dermatopathol 2001;23:419-426.

470. Santa-Cruz DJ, Kyriakos M. Aneurysmal ("angiomatoid") fibrous histiocytoma of the skin. Cancer 1981;47:2053-2061.

471. Calonje E, Fletcher CD. Aneurysmal benign fibrous histiocytoma: clinicopathological analysis of 40 cases of a tumour frequently misdiagnosed as a vascular neoplasm. Histopathology 1995;26:323-331.

472. Zelger BW, Zelger BG, Steiner H, Ofner D. Aneurysmal and hemangiopericytoma-like fibrous histiocytoma. J Clin Pathol 1996;49:313-318.

473. Sheehan KM, Leader MB, Sexton S, Cunningham F, Leen E. Recurrent aneurysmal fibrous histiocytoma. J Clin Pathol 2004;57:312-314.

474. Guillou L, Gebhard S, Salmeron M, Coindre JM. Metastasizing fibrous histiocytoma of the skin: a clinicopathologic and immunohistochemical study of three cases. Mod Pathol 2000:13:654-660.

475. Bisceglia M, Attino V, Bacchi CE. Metastasizing 'benign" fibrous histiocytoma of the skin: a report of two additional cases and review of the literature. Adv Anat Pathol 2006;13:89-96.

476. Botrus G, Sciot R, Debiec-Rychter M. Cutaneous aneurysmal fibrous histiocytoma with a t(12;19)(p12;q13) as the sole cytogenetic abnormality. Cancer Genet Cytogenet 2006;164:155-158.

477. Calonje E, Mentzel T, Fletcher CD. Cellular benign fibrous histiocytoma. Clinicopathologic analysis of 74 cases of a distinctive variant of cutaneous fibrous histiocytoma. Am J Surg Pathol 1994;18:668-676.

478. Colome-Grimmer MI, Evans HL. Metastasizing cellular dermatofibroma. A report of two cases. Am J Surg Pathol 1996;20:1361-1367.

479. Osborn M, Mandys V, Beddow E, et al. Cystic fibrohistiocytic tumors presenting in the lung: primary of metastatic disease? Histopathology 2003;43:556-562.

480. Gu M, Sohn K, Kim D, Kim B. Metastasizing dermatofibroma in lung. Ann Diagn Pathol 2007;11:64-67.

481. Volpicelli ER, Fletcher CD. Desmin and CD34 positivity in cellular fibrous histiocytoma: an immunohistochemical analysis of 100 cases. J Cutan Pathol 2012;39:747-752.

482. Iwata J, Fletcher CD. Lipidized fibrous histiocytoma: clinicopathologic analysis of 22 cases. Am J Dermatopathol 2000;22:126-134.

483. Wagamon K, Somach SC, Bass J, et al. Lipidized dermatofibromas and their relationship to serum lipids. J Am Acad Dermatol 2006;54:494-498.

484. Fukamizu H, Oku T, Inoue K, Matsumoto K, Okayama H, Tagami H. Atypical pseudosarcomatous cutaneous fibrous histiocytoma. J Cutan Pathol 1983;10:327-333.

485. Leyva WH, Santa Cruz DJ. Atypical cutaneous fibrous histiocytoma. Am J Dermatopathol 1986;8:467-471.

486. Tamada S, Ackerman AB. Dermatofibroma with monster cells. Am J Dermatopathol 1987;9:380-387.

487. Beham A, Fletcher CD. Atypical "pseudosarcomatous" variant of cutaneous benign fibrous histiocytoma: Report of eight cases. Histopathology 1990;17:167-169.

488. Kaddu S, McMenamin ME, Fletcher CD. Atypical fibrous histiocytoma of the skin: clinicopathologic analysis of 59 cases with evidence of infrequent metastasis. Am J Surg Pathol 2002;26:35-46.

Non-Neural Granular Cell Tumor

489. Val-Bernal JF, Mira C. Dermatofibroma with granular cells. J Cutan Pathol 1996;23:562-565.

490. Zelger BG, Steiner H, Kutzner H, Rütten A, Zelger B. Granular cell dermatofibroma. Histopathology 1997;31:258-262.

491. Soyer HP, Metze D, Kerl H. Granular cell dermatofibroma. Am J Surg Pathol 1997;19:168-173.

492. LeBoit PE, Barr RJ, Burall S, Metcalf JS, Yen TS, Wick MR. Primitive granular-cell tumor and other cutaneous granular-cell neoplasms of apparent nonneural origin. Am J Surg Pathol 1991;15:48-58.

493. Lazar AJ, Fletcher CD. Primitive nonneural granular cell tumors of skin. Clinicopathologic analysis of 13 cases. Am J Surg Pathol 2005;29:927-934.

Neurothekeoma

494. Pulitzer DR, Reed RJ. Nerve-sheath myxoma (perineurial myxoma). Am J Dermatopathol 1985;7:409-421.

495. Scheithauer BW, Woodruff JM, Erlandson, RA. Tumors of the peripheral nervous system. AFIP Atlas of Tumor Pathology, 3rd Series, Fascicle 24. Washington, DC: American Registry of Pathology; 1999:219-282.

496. Fullen DR, Lowe L, Su LD. Antibody to S100a6 protein is a sensitive immunohistochemical marker for neurothekeoma. J Cutan Pathol 2003;30:118-122.

497. Jaffer S, Ambrosini-Spaltro A, Mancini AM, Eusebi V, Rosai J. Neurothekeoma and plexiform fibrohistiocytic tumor: mere histologic resemblance or histogenetic relationship? Am J Surg Pathol 2009;33:905-913.

498. Fetsch JF, Laskin WB, Miettinen M. Nerve sheath myxoma: a clinicopathologic and immunohistochemical analysis of 57 norphologically distinctive, S-100 protein- and GFAP-positive, myxoid peripheral nerve sheath tumors with a predilection for the extremities and a high local recurrence rate. Am J Surg Pathol 2005;29:1615-1624.

499. Fetsch JF, Laskin WB, Hallman JR, Lupton GP, Miettinen M. Neurothekeoma: an analysis of 178 tumors with detailed immunohistochemical data and long-term patient follow-up information. Am J Surg Pathol 2007;31:1103-1114.

500. Hornick JL, Fletcher CD. Cellular neurothekeoma: detailed characterization in a series of 133 cases. Am J Surg Pathol 2007;31:329-340.

501. Laskin WB, Fetsch JF, Miettinen M. The "neurothekeoma": immunohistochemical analysis distinguishes the true nerve sheath myxoma from its mimics. Hum Pathol 2000;31:1230-1241.

502. Zelger BG, Steiner H, Kutzner H, Maier H, Zelger B. Cellular 'neurothekeoma': an epithelioid variant of dermatofibroma? Histopathology 1998;32:414-422.

503. Moosavi C, Jha P, Fanburg-Smith JC. An update on plexiform fibrohistiocytic tumor and addition of 66 new cases from the Armed Forces Institute of Pathology, in honor of Franz M. Enzinger, MD. Ann Diagn Pathol 2007;11:313-319.

504. Requena L, Sangüeza OP. Benign neoplasms with neural differentiation: a review. Am J Dermatopathol 1995;17:75-96.

505. Gallager RL, Helwig EB. Neurothekeoma—a benign cutaneous tumor of neural origin. Am J Clin Pathol 1980;74:759-764.

506. Busam KJ, Mentzel T, Colpaert C, Barnhill RL, Fletcher CD. Atypical or worrisome features in cellular neurothekeoma: a study of 10 cases. Am J Surg Pathol 1998;22:1067-1072.

507. Page RN, King R, Mihm Jr MC, Googe PB. Microphthalmia transcription factor and NKI/C3 expression in cellular neurothekeoma. Mod Pathol 2004;17:230-234.

508. Argenyi ZB, LeBoit PE, Santa Cruz D, Swanson PE, Kutzner H. Nerve sheath myxoma (neurothekeoma) of the skin: light microscopic and immunohistochemical reappraisal of the cellular variant. J Cutan Pathol 1993;20:294-303.

509. Angevall L, Kindblom LG, Haglid K. Dermal nerve sheath myxoma. A light and electron microscopic, histochemical and immunohistochemical study. Cancer 1984;53:1752-1759.

510. Blumberg AK, Kay S, Adelaar RS. Nerve sheath myxoma of digital nerve. Cancer 1989;63:1215-1218.

511. Webb JN. The histogenesis of nerve sheath myxoma: report of a case with electron microscopy. J Pathol 1979;127:35-37.

512. Yamamoto H, Kawana T. Oral nerve sheath myxoma. Report of a case with findings of ultrastructural and immunohistochemical studies. Acta Pathol Jpn 1988;38:121-127.

Plexiform Fibrohistiocytic Tumor

513. Fetsch JF, Laskin WB, Hallman JR, Lupton GP, Miettinen M. Neurothekeoma: an analysis of 178 tumors with detailed immunohistochemical data and long-term patient follow-up information. Am J Surg Pathol 2007;31:1103-1114.

514. Hornick JL, Fletcher CD. Cellular neurothekeoma: detailed characterization in a series of 133 cases. Am J Surg Pathol 2007;31:329-340.

515. Enzinger FM, Zhang R. Plexiform fibrohistiocytic tumor presenting in children and young adults. An analysis of 65 cases. Am J Surg Pathol 1988;12:818-826.

516. Hollowood K, Holley MP, Fletcher CD. Plexiform fibrohistiocytic tumour: clinicopathological, immunohistochemical and ultrastructural analysis in favour of a myofibroblastic lesion. Histopathology 1991;19:503-513.

517. Moosavi C, Jha P, Fanburg-Smith JC. An update on plexiform fibrohistiocytic tumor and addition of 66 new cases from the Armed Forces Institute of Pathology, in honor of Franz M. Enzinger, MD. Ann Diagn Pathol 2007;11:313-319.

518. Remstein ED, Arndt CA, Nascimento AG. Plexiform fibrohistiocytic tumor: clinicopathologic analysis of 22 cases. Am J Surg Pathol 1999;23:662-670.

519. Taher A, Pushpanathan C. Plexiform fibrohistiocytic tumor: a brief review. Arch Pathol Lab Med 2007;131:1135-1138.

520. Salomao DR, Nascimento AG. Plexiform fibrohistiocytic tumor with systemic metastases: a case report. Am J Surg Pathol 1997;21:469-476.

521. Smith S, Fletcher CD, Smith MA, Gusterson BA. Cytogenetic analysis of a plexiform fibrohistiocytic tumor. Cancer Genet Cytogenet 1990;48:31-34.

522. Redlich GC, Montgomery KD, Allgood GA, Joste NE. Plexiform fibrohistiocytic tumor with a clonal cytogenetic anomaly. Cancer Genet Cytogenet 1999;108:141-143.

523. Michal M, Fanburg-Smith JC. Plexiform xanthomatous tumor: a report of 20 cases in 12 patients. Am J Surg Pathol 2002;26:1302-1311.

Superficial Acral Fibromyxoma

524. Al-Daraji WI, Miettinen M. Superficial acral fibromyxoma: a clinicopathological analysis of 32 tumors including 4 in the heel. J Cutan Pathol 2008;35:1020-1026.

525. Fetsch JF, Laskin WB, Miettinen M. Superficial acral fibromyxoma: a clinicopathologic and immunohistochemical analysis of 37 cases of a distinctive soft tissue tumor with a predilection for the fingers and toes. Hum Pathol 2001; 32:704-714.

525a. Hollmann TJ, Bovée JV, Fletcher CD. Digital fibromyxoma (superficial acral fibromyxoma): a detailed characterization of 124 cases. Am J Surg Pathol 2012;36:789-798.

526. Lisovsky M, Hoang MP, Dresser KA, Kapur P, Bhawan J, Mahalingam M. Apolipoprotein D in CD34-positive and CD34-negative cutaneous neoplasms: a useful marker in differentiating superficial acral fibromyxoma from dermatofibrosarcoma protuberans. Mod Pathol 2008;21:31-38.

527. Luzar B, Calonje E. Superficial acral fibromyxoma: clinicopathological study of 14 cases with emphasis on a cellular variant. Histopathology 2009;54:375-377.

528. Misago N, Ohkawa T, Yanai T, Narisawa Y. Superficial acral fibromyxoma on the tip of the big toe: expression of CD10 and nestin. J Eur Acad Dermatol Venereol 2008;22:255-257.

529. Prescott RJ, Husain EA, Abdellaoui A, et al. Superficial acral fibromyxoma: a clinicopathological study of new 41 cases from the U.K.: should myxoma (NOS) and fibroma (NOS) continue as part of 21-century reporting? Br J Dermatol 2008;159:1315-1321.

530. Tardío JC, Burtrón M, Martín-Fragueiro LM. Superficial acral fibromyxoma: report of 4 cases with CD10 expression and lipomatous component, two previously underrecognized features. Am J Dermatopathol 2008;30:431-435.

531. Varikatt W, Soper J, Simmons G, Dave C, Munk J, Bonar F. Superficial acral fibromyxoma: a report of two cases with radiological findings. Skeletal Radiol 2008;37:499-503.

Superficial Angiomyxoma

532. Allen PW, Dymock RB, MacCormac LB. Superficial angiomyxomas with and without epithelial components. Report of 30 tumors in 28 patients. Am J Surg Pathol 1988;12:519-530.

533. Calonje E, Guerin D, McCormick D, Fletcher CD et al. Superficial angiomyxoma: clinico-pathologic analysis of a series of distinctive but poorly recognized cutaneous tumors with tendency for recurrence. Am J Surg Pathol 1999;23:910-917.

534. Fetsch JF, Laskin WB, Tavassoli FA. Superficial angiomyxoma (cutaneous myxoma): a clinicopathologic study of 17 cases arising in the genital region. Int J Gynecol Pathol 1997; 16:325-334.

535. Boikos SA, Stratakis CA. Carney complex: pathology and molecular genetics. Neuroendocrinology 2006;83:189-199.

536. Kacerovska D, Sima R, Michal M, et al. Carney complex: a clinicopathologic and molecular biological study of a sporadic case, including extracutaneous and cutaneous lesions and a novel mutation of the PRKAR1A gene. J Am Acad Dermatol 2009;61:80-87.

537. Mateus C, Palangie A, Franck N, et al. Heterogeneity of skin manifestations in patients with Carney complex. J Am Acad Dermatol 2008;59:801-810.

538. Stratakis CA, Kirschner LS, Carney JA. Clinical and molecular features of the Carney complex: diagnostic criteria and recommendations for patient evaluation. J Clin Endocrinol Metab 2001;86:4041-4046.

539. Stratakis CA, Horvath A. Carney complex. In: Pagon RA, Bird TC, Dolan CR, et al, eds. GeneReviews [Internet]. Seattle (WA): University of Washington, Seattle; 1993-2003 Feb 05 [updated 2010 Jun 22].

540. Carney JA, Headington JT, Su WP. Cutaneous myxomas. A major component of the complex of myxomas, spotty pigmentation, and endocrine overactivity. Arch Dermatol 1986;122:790-798.

541. Koopman RJ, Happle R. Aytosomal dominant transmission of the NAME syndrome (nevi, atrial myxoma, mucinosis of the skin and endocrine overactivity). Hum Genet 1991;86:300-304.

542. Rhodes AR, Silverman RA, Harrist TJ, Perez-Atayde AR. Mucocutaneous lentigines, cardiomuco-cutaneous myxomas, and multiple blue nevi: the "LAMB" syndrome. J Am Acad Dermatol 1984;10:72-82.

543. Boikos SA, Stratakis CA. Carney complex: the first 20 years. Curr Opin Oncol 2007;19:24-29.

544. Ferreiro JA, Carney JA. Myxomas of the external ear and their significance. Am J Surg Pathol 1994;18:274-280.

545. Kirschner LS, Carney JA, Pack SD, et al. Mutations of the gene encoding the protein kinase A type I-alpha regulatory subunit in patients with the Carney complex. Nat Genet 2000;26:89-92.

546. Wilkes D, Charitakis K, Basson CT. Inherited disposition to cardiac myxoma development. Nat Rev Cancer 2006;6:157-165.

547. Horvath A, Bossis I, Glatzakis C, et al. Large deletions of the PRKAR1A gene in Carney complex. Clin Cancer Res 2008;14:388-395.

548. Bertherat J, Horvath A, Groussin L, et al. Mutations in regulatory subunit type 1A of cyclic adenosine 5'-monophosphate-dependent protein kinase (PRKAR1A): phenotype analysis in 353 patients and 80 different genotypes. Clin Endocrinol Metab 2009;94:2085-2091.

549. Cazabat L, Ragazzon B, Groussin L, Bertherat J. PRKAR1A mutations in primary pigmented nodular adrenocortical disease. Pituitary 2006; 9:211-219.

550. Horvath A, Bertherat J, Groussin L, et al. Mutations and polymorphisms in the gene encoding regulatory subunit type 1-alpha of protein kinase A (PRKAR1A): an update. Hum Mutat 2010;31:369-379.

551. Kirschner LS, Sandrini F, Monbo J, Lin JP, Carney JA, Stratakis CA. Genetic heterogeneity and spectrum of mutations of the PRKAR1A gene in patients with the Carney complex. Hum Mol Genet 2000;9:3037-3046.

552. Johnson WC, Helwig EB. Cutaneous focal mucinosis. A clinicopathological and histochemical study. Arch Dermatol 1966;93:13-20.

553. Wilk M, Schmoeckel C. Cutaneous focal mucinosis—a histopathological and immunohistochemical analysis of 11 cases. J Cutan Pathol 1994;21:446-452.

554. Johnson WC, Graham JH, Helwig EB. Cutaneous myxoid cyst. A clinicopathological and histochemical study. JAMA 1965;191:15-20.

555. Sonnex TS. Digital myxoid cysts: a review. Cutis 1986;37:89-94.

556. Fetsch JF, Laskin WB, Miettinen M. Nerve sheath myxoma: a clinicopathologic and immunohistochemical analysis of 57 morphologically distinctive, S-100 protein- and GFAP-positive, myxoid peripheral nerve sheath tumors with a predilection for the extremities and a high local recurrence rate. Am J Surg Pathol 2005;29:1615-1624.

557. Fetsch JF, Laskin WB, Hallman JR, Lupton GP, Miettinen M. Neurothekeoma: an analysis of 178 tumors with detailed immunohistochemical data and long-term patient follow-up information. Am J Surg Pathol 2007;31:1103-1114.

558. Gallager RL, Helwig EB. Neurothekeoma—a benign cutaneous tumor of neural origin. Am J Clin Pathol 1980;74:759-764.

Intramuscular Myxoma

559. Wirth WA, Leavitt D, Enzinger FM. Multiple intramuscular myxomas. Another extraskeletal manifestation of fibrous dysplasia. Cancer 1971;27:1167-1173.

560. Ireland DC, Soule EH, Ivins JC. Myxoma of the somatic soft tissues. A report of 58 patients, 3 with multiple tumors and fibrous dysplasia of the bone. Mayo Clin Proc 1973;48:401-410.

561. Szendroi M, Rahoty P, Antal I, Kiss J. Fibrous dysplasia associated with intramuscular myxoma (Mazabraud's syndrome): a long term follow-up of three cases. J Cancer Res Clin Oncol 1998;124:401-406.

562. Faivre L, Nivelon-Chevallier A, Kottler ML, et al. Mazabraud syndrome in two patients: clinical overlap with McCune-Albright syndrome. Am J Med Genet 2001;99:132-136.

563. Nielsen GP, O'Connell JX, Rosenberg AE. Intramuscular myxoma: a clinicopathologic study of 51 cases with emphasis on hypercellular and hypervascular variants. Am J Surg Pathol 1998;22:1222-1227.

564. van Roggen JF, McMenamin ME, Fletcher CD. Cellular myxoma of soft tissue: a clincopathologic study of 38 cases confirming indolent behaviour. Histopathology 2001;39:287-297.

565. Miettinen M, Hockerstedt K, Reitamo J, Totterman S. Intramuscular myxoma—a clinicopathological study of twenty-three cases. Am J Clin Pathol 1985;84:265-272.

566. Hashimoto H, Tsuneyoshi M, Daimaru Y, Enjoji M, Shinohara N. Intramuscular myxoma. A clinicopathologic, immunohistochemical, and electron microscopic study. Cancer 1986;58:740-747.

567. Okamoto S, Hisaoka M, Ushijima M, Nakahara S, Toyoshima S, Hashimoto H. Activating Gs(alpha) mutation in intramuscular myxomas with and without fibrous dysplasia of bone. Virchows Arch 2000;437:133-137.

568. Malchoff CD, Reardon G, Macgillivray DC, Yamase H, Rogol AD, Malchoff DM. An unusual presentation of McCune-Albright syndrome confirmed by an activating mutation of the Gs alpha-subunit from a bone lesion. J Clin Endocr Metab 1994;78:803-806.

569. Shenker A, Weinstein LS, Sweet DE, Spiegel AM. An activating Gs alpha mutation is present in fibrous dysplasia of bone in the McCune-Albright syndrome. J Clin Endocr Metab 1994;79:750-755.

570. Bancroft LW, Kransdorf MJ, Menke DM, O'Connor MI, Foster WC. Intramuscular myxoma: characteristic MR imaging features. Am J Roengenol 2002;178:1255-1259.

571. Murphey MD, McRae GA, Fanburg-Smith JC, Temple HT, Levine AM, Aboulafia AJ. Imaging of soft-tissue myxoma with emphasis on CT and MR and comparison of radiologic and pathologic findings. Radiology 2002;225:215-224.

572. Enzinger FM. Intramuscular myxoma; a review and follow-up study of 34 cases. Am J Clin Pathol 1965;43:104-110.

573. Kindblom LG, Stener B, Angervall L. Intramuscular myxoma. Cancer 1974;34:1737-1744.

Juxta-articular Myxoma

574. Meis JM, Enzinger FM. Juxta-articular myxoma: a clinical and pathologic study of 65 cases. Hum Pathol 1992;23:639-646.

575. Minkoff J, Stecker S, Irizarry J, Whiteman M, Woodhouse S. Juxta-articular myxoma: a rare cause of painful restricted motion of the knee. Arthroscopy 2003;19:E6-13.

576. Okamoto S, Hisaoka M, Meis-Kindblom JM, Kindblom LG, Hashimoto H. Juxta-articular myxoma and intramuscular myxoma are two distinct entities. Activating Gs alpha mutation at Arg 201 codon does not occur in juxta-articular myxoma. Virchows Arch 2002;440:12-15.

577. Sciot R, Dal Cin P, Samson I, van den Berghe H, van Damme B. Clonal chromosomal changes in juxta-articular myxoma. Virchows Arch 1999;434:177-180.

Aggressive Angiomyxoma

578. Clatch RJ, Drake WK, Gonzalez JG. Aggressive angiomyxoma in men. A report of two cases associated with inguinal hernias. Arch Pathol Lab Med 1993;117:911-913.

579. Iezzoni JC, Fechner RE, Wong LS, Rossai J. Aggressive angiomyxoma in males. A report of four cases. Am J Clin Pathol 1995;104:391-396.

580. McCluggage WG, Patterson A, Maxwell P. Aggressive angiomyxoma of pelvic parts exhibits oestrogen and progesterone receptor positivity. J Clin Pathol 2000;53:603-605.

581. Tsang WY, Chan JK, Lee KC, Fisher C, Fletcher CD. Aggressive angiomyxoma. A report of four cases occurring in men. Am J Surg Pathol 1992;16:1059-1065.

582. Chan IM, Hon E, Ngai SW, Ng TY, Wong LC. Aggressive angiomyxoma in females: is radical resection the only option? Acta Obstet Gynecol Scand 2000;79:216-220.

583. Fetsch JF, Laskin WB, Lefkowitz M, Kindblom LG, Meis-Kindblom JM. Aggressive angiomyxoma: a clinicopathologic study of 29 female patients. Cancer 1996;78:79-90.

584. Granter SR, Nucci MR, Fletcher CD. Aggressive angiomyxoma: reappraisal of its relationship to angiomyofibroblastoma in a series of 16 cases. Histopathology 1997;30:3-10.

585. White J, Chan YF. Aggressive angiomxyoma of the vulva in an 11-year-old girl. Pediatr Pathol 1994;14:27-37.

586. Steeper TA, Rosai J. Aggressive angiomyxoma of the female pelvis and perineum. Report of nine cases of a distinctive type of gynecologic soft-tissue neoplasm. Am J Surg Pathol 1983;7:463-475.

587. Chien AJ, Freeby JA, Win TT, Gadwood KA. Aggressive angiomyxoma of the female pelvis: sonographic, CT, and MR findings. AJR Am J Roentgenol 1998;171:530-531.

588. Outwater EK, Marchetto BE, Wagner BJ, Siegelman ES. Aggressive angiomyxoma: findings on CT and MR imaging. AJR Am J Roentgenol 1999;172:435-438.

589. Davani M, Chablani VN, Saba PR. Aggressive angiomyxoma of pelvic soft tissues: MR imaging appearance. AJR Am J Roentgenol 1998; 170:1113-1114.

590. Skálová A, Michal M, Hušek K, Zámecník M, Leivo I. Aggressive angiomyxoma of the pelvioperineal region. Immunohistochemical and ultrastructural study of seven cases. Am J Dermatopathol 1993;15:446-451.

591. Fine BA, Munoz AK, Litz CE, Gershenson DM. Primary medical management of recurrent aggressive angiomyxoma of the vulva with a gonadotrophin-releasing hormone agonist. Gynecol Oncol 2001;81:120-122.

592. Nucci MR, Castrillon DH, Bai H, et al. Biomarkers in diagnostic obstetric and gynecologic pathology: a review. Adv Anat Pathol 2003;10:55-68.

593. Medeiros F, Erickson-Johnson MR, Keeney GL, et al. Frequency and characterization of HMGA2 and HMGA1 rearrangements in mesenchymal tumors of the lower genital tract. Genes Chromosomes Cancer 2007;46:981-990.

594. Micci F, Panagopoulos I, Bjerkehagen B, Heim S. Deregulation of HMGA2 in an aggressive angiomyxoma with t(11;12)(q23;q15). Virchows Arch 2006;448:838-842.

595. Nucci MR, Weremowicz S, Neskey DM, et al. Chromosomal translocation t(8;12) induces aberrant HMGIC expression in aggressive angiomyxoma of the vulva. Genes Chromosomes Cancer 2001;32:172-176.

596. Rawlinson NJ, West WW, Nelson M, Bridge JA. Aggressive angiomyxoma with t(12;21) and HMGA2 rearrangement: report of a case and review of the literature. Cancer Genet Cytogenet 2008;181:119-124.

597. Tsuji T, Yoshinaga M, Inomoto Y, Taguchi S, Douchi T. Aggressive angiomyxoma of the vulva with a sole t(5;8)(p15;q22) chromosome change. Int J Gynecol Pathol 2007;26:494-496.

598. Altchek A, Deligdisch L, Norton K, Gordon R, Greco MA, Magid MS. Prepubertal unilateral fibrous hyperplasia of the labium majus: report of eight cases and review of the literature. Obstet Gynecol 2007;110:103-108.

599. Iwasa Y, Fletcher CD. Distinctive prepubertal vulval fibroma: a hitherto unrecognized mesenchymal tumor of prepubertal girls: analysis of 11 cases. Am J Surg Pathol 2004;28:1601-1608.

600. Vargas SO, Kozakewich HP, Boyd TK, et al. Childhood asymmetric labium majus enlargement: mimicking a neoplasm. Am J Surg Pathol 2005;29:1007-1016.

601. Vang R, Connelly JH, Hammill HA, Shannon RL. Vulvar hypertrophy with lymphedema. A mimicker of aggressive angiomyxoma. Arch Pathol Lab Med 2000;124:1697-1699.

602. McCluggage WG, Jamieson T, Dobbs SP, Grey A. Aggressive angiomyxoma of the vulva: Dramatic response to gonadotropin-releasing hormone agonist therapy. Gynecol Oncol 2006; 100:623-625.

603. Blandamura S, Cruz J, Faure Vergara L, Machado Puerto I, Ninfo V. Aggressive angiomyxoma: a second case of metastasis with patient's death. Hum Pathol 2003;34:1072-1074.

604. Siassi RM, Papadopoulos T, Matzel KE. Metastasizing aggressive angiomyxoma. N Engl J Med 1999;341:1772.

Angiomyofibroblastoma

605. Nielsen GP, Rosenberg AE, Young RH, Dickersin GR, Clement PB, Scully RE. Angiomyofibroblastoma of the vulva and vagina. Mod Pathol 1996;9:284-291.

606. Cao D, Srodon M, Montgomery EA, Kurman RJ. Lipomatous variant of angiomyofibroblastoma: report of two cases and review of the literature. Int J Gynecol Pathol 2005;24:196-200.

607. Fletcher CD, Tsang WY, Fisher C, Lee KC, Chan JK. Angiomyofibroblastoma of the vulva. A benign neoplasm distinct from aggressive angiomyxoma. Am J Surg Pathol 1992;16:373-382.

608. Horiguchi H, Matsui-Horiguchi M, Fujiwara M, et al. Angiomyofibroblastoma of the vulva: report of a case with immunohistochemical and molecular analysis. Int J Gynecol Pathol 2003;22:277-284.

609. Laskin WB, Fetsch JF, Tavassoli FA. Angiomyofibroblastoma of the female genital tract: analysis of 17 cases including a lipomatous variant. Hum Pathol 1997;28:1046-1055.

610. Sasano H, Date F, Yamamoto H, Nagura H. Angiomyofibroblastoma of the vulva: case report with immunohistochemical, ultrastructural and DNA ploidy studies and a review of the literature. Pathol Int 1997;47:647-650.

611. Fukunaga M, Nomura K, Matsumoto K, Doi K, Endo Y, Ushigome S. Vulval angiomyofibroblastoma. Clinicopathologic analysis of six cases. Am J Clin Pathol 1997;107:45-51.
612. Nucci MR, Castrillon DH, Bai H, et al. Biomarkers in diagnostic obstetric and gynecologic pathology: a review. Adv Anat Pathol 2003;10:55-68.
613. Medeiros F, Erickson-Johnson MR, Keeney GL, et al. Frequency and characterization of HMGA2 and HMGA1 rearrangements in mesenchymal tumors of the lower genital tract. Genes Chromosomes Cancer 2007;46:981-990.
614. Ganesan R, McCluggage WG, Hirschowitz L, Rollason TP. Superficial myofibroblastoma of the lower female genital tract: report of a series including tumours with a vulvar location. Histopathology 2005;46:137-143.
615. Laskin WB, Fetsch JF, Tavassoli FA. Superficial cervicovaginal myofibroblastoma: fourteen cases of a distinctive mesenchymal tumor arising from the specialized subepithelial stroma of the lower female genital tract. Hum Pathol 2001;32:715-725.
616. Nielsen GP, Young RH, Dickersin GR, Rosenberg AE. Angiomyofibroblastoma of the vulva with sarcomatous transformation ("angiomyofibrosarcoma"). Am J Surg Pathol 1997;21:1104-1108.

Cellular Angiofibroma

617. Flucke U, van Krieken JH, Mentzel T. Cellular angiofibroma: analysis of 25 cases emphasizing its relationship to spindle cell lipoma and mammary-type myofibroblastoma. Mod Pathol 2011;24: 82-89.
618. Hameed M, Clarke K, Amer HZ, Mahmet K, Aisner S. Cellular angiofibroma is genetically similar to spindle cell lipoma; a case report. Cancer Genet Cytogenet 2007;177:131-134.
619. Iwasa Y, Fletcher CD. Cellular angiofibroma: clinicopathologic and immunohistochemical analysis of 51 cases. Am J Surg Pathol 2004; 28:1426-1435.
620. Laskin WB, Fetsch JF, Mostofi FK. Angiomyofibroblastomalike tumor of the male genital tract: analysis of 11 cases with comparison to female angiomyofibroblastoma and spindle cell lipoma. Am J Surg Pathol 1998;22:6-16.
621. Maggiani F, Debiec-Rychter M, Vanbockrijck M, Sciot R. Cellular angiofibroma: another mesenchymal tumour with 13q14 involvement, suggesting a link with spindle cell lipoma and (extra)-mammary myofibroblastoma. Histopathology 2007;51:410-412.
622. Nucci MR, Granter SR, Fletcher CD. Cellular angiofibroma: a benign neoplasm distinct from angiomyofibroblastoma and spindle cell lipoma. Am J Surg Pathol 1997;21:636-644.
623. Kandil DH, Kida M, Laub DR, Cooper K. Sarcomatous transformation in a cellular angiofibroma: a case report. J Clin Pathol 2009;62:945-947.
624. Chen E, Fletcher CD. Cellular angiofibroma with atypia or sarcomatous transformation: clinicopathologic analysis of 13 cases. Am J Surg Pathol 2010;34:707-714.
625. McCluggage WG, Perenyei M, Irwin ST. Recurrent cellular angiofibroma of the vulva. J Clin Pathol 2002;55:477-479.
626. Curry JL, Olejnik JL, Wojcik EM. Cellular angiofibroma of the vulva with DNA ploidy analysis. Int J Gynecol Pathol 2001;20:200-203.
627. Medeiros F, Erickson-Johnson MR, Keeney GL, et al. Frequency and characterization of HMGA2 and HMGA1 rearrangements in mesenchymal tumors of the lower genital tract. Genes Chromosomes Cancer 2007;46:981-990.

3 FIBROBLASTIC/MYOFIBROBLASTIC NEOPLASMS WITH VARIABLE BIOLOGIC POTENTIAL

This chapter includes malignant and potentially malignant fibroblastic/myofibroblastic neoplasms. Most tumors of this group carry the designation "malignant," although the spectrum ranges from histologically and clinically benign to overt sarcoma (solitary fibrous tumor). We consider undifferentiated sarcomas (malignant fibrous histiosarcoma) as part of the fibroblastic group because they are closely related to and overlap with myxofibrosarcoma. "Fibrohistiocytic tumors" are just variants of fibroblastic/myofibroblastic neoplasms.

SOLITARY FIBROUS TUMOR

Definition. *Solitary fibrous tumor* is a fibroblastic neoplasm typically consisting of CD34-positive spindle cells with variable interstitial collagen and often a hemangiopericytoma-like vascular pattern. It is analogous to similarly named pleural tumors and closely related, if not identical, to *hemangiopericytoma of peripheral soft tissues*.

General Considerations. Solitary fibrous tumors include a spectrum of tumors that vary from benign to overt sarcoma, although malignant examples are rare (5 to 10 percent). This tumor is identical to pleural tumors previously designated fibrous mesothelioma or localized fibrous tumor (1). It is virtually identical to hemangiopericytoma of soft tissues, although tumors with more spindled and fibrous features have been generally classified as solitary fibrous tumors and those composed of oval cells with a prominent staghorn vasculature have been previously considered hemangiopericytomas (2,3).

Solitary fibrous tumors are reported in a wide variety of soft tissue locations and in different parenchymal organs. Histologic variants include *giant cell angiofibroma* and *lipomatous solitary fibrous tumor/hemangiopericytoma*. This text concentrates on solitary fibrous tumors in soft tissue locations. Hemangiopericytoma/solitary fibrous tumors in the pleura, lung, other parenchymal organs, and central nervous system are excluded.

Clinical Features. Solitary fibrous tumor occurs in adult patients of all ages. In peripheral soft tissues, the variety of locations includes the extremities (especially thigh), buttock, trunk wall, and head and neck. Tumors variably involve the subcutis and deeper intramuscular tissues. Tumor size varies from less than 1 cm to larger than 10 cm. Small tumors are often diagnosed in the head and neck area, such as the orofacial region, and sometimes in superficial peripheral soft tissues. The nasal passages and orbit are among the more common locations in the head. Approximately one third of tumors occur in body cavities, especially in the pelvis, where they often are large (20 to 30 cm or more) and more often manifest as a malignancy (4–11). Solitary fibrous tumors in the mediastinum are probably related to the pleural examples (12). "Cutaneous" solitary fibrous tumors usually also involve the subcutis (13). Large tumors (especially pleural and abdominal/retroperitoneal) are sometimes associated with paraneoplastic hypoglycemia due to the production of insulin-like growth factor 1 or 2 by the tumor (14–16).

Gross Findings. The tumors vary greatly in size, from 1 cm to over 30 cm, and the largest examples typically occur in the body cavities. Solitary fibrous tumor is typically well circumscribed but unencapsulated. Large tumors may contain cysts. Some peritoneal examples are attached with a narrow pedicle to the outer surface of liver or intestines. On sectioning, the tissue is homogeneously firm and gray-white or pale tan and may show trabeculation (fig. 3-1). Malignant tumors may appear softer and contain areas of gross necrosis.

Microscopic Findings. The tumor cells consist of uniform spindled cells in a variably collagenous or occasionally myxoid matrix, in which cellular and hyalinized areas alternate in irregular patterns (fig. 3-2). A hemangiopericytoma-like vascular pattern with a complex "antler" or

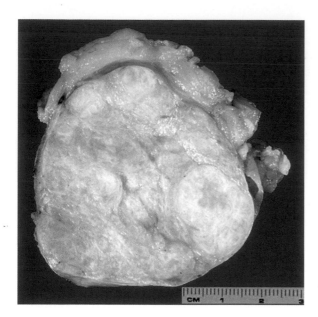

Figure 3-1

SOLITARY FIBROUS TUMOR

Grossly, solitary fibrous tumor forms a circumscribed mass. On sectioning, this fixed specimen shows a pale tan to off-white cut surface.

"staghorn-like" profile is present in most cases, at least in some areas. Cellular areas with focal epithelioid morphology, sometimes with a trabecular arrangement, may be present.

The tumor cells have indistinct cytoplasm and oval nuclei, usually with inconspicuous nucleoli. Mitotic activity is low (less than 2 to 3 mitoses per 10 high-power fields) in most cases. The mitotic rate threshold of 4 per 10 fields is often used for solitary fibrous tumors, and this threshold was initially established for hemangiopericytoma. Some cases with conventional histology contain mitotically active foci. Their significance is uncertain at the present in the absence of follow-up studies.

Variants containing cystic or angiectoid spaces that are focally lined by multinucleated giant cells are designated as *giant cell angiofibroma* (fig. 3-2A). Originally reported in the orbit, this variant has subsequently been seen in peripheral soft tissues (17–19).

The *lipomatous variant* (also designated *lipomatous hemangiopericytoma*) contains a nonatypical lipomatous component intermingling with the solitary fibrous tumor component (fig. 3-3B). In most cases, this component is focal,

but rarely, it forms a dominant portion of the tumor. Otherwise these tumors are clinicopathologically similar to ordinary solitary fibrous tumors, although cases with mitotic rates over the threshold of 4 per 10 high-power fields have been reported (20–22). A malignant adipose tissue component histologically corresponding to atypical lipomatous tumor/well-differentiated liposarcoma has been reported in this variant and shown to be MDM2 negative (23).

Some solitary fibrous tumors show overtly sarcomatous features with high mitotic activity. The transition from histologically benign to malignant areas is observed, and sometimes referred to as "dedifferentiation" (24). These tumors typically also show significant nuclear atypia and sometimes coagulative tumor necrosis (fig. 3-3C,D).

Special Studies. Immunohistochemically, the tumor cells are positive for CD34, CD99, and bcl-2, and sometimes focally for α-smooth muscle actin. They are generally negative for desmin, S-100 protein, and epithelial membrane antigen (EMA). Some examples, especially malignant ones, contain desmin- and keratin-positive cells. Nuclear positivity for β-catenin, better known for desmoid tumor, is reportedly common (40 percent) (22,25–28). The percent of Ki67-positive nuclei is low in conventional examples (1 to 2 percent), but is often over 5 percent in atypical and malignant variants; a definitive cutoff value for diagnostic use has not yet been developed. The different histologic variants are all immunohistochemically similar.

Genetics. Genetic studies so far have not shown consistently recurrent tumor type-specific changes (29). However, recurrent 4q13 involvement has been reported (30,31). The *NAB2-STAT6* gene fusion has been recently established as a recurrent genetic change in solitary fibrous tumor (32,33).

Differential Diagnosis. Monophasic spindle cell synovial sarcoma is typically a more homogeneous and highly cellular spindle cell proliferation. It almost invariable shows immunoreactivity for keratins, EMA, or both, and is almost never CD34 positive.

Many other tumors may have a hemangiopericytoma-like vascular pattern. Sarcomas with such features include monophasic and poorly differentiated synovial sarcoma, mesenchymal

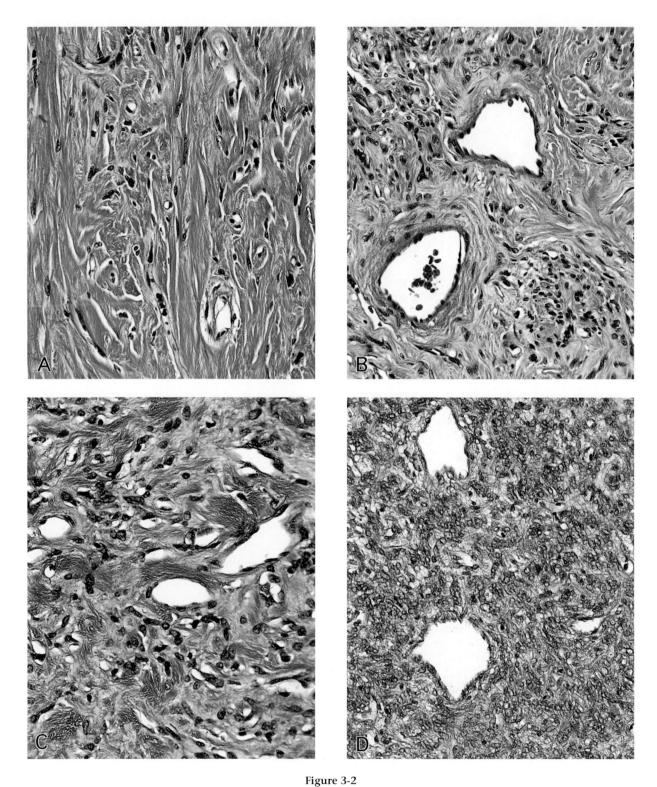

Figure 3-2

SOLITARY FIBROUS TUMOR

A–C: A bland spindled to ovoid fibroblastic proliferation is seen in a variably collagenous matrix; often, a hemangioperi-cytoma-like vascular pattern is present.

D: A more cellular example of solitary fibrous tumor with a hemangiopericytoma-like pattern.

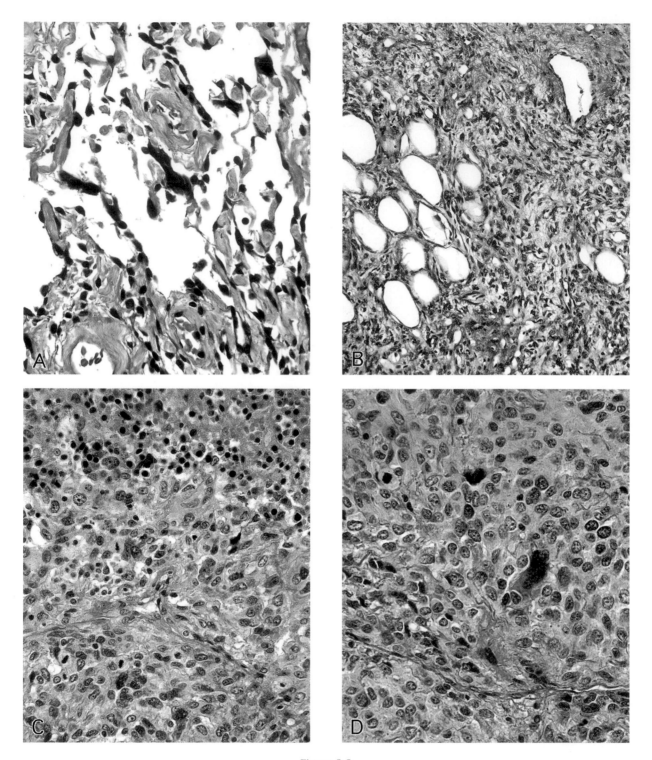

Figure 3-3

VARIANTS OF SOLITARY FIBROUS TUMOR

A: A giant cell angiofibroma variant contains pseudovascular spaces lined by multinucleated tumor cells.

B: A lipomatous variant contains a nonatypical fatty component.

C,D: Histologically malignant variants are recognized by cytologic atypia, increased mitotic rate, and sometimes, coagulative tumor necrosis.

chondrosarcoma, and myxoid/round cell liposarcoma. Among epithelial tumors, some thymomas and (follicular) thyroid carcinomas have a hemangiopericytoma-like vascular pattern as well (34). Infantile hemangiopericytomas are for the most part closely related to infantile myofibromas (35).

Treatment and Prognosis. Although solitary fibrous tumors may be malignant and metastatic, local recurrences have been more common than distant metastases. Either of these can occur long after the primary tumor is diagnosed, even 10 to 20 years later. Current information is insufficient for formulating the site, tumor size, or mitosis rate-specific criteria for the risk of clinically malignant behavior. However, the threshold of 4 mitoses per 10 high-power fields, as originally identified as Enzinger and Smith for soft tissue hemangiopericytoma (2), is commonly used for solitary fibrous tumor (3). Also, tumors with atypia, mitotic activity, or size over 5 cm should be approached with caution, until more precise criteria to define tumor behavior become available. Complete excision and long-term follow-up are generally indicated.

DERMATOFIBROSARCOMA PROTUBERANS

Definition. *Dermatofibrosarcoma protuberans* (DFSP) is a fibroblastic neoplasm of low malignant potential that usually arises in the dermis and is composed of spindle cells, often arranged in monotonous, tight storiform arrays with infiltrative growth. Rare examples (1 to 5 percent) contain scattered melanin-laden pigmented cells (*pigmented DFSP*). Fibrosarcomatous or pleomorphic sarcomatous transformation occurs in 7 to 16 percent of cases (36–40).

General Considerations. DFSP and *giant cell fibroblastoma* are closely related entities (41–44). The latter is often viewed as a special variant of dermatofibrosarcoma protuberans that is predominantly encountered during childhood. Many tumors exhibiting hybrid features have been documented over the past 20 years. Fibrosarcomatous transformation occurs in both settings, and careful evaluation for this potentially adverse prognostic finding is warranted.

Clinical Features. DFSP often has its onset in early to mid adult life, but pediatric patients (43,45–47) and the elderly (48–50) are also affected. The process initially manifests as a small cutaneous plaque-like lesion that, over time, progresses to form a protuberant multinodular mass (48–50). The growth rate often varies, with long intervals of relative stasis, separated by periods of slow or more rapid enlargement. Because early tumor progression is frequently slow, patients often delay seeking medical attention for years after the onset of disease (50). Pain or tenderness, rapid growth, and ulceration are the most common presenting complaints.

DFSP has a strong predilection for the trunk and limb girdle regions, but also occurs with some frequency in the head and neck area and elsewhere on the extremities (36,51–54). Acral sites are only rarely affected. Conventional DFSP affects males slightly more often than females (36,48,49,53,55), but several series suggest women may be somewhat more prone to develop fibrosarcomatous transformation (37,39,51,56,57).

Gross Findings. The gross appearance varies with the duration and size of the tumor. Early lesions form dermal-based plaques, whereas advanced tumors form solitary or multinodular, elevated masses that sometimes ulcerate (fig. 3-4). The tumors usually have a firm consistency. The cut surface generally reveals a solid, fairly homogeneous mass with an off-white to tan color. Some tumors contain myxoid foci, intralesional hemorrhage, or pigmented areas with slate gray or even black pigmentation (see fig. 3-9A). Necrosis is only rarely evident. Many tumors on casual review have a deceptively well-marginated appearance, although closer gross examination sometimes discloses infiltration of adjacent subcutaneous fat, extension along a fascia plane, or involvement of underlying skeletal muscle.

Microscopic Findings. Most examples of DFSP arise in the dermis and subsequently spread into the subcutis, occasionally involving deeper structures. Histologically, the tumors are composed of fairly uniform, mildly atypical, spindled fibroblast-like cells, often arranged in a monotonous, tight, storiform growth pattern (figs. 3-5–3-7). The mitotic rates are variable but are usually low. Secondary elements, such as lymphocytes, giant cells, and xanthoma cells, are rarely encountered. Hemorrhage, hemosiderin deposition, and necrosis are also uncommon. The overlying epidermis is usually

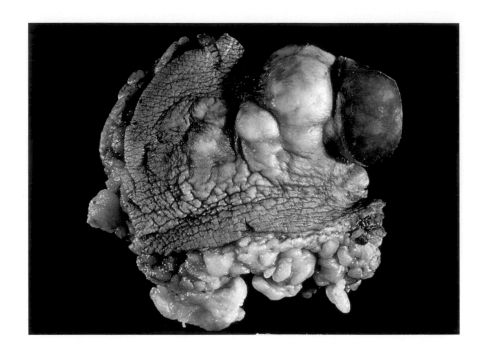

Figure 3-4

DERMATOFIBROSARCOMA PROTUBERANS

An advanced case.

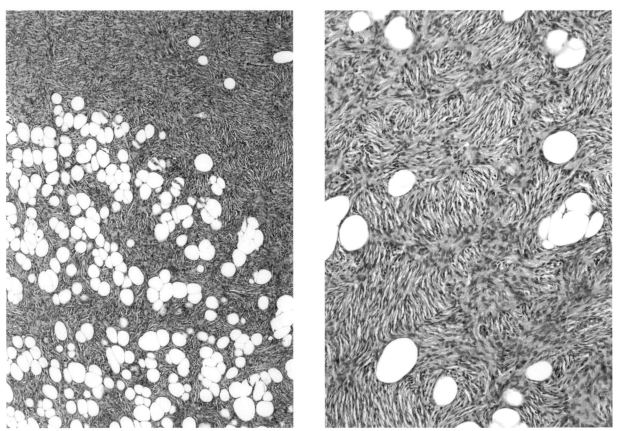

Figure 3-5

DERMATOFIBROSARCOMA PROTUBERANS

Left, Right: The monotonous, tight, storiform growth infiltrates and entraps subcutaneous fat.

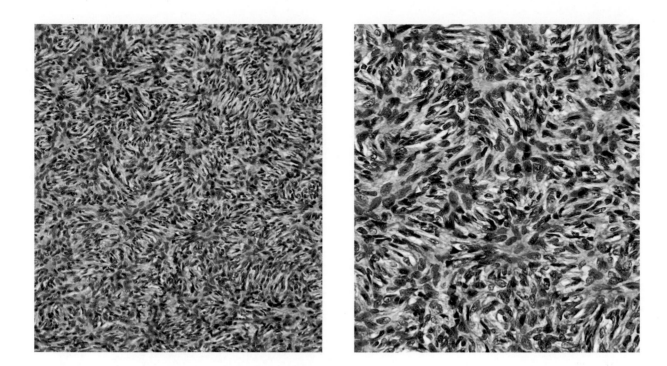

Figure 3-6

DERMATOFIBROSARCOMA PROTUBERANS

Left, Right: A fairly uniform population of mildly atypical spindled cells with monotonous, tight, storiform growth.

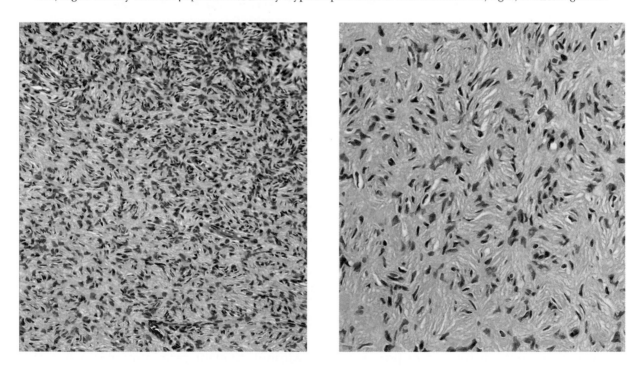

Figure 3-7

DERMATOFIBROSARCOMA PROTUBERANS

The tumor transitions from moderately high cellularity to lower cellularity due to increased collagen deposition (left). Some foci of tumor may have even lower cellularity than illustrated in figure (right).

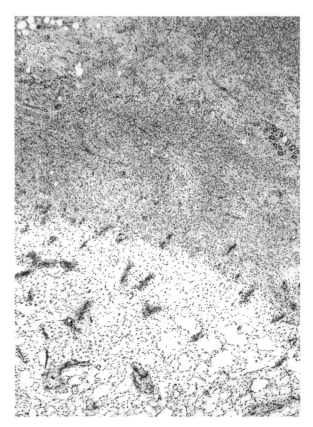 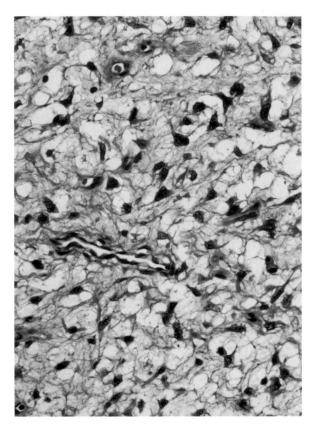

Figure 3-8

DERMATOFIBROSARCOMA PROTUBERANS WITH MYXOID CHANGE
Left, Right: Myxoid areas often lack storiform growth.

attenuated, in contrast with the acanthotic appearance characteristically associated with fibrous histiocytomas.

A frequent finding of diagnostic importance is the entrapment of skin adnexa and fat within the tumor. A myxoid matrix is present in some examples and, in rare instances, is a dominant feature (fig. 3-8), often associated with a prominent microvasculature, stellate cell morphology, and a random nonstoriform cellular distribution (55,58–61). Approximately 1 to 5 percent of cases (the so-called *Bednar tumors*) contain melanin-laden spindled, tadpole-shaped, epithelioid, or dendritic cells (fig. 3-9) (46,47,55,62,63). These cells are lightly or darkly pigmented, and may be sparsely distributed or present in substantial numbers.

Additional findings include zonal atrophy with increased collagen deposition (sometimes with a hyalinized keloidal appearance) (fig. 3-7,

right), and foci with myoid morphology (fig. 3-10) (64). The latter may be caused by tumor cells exhibiting myofibroblastic differentiation, but more often, is a secondary vascular-related (myointimal) change.

A small percentage of DFSPs (probably less than 10 percent) contain areas with solid fascicular growth, morphologically indistinguishable from classic adult-type fibrosarcoma (fig. 3-11) (36,39,40,51,65). These lesions are referred to as *DFSP with fibrosarcomatous transformation*. The minimum criteria for diagnosis have varied from one published series to the next: some authors require the fibrosarcomatous element to comprise 5 to 10 percent of the tumor area (without stipulating a minimum size, but with the understanding it must be more than a rare microscopic focus) (36,40,51,56); others require the fibrosarcomatous element to make up 25 to 30 percent of the tumor area (57,66) or for it to

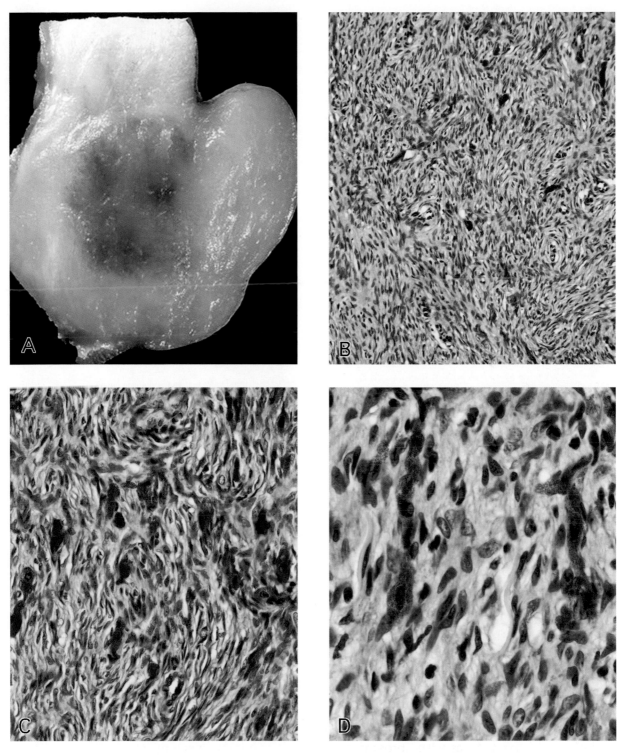

Figure 3-9

PIGMENTED DERMATOFIBROSARCOMA PROTUBERANS (BEDNAR TUMOR)

A: Gross specimen.

B–D: The scattered melanin-laden cells are spindle-, tadpole-, and stellate-shaped and epithelioid. The pigmented cells may be sparsely distributed or present in considerable numbers.

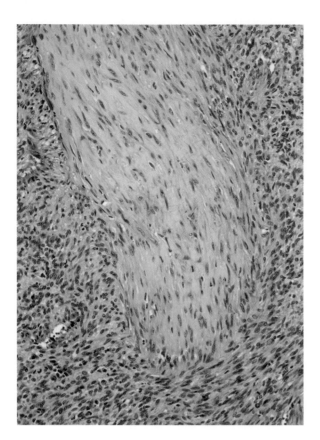
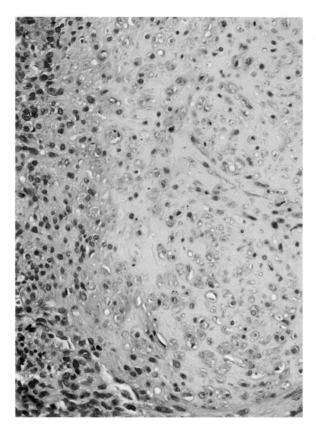

Figure 3-10

DERMATOFIBROSARCOMA PROTUBERANS

Left, Right: Myxoid nodules with this appearance are vascular (myointimal) derived.

be 1 cm or larger in size (37). The fibrosarcomatous component often arises in the subcutis, and frequently (although not always) has greater cytologic atypia, increased cellularity, and more mitotic activity than adjacent classic areas of DFSP with storiform growth (38,39,51,56,66). In fewer than 1 percent of cases, DFSPs contain foci with substantial pleomorphism, mimicking malignant fibrous histiocytoma (pleomorphic undifferentiated sarcoma) (39,49).

Special Studies. The typical spindled tumor cells of DFSP are immunoreactive for CD34 (fig. 3-12) (39,43,51,59,60) and negative for S-100 protein, keratins, EMA, factor XIIIa, desmin, and CD117 (52,67). Focal actin expression is sometimes observed. Areas with fibrosarcomatous transformation often have diminished CD34 (fig. 3-10) (38–40) and increased p53 (51) expression. The melanin-laden spindled and dendritic cells present in pigmented tumors (Bednar tumor) are immunoreactive for S-100

protein, melan A, and HMB-45 (best observed with a red chromogen stain if the cells have not been bleached).

Genetics. DFSP generally harbors either a supernumerary ring chromosome with low amplification of sequences from chromosomes 17 and 22, or it contains a linear t(17;22) translocation (41,42,67–70). Approximately 80 percent of tumors from adult patients contain ring chromosomes, but tumors from pediatric patients consistently feature a linear balanced or unbalanced translocation (42). Both genetic events produce a *COL1A1/PDGFß* fusion gene (42,71). There is wide variation in the breakpoint on the *COL1A1* gene (located on chromosome 17) but consistent involvement of exon 2 on the *PDGFß* gene (located on chromosome 22) (42,67). The resultant chimeric protein product is processed to mature PDGF-ββ, which causes continuous autocrine and paracrine activation of the PDGFRß protein-tyrosine kinase, promoting

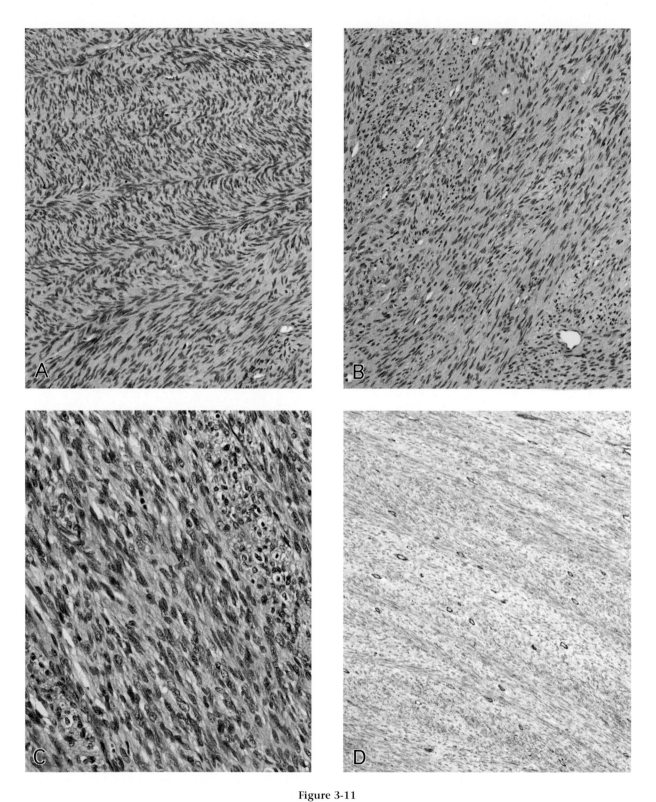

Figure 3-11

DERMATOFIBROSARCOMA PROTUBERANS WITH FIBROSARCOMATOUS TRANSFORMATION

The fibrosarcomatous element may have a herringbone (A) or fascicular (B,C) growth pattern. This element often has diminished immunoreactivity for CD34 (D).

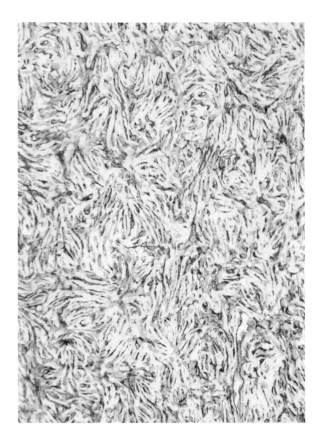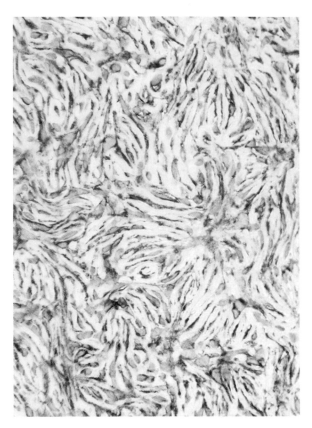

Figure 3-12

CONVENTIONAL DERMATOFIBROSARCOMA PROTUBERANS

Left, Right: CD34 immunoreactivity is seen.

cell proliferation and tumor growth (71,72). Mutagenesis experiments suggest unprocessed chimeric COL1A1-PDGFB also has the capacity to stimulate cell growth (42,71).

Various additional numerical (especially trisomies 8 and 5) and structural abnormalities may accompany the *COL1A1-PDGFB* rearrangement (42). There are also rare case reports that describe dermatofibrosarcoma protuberans-like neoplasms that lack a ring chromosome or t(17;22), suggesting that genes other than *COL1A1* or *PDGFB* are potentially involved in a small subset of cases (42,73).

Differential Diagnosis. Key considerations in the differential diagnosis of DFSP include fibrous histiocytoma variants, diffuse and pigmented (melanotic) neurofibromas, and superficial malignant peripheral nerve sheath tumor. Fibrous histiocytomas are often associated with epidermal acanthosis, frequently displace (rather than entrap) regional structures, and commonly contain an admixture of multinucleated giant cells, xanthoma cells, and siderophages (74). They have a more random storiform growth pattern than DFSP or a fascicular pattern (cellular fibrous histiocytoma), and they are usually (more than 95 percent) CD34 negative, except for a peripheral rim (75).

Diffuse neurofibromas infiltrate and entrap regional structures, and may have areas with vague storiform growth. On rare occasion, diffuse neurofibromas also contain pigmented cells, morphologically indistinguishable from the melanin-laden cells encountered in pigmented DFSP. In contrast with DFSP, however, diffuse neurofibromas contain a neoplastic population of S-100 protein–positive Schwann cells. CD34 should not be used as the sole means of discriminating between diffuse neurofibroma and DFSP, because the former commonly contains a prominent subpopulation of CD34-positive fibroblasts.

Superficial malignant peripheral nerve sheath tumors are largely recognized by documenting origin from a nerve trunk, the presence of S-100 protein immunoreactivity, and, in some instances, a positive history of neurofibromatosis type 1 (NF1). The monotonous, tight, storiform growth pattern of a conventional DFSP is absent, and some examples contain areas with epithelioid morphology, geographic necrosis, perivascular hypercellularity, and a glomeruloid-like vascular proliferation.

For DFSPs with abundant myxoid matrix, the differential diagnosis includes myxofibrosarcoma and myxoid liposarcoma. Myxofibrosarcomas tend to have greater variability in cell distribution, often with zonal perivascular hypercellularity, and even when of low histologic grade, have more atypia and pleomorphism than myxoid DFSP. Myxoid liposarcomas often involve the subcutis, but they almost never present as dermal-based tumors, and they characteristically contain a complex microvascular network and scattered lipoblasts.

The most common source of a fibrosarcomatous pattern in the skin or subcutis of an adult patient is DFSP (i.e., DFSP with fibrosarcomatous transformation). This should always be considered before entertaining the possibility of a stand-alone diagnosis of superficial adult-type fibrosarcoma.

Treatment and Prognosis. DFSP is a tumor of "indeterminate" or low malignant potential. Probably less than 3 percent of conventional examples give rise to metastases (36,54,55,66,76). When fibrosarcomatous transformation is present, however, the risk of metastasis increases to 10 to 15 percent (40,51,66). An increased risk of metastasis is also believed to be present when malignant fibrous histiocytoma-like areas are detected (40), but this is so rare that it has not yet been adequately studied.

A wide local excision is the generally recommended treatment for DFSP, because invasion beyond gross margins is common, and there is a strong propensity for recurrence when inadequately excised (49,50,54,76). The overall recurrence rate for excisions with undefined or conservative surgical margins is 44 percent (range, 26 to 60 percent in various series), compared to 20 percent for wide margins (range, 0 to 60 percent in various series) (77). A 2- to 3-cm margin of

normal-appearing tissue, with the inclusion of underlying fascia, has been advocated by some to minimize the risk of recurrence (43,53,54,76,77). For children 5 years of age or younger, including neonates, a narrower tumor-free margin has been suggested (43). A growing number of patients have been successfully treated with Mohs micrographic surgery (53,77–79), which helps minimize unnecessary removal of normal tissue, and therefore, is an important consideration in delicate anatomic sites.

Long-term follow-up is required for all patients, and periodic screening for metastases (chest X ray and other modalities) is indicated when increased risk is documented. Imatanib mesylate, a potent inhibitor of several protein-tyrosine kinases, including PDGF receptors, has had a beneficial effect for some patients with locally advanced or metastatic disease (42,53).

GIANT CELL FIBROBLASTOMA

Definition. *Giant cell fibroblastoma* is a borderline/low malignant potential neoplasm that characteristically involves the dermis and subcutis. It contains bland to mildly atypical stellate- and spindle-shaped cells admixed with varying numbers of multinucleated tumor giant cells that often line angiectoid (pseudovascular) spaces. Giant cell fibroblastoma is closely related to DFSP, so that features of it or its variants may be present. *Juvenile dermatofibrosarcoma protuberans* is a synonym.

General Considerations. Giant cell fibroblastoma is often regarded as a juvenile variant of DFSP (80). Both tumors share a similar anatomic distribution, superficial location, and strong tendency for local recurrence if incompletely excised. Examples with overlapping morphologic features are well documented (81–85), and both tumor types contain a t(17;22) cytogenetic abnormality (86–89). While most tumors with a giant cell fibroblastoma morphology occur in the pediatric population, rare examples are reported in adults. A tumor initially classified as giant cell fibroblastoma may show partial or even "pure" DFSP morphology in a recurrence (90–94).

Clinical Features. There is a greater than 2 to 1 male predominance and a strong predilection for the first decade of life. The median age for patients ranges from 3 to 6 years in the largest series (80,83,95). More than 60 percent

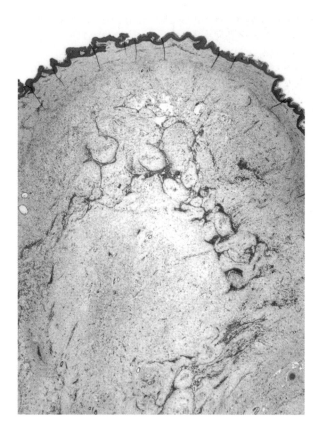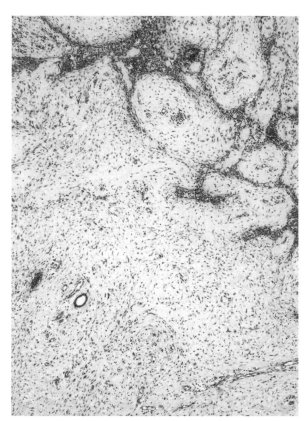

Figure 3-13

GIANT CELL FIBROBLASTOMA

Left, Right: The tumor involves dermal and subcutaneous tissue. Random growth pattern of the tumor cells, abundant myxocollagenous matrix, mild vascular accentuation, and focally prominent angiectoid (pseudovascular) spaces are seen.

of patients are younger than 10 years old and more than 75 percent are less than 20 years old (95). Examples in adults are well documented but notably uncommon. The oldest patient thus far reported was 64 years old (96).

The tumors tend to be slow growing and nontender. They are fixed to the overlying skin and have a firm to rubbery consistency. Some examples form a protuberant or polypoid mass. The lesions occur over a wide anatomic distribution, but most involve the trunk and the proximal portions of the extremities (especially the thigh) (80,83).

Gross Findings. Gross examination generally reveals an ill-defined, gray-white to tan mass involving the skin and subcutis. Some examples have a mucoid cut surface. Tumors range from less than 1 cm to 8 cm or larger (mean, 3.5 cm) (80,97). Infrequently, extension into underlying skeletal muscle occurs.

Microscopic Findings. Most tumors involve both the skin and subcutis (fig. 3-13), and a small percentage of cases extend into underlying skeletal muscle. The process is poorly demarcated, and features delicate, mononucleated and multinucleated, stellate- and spindle-shaped cells, admixed with larger multinucleated tumor giant cells (figs. 3-14, 3-15). The latter often have abundant amphophilic cytoplasm and a wreath-like nuclear arrangement. Loose myxocollagenous matrix with a mildly accentuated capillary network predominates, but areas with more densely organized collagen may be present. The cells tend to be uniformly distributed in a random or vague storiform arrangement, and there is entrapment of skin adnexa, fat, and other regional structures. Scattered foci with increased myxoid matrix may be present, and these are frequently bordered by tumor giant cells (80,89,96,98), giving rise to the so-called

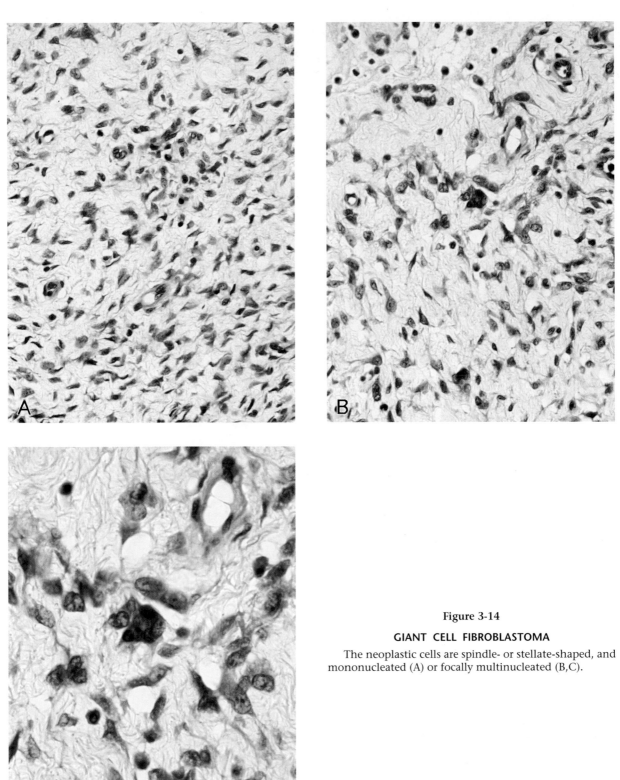

Figure 3-14

GIANT CELL FIBROBLASTOMA

The neoplastic cells are spindle- or stellate-shaped, and mononucleated (A) or focally multinucleated (B,C).

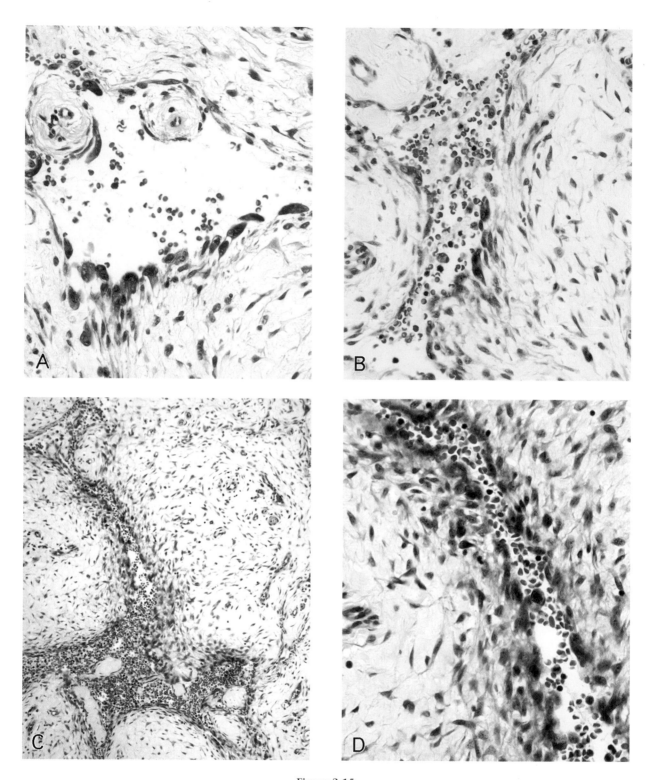

Figure 3-15

GIANT CELL FIBROBLASTOMA

A–D: The angiectoid (pseudovascular) spaces are often bordered by multinucleated tumor cells. Unadulterated spaces may have only myxoid matrix, but more often, because of capillary shearing and bleeding, they contain varying numbers of lymphocytes and red blood cells. The lining cells are not endothelial cells, and there is no accompanying smooth muscle coat.

angiectoid (pseudovascular) spaces. Unadulterated angiectoid spaces are typically hyaluronic acid rich and paucicellular, but may develop an appearance closely resembling an ectatic vascular channel (figs. 3-13, 3-15). A mild patchy lymphoplasmacytic inflammatory infiltrate is often present. Mitotic figures are uncommon, and atypical mitotic figures are absent.

Hybrid tumors containing foci with well-developed storiform growth and classic DFSP morphology are well-documented (82,83,88, 89,93). Rare examples contain pigmented cells, as described in pigmented DFSP (Bednar tumor) (85,95). We have seen two hybrid tumors with a well-developed fascicular pattern, consistent with low-grade fibrosarcomatous transformation, and this rare finding has been documented by others (93–95).

Special Studies. The neoplastic cells are immunoreactive for CD34, and are negative for S-100 protein, HMB-45, factor XIIIa, factor VIIIrAg, smooth muscle actin, desmin, and keratins (83,89,93,95).

Genetics. Giant cell fibroblastoma has a chromosomal t(17;22), +/- der(22) that results in the formation of a *COL1A1/PDGFß* chimeric gene, similar to that encountered in DFSP (87,89,99–101). Giant ring chromosomes are typically absent (100). In one study, histologic transitioning of giant cell fibroblastoma to DFSP was associated with *COL1A1/PDGFß* genomic gains (87).

Differential Diagnosis. The differential diagnosis includes myxofibrosarcoma (myxoid malignant fibrous histiocytoma), myxoid liposarcoma, and an unusual atypical vascular neoplasm, all of which are uncommon in the pediatric population. Myxofibrosarcoma is usually a deep-seated or fascial-based neoplasm that only infrequently affects the dermis. This entity generally has greater mitotic activity than giant cell fibroblastoma, and it often contains atypical mitotic figures. Myxoid liposarcoma typically contains identifiable lipoblasts, and lacks the multinucleated tumor giant cells characteristically present in giant cell fibroblastoma.

The angiectoid (pseudovascular) spaces in giant cell fibroblastoma may initially suggest a vascular neoplasm. This is especially true when blood elements have accumulated within these spaces. This consideration can be dismissed, however, by noting the nonvasoformative stellate and spindled tumor cells elsewhere in the neoplasm, lack of any smooth muscle element associated with the angiectoid spaces, and appearance of the multinucleated tumor giant cells that commonly border the spaces. The tumor cells of giant cell fibroblastoma are CD34 positive but factor VIIIrAg and CD31 negative (83,89,96,99,102).

Treatment and Prognosis. Giant cell fibroblastoma has a recurrence rate that approximates 50 percent when managed by simple local excision (80,83,97). As a result, wide local excision is generally preferable when this can be accomplished with minimal morbidity. Long-term follow-up is indicated, as it sometimes takes several years for a recurrence to become clinically apparent. To date, there are no reports of a tumor with a pure giant cell fibroblastoma morphology giving rise to metastases.

LOW-GRADE FIBROMYXOID SARCOMA

Definition. *Low-grade fibromyxoid sarcoma* (LGFMS) is a fibroblastic sarcoma typically occurring in young adults with a bland appearance but with metastatic potential. The tumor is characterized by focal hypercellularity and vascularity and genetically by a *FUS-CREB3L2/1* fusion. High-grade transformation is possible.

Clinical Features. The tumor occurs predominantly in young and middle-aged adults between the ages of 25 and 45, and also in children; there is a mild male predominance. It usually forms an intramuscular mass, which is often large, but rare distal examples in hands and those that involve superficial soft tissues are usually smaller. The most common sites of presentation are the thigh and buttocks, inguinal area, shoulder region, and chest wall. LGFMS has also been reported in the retroperitoneum and mesentery (103–107).

The clinical course is typically slow. Local recurrences occur over a long time span, up to 50 years. Lung metastases often develop after a long period of repeated local recurrences. In some cases, the pulmonary metastases are diagnosed before the detection of a large, occult primary soft tissue tumor involving the buttock or abdominal soft tissues.

Gross Findings. The tumor usually ranges from 3 to 10 cm, but can be larger than 15 cm. It is firm and rubbery, but may be have a

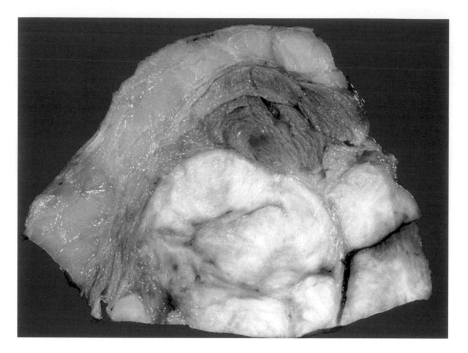

Figure 3-16

LOW-GRADE FIBROMYXOID SARCOMA

The off-white tumor tissue has a mucoid character.

mucoid appearance on sectioning (fig. 3-16). Although this tumor may appear well-circumscribed, microscopically it typically infiltrates skeletal muscle.

Microscopic Findings. Histologically, the tumor is often multinodular. The nodules typically have myxoid areas intermingled with dense fibrous tissue. The cellular nodules are mildly hypervascular and sometimes show perivascular hypercellularity. Some tumors are more collagenous and have fibromatosis or a neurofibroma-like appearance. In other areas, the tumor has a storiform appearance (fig. 3-17). Mitotic activity is typically very low, but focal necrosis may be present.

A histologic variant of LGFMS, originally reported as *hyalinizing spindle cell tumor with giant rosettes* contains mildly epithelioid tumor cells arranged in giant rosettes around dense collagen. This variant is otherwise histologically as well immunohistochemically and genetically similar to the usual form of LGFMS (fig. 3-17D) (107–109).

Perivascular hypercellularity may be present (fig. 3-18A). In some cases, LGFMS undergoes transformation to a higher histologic grade, with sheets or streaks of ovoid cells in a fibrosclerosing matrix, and this pattern may closely resemble the histology of sclerosing epithelioid fibrosarcoma (fig. 3-18B) (103,106). Osseous metaplasia may be a focal finding, and an osteosarcomatous or fibrosarcomatous (fig. 3-18C) morphology may develop during morphologic tumor progression. Pulmonary metastases often show a more cellular, epithelioid appearance (fig. 3-18D).

Special Studies. LGFMS is typically immunohistochemically positive for MUC4, and focally positive for EMA. Focal positivity for smooth muscle actin and CD34 positivity are possible. These tumors are negative for desmin, S-100 protein, and keratins (103,109,110).

Genetics. Characteristic gene fusions *FUS-CREB3L2* or rarely *FUS-CREB3L1* occur in most cases. The former corresponds with t(7;16) (q34;p11) translocation (111,112). Polymerase chain reaction (PCR)-based fusion transcript assays (113) and interphase fluorescence in situ hybridization (FISH) for *FUS* gene rearrangements help in the differential diagnosis of LGFMS and other fibroblastic tumors, but the *FUS* gene is also rearranged in myxoid liposarcoma (114,115).

Differential Diagnosis. Prior to its description, many LGFMSs were undoubtedly diagnosed as benign tumors, with diagnoses ranging from fibroma and neurofibroma variants to fibromatosis and deep fibrous histiocytoma. A higher cellularity, widespread mild nuclear atypia, multinodular fibromyxoid character, and alternating fibrous and myxoid areas allow distinction from these benign fibroblastic tumors and also from desmoid fibromatosis.

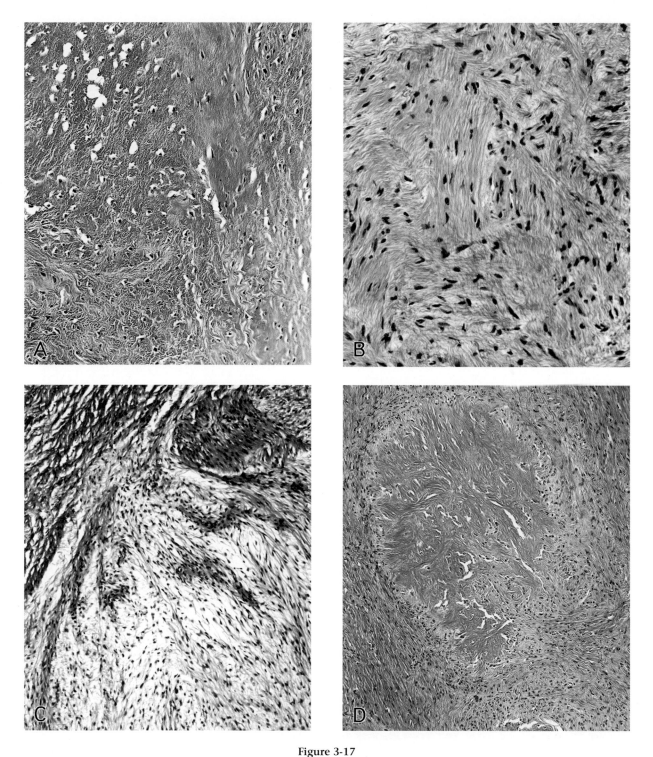

Figure 3-17

LOW-GRADE FIBROMYXOID SARCOMA

A: The fibrous matrix dominates the tumor.

B: The tumor shows only moderate cellularity with limited atypia.

C: Alternating fibrous and myxoid areas are typical of this tumor.

D: A low-grade fibromyxoid sarcoma variant with giant hyaline rosettes and a collagen core. The rosettes are surrounded by epithelioid fibroblasts.

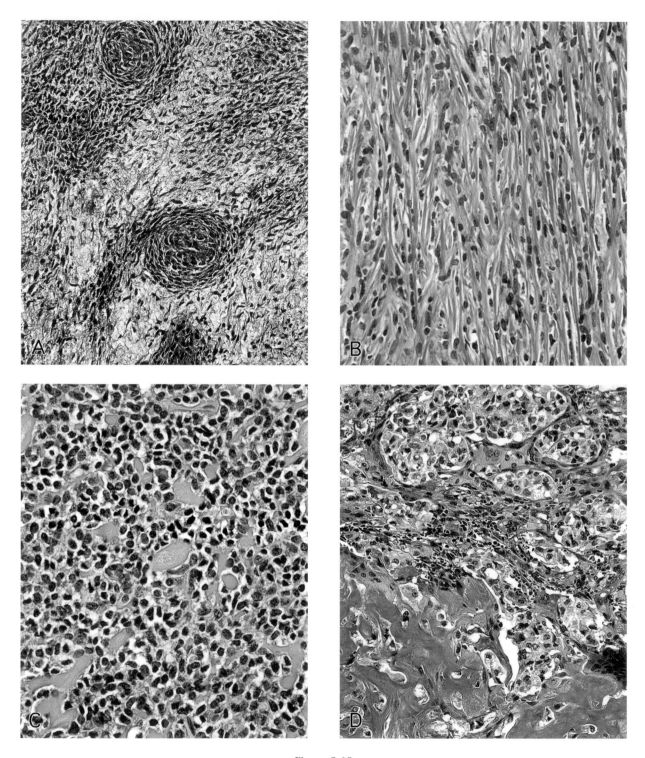

Figure 3-18

LOW-GRADE FIBROMYXOID SARCOMA

A: Perivascular hypercellularity.
B: A more cellular example with features similar to sclerosing epithelioid fibrosarcoma.
C: A highly cellular example representing tumor progression.
D: Lung metastasis with epithelioid histology.

Low-grade myxofibrosarcoma (low-grade myxoid malignant fibrous histiocytoma) differs from LGFMS by a more prominent vascular pattern, often with perivascular hypercellular zones, and the presence of greater nuclear atypia with common focal pleomorphism.

Treatment and Prognosis. LGFMS is treated with complete excision and follow-up. Incomplete excision results in a high rate of local recurrences, which may become uncontrollable over time. The reported frequency of metastases has varied from 6 to 40 percent, and in many cases, the metastases are delayed 10 to 15 years or more after the initial surgery. The lower estimates of metastatic frequency have been based on very short follow-up, while the higher estimates were observed in cancer hospital series with a bias for more aggressive tumors, so that the true metastatic rate is probably between these estimates.

Considering their often low-grade nature, surgery for pulmonary metastases, even if multiple, is often beneficial and many patients live long even after their development. Smaller primary tumor size (under 5 cm) is a favorable feature, whereas high-grade transformation is an ominous prognostic sign. Often, however, the development of metastases is not predictable by tumor morphology (105).

SCLEROSING EPITHELIOID FIBROSARCOMA

Definition. *Sclerosing epithelioid fibrosarcoma* (SEF) is a fibrosarcoma variant typically composed of corded spindle cells in a fibrosclerosing matrix. It is often of high histologic grade. In part, it includes tumors that appear to be progression variants of LGFMS.

General Comments. Although originally reported as an independent entity (116–118), subsequent studies have shown that the same histologic features are seen in LGFMS progression forms. Many of these tumors also have the same gene fusions and show MUC4 immunoreactivity similar to LGFMS (119–121). Nevertheless, a number of tumors remain that do not have histologic, immunohistochemical, or genetic features of LGFMS and these are classified under SEF. Because older series did not rigorously exclude LGFMS, their data are at least moderately contaminated with LGFMS cases.

Clinical Features. Tumors reported as SEF occur in a wide age range (14 to 87 years), with a mean age between 40 and 45 years and no sex predilection. Most SEFs are located in deep soft tissues of the proximal parts of the extremities, trunk, and head and neck region. Nearly half are 10 cm or larger (116–118).

The tumors behave as fully malignant sarcomas causing death in over half the patients. The most common metastatic sites are the lung and bone. In some cases, the metastases develop in less than 2 years, whereas in other cases, they develop 10 or more years after resection of the primary lesion.

Gross Findings. SEF forms a large oval or discoid mass measuring 2 to 15 cm. It has a fleshy to hard consistency on sectioning, often with necrosis.

Microscopic Findings. The microscopically distinctive feature is the presence of oval to epithelioid cells with pericellular clearing in a dense collagenous matrix (fig. 3-19). Mitotic activity varies from 0 to 15 mitoses per 10 high-power fields. The tumor may have areas of conventional fascicular fibrosarcoma.

Special Studies. Immunohistochemically, the tumor cells are usually negative for muscle-specific actins, desmin, CD34, S-100 protein, and keratins. Weak positivity for EMA and occasional keratin positivity with AE1/AE3 and CAM5.2 antibodies are reported (116).

Differential Diagnosis. LGFMS is ruled out by its histologic, immunohistochemical, and genetic features. We consider MUC4-positive examples and those containing LGFMS fusions examples of LGFMS.

Immunohistochemical studies for desmin and myogenin are necessary to rule out sclerosing spindle cell rhabdomyosarcoma, which may contain areas histologically resembling SEF. Sclerosing metaplastic carcinoma and malignant mixed tumor/myoepithelioma are ruled out by immunohistochemistry for epithelial markers (extensive keratin positivity) and by clinicopathologic correlation. Solitary fibrous tumor may have a somewhat similar histologic pattern but is consistently CD34 positive.

Treatment and Prognosis. SEF is usually a high-grade sarcoma with significant potential for distant metastases. The treatment, therefore, often includes multimodality components of oncology, in addition to surgery.

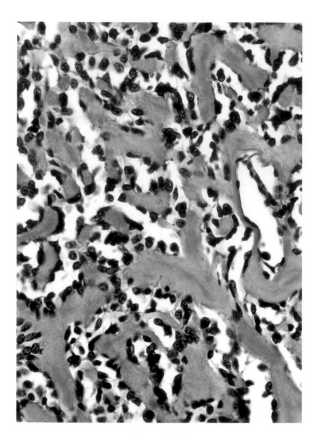

Figure 3-19

SCLEROSING EPITHELIOID FIBROSARCOMA

Cords of slightly epithelioid tumor cells have collagenous cores.

INFLAMMATORY MYOFIBROBLASTIC TUMOR

Definition. *Inflammatory myofibroblastic tumor* (IMFT) is a distinctive myofibroblastic neoplasm featuring spindled or ganglion-like cells with abundant cytoplasm in an inflammatory lymphoplasmacytic background. Anaplastic lymphoma kinase (ALK) positivity and ALK-involving gene fusions are present. *Inflammatory fibrosarcoma, inflammatory pseudosarcomatous fibromyxoid tumor,* and *inflammatory pseudotumor* are synonyms.

General Comments. Different designations have been applied to various subsets of IMFT, but the designation "inflammatory pseudotumor" has been also applied to reactive fibroinflammatory processes, so that this term should no longer be used for IMFT. Many visceral examples have been designated as leiomyosarcomas or gastrointestinal stromal tumors in the past,

especially when located in the gastrointestinal and genitourinary tracts. The definition of this entity is still controversial, as some investigators have accepted a substantial number of cases without ALK expression or *ALK* gene rearrangements under the umbrella of IMFT.

Clinical Features. IMFT usually occurs in children and young adults. The most common soft tissue sites are the intra-abdominal soft tissues, especially omentum and mesenteries. Abdominal IMFTs are often large masses that may cause intestinal obstruction. Occurrence of multiple lesions is not rare. Fifteen to 30 percent of patients have constitutional inflammation and cytokine-related symptoms that abate after tumor removal but may reappear upon tumor recurrence. They include fever, malaise, and weight loss, and children may experience growth retardation. Pathologic laboratory findings include anemia (normochromic or hypochromic, microcytic), leukocytosis, thrombocytosis, elevated erythrocyte sedimentation rate, and polyclonal hypergammaglobulinemia. Visceral involvement is common, especially in the urinary bladder, lung, and gastrointestinal tract (122–127). Occurrence in peripheral soft tissue is rare, but occasional cases occur in the head and neck region.

Gross Findings. The abdominal and pelvic lesions have a wide size range of 1 to 20 cm (median, 10 cm). Multiple tumor nodules are common and show a lobular, multinodular, sometimes whorled texture on sectioning. The tumor tissue is gray-white or tan-pink. The cut surface is usually rubbery, but may be focally myxoid (fig. 3-20).

Microscopic Findings. Histologically, IMFT is composed of a mixture of spindle or polygonal cells, (myo)fibroblasts, plasma cells, and lymphocytes in varying proportions (fig. 3-21). Some lesions contain eosinophils and neutrophils. The spindle cells may show a dense storiform or fascicular arrangement, with few inflammatory cells in between, or there may be an extensive inflammatory infiltrate and a scant neoplastic component. Myxoid, paucicellular areas, with a rich network of delicate capillaries or foci with dense fibrosis are common. Calcifications have been reported but are rare in our experience.

The spindle cells have typically oval to elongated nuclei, variably prominent eosinophilic

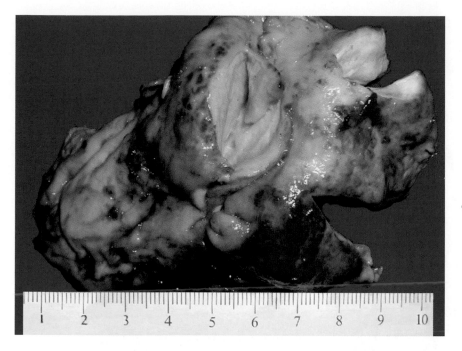

Figure 3-20

INFLAMMATORY MYOFIBROBLASTIC TUMOR

The tumor is a solid, homogeneous, fleshy whitish mass.

nucleoli, and amphophilic, often abundant cytoplasm, creating some resemblance to skeletal muscle cells or ganglion cells (fig. 3-21). There is a histologic spectrum that includes relatively bland and paucicellular sclerotic lesions at one end, and more highly cellular and atypical lesions at the other. Mitotic frequency varies but is generally low, and necrosis is rare. It has been suggested that tumors with a high content of large ganglion-like cells behave more aggressively (128). Vascular invasion may occur, but this has no adverse prognostic significance.

Special Studies. The ample cytoplasmic myofibroblasts often show positivity for ALK (fig. 3-22), although the percentage of positive cases varies in different studies. Some specific fusion types are associated with nuclear membrane-associated ALK positivity. Immunohistochemical evaluation of ALK expression is useful in the differential diagnosis, since inflammatory pseudotumors are usually ALK negative, although positivity has been reported in rhabdomyosarcoma and leiomyosarcoma, indicating that an immunohistochemical panel addressing these different diagnostic possibilities is necessary.

IMFTs are also variably positive for muscle actin (HHF-35), α-smooth muscle actin (fig. 3-22), and sometimes for desmin, although cases with primitive nonmyoid phenotypes have also been reported. Keratin positivity for AE1/AE3

cocktail and CAM5.2 antibodies is common, especially in abdominal and urinary bladder tumors (126,127). The tumor cells are negative for myoglobin, MyoD1/myogenin, S-100 protein, and KIT (CD117).

Genetics. *ALK* (at 2p23) gene rearrangements in the form of fusion translocations are typical of IMFT, and FISH analysis of *ALK* gene split rearrangements using a break-apart probe is the most practical way to evaluate IMFTs (129,130). Application of PCR-based tests is more difficult because of varying translocation partners. These assays specify the fusion type, however, which may have clinicopathologic importance (Table 3-1) (131–137). Some fusions (*TMPM3-ALK* and *TPM4-ALK*) are identical to those seen in anaplastic large cell lymphoma, so the diagnosis is made by multiparameter immunohistochemical analysis.

Differential Diagnosis. The childhood lesions may both clinically and histologically resemble embryonal rhabdomyosarcoma. The extensive inflammatory background, however, differs. The large cytoplasmic cells are always negative for MyoD1/myogenin.

IMFT should be also separated from specific and nonspecific inflammatory pseudotumors, well-differentiated or dedifferentiated liposarcoma with an inflammatory component, and malignant fibrous histiocytoma. Caution is needed when making a diagnosis of IMFT in

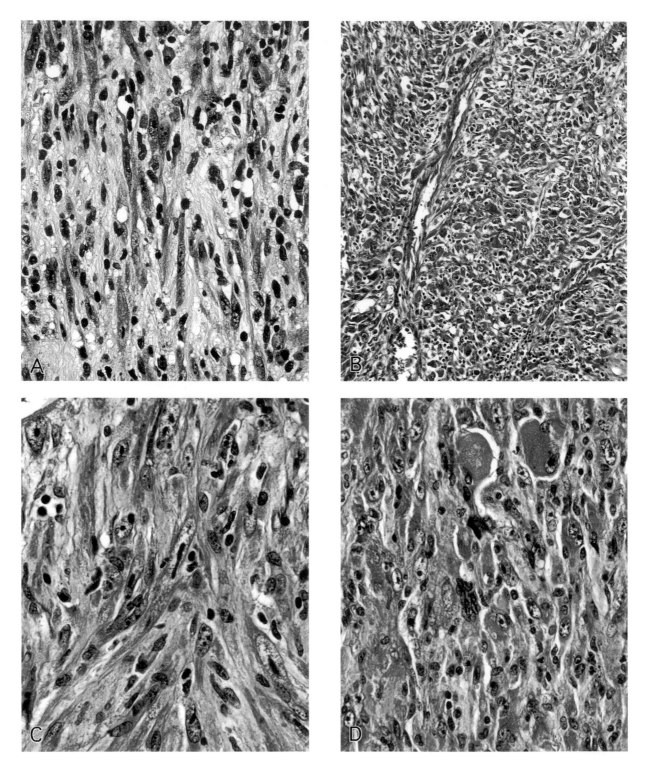

Figure 3-21

INFLAMMATORY MYOFIBROBLASTIC TUMOR

A–C: Elongated spindled neoplastic cells and a mixed inflammatory, especially lymphoplasmacytic, infiltration.

C,D: Some examples contain increased numbers of ganglion-like cells, and these tumors may behave more aggressively.

an older adult, as many dedifferentiated liposarcomas superficially resemble IMFT in their content of a prominent inflammatory background. Immunohistochemistry for MDM2 is useful, as dedifferentiated liposarcomas often show extensive nuclear positivity.

Leiomyosarcomas typically have eosinophilic, fibrillary cytoplasm not seen in IMFT. Gastrointestinal stromal tumors (GISTs) have a more homogeneous cellular composition, almost exclusively present in adults over 40 years of age, and are almost always KIT positive. It is likely that some early childhood tumors reported as GISTs are abdominal IMFTs.

Ultimately, genetic correlation with *ALK* gene rearrangements or specific fusions is diagnostic. ALK positivity is useful in the differential diagnosis, but is not specific for IMFT, and also may be absent or undetectable in some *ALK* fusion variants (see below).

Treatment and Prognosis. In general, the prognosis of patients with IMFT is good. Abdominal tumors recur in 25 percent of cases. Pulmonary and brain metastases developed in 10 percent of patients in tumors reported as inflammatory fibrosarcomas (125,126). A variant predominantly composed of epithelioid ganglion-like cells is more aggressive (128). Surgery is the main treatment modality. Recurrent or metastatic cases have been treated with a new ALK tyrosine kinase inhibitor, crizotinib (138).

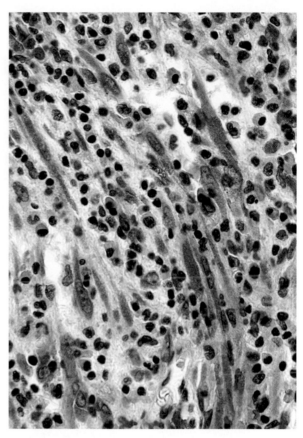

Figure 3-22

INFLAMMATORY MYOFIBROBLASTIC TUMOR

The tumor cells show strong cytoplasmic positivity for anaplastic lymphoma kinase (ALK).

Table 3-1

GENE FUSIONS AND ASSOCIATED DEMOGRAPHY OF INFLAMMATORY MYOFIBROBLASTIC TUMORS

Fusion Partners	Expected Translocation	Tumor Location	Age	Sex	Ref.
TPM3-ALK	t(1;2)(q21;p23)*	abdomen	23 yrs.	female	131
		lung	30 yrs.	female	
TPM4-ALK	t(2;19)(p23;p13)*	abdomen	1 yrs.	male	131
CLTC-ALK	t(2;17)(p23;q11)	neck	3 yrs.	female	132
CARS-ALK	t(2;11)(p23;p15)	cervical paraspinal	10 yrs.	male	133
		pelvis	37 yrs.	male	
ATIC-ALK	t(2;2)(p23;q35)	urinary bladder	46 yrs.	male	134
RANBP2-ALK	t(2;2)(p23;q12)	base of mesentery	7 mos.	male	135
		abdomen	7 yrs.	male	
SEC31L1-ALK	t(2;4)(p23;q21)*	omentum	23 yrs.	male	136
PPFIBP1-ALK	t(2;12)(p23;p12)	lung	34 yrs.	female	137
		lung	45 yrs.	male	

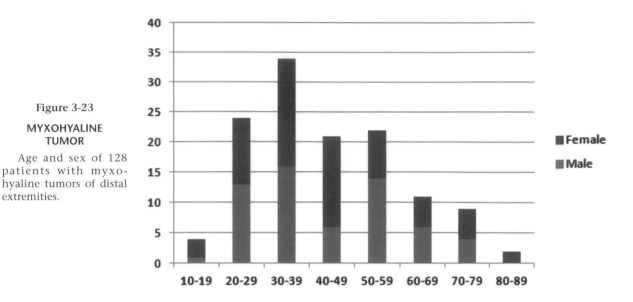

Figure 3-23

MYXOHYALINE TUMOR

Age and sex of 128 patients with myxohyaline tumors of distal extremities.

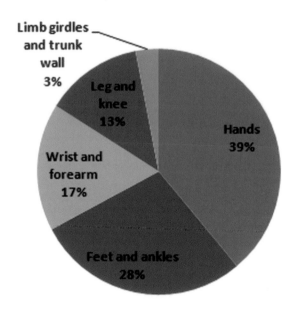

Figure 3-24

MYXOHYALINE TUMOR

Anatomic distribution of 131 myxohyaline tumors of distal extremities.

INFLAMMATORY MYXOHYALINE TUMOR OF DISTAL EXTREMITIES (ACRAL MYXO-INFLAMMATORY FIBROBLASTIC SARCOMA)

Definition. *Inflammatory myxohyaline tumor of distal extremities* is a borderline to low-grade malignant fibroblastic proliferation typically occurring in fingers and hands, or rarely, in feet and ankles. It has a prominent inflammatory component and variable numbers of epithelioid tumor cells with abundant cytoplasm, large nuclei, and inclusion-like nucleoli but lacks widespread nuclear atypia and atypical mitoses. An alternative name is *myxoinflammatory fibroblastic sarcoma*.

Clinical Features. The tumor occurs in adults with a median age of 44 to 53 years and equal occurrence in men and women (fig. 3-23). At least two thirds of cases occur in the distal extremities: fingers, hands, feet, and ankle. Wrist and forearm, and lower leg and knee region are less common sites, and occurrence in limb girdles of the trunk wall is exceptional (fig. 3-24). The median duration of symptoms is 1 year, but some patients have a longer history of a mass. The tumor has a predilection for the dorsal aspect of the hands and feet, where it typically forms an ill defined, raised mass that is much wider than deep and may clinically resemble inflammation or infection more than a discrete tumor (139–141).

Gross Findings. The tumor typically measures 1 to 5 cm, with the median size around 3 cm. It is usually poorly circumscribed and may have a mucoid character.

Microscopic Findings. Histologically, the tumor is distinctive for a multinodular pattern at a low magnification (fig. 3-25A). There is a variably prominent mixed inflammatory infiltrate composed of lymphocytes, plasma cells, neutrophils,

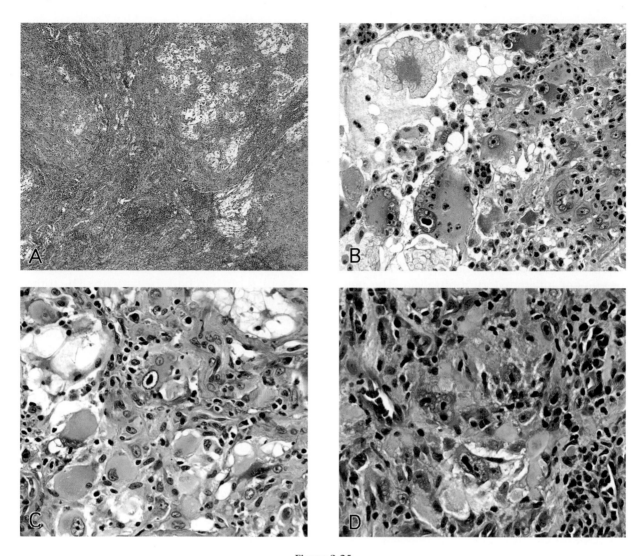

Figure 3-25

INFLAMMATORY MYXOHYALINE TUMOR

A: A multinodular subcutaneous infiltration is associated with a prominent lymphoid infiltration and areas of fibrosis.

B–D: Higher magnification reveals large epithelioid cells with large nuclei and prominent inclusion-like nucleoli, and pseudolipoblast-like cells as lesional components. There are also intermingled inflammatory cells.

and eosinophils in a variably myxoid and collagenous background. Germinal centers may be present, especially in the periphery.

The neoplastic cells often have an epithelioid appearance, although a spindle cell component may also be present. Large atypical ganglion-like cells with abundant cytoplasm and large nuclei with prominent, eosinophilic nucleoli are typical. These cells superficially resemble Hodgkin cells or viral inclusion bodies. Vacuolated polygonal fibroblasts with intracellular mucin accumulation ("pseudolipoblasts") are also common (fig.

3-25C,D). Mitotic activity is scant, and atypical mitoses are not generally present.

Special Studies. The immunohistochemical features are nonspecific. High numbers of histiocytes are demonstrated with stains for CD68 and CD163, but the large epithelioid cells are negative, especially for the more histiocyte-specific CD163. In 10 to 15 percent of cases, large atypical cells are focally keratin and EMA positive. Studies for CD15 and CD30, microorganisms (bacteria by gram and acid-fast stains, and Grocott methenamine silver for fungi) are negative. The tumor cells are negative for desmin, smooth muscle actin, CD34, and S-100 protein. PCR-based assays for cytomegalovirus and Epstein-Barr-virus are negative (140).

Genetics. An unbalanced translocation t(1;10)(p22;q24) and 3p amplification involving the *VGLL3* gene seem to be recurrent genetic changes (143–146). At the molecular genetic level, the translocation maps to the *TGFBR3* gene at 1p22 and near the *MGEA5* locus at 10q24, but its precise genomic structure is presently unknown. The same translocation also occurs in hemosiderotic fibrolipomatous tumor (145,146).

Differential Diagnosis. This tumor can be confused with proliferative synovitis because of the prominent inflammatory infiltration. The presence of atypical cells with prominent eosinophilic nucleoli is a distinctive feature and differentiates this tumor as well from ganglion cyst and other benign fibromyxoid proliferations. The potential occurrence of keratin-positive cells may lead to confusion with epithelioid sarcoma, which contains sheets of keratin-positive cells and additionally shows loss of INI1 in most cases.

Myxoid malignant fibrous histiocytoma (MFH)/myxofibrosarcoma contains a greater number of atypical cells, often in solid sheets. We believe that tumors with solid sheets of atypical cells and numerous atypical mitotic figures should be classified as myxoid MFH rather than inflammatory myxohyaline tumor. The Reed-Sternberg–like cells are not specific for a myxohyaline tumor and can occur in sarcomas, such as MFH and myxofibrosarcoma. Cases with hybrid features of myxohyaline tumor and hemosiderotic fibrolipomatous tumor have been reported and some authors believe that these entities are closely related (142).

Treatment and Prognosis. Tumor behavior is variable, with a high rate of local, often multiple, recurrences. We have seen isolated proximal locoregional recurrences but no distant metastases. Two series had no metastases (140,141), and one series had documented lymph node metastasis in one patient and a histologically undocumented pulmonary lesion in another (139). Another series reported a rapidly metastasizing lesion, but it is unclear whether lesion types with a higher biologic potential were excluded (147).

Complete excision should be performed whenever this can be achieved in a function-preserving manner. Recently, good results were obtained with a combination of conservative excision and postoperative radiation, and this could obviate the frequent finger or ray amputations used in the past (148).

INFANTILE FIBROSARCOMA (CONGENITAL FIBROSARCOMA)

Definition. *Infantile fibrosarcoma*, also termed *congenital fibrosarcoma*, is a fibrosarcoma variant that occurs in newborns or infants and is characterized by an *ETV6-NTRKC* gene fusion.

Clinical Features. The tumor is rare and usually arises during the first year of life; it is present at birth in half the patients. The tumor is sometimes diagnosed in fetuses and may be responsible for intrauterine death in some cases. There is a 3 to 2 male predominance. The tumor mainly affects the distal parts of the upper and lower extremities: hands, forearm, ankle, and feet, but isolated cases have been reported in the intestines. The tumor grows rapidly and forms a poorly circumscribed mass that can measure 10 cm or more (149–154).

Gross Features. Infantile fibrosarcoma varies from a small nodule to a bulky exophytic tumor, with a mean size of 4 cm in the largest series. On sectioning, the tumor may appear hemorrhagic, but solid pale tan or fleshy areas are often present (fig. 3-26). Larger tumors often are necrotic.

Microscopic Features. Histologically, infantile fibrosarcoma varies from a well-differentiated collagen-forming fibrosarcomatous pattern to a highly cellular noncollagenous spindle cell tumor arranged in fascicles or diffuse sheets (fig. 3-27). Some tumors are composed of oval cells. A prominent vascular pattern, often with dilated and engorged vessels, is a common feature. Mitotic activity is often high. Malignant fibrous histiocytoma-like pleomorphic transformation may occur and result in a poor prognosis (155).

Special Studies. Immunohistochemically, infantile fibrosarcoma is positive for vimentin, and variably for actins. Negative results have been obtained for desmin, keratins, EMA, and S-100 protein. Actin positivity correlates with the myofibroblastic-fibroblastic differentiation detected on ultrastructural studies (156,157).

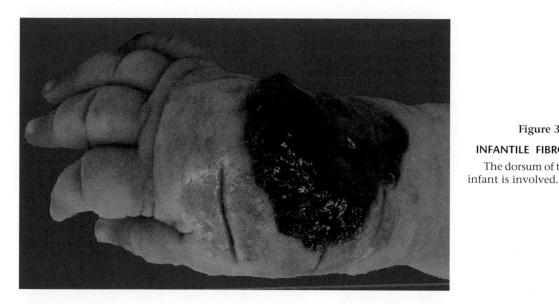

Figure 3-26

INFANTILE FIBROSARCOMA

The dorsum of the hand of an infant is involved.

Large studies on genetically verified cases are not available.

Genetics. A reciprocal translocation t(12;15) (p13;q25) resulting in the fusion of the *ETV6* and *NTRK3* genes is present in most cases (158–161). Notably, the same fusion occurs in the cellular (but not the typical) variant of mesoblastic nephroma and secretory carcinoma of the breast (162–165).

Trisomy of chromosome 11, along with variable trisomies of chromosomes 17 and 20 and occasionally of 8 and 10, occur as nonrandom cytogenetic changes with possible differential diagnostic value (162,166).

Differential Diagnosis. Spindle cell and poorly differentiated embryonal rhabdomyosarcoma have to be ruled out, especially in genital and pelvic tumors. Immunohistochemistry is required for this in every case, and a wide panel of markers, including desmin and skeletal muscle transcriptional regulators (MyoD1, myogenin), should be evaluated. The intratumoral hemorrhage seen in some cases should not be mistaken for a vascular tumor.

Dermatofibrosarcoma protuberans and giant cell fibroblastoma can be recognized by their variably storiform architecture, giant cells, and superficial and subcutaneous fat involvement. Testing for tumor-specific translocations is useful in problem cases.

Treatment and Prognosis. Because of its relatively good prognosis despite the ominous clinical and histologic features, conservative function-preserving primary surgery is now advocated as much as possible, although complete excision is an ideal goal (167). Chemotherapy may obviate amputations in some cases in which this would be otherwise required for complete removal (168).

Infantile fibrosarcoma is prone to local recurrences, but distant metastases to lung and other sites (brain, liver) occur in only 5 to 10 percent of patients. Large head and neck, truncal, or proximal extremity tumors are associated with a higher mortality rate.

ADULT FIBROSARCOMA AND MYOFIBROBLASTIC SARCOMA

Definition. *Adult fibrosarcoma* is a collagen-forming nonpleomorphic spindle cell sarcoma occurring after the age of 10 years that cannot be classified into any other category (i.e., malignant peripheral nerve sheath tumor, synovial sarcoma, solitary fibrous tumor, low-grade fibromyxoid sarcoma [LGFMS], cellular desmoid tumor, dermatofibrosarcoma protuberans [DFSP] with fibrosarcomatous transformation, or dedifferentiated liposarcoma).

Myofibroblastic sarcoma is a spindle cell sarcoma with an immunohistochemically or ultrastructurally documented myofibroblastic phenotype.

General Comments. Today, adult fibrosarcoma is a rare diagnosis and one of exclusion.

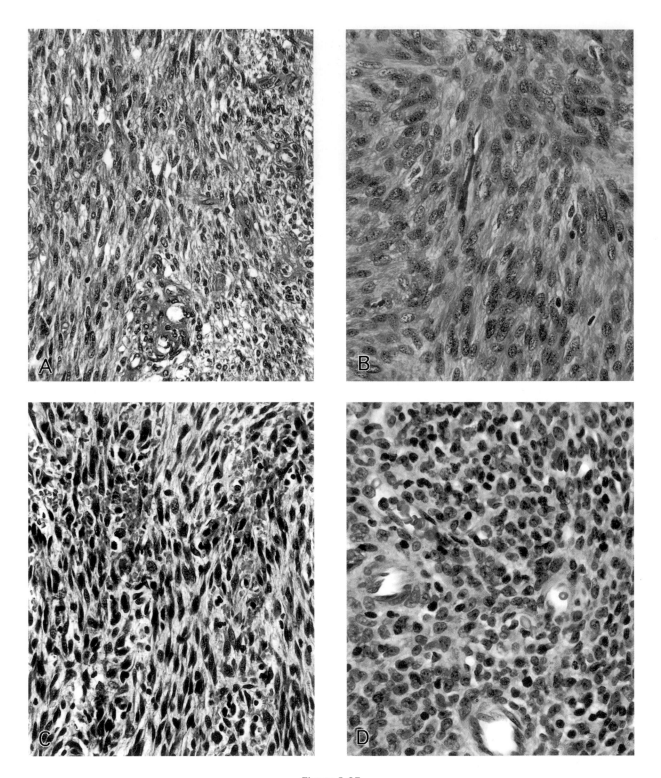

Figure 3-27

INFANTILE FIBROSARCOMA

A–C: The tumor is composed of uniform, mildly to moderately atypical spindle cells with oval to fusiform nuclei. A prominent vascular pattern and intratumoral hemorrhage are common findings.

D: Some examples are composed of oval, less-differentiated cells.

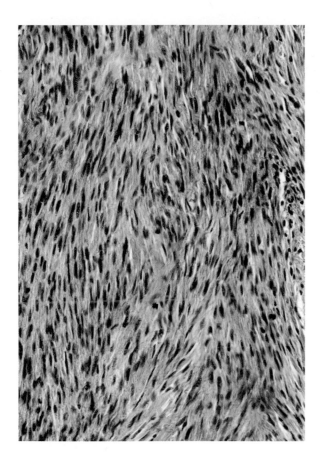 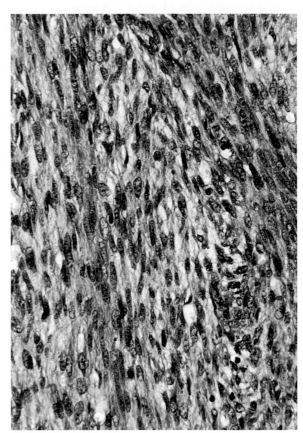

Figure 3-28

ADULT FIBROSARCOMA

Left, Right: Fascicles of moderately atypical spindle cells with elongated or spindle-shaped nuclei are in a variably collagenous matrix.

It is likely that many superficial fibrosarcomas are DFSP-derived fibrosarcomas, based on the presence of a *COLIA1-PDGF* fusion transcript in many such tumors (169). Most fibroblastic sarcomas have at least some pleomorphic and myxoid features, and are therefore usually classified as myxofibrosarcomas or malignant fibrous histiocytomas.

Because published older series on adult fibrosarcomas predate the present classification and emergence of diagnoses such as LGFMS, it is difficult to project the old data into the current classification.

Clinical Features. More recent series of adult fibrosarcomas indicate preferential occurrence in the deep soft tissues of the extremities or trunk of middle-aged adults (170). A recent series, employing strict criteria and stringent exclusion of other entities, found that fewer than 20 percent of cases originally classified as

fibrosarcoma fulfilled those stringent criteria. These tumors occur in an age range of 6 to 74 years (median, 50 years), with a male predominance. Half of the tumors involve the lower extremities (especially thigh), and half the head and neck, trunk, and upper extremities. Fifty percent of patients die of disease (171).

Microscopic Findings. Histologically typical are fascicles of spindle cells in a variably collagenous matrix (fig. 3-28). The most stringent reclassification studies have accepted only focal smooth muscle actin positivity. The tumors are negative for all other mesenchymal markers, including CD34, desmin, EMA, MyoD1, and S-100 protein.

Myofibroblastic sarcoma (myofibrosarcoma) is a designation given to fibrosarcoma with myofibroblastic differentiation, as defined by the histologic appearance: spindled cells with amphophilic abundant "myoid" cytoplasm and smooth muscle actin positivity. Electron microscopy shows myofibroblastic features with partial basement membranes, focal clusters of actin filaments, and attachment plaques at the cell membrane. The reported tumors have been mostly low-grade sarcomas presenting in a variety of locations (172,173). Many myxofibrosarcomas and malignant fibrous histiocytomas contain focal smooth muscle actin positivity, indicating focal myofibroblastic differentiation and therefore potentially qualifying as myofibroblastic sarcomas. It is not known whether myofibroblastic differentiation in this context has specific clinical significance.

MYXOFIBROSARCOMA

Definition. *Myxofibrosarcoma* is a fibroblastic sarcoma characterized by a myxoid nodular appearance, variable nuclear pleomorphism, and curvilinear vasculature.

General Considerations. The term myxofibrosarcoma was first used by Scandinavian investigators to focus attention on the myxoid and fibroblastic elements of the tumor (174). At the same time, Weiss and Enzinger (175) published their experience with this neoplasm, but preferred the term *myxoid malignant fibrous histiocytoma* (MFH) to distinguish if from the more aggressive storiform-pleomorphic MFH group (175). They applied strict diagnostic criteria to define myxoid MFH, which was defined as having a greater than 50 percent hypocellular myxoid component, representing mainly lower-grade lesions, with better outcome, including a significantly lower metastatic rate, compared to the more solid, pleomorphic MFH (175).

The definition of myxoid MFH/myxofibrosarcoma has evolved over the years to encompass higher-grade tumors with a less pronounced myxoid component. As such, Mentzel at al. (176) defined myxofibrosarcoma as a tumor with at least 10 percent myxoid areas, recognizing that these lesions show a spectrum between a "hypocellular, mainly myxoid, and purely spindle-cell appearance (low-grade neoplasms) to high-grade, pleomorphic (MFH-like) lesions with multinucleated giant cells, high mitotic activity, and areas of necrosis." In fact, the latest World Health Organization (WHO) classification of soft tissue tumors suggests that the presence of any distinctive low-grade tumor with curvilinear vessels is what separates the higher-grade myxofibrosarcoma from the heterogeneous group of pleomorphic MFH-like lesions, with no minimal percent required for the myxoid component. Thus, the distinction between mostly solid, high-grade myxofibrosarcoma with only minimal myxoid changes and pleomorphic MFH/undifferentiated pleomorphic sarcoma (UPS) remains arbitrary. Loosening these diagnostic criteria obscures the boundaries between myxofibrosarcoma and MFH, including their differences in clinical behavior. Many soft tissue experts (including the authors of this Fascicle) believe that there is a morphologic continuum between high-grade myxofibrosarcoma and MFH/undifferentiated pleomorphic sarcoma, and that their separation is artificial. As a significant number of pleomorphic MFHs (exhibiting some but less than 50 percent myxoid component) are now reclassified as high-grade myxofibrosarcoma, and the diagnosis of pleomorphic MFH/UPS, once the most common adult soft tissue sarcoma, has become rare or its existence even denied altogether (177).

Although there is full agreement on the fibroblastic lineage of myxofibrosarcoma, based on numerous ultrastructural studies (178–180), there is no electron microscopic evidence of fibroblastic differentiation in the storiform-pleomorphic MFH/UPS (181).

Clinical Features. Myxofibrosarcoma is the most common sarcoma affecting limbs and limb girdles of older patients, with a peak incidence in the sixth and seventh decades (174,176,182, 183); involvement of trunk, head and neck, and hands and feet is less common. Intra-abdominal and retroperitoneal occurrence is very uncommon, as most lesions with myxofibrosarcoma-like features in these locations are dedifferentiated liposarcomas (184,185).

Clinically, the primary lesion presents as a predominantly deep or subcutaneous multinodular growth. Occasionally, it may be centered in the dermis (186). Myxofibrosarcoma often extends along fascial planes, well beyond the apparent tumor border, as radiologically seen in 60 percent of cases (fig. 3-29) (187,188).

Gross Findings. Grossly, myxofibrosarcoma is characteristically nodular, with either a single circumscribed mass or several closely packed

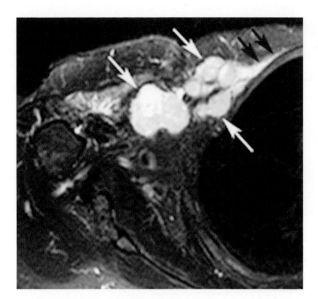

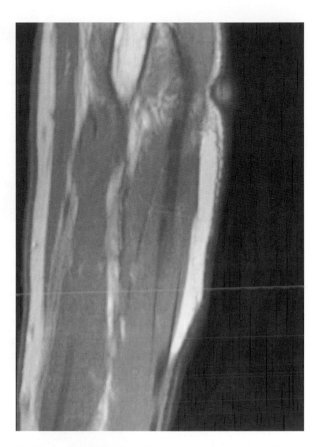

Figure 3-29

MYXOFIBROSARCOMA

Axial fat-suppressed T2-weighted magnetic resonance image (MRI) of two locally recurrent low-grade tumors showing the following: mixed multinodular (white arrows) and infiltrative growth, with the characteristic "tail" sign (red arrows) (above), and the typical superficial spreading along the subcutaneous tissue (right).

nodules, which range in size from a few millimeters to several centimeters. The tumors are soft, gelatinous to rubbery, and tan-white, and often show a bulging surface on cut section (174,175). The growth pattern is either expansile, circumscribed, or multinodular.

The tumor frequently displays infiltrative borders, with anatomically deceptive boundaries and extension into the dermis and skeletal muscles (fig. 3-30) (183,186). The low-grade myxoid lesions, in particular, have a propensity to spread along septal and fascial planes, showing a more infiltrative nature with loss of nodularity (175,176,183). Necrosis and hemorrhage are more common in higher-grade lesions (fig. 3-31).

Microscopic Findings. Microscopically, the tumors are composed of fusiform cells, with indistinct cell borders and vacuolated or slightly eosinophilic cytoplasm (fig. 3-32A). The cytoplasmic vacuolization may be focally pronounced to mimic lipoblasts, so-called pseudolipoblasts (fig. 3-32B). Nuclear pleomorphism of varying degree, with hyperchromatic, smudgy chromatin and marked variations in size and shape of the nuclei, within often mul-

tilobated and/or multinucleated tumor cells, is characteristic (fig. 3-32C). The lesional cells are arranged haphazardly or in loose storiform or short intersecting fascicles and embedded in a variably myxoid or fibromyxoid matrix rich in elongated, curvilinear capillaries with perivascular cell condensation (fig. 3-33). The solid, nonmyxoid components typically exhibit a higher degree of nuclear pleomorphism and increased mitotic activity, and are indistinguishable from the pleomorphic MFH/UPS (fig. 3-34A). The progression from the low-grade myxoid component to the higher-grade solid areas is either abrupt or gradual (fig. 3-34B,C).

Special Studies. Tumor cells show variable reactivity for CD34 and smooth muscle actin, with the latter reflecting a myofibroblastic component. Sporadic cells may be positive for desmin and keratins, but the tumor is negative for S-100 protein.

Genetics. Myxofibrosarcomas show a highly complex karyotype, with extensive intratumoral heterogeneity without recurrent numerical or structural aberrations. Triploid and tetraploid ranges are noted in most cases, including in

197

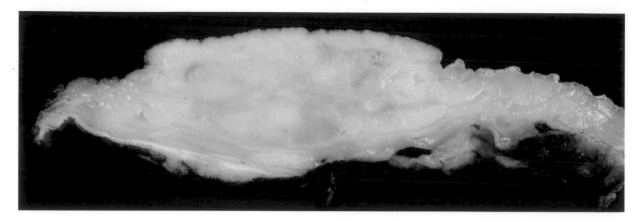

Figure 3-30

MYXOFIBROSARCOMA

Deceptive gross appearance within the subcutaneous tissue of the lower leg, with vague multinodular as well as more infiltrative growth, extending microscopically to multiple margins. The lesion appears to be confined to the fascial plane.

Figure 3-31

MYXOFIBROSARCOMA

Gross appearance of a subcutaneous high-grade tumor showing a heterogeneous mass, with distinct gelatinous, myxoid components, as well as more fleshy, higher-grade areas and necrosis.

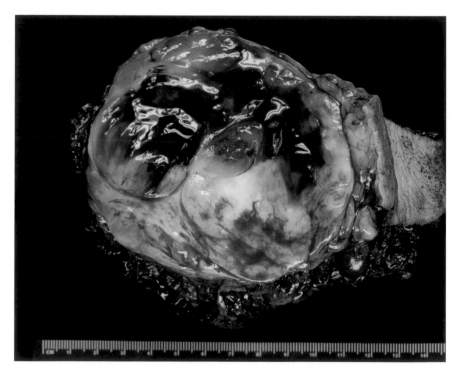

low-grade lesions (189,190). However, progression in histologic grade has been associated with an increase in cytogenetic aberrations (191). A diverse pattern of NF1 aberrations, including point mutations and deletions, is present in 10 percent of tumors (192).

Differential Diagnosis. At the low-grade end of the spectrum, myxofibrosarcomas may be difficult to distinguish from a cellular myxoma. Myxomas are typically hypovascular and lack the distinctive curvilinear vasculature and degree of cytologic atypia displayed by myxofibrosarcomas. In challenging diagnostic cases, molecular studies can be applied, since in contrast to cellular myxoma, no activating missense mutations at Arg201 codon of the *GNAS1* gene, encoding the alpha subunit of Gs, are demonstrated in myxofibrosarcomas (193).

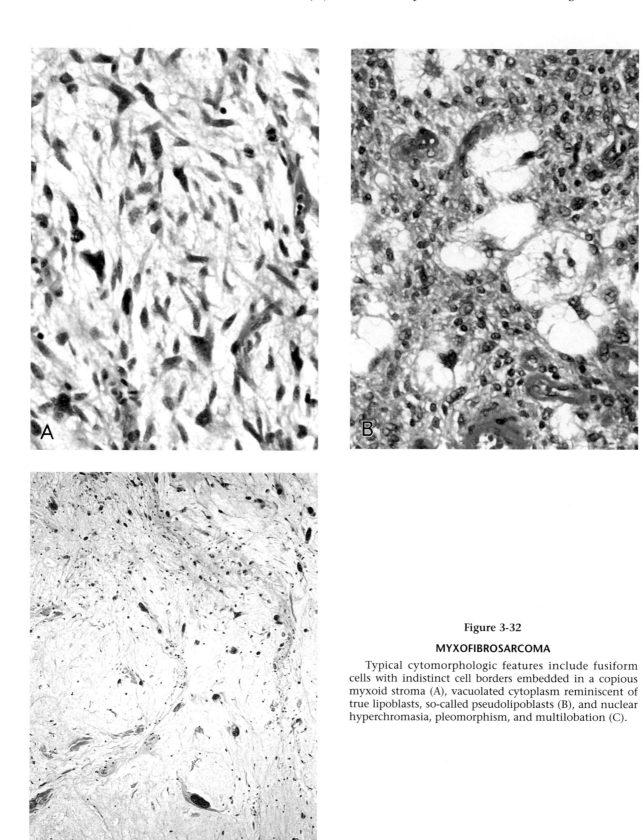

Figure 3-32

MYXOFIBROSARCOMA

Typical cytomorphologic features include fusiform cells with indistinct cell borders embedded in a copious myxoid stroma (A), vacuolated cytoplasm reminiscent of true lipoblasts, so-called pseudolipoblasts (B), and nuclear hyperchromasia, pleomorphism, and multilobation (C).

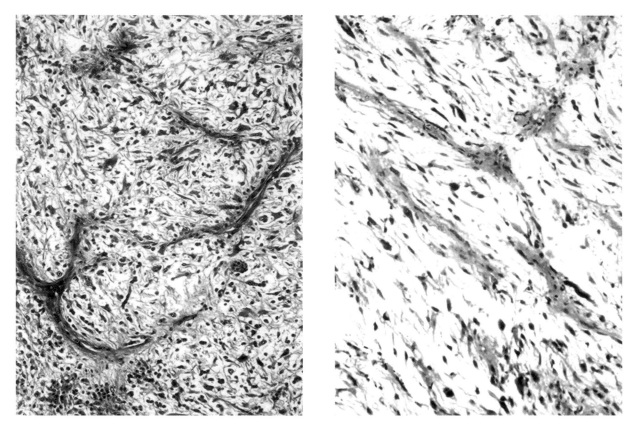

Figure 3-33

MYXOFIBROSARCOMA

Left, Right: Distinctive histologic features include curvilinear vessels, which have thicker walls with conspicuous pericytic cells, as well as perivascular condensation of tumor cells.

Low-grade myxofibrosarcomas may resemble myxoid liposarcoma, particularly in a limited, small biopsy sample; however, the degree of spindling, hyperchromasia, and nuclear pleomorphism is significantly higher in myxofibrosarcomas. Furthermore, the chicken-wire capillary network seen in myxoid liposarcoma is very delicate, lacking the perivascular condensations of myxofibrosarcoma tumor cells.

At the high-grade end of the spectrum, myxofibrosarcomas may be confused with a pleomorphic liposarcoma. The presence of pleomorphic lipoblasts confirms a diagnosis of pleomorphic liposarcoma. In the retroperitoneum, dedifferentiated liposarcoma may resemble myxofibrosarcomas. Nuclear immunoreactivity or gene amplification by FISH for MDM2 and immunohistochemistry for CDK4 help establish the diagnosis of dedifferentiated liposarcoma.

Treatment and Prognosis. The therapy of choice for primary myxofibrosarcoma is wide surgical resection. The role of postoperative radiation with positive surgical margins remains controversial (194,195). Myxofibrosarcoma often has an indolent course, but with a high propensity for local recurrence, ranging from 55 to 63 percent (175,176,182,183). The rate of local recurrence is independent of the histologic grade and the depth of tumor invasion (176,183). The characteristic growth pattern is horizontal spread along fascial planes (fig. 3-35A), with extension to the dermis (fig. 3-35B) and well beyond the primary mass, infiltrating the subcutaneous tissues (fig. 3-35C) or muscle, which likely, or at least partly, accounts for its propensity for multiple recurrences. Myxofibrosarcoma tends to become progressively higher in grade as recurrences occur; therefore, even low-grade tumors must

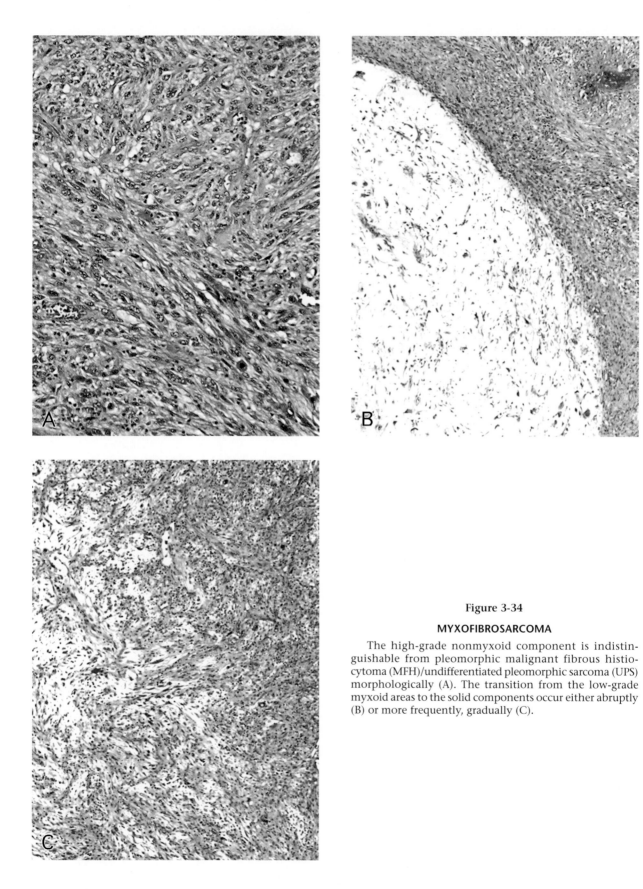

Figure 3-34

MYXOFIBROSARCOMA

The high-grade nonmyxoid component is indistinguishable from pleomorphic malignant fibrous histiocytoma (MFH)/undifferentiated pleomorphic sarcoma (UPS) morphologically (A). The transition from the low-grade myxoid areas to the solid components occur either abruptly (B) or more frequently, gradually (C).

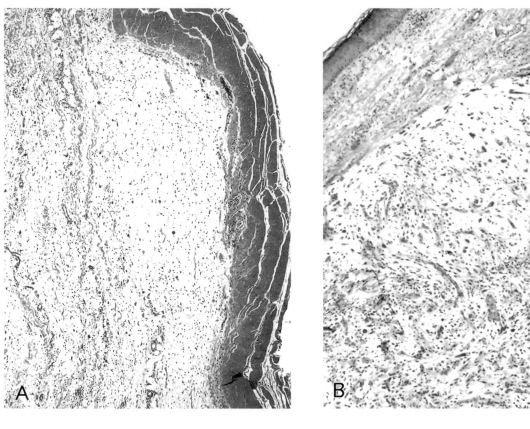

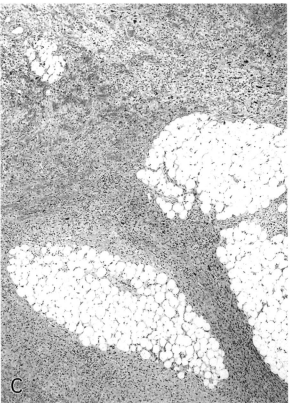

Figure 3-35

MYXOFIBROSARCOMA

The distinctive pattern of local invasion of low-grade myxofibrosarcoma includes horizontal spread of the tumor along the fascial plane, and even in the case of large size tumors, the fascia is often spared and the tumor remains superficially located (A). The tumor also may extend to involve dermis (B) and typically spreads away from the grossly identified nodular mass, showing diffusely infiltrative growth within subcutaneous fat (C).

be diligently followed and monitored for local recurrence (176,183). Progression to higher grade increases the risk of distant metastasis from 16 percent to as high as 23 percent (176). Metastases are also seen in larger (over 10 cm) and deep-seated tumors (175), but are still less common than in other high-grade sarcomas. Recurrence within 12 months of original resection is associated with a higher mortality rate (176). The nonmyxoid histology seen in fewer than 75 percent of the tumors seems to be associated with decreased disease-specific survival (188).

MALIGNANT FIBROUS HISTIOCYTOMA/UNDIFFERENTIATED PLEOMORPHIC SARCOMA

Definition. *Malignant fibrous histiocytoma /undifferentiated pleomorphic sarcoma* (MFH/UPS) is a pleomorphic sarcoma that lacks a specific line of differentiation after judicious sampling and application of ancillary techniques. Despite a remarkable heterogeneity in morphologic appearance, the lesions share a high degree of nuclear pleomorphism and often show a storiform growth pattern.

General Considerations. The term malignant fibrous histiocytoma was coined by Stout and associates in the 1960s to encompass pleomorphic soft tissue sarcomas presumably derived from histiocytes that are capable of fibroblastic transformation (196,197). However, recent, more critical clinicopathologic, ultrastructural, and immunohistochemical studies have shown that MFH is not derived from histiocytic "facultative fibroblasts" and many neoplasms so diagnosed actually are pleomorphic subtypes of other sarcomas (198,199). Thus, with the application of immunohistochemical studies to clinical practice, it has been suggested that most pleomorphic sarcomas show a definable line of differentiation, including pleomorphic variants of leiomyosarcoma, liposarcoma, rhabdomyosarcoma, and myxofibrosarcoma. As such, the incidence of MFH has sharply fallen from the most common soft tissue sarcoma in adults to only a small subset (5 to 13 percent) of pleomorphic sarcomas (198,200,201).

In the 2002 WHO classification of soft tissue and bone tumors, the term undifferentiated pleomorphic sarcoma was introduced and used interchangeably with pleomorphic MFH, which defines a small group of tumors that by current methodology shows no detectable line of differentiation. The decreased incidence in the diagnosis of pleomorphic MFH/UPS can also be explained by the fact that a significant number of formerly diagnosed pleomorphic MFHs, exhibiting some but less than 50 percent myxoid component, are now reclassified as high-grade myxofibrosarcoma (see previous section). To reflect the fall in its popularity, at the recent 2012 WHO consensus meeting, the MFH/UPS group lost its own category and was lumped with other undifferentiated soft tissue sarcomas (USTS), including tumors that show predominantly a small blue round cell, spindle, or epithelioid phenotype. One of the main arguments supporting that MFH/UPS is a waste-basket diagnosis is that many other soft tissue tumors share the ubiquitous storiform-pleomorphic pattern, including pleomorphic liposarcoma and dedifferentiated liposarcoma, among the most common. Thorough sampling of these tumors usually provides evidence of the better-differentiated areas, such as the presence of a lipomatous component. This has been the case in retroperitoneum/intra-abdominal locations, but it is still debatable for extremity locations.

Clinical Features. MFH/UPS tends to occur in the extremities, more often in the lower limbs, of elderly patients (peak incidence in the sixth and seventh decades). The lesions are typically deep seated and present as progressively enlarging masses. A few patients present with disseminated disease, mostly to the lungs, at diagnosis.

Gross and Microscopic Findings. The gross appearance is typically heterogeneous, with areas of gelatinous, firm, and fleshy components, admixed with areas of necrosis and cystic hemorrhagic change (fig. 3-36). Microscopically, the lesions also show a variegated appearance, from tumor to tumor, and within different areas of the tumor (fig. 3-37). They all, however, have in common a high degree of nuclear pleomorphism, often with multinucleated and bizarre giant cells, with dense hyperchromatic nuclei (fig. 3-38). The nonpleomorphic cellular component exhibits a variable cytomorphology, ranging from spindle to more epithelioid (figs. 3-39, 3-40). The spindle cells are typically arranged in a storiform pattern or intersect in short fascicles,

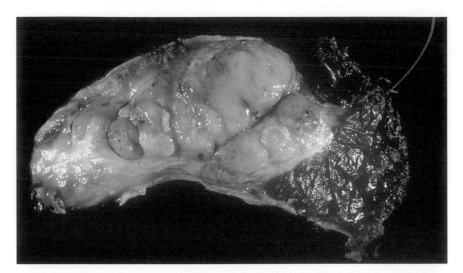

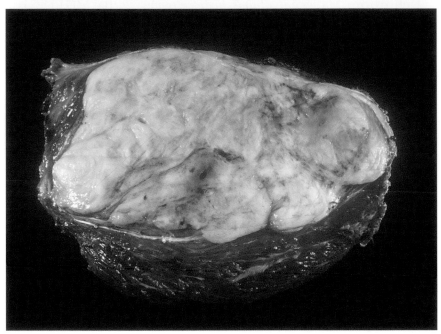

Figure 3-36

MALIGNANT FIBROUS HISTIOCYTOMA/ UNDIFFERENTIATED PLEOMORPHIC SARCOMA

Top, Bottom: A large, multi_nodular mass, with a fleshy, tan-yellow cut surface, has chalky areas of necrosis involving sub-cutis and skeletal muscle.

and show a modest amount of amphophilic to pale eosinophilic cytoplasm. The nuclei are fusiform, with open or vesicular chromatin and inconspicuous nucleoli (figs. 3-37, 3-39). The epithelioid/histiocytoid cells display moderate to abundant eosinophilic or vacuolated cytoplasm and eccentric nuclei (fig. 3-40). In some cases, the histiocytoid cells have more basophilic cyto-plasm and open chromatin with large, virocyte-like nucleoli (fig. 3-40C). Occasional osteoclast-type giant cells may be seen scattered, although rarely represent a predominant feature (figs. 3-37B, 3-38B). The extracellular stroma varies

from myxoid to more often densely sclerotic (fig. 3-37D). Areas of necrosis and increased mitotic activity, including atypical mitotic figures, are typically present (fig. 3-38).

Special Studies. A wide panel of immuno-histochemical studies is required in the work-up of a MFH/UPS lesion, in order to exclude other nonmesenchymal neoplasms such as carcinoma, melanoma, or lymphoma. Immuno-histochemical stains are not helpful for distin-guishing between other mesenchymal lesions sharing a pleomorphic phenotype, since MFH shows mainly fibroblastic and myofibroblastic

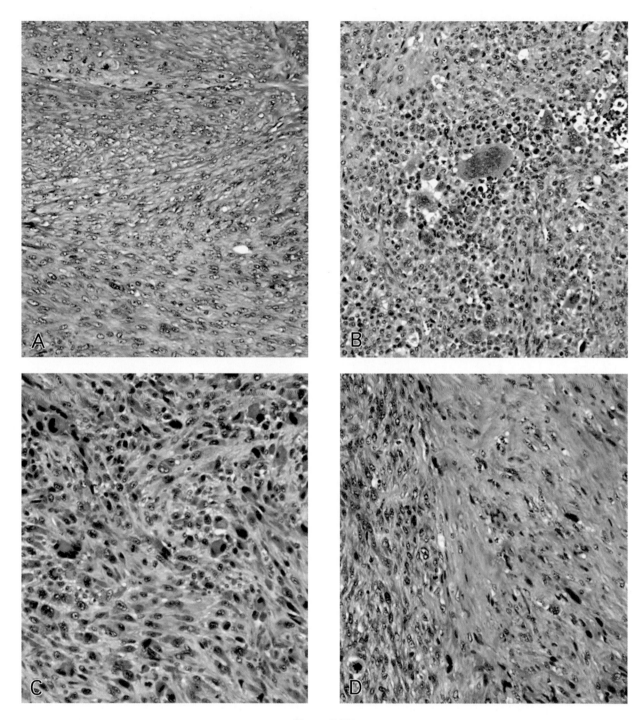

Figure 3-37

MALIGNANT FIBROUS HISTIOCYTOMA/UNDIFFERENTIATED PLEOMORPHIC SARCOMA

The microscopic appearance is characterized typically by marked heterogeneity, with a wide range of morphologies within the same tumor (59-year-old man with a large thigh mass).

A: Spindle cell areas with bland nuclei, arranged in long, intersecting fascicles reminiscent of fibrosarcoma or desmoid-like morphology.

B: Rounded, primitive cells with scattered multinucleated, osteoclast-type giant cells.

C: Pleomorphic and histiocytoid cells with eccentric and multilobated nuclei.

D: Sclerotic areas.

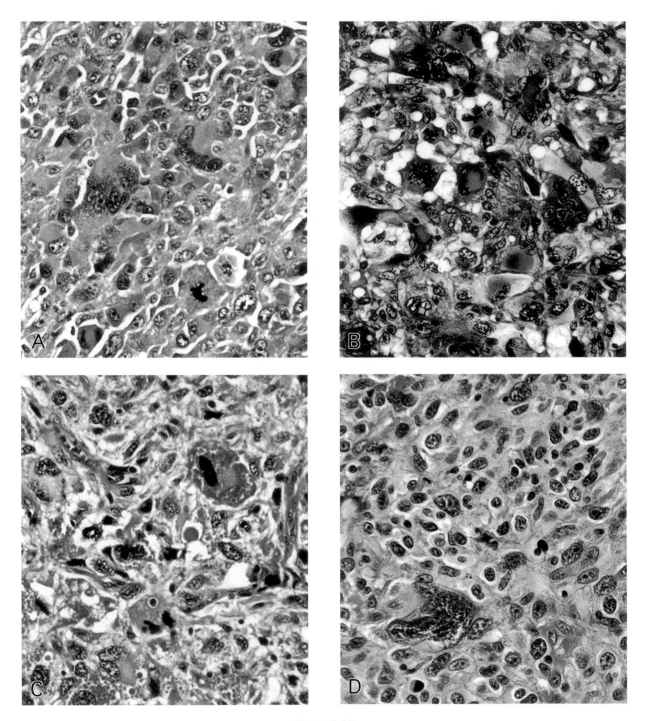

Figure 3-38

MALIGNANT FIBROUS HISTIOCYTOMA/UNDIFFERENTIATED PLEOMORPHIC SARCOMA

Marked nuclear pleomorphism is the hallmark microscopic feature.

A: Multinucleated, bizarre tumor cells with abundant eosinophilic cytoplasm and atypical mitoses.

B: Rare osteoclast-type giant cells are intermixed with the multinucleated, pleomorphic tumor cells.

C: Pleomorphic tumor cells may show occasionally abundant eosinophilic globules, most likely representing dilated phagolysosomes.

D: The bizarre, multilobated tumor cells sometimes represent a focal finding, admixed with short fusiform cells with open, vesicular chromatin.

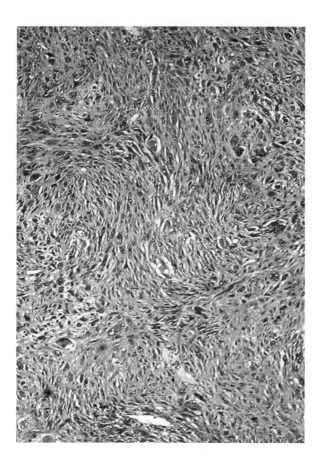 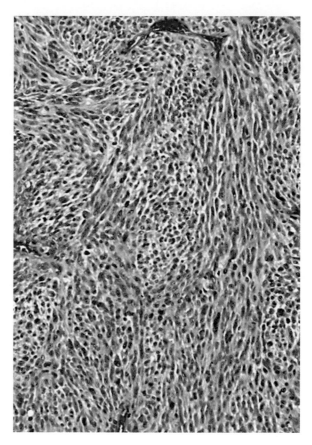

Figure 3-39

MALIGNANT FIBROUS HISTIOCYTOMA/UNDIFFERENTIATED PLEOMORPHIC SARCOMA

Left: The spindle cell component is present in different proportions, and often arranged in a storiform, pin-wheel growth pattern.

Right: Occasionally, a herring-bone arrangement, reminiscent of an adult-type fibrosarcoma, is noted.

differentiation, with common vimentin and focal actin reactivity.

The expression of muscle markers, including actin or desmin, has been shown in a subset of pleomorphic MFHs, with suggested prognostic implications (see below). So-called histiocytic markers, such as CD68 and MAC56, show positivity in a significant number of cells, but are of no diagnostic value. In retroperitoneal locations, MDM2 and CDK4 immunoreactivities in MFH/UPS-like tumors are able to exclude this diagnosis and confirm a dedifferentiated liposarcoma.

Genetics. The tumors are associated with a highly complex karyotype, and numerous but non-recurrent structural aberrations (202). Cytogenetic signs of amplification, ring chromosomes, and double minutes are often seen.

The TP53 and RB1 pathways are inactivated in virtually all tumors (203,204).

Differential Diagnosis. MFH/UPS is a diagnosis by exclusion, and sarcomatoid carcinoma (extensive keratin expression), melanoma (S-100 positive), and specific sarcoma types have to be excluded by detailed histologic examination and immunohistochemistry. The diagnosis of lipoblast-poor pleomorphic liposarcoma can be confirmed only after identifying focal lipoblasts. Dedifferentiated liposarcoma is substantiated by the presence of well-differentiated liposarcoma or *MDM2/CDK4* gene amplification. Pleomorphic leiomyosarcoma is typically confirmed by the presence of residual differentiated areas by extensive sampling, or by diffuse positivity of at least two muscle markers, such as desmin or caldesmon. The focal expression of actins or

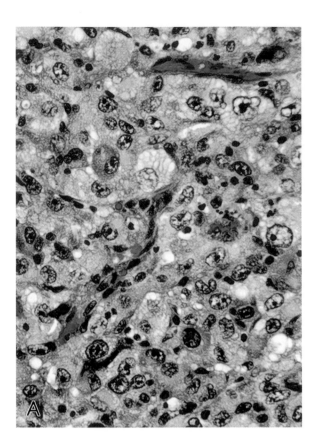

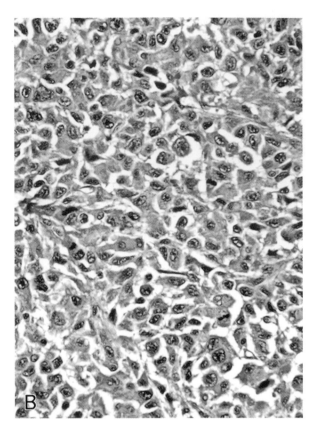

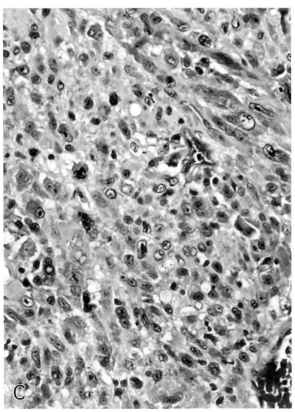

Figure 3-40

**MALIGNANT FIBROUS HISTIOCYTOMA/
UNDIFFERENTIATED PLEOMORPHIC SARCOMA**

The epithelioid or histiocytoid cell component is a consistent cellular phenotype. The cytomorphologic appearance ranges from solid sheets of large histiocytoid cells with vacuolated eosinophilic cytoplasm intermixed with a chronic inflammatory infiltrate (A); discohesive sheets of epithelioid cells with dense eosinophilic cytoplasm and eccentric nuclei with vesicular chromatin and only slight pleomorphism (B); and histiocytoid cells with basophilic cytoplasm and virocyte-like nucleoli, reminiscent of Reed-Sternberg cells (C).

desmin is more in keeping with MFH/UPS with myofibroblastic differentiation.

Treatment and Prognosis. The primary treatment is surgical. The ability to gain negative margins in these lesions can be challenging. In metastatic settings, MFH/UPS may respond to doxorubicin-, ifosfamide-, or gemcitabine-docetaxel-type regimes. Patients have a substantial risk of metastatic disease, with a disease-specific survival rate of approximately 60 percent at 10 years.

Large size (over 10 cm), deep-seated location, and high grade are all unfavorable prognostic markers. Myoid differentiation (defined as positivity for at least one muscle marker) is an independent indicator of adverse prognosis in adult patients with pleomorphic sarcomas in general, including MFH/UPS of the extremity (198,205,206).

PLEOMORPHIC HYALINIZING ANGIECTATIC TUMOR

Definition. *Pleomorphic hyalinizing angiectatic tumor* (PHAT) is a pleomorphic mesenchymal neoplasm of low malignant potential.

Clinical Features. PHAT occurs in adults of all ages. The median reported patient age is 54 years, with a mild female predominance. The tumor most commonly occurs in the distal lower extremity: foot, ankle, and lower leg. The tumor is also reported in the trunk and upper extremity. It is usually subcutaneous, but rare examples are intramuscular. The tumor size varies from a nodule smaller than 1 cm to a large mass over 30 cm, with a median size of 5 to 6 cm (207–209).

Gross and Microscopic Findings. Grossly, PHAT may be circumscribed or with diffuse borders. On sectioning, the tumor varies form whitish tan to red-purple.

Histologically distinctive is the presence of clusters of dilated blood vessels that often contain luminal thrombosis and fibrinous or hyaline material in walls resembling the vascular changes commonly seen in schwannoma (fig. 3-41). The cellular element often infiltrates the subcutaneous fat and is spindled to epithelioid and pleomorphic. Focal cytoplasmic hemosiderin pigment may be present, giving the cytoplasm a brownish appearance. Moderate nuclear pleomorphism and intranuclear vacuolization

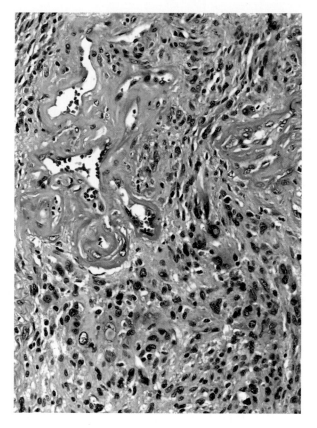

Figure 3-41

PLEOMORPHIC HYALINIZING ANGIECTATIC TUMOR

The tumor is characterized by ovoid to pleomorphic mesenchymal cells with intranuclear pseudoinclusions. The vascular hyalinizing changes resemble those seen in schwannoma.

(cytoplasmic inclusions) are often detected. The mitotic rate is low, and the presence of high mitotic activity and atypical mitoses should prompt an alternative diagnosis (sarcoma). A series describing spindle cell proliferations with similar vascular changes suggested that these may represent precursors to PHAT (209).

Immunohistochemically the tumor cells are often positive for CD34 but are negative for S-100 protein, smooth muscle actin, and desmin.

Differential Diagnosis. Pleomorphic mesenchymal neoplasms with marked nuclear atypia and mitotic activity, especially if atypical mitoses are present, are better considered myxofibrosarcomas or pleomorphic undifferentiated sarcomas (MFH). Negativity for S-100 protein helps to separate this tumor from schwannoma with nuclear atypia.

Treatment and Prognosis. Complete excision with negative margins should be performed whenever possible, as the tumor has a significant potential to recur after simple excision. Recurrences may develop long (over 10 years) after primary surgery so that long-term follow-up is necessary. Metastases have not been reported. Several reports describe similarities or conversions between PHAT and myxofibrosarcoma, so that PHAT may be a precursor lesion or closely related to the latter (210–212).

GIANT CELL TUMOR OF SOFT PARTS AND GIANT CELL MALIGNANT FIBROUS HISTIOCYTOMA

Definition. *Giant cell tumor of soft parts* is a lobulated mesenchymal tumor distinct from tenosynovial giant cell tumor and rich in osteoclastic giant cells. It often contains metaplastic bone, with minimal or no low-grade malignant features. *Malignant giant cell tumor of soft parts* is synonymous with giant cell type of *malignant fibrous histiocytoma* (MFH, undifferentiated high-grade sarcoma) and contains numerous osteoclastic giant cells with an often multinodular histologic pattern.

General Comments. Giant cell tumors of soft parts and giant cell type of MFH belong to a spectrum of giant cell-rich tumors in which the essential neoplastic component is fibroblastic or myofibroblastic. The benign end of this spectrum is classified as giant cell tumor of soft parts, which is a benign tumor with a potential to recur. It has been likened to giant cell tumor of bone. In contrast, giant cell tumors with significant stromal nuclear atypia and mitotic activity, comparable to other intermediate- to high-grade sarcomas, are classified as giant cell MFH (malignant giant cell tumor of soft parts).

Clinical Features. Giant cell tumor of soft parts occurs in a wide age range, including children. Collective data from the larger series suggest a mild male predominance (213–215). Most of these tumors occur in the extremities: arm, thigh, knee, and leg are the most common locations, but examples have also been reported from the hands and feet. Trunk wall and body cavities (retroperitoneum) are rare locations. Approximately 60 percent of the tumors are subcutaneous or dermal, and 40 percent are deep to the superficial fascia. By definition, origin from bone (giant cell tumor of the bone) has to be ruled out (213–216).

Giant cell MFH typically occurs in older adults and usually presents as a deep, often large (over 5-10 cm) intramuscular mass (217,218).

Gross Findings. Giant cell tumor of soft parts typically forms a circumscribed nodule or larger mass measuring 1 to 10 cm. The median sizes in the four published series are 2 to 4 cm (213–216). The cut surface appears reddish or gray and varies from fleshy to rubbery. Most tumors are subcutaneous (213–216).

Microscopic Findings. Histologically typical is a multinodular pattern with fibrous septa dividing the tumor into cellular lobules; a peripheral rim of metaplastic bone may be present. The cellular areas are conspicuously rich in evenly distributed osteoclast-like giant cells. There is a mononuclear element, which may be composed of round, oval, or spindled cells. Atypia is limited in this component, and bizarre giant cells do not occur (fig. 3-42). The mitotic rate varies widely, averaging 3 mitoses per 10 high-power fields, but may be as high as over 30 mitoses. Necrosis is uncommon, but vascular invasion is often detected and has no adverse significance in this tumor.

Giant cell MFH also forms a multinodular mass. It consists of osteoclastic giant cells and admixed stromal cells that show high-grade nuclear atypia and significant mitotic activity, including atypical mitotic figures (fig. 3-43). Tumor necrosis and hemorrhage are common (217,218).

Differential Diagnosis. Tenosynovial giant cell tumor (giant cell tumor of tendon sheath) is a clinically and pathologically distinctive tumor that should be separated from this group. These tumors are almost always benign. They typically show an admixture of osteoclastic giant cells and small epithelioid neoplastic cells in a variably sclerosing stroma that often contains numerous xanthoma cells. Tumors that contain osteoid associated with malignant cells (malignant osteoid formation) are better classified as (extraskeletal) osteosarcomas. Osteoclastic giant cells may be present in many other tumors, such as certain carcinomas (for example, pancreatic). These have to be ruled out, especially in the organ-based tumors.

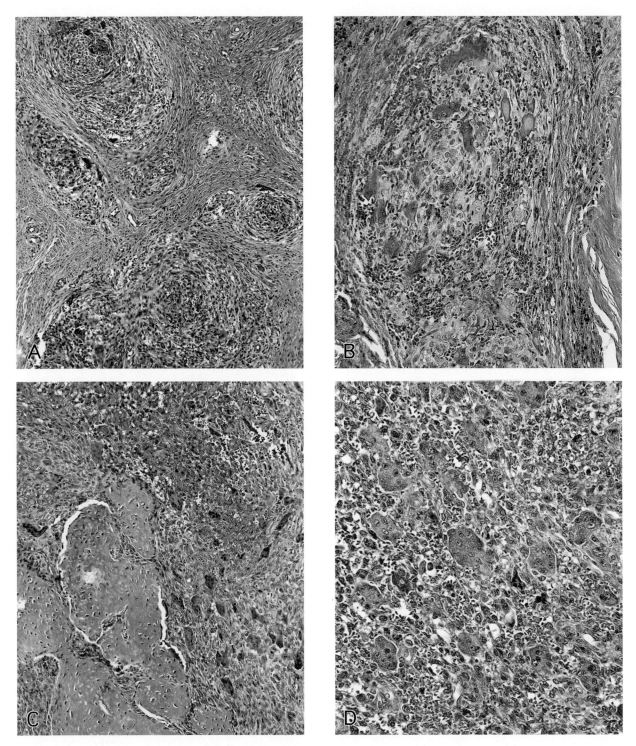

Figure 3-42

GIANT CELL TUMOR OF SOFT PARTS

A: The tumor is often multinodular.

B: The individual nodules are composed of bland mononuclear cells and multinucleated osteoclast-like giant cells.

C,D: Focal osteoid is often present.

D: The overall appearance may resemble that of giant cell tumor of bone.

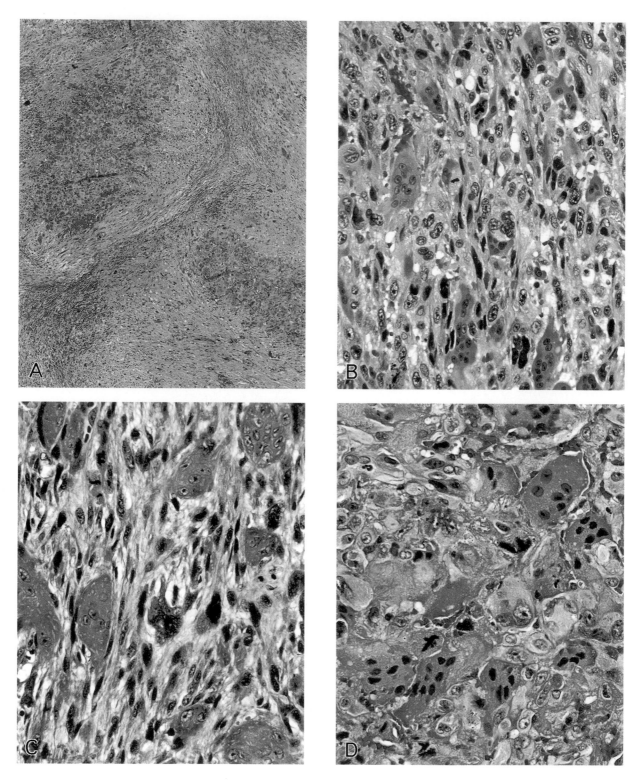

Figure 3-43

GIANT CELL MALIGNANT FIBROUS HISTIOCYTOMA

Like giant cell tumor of soft parts, this tumor also forms a multinodular mass (A), but in contrast, contains a highly atypical mononuclear neoplastic cellular population, often with atypical mitoses (B–D).

Treatment and Prognosis. Tumors with limited nuclear atypia have an excellent prognosis, with potential for local recurrence after an incomplete excision. None of the patients in current series have extensive long-term follow-up, and further studies are needed to confirm the biologic potential of these lesions. This especially applies to large and deep tumors.

Giant cell MFH is generally a high-grade tumor with significant potential for both local recurrence and distant metastasis. Its treatment is similar to that for other MFHs.

REFERENCES

Solitary Fibrous Tumor

1. England DM, Hochholzer L, McCarthy MJ. Localized benign and malignant fibrous tumors of the pleura. A clinicopathologic review of 223 cases. Am J Surg Pathol 1989;13:640-658.
2. Enzinger FM, Smith BH. Hemangiopericytoma. An analysis of 106 cases. Hum Pathol 1976;7:61-82.
3. Nascimento AG. Solitary fibrous tumor: A ubiquitous neoplasm of mesenchymal differentiation. Adv Anat Pathol 1996;3:388-395.
4. Nielsen GP, O'Connell JX, Dickersin GR, Rosenberg AE. Solitary fibrous tumor of soft tissue: a report of 15 cases, including 5 malignant examples with light microscopic, immunohistochemical and ultrastructural data. Mod Pathol 1997;10:1028-1037.
5. Fukunaga M, Naganuma H, Nikaido T, Harada T, Ushigome S. Extrapleural solitary fibrous tumor: a report of seven cases. Mod Pathol 1997;10:443-450.
6. Vallat-Decouvelaere AV, Dry SM, Fletcher CD. Atypical and malignant solitary fibrous tumors in extrathoracic locations: evidence of their comparability to intra-thoracic tumors. Am J Surg Pathol 1998;22:1501-1511.
7. Brunnemann RB, Ro JY, Ordonez NG, Mooney J, El-Naggar AK, Ayala AG. Extrapleural solitary fibrous tumor: a clinicopathologic study of 24 cases. Mod Pathol 1999;12:1034-1042.
8. Hasegawa T, Matsuno Y, Shimoda T, Hasegawa F, Sano T, Hirohashi S. Extrathoracic solitary fibrous tumors: their histological variability and potentially aggressive behavior. Hum Pathol 1999;30:1464-1473.
9. Morimitsu Y, Nakajima M, Hisaoka M, Hashimoto H. Extrapleural solitary fibrous tumor: clinicopathologic study of 17 cases and molecular analysis of the p53 pathway. APMIS 2000;108:617-625.
10. Alawi F, Stratton D, Freedman PD. Solitary fibrous tumor of oral soft tissues: a clinicopathologic and immunohistochemical study of 16 cases. Am J Surg Pathol 2001;25:900-910.
11. Bernardini FP, de Conciliis C, Schneider S, Kersten RC, Kulwin DR. Solitary fibrous tumor of the orbit: is it rare? Report of a case series and review of literature. Ophthalmology 2003;110:1442-1448.
12. Witkin GB, Rosai J. Solitary fibrous tumor of the upper respiratory tract. A report of six cases. Am J Surg Pathol 1991;15:842-848.
13. Erdag G, Qureshi HS, Patterson JW, Wick MR. Solitary fibrous tumor of the skin: a clinicopathologic study of 10 cases and review of the literature. J Cutan Pathol 2007;34:844-850.
14. Strom EH, Skjorten F, Aarseth LB, Haug E. Solitary fibrous tumor of the pleura. An immunohistochemical, electron microscopic and tissue culture study of a tumor producing insulin-like growth factor I in a patient with hypoglycemia. Pathol Res Pract 1991;187:109-113.
15. Fukasawa Y, Takada A, Tateno M, et al. Solitary fibrous tumor of the pleura causing recurrent hypoglycemia by secretion of insulin-like growth factor II. Pathol Int 1998;48:47-52.
16. Hajdu M, Singer S, Maki RG, Schwartz GK, Keohan ML, Antonescu CR. IFG2-over-expression in solitary fibrous tumors in independent of anatomical location is related to loss of imprinting. J Pathol 2010;221:300-307.
17. Dei Tos A, Seregard S, Calonje E, Chan JK, Fletcher CD. Giant cell angiofibroma. A distinctive orbital tumor in adults. Am J Surg Pathol 1995;19:1286-1293.
18. Guillou L, Gebhard S, Coindre JM. Orbital and extraorbital giant cell angiofibroma: a giant cell-rich variant of solitary fibrous tumor? Clinicopathologic, immunohistochemical, and ultrastructural analysis of a series in favor of a unifying concept. Am J Surg Pathol 2000;24:971-979.
19. Thomas R, Banerjee SS, Eyden BP, et al. A study of four cases of giant cell angiofibroma with documentation of some unusual features. Histopathology 2001;39:390-396.

20. Nielsen GP, Dickersin GR, Provenzal JM, Rosenberg AE. Lipomatous hemangiopericytoma. A histologic, ultrastructural and immunohistochemical study of a unique variant of hemangiopericytoma. Am J Surg Pathol 1995;19:748-756.

21. Folpe AL, Devaney K, Weiss SW. Lipomatous hemangiopericytoma: a rare variant of hemangiopericytoma that may be confused with liposarcoma. Am J Surgical Pathol 1999;23:1201-1207.

22. Guillou L, Gebhard S, Coindre JM. Lipomatous hemangiopericytoma: a fat-containing variant of solitary fibrous tumor? Clinicopathologic, immunohistochemical, and ultrastructural analysis of a series in favor of a unifying concept. Hum Pathol 2000;31:1108-1115.

23. Lee JC, Fletcher CD. Malignant fat-forming solitary fibrous tumor (so-called "lipomatoud hemangipericytoma"): clinicopathologic analysis of 14 cases. Am J Surg Pathol 2011;35:1177-1185.

24. Mosquera JM, Fletcher CD. Expanding the spectrum of malignant progression in solitary fibrous tumors: a study of 8 cases with a dsicrete anaplastic component—is this dedifferentiated SFT? Am J Surg Pathol 2009;33:1314-1321.

25. van de Rijn M, Lombard CM, Rouse RV. Expression of CD34 by solitary fibrous tumors of the pleura, mediastinum, and lung. Am J Surg Pathol 1994;18:814-820.

26. Flint A, Weiss SW. CD-34 and keratin expression distinguishes solitary fibrous tumor (fibrous mesothelioma) of pleura from desmoplastic mesothelioma. Hum Pathol 1995;26:428-431.

27. Chilosi M, Facchetti F, DeiTos AP, et al. bcl-2 expression in pleural and extrapleural solitary fibrous tumours. J Pathol 1997;181:362-367.

28. Ng TL, Gown AM, Barry TS, et al. Nuclear beta-catenin in mesenchymal tumors. Mod Pathol 2005;18:68-74.

29. Dal Cin P, Pauwels P, Van Den Berghe H. Solitary fibrous tumor of the pleura with t(4;15)(q13;q26). Histopathology 1999;35:94-95.

30. Debiec-Rychter M, de Wever I, Hagemeijer A, Sciot R. Is 4q13 a recurring breakpoint in solitary fibrous tumors? Cancer Genet Cytogenet 2001;131:69-73.

31. Donner LR, Silva MT, Dobin SM. Solitary fibrous tumor of the pleura: a cytogenetic study. Cancer Genet Cytogenet 1999;111:169-171.

32. Robinson DR, Wu YM, Kalyana-Sundaram S, et al. Identification of recurrent NAB2-STAT6 gene fusions in solitary fibrous tumor by integrative sequencing. Nat Genet 2013;45:180-185.

33. Chmielecki J, Crago AM, Rosenberg M, et al. Whole-exome sequencing identifies a recurrent NAB2-STAT6 fusion in solitary fibrous tumors. Nat Genet 2013;45:131-132.

34. Tsuneyoshi M, Daimaru Y, Enjoji M. Malignant hemangiopericytoma and other sarcomas with hemangiopericytoma-like pattern. Pathol Res Pract 1984;178:446-453.

35. Mentzel T, Calonje E, Nascimento AG, Fletcher CD. Infantile hemangiopericytoma versus infantile myofibromatosis. Study of a series suggesting a continuous spectrum of infantile myofibroblastic lesions. Am J Surg Pathol 1994;18:922-930.

Dermatofibrosarcoma Protuberans

36. Bowne WB, Antonescu CR, Leung DH, et al. Dermatofibrosarcoma protuberans. A clinicopathologic analysis of patients treated and followed at a single institution. Cancer 2000;88:2711-2720.

37. Connelly JH, Evans HL. Dermatofibrosarcoma protuberans. A clinicopathologic review with emphasis on fibrosarcomatous areas. Am J Surg Pathol 1992;16:921-925.

38. Goldblum JR. CD34 positivity in fibrosarcomas which arise in dermatofibrosarcoma protuberans. Arch Pathol Lab Med 1995;119:238-241.

39. Goldblum JR, Reith JD, Weiss SW. Sarcomas arising in dermatofibrosarcoma protuberans: a reappraisal of biologic behavior in eighteen cases treated by wide local excision with extended clinical follow up. Am J Surg Pathol 2000;24:1125-1130.

40. Mentzel T, Beham A, Katenkamp D, Dei Tos AP, Fletcher CD. Fibrosarcomatous ("high-grade") dermatofibrosarcoma protuberans: clinicopathologic and immunohistochemical study of a series of 41 cases with emphasis on prognostic significance. Am J Surg Pathol 1998;22:576-587.

41. Sandberg AA, Bridge JA. Updates on the cytogenetics and molecular genetics of bone and soft tissue tumors. Dermatofibrosarcoma protuberans and giant cell fibroblastoma. Cancer Genet Cytogenet 2003;140:1-12.

42. Sirvent N, Maire G, Pedeutour F. Genetics of dermatofibrosarcoma protuberans family of tumors: from ring chromosomes to tyrosine kinase inhibitor treatment. Genes Chromosomes Cancer 2003;37:1-19.

43. Terrier-Lacombe MJ, Guillou L, Maire G, et al. Dermatofibrosarcoma protuberans, giant cell fibroblastoma, and hybrid lesions in children: clinicopathologic comparative analysis of 28 cases with molecular data—a study from the French Federation of Cancer Centers Sarcoma Group. Am J Surg Pathol 2003;27:27-39.

44. Vanni R, Faa G, Dettori T, Dumanski JP, O'Brien KP. A case of dermatofibrosarcoma protuberans of the vulva with a COL1A1/PDGFB fusion identical to a case of giant cell fibroblastoma. Virchows Arch 2000;437:95-100.

45. Checketts SR, Hamilton TK, Baughman RD. Congenital and childhood dermatofibrosarcoma: a case report and review of the literature. J Am Acad Dermatol 2000;42:907-913.

46. Maire G, Fraitag S, Galmiche L, et al. A clinical, histologic, and molecular study of 9 cases of congenital dermatofibrosarcoma protuberans. Arch Dermatol 2007;143:203-210.

47. McKee PH, Fletcher CD. Dermatofibrosarcoma protuberans presenting in infancy and childhood. J Cutan Pathol 1991;18:241-246.

48. Burkhardt BR, Soule EH, Winkelmann RK, Ivins JC. Dermatofibrosarcoma protuberans. Study of fifty-six cases. Am J Surg 1966;111:638-644.

49. McPeak CJ, Cruz T, Nicastri AD. Dermatofibrosarcoma protuberans: an analysis of 86 cases—five with metastasis. Ann Surg 1967;166:803-816.

50. Taylor HB, Helwig EB. Dermatofibrosarcoma protuberans. A study of 115 cases. Cancer 1962;15:717-725.

51. Abbott JJ, Oliveira AM, Nascimento AG. The prognostic significance of fibrosarcomatous transformation in dermatofibrosarcoma protuberans. Am J Surg Pathol 2006;30:436-443.

52. Alvarez-Canas MC, Mayorga M, Fernandez F, et al. Dermatofibrosarcoma protuberans of the vulva: clinico-pathological, immunohistochemical and flow cytometric study of a case. Acta Obstet Gynecol Scand 1996;75:82-85.

53. McArthur G. Dermatofibrosarcoma protuberans: recent clinical progress. Ann Surg Oncol 2007;14:2876-2886.

54. Roses DF, Valensi Q, LaTrenta G, Harris MN. Surgical treatment of dermatofibrosarcoma protuberans. Surg Gynecol Obstet 1986;162:449-452.

55. Fletcher CD, Evans BJ, Macartney JC, Smith N, Wilson Jones E, McKee PH. Dermatofibrosarcoma protuberans: a clinicopathologic and immunhistochemical study with a review of the literature. Histopathology 1985;9:921-938.

56. Díaz-Cascajo C, Weyers W, Borrego L, Iñarrea JB, Borghi S. Dermatofibrosarcoma protuberans with fibrosarcomatous areas: a clinico-pathologic and immunohistochemical study in four cases. Am J Dermatopathol 1997;19:562-567.

57. Wrotnowski U, Cooper PH, Shmookler BM. Fibrosarcomatous change in dermatofibrosarcoma protuberans. Am J Surg Pathol 1988;12:287-293.

58. Frierson HF, Cooper PH. Myxoid variant of dermatofibrosarcoma protuberans. Am J Surg Pathol 1983;7:445-450.

59. Mentzel T, Schärer L, Kazakov DV, Michal M. Myxoid dermatofibrosarcoma protuberans: clinicopathologic, immunohistochemical, and molecular analysis of eight cases. Am J Dermatopathol 2007;29:443-448.

60. Reimann JD, Fletcher CD. Myxoid dermatofibrosarcoma protuberans: a rare variant analyzed in a series of 23 cases. Am J Surg Pathol 2007;31:1371-1377.

61. Zámecnik M, Michal M. Myxoid variant of dermatofibrosarcoma protuberans with fibrosarcomatous areas. Zentralbl Pathol 1993;139:373-376.

62. Dupree WB, Langloss JM, Weiss SW. Pigmented dermatofibrosarcoma protuberans (Bednar tumor). A pathologic, ultrastructural, and immunohistochemical study. Am J Surg Pathol 1985;9:630-639.

63. Fletcher CD, Theaker JM, Flanagan A, Krausz T. Pigmented dermatofibrosarcoma protuberans (Bednar tumour): melanocytic colonization or neuroectodermal differentiation? A clinicopathological and immunohistochemical study. Histopathology 1988;13:631-643.

64. Calonje E, Fletcher CD. Myoid differentiation in dermatofibrosarcoma protuberans and its fibrosarcomatous variant: clinicopathologic analysis of 5 cases. J Cutan Pathol 1996;23:30-36.

65. Ghorbani RP, Malpica A, Ayala AG. Dermatofibrosarcoma protuberans of the vulva: clinicopathologic and immunohistochemical analysis of four cases, one with fibrosarcomatous change, and review of the literature. Int J Gynecol Pathol 1999;18:366-373.

66. Ding J, Hashimoto H, Enjoji M. Dermatofibrosarcoma protuberans with fibrosarcomatous areas. A clinicopathologic study of nine cases and a comparison with allied tumors. Cancer 1989;64:721-729.

67. Gökden N, Dehner LP, Zhu X, Pfeifer JD. Dermatofibrosarcoma protuberans of the vulva and groin: detection of COL1A1-PDGFB fusion transcripts by RT-PCR. J Cutan Pathol 2003;30:190-195.

68. Minoletti F, Miozzo M, Pedeutour F, et al. Involvement of chromosomes 17 and 22 in dermatofibrosarcoma protuberans. Genes Chromosomes Cancer 1995;13:62-65.

69. Pedeutour F, Simon MP, Minoletti F, et al. Ring 22 chromosomes in dermatofibrosarcoma protuberans are low-level amplifiers of chromosome 17 and 22 sequences. Cancer Res 1995;55:2400-2403.

70. Pedeutour F, Simon MP, Minoletti F, et al. Translocation, t(17;22)(q22;q13), in dermatofibrosarcoma protuberans: a new tumor-associated chromosome rearrangement. Cytogenet Cell Genet 1996;72:171-174.

71. Simon MP, Navarro M, Roux D, Pouysségur J. Structural and functional analysis of a chimeric protein COL1A1-PDGFB generated by the translocation t(17;22)(q22;q13.1) in dermatofibrosarcoma protuberans (DP). Oncogene 2001;20:2965-2975.

215

72. Shimizu A, O'Brien KP, Sjöblom T, et al. The dermatofibrosarcoma protuberans-associated collagen type I alpha1/platelet-derived growth factor (PDGF) B-chain fusion gene generates a transforming protein that is processed to functional PDGF-BB. Cancer Res 1999;59:3719-3723.

73. Bianchini L, Maire G, Guillot B, et al. Complex t(5;8) involving the CSPG2 and PTK2B genes in a case of dermatofibrosarcoma protuberans without the COL1A1-PDGFB fusion. Virchows Arch 2008;452:689-696.

74. Kamino H, Jacobson M. Dermatofibroma extending into the subcutaneous tissue. Differential diagnosis from dermatofibrosarcoma protuberans. Am J Surg Pathol 1990;14:1156-1164.

75. Kutzner H. Expression of the human progenitor cell antigen CD34 (HPCA-1) distinguishes dermatofibrosarcoma protuberans from fibrous histiocytoma in formalin-fixed, paraffin-embedded tissue. J Am Acad Dermatol 1993;28:613-617.

76. Rutgers EJ, Kroon BB, Albus-Lutter CE, Gortzak E. Dermatofibrosarcoma protuberans: treatment and prognosis. Eur J Surg Oncol 1992;18:241-248.

77. Gloster HM Jr, Harris KR, Roenigk RK. A comparison between Mohs micrographic surgery and wide surgical excision for the treatment of dermatofibrosarcoma protuberans. J Am Acad Dermatol 1996;35:82-87.

78. DuBay D, Cimmino V, Lowe L, Johnson TM, Sondak VK. Low recurrence rate after surgery for dermatofibrosarcoma protuberans: a multidisciplinary approach from a single institution. Cancer 2004;100:1008-1016.

79. Snow SN, Gordon EM, Larson PO, Bagheri MM, Bentz ML, Sable DB. Dermatofibrosarcoma protuberans: a report on 29 patients treated by Mohs micrographic surgery with long-term follow-up and review of the literature. Cancer 2004;101:28-38.

Giant Cell Fibroblastoma

80. Shmookler BM, Enzinger FM, Weiss SW. Giant cell fibroblastoma. A juvenile form of dermatofibrosarcoma protuberans. Cancer 1989;64:2154-2161.

81. Beham A, Fletcher CD. Dermatofibrosarcoma protuberans with areas resembling giant cell fibroblastoma: report of two cases. Histopathology 1990;17:165-167.

82. Galinier P, Scheiner C, Bardot J, et al. Giant-cell fibroblastoma and dermatofibrosarcoma protuberans: the same tumoral spectrum? Report of two cases of association in chidren. Eur J Pediatr Surg 2000;10:390-394.

83. Maeda T, Hirose T, Furuya K, Shirakawa K, Kobayashi K. Giant cell fibroblastoma associated with dermatofibrosarcoma protuberans: a case report. Mod Pathol 1998;11:491-495.

84. Michal M, Zamecnik M. Giant cell fibroblastoma with a dermatofibrosarcoma protuberans component. Am J Dermatopathol 1992;14:549-552.

85. Zámecník M, Michal M. Giant-cell fibroblastoma with pigmented dermatofibrosarcoma protuberans component. Am J Surg Pathol 1994;18:736-740.

86. Dal Cin P, Polito P, Van Eyken P, et al. Anomalies of chromosomes 17 and 22 in giant cell fibroblastoma. Cancer Genet Cytogenet 1997;97:165-166.

87. Macarenco RS, Zamolyi R, Nascimento AG, et al. Genomic gains of COL1A1-PDFGB occur in the histologic evolution of giant cell fibroblastoma into dermatofibrosarcoma protuberans. Genes Chromosomes Cancer 2008;47:260-265.

88. Rubin BP, Fletcher JA, Fletcher CD. The histologic, genetic, and biologic relationships between dermatofibrosarcoma protuberans and giant cell fibroblastoma: an unexpected story. Adv Anat Pathol 1997;4:336-341.

89. Terrier-Lacombe MJ, Guillou L, Maire G, et al. Dermatofibrosarcoma protuberans, giant cell fibroblastoma, and hybrid lesions in children: clinicopathologic comparative analysis of 28 cases with molecular data. A study from the French Federation of Cancer Centers Sarcoma Group. Am J Surg Pathol 2003;27:27-39.

90. Alguacil-Garcia A. Giant cell fibroblastoma recurring as dermatofibrosarcoma protuberans. Am J Surg Pathol 1991;15:798-801.

91. Allen PW, Zwi J. Giant cell fibroblastoma transforming into dermatofibrosarcoma protuberans. Am J Surg Pathol 1992;16:1127-1129.

92. Coyne J, Kaftan SM, Craig RD. Dermatofibrosarcoma protuberans recurring as a giant cell fibroblastoma. Histopathology 1992;21:184-187.

93. Goldblum JR. Giant cell fibroblastoma: a report of three cases with histologic and immunohistochemical evidence of a relationship to dermatofibrosarcoma protuberans. Arch Pathol Lab Med 1996;120:1052-1055.

94. Pitt MA, Coyne JD, Harris M, et al. Dermatofibrosarcoma protuberans recurring as a giant cell fibroblastoma with subsequent fibrosarcomatous change. Histopathology 1994;24:197-198.

95. Jha P, Moosavi C, Fanburg-Smith JC. Giant cell fibroblastoma: an update and addition of 86 new cases from the Armed Forces Institute of Pathology, in honor of Dr. Franz M. Enzinger. Ann Diagn Pathol 2007;11:81-88.

96. Fletcher CD. Giant cell fibroblastoma of soft tissue: a clinicopathological and immunohistochemical study. Histopathology 1988;13:499-508.

97. Kanai Y, Mukai M, Sugiura H, et al. Giant cell fibroblastoma. A case report and immunohistochemical comparison with ten cases of dermatofibrosarcoma protuberans. Acta Pathol Jpn 1991;41:552-560.

98. Dymock RB, Allen PW, Stirling JW, Gilbert EF, Thornbery JM. Giant cell fibroblastoma. A distinctive, recurrent tumor of childhood. Am J Surg Pathol 1987;11:263-271.

99. Dal Cin P, Sciot R, de Wever I, et al. Cytogenetic and immunohistochemical evidence that giant cell fibroblastoma is related to dermatofibrosarcoma protuberans. Genes Chromosomes Cancer 1996;15:73-75.

100. Maire G, Martin L, Michalak-Provost S, et al. Fusion of *COL1A1* exon 29 with *PDGFB* exon 2 in a der(22)t(17;22) in a pediatric giant cell fibroblastoma with a pigmented Bednar tumor component. Evidence for age-related chromosomal pattern in dermatofibrosarcoma protuberans and related tumors. Cancer Genet Cytogenet 2002;134:156-161.

101. Simon MP, Pedeutour F, Sirvent N, et al. Deregulation of the platelet-derived growth factor B-chain gene via fusion with collagen gene COL1A1 in dermatofibrosarcoma protuberans and giant-cell fibroblastoma. Nat Genet 1997;15:95-98.

102. Abdul-Karim FW, Evans HL, Silva EG. Giant cell fibroblastoma: a report of three cases. Am J Clin Pathol 1985;83:165-170.

Low-Grade Fibromyxoid Sarcoma

103. Guillou L, Benhattar J, Gengler C, et al. Translocation-positive low-grade fibromyxoid sarcoma: clinicopathologic and molecular analysis of a series expanding the morphologic spectrum and suggesting a potential relationship with sclerosing epithlioid fibrosarcoma: a study from the French sarcoma group. Am J Surg Pathol 2007;31:1887-1402.

104. Oda Y, Takahira T, Kawaguchi K, et al. Low-grade fibromyxoid sarcoma versus low-grade myxofibrosarcoma in the extremities and trunk. A comparison of clinicopathological and immunohistochemical features. Histopathology 2004;45:29-38.

105. Evans HL. Low-grade fibromyxoid sarcoma: a clinicopathologic study of 33 cases with a long-term follow-up. Am J Surg Pathol 2011;35:1450-1462.

106. Rekhi B, Deshmukh M, Jambhekar NA. Low-grade fibromyxoid sarcoma: a clinicopathologic study of 18 cases, including histopathologic relationship with clerosing epithelioid fibrosarcoma in a subset of cases. Ann Diagn Pathol 2011;15:303-311.

107. Hisaoka M, Matsuyama A, Aoki T, Sakamoto A, Yokoyama K. Low-grade fibromyxoid sarcoma with prominent giant rosettes and heterotopic ossification. Pathol Res Pract 2012;208:557-560.

108. Lane KL, Shannon RJ, Weiss SW. Hyalinizing spindle cell tumor with giant rosettes. a distinctive tumor closely resembling low-grade fibromyxoid sarcoma. Am J Surg Pathol 1997;21:1481-1488.

109. Reid R, Chandu de Silva MV, Paterson L, Ryan E, Fisher C. Low-grade fibromyxoid sarcoma and hyalinizing spindle cell tumor with giant rosettes share a common t(7;16)(q34;p11) translocation. Am J Surg Pathol 2003;27:1229-1236.

110. Doyle LA, Möller E, Dal Cin P, Fletcher CD, Mertens F, Hornick JL. MUC4 is a highly sensitive and specific marker for low-grade fibromyxoid sarcoma. Am J Surg Pathol 2011;35:733-741.

111. Panagopoulos I, Storlazzi CT, Fletcher CD, et al. The chimeric FUS/CREB312 gene is specific for low-grade fibromyxoid sarcoma. Genes Chrosom Cancer 2004;40:218-228.

112. Mertens F, Fletcher CD, Antonescu CR, et al. Clinicopathologic and molecular genetic characterization of low-grade fibromyxoid sarcoma, and cloning of a novel FUS/CREB3L1 fusion gene. Lab Invest 2005;85:408-415.

113. Matsuyama A, Hisaoka M, Shimajiri S, et al. Molecular detection of FUS-CREB3L2 fusion transcripts in low-grade fibromyxoid sarcoma using formalin-fixed, paraffin-embedded tissue specimens. Am J Surg Pathol 2006;30:1077-1084.

114. Downs-Kelly F, Goldblum JR, Patel RM, et al. The utility of fluorescence in-situ hybridization (FISH) in the diagnosis of myxoid soft tissue neoplasms. Am J Surg Pathol 2008;32:8-13.

115. Patel RM, Downs-Kelly E, Dandekar MN, et al. FUS (16p11) Gene rearrangement as detected by fluorescence in-situ hybridization in cutaneous low-grade fibromyxoid sarcoma: a potential diagnostic tool. Am J Dermatopathol 2011;33:140-143.

Sclerosing Epithelioid Fibrosarcoma

116. Meis-Kindblom JM, Kindblom LG, Enzinger FM. Sclerosing epithelioid fibrosarcoma. A variant of fibrosarcoma simulating carcinoma. Am J Surg Pathol 1995;19:979-993.

117. Eyden BP, Manson C, Banerjee SS, Roberts IS, Harris M. Sclerosing epithelioid fibrosarcoma: a study of five cases emphasizing diagnostic criteria. Histopathology 1998;33:354-360.

118. Antonescu C, Rosenblum MK, Pereira P, Nascimento AG, Woodruff JM. Sclerosing epithelioid fibrosarcoma. A study of 16 cases and confirmation of a clinicopathologic entity. Am J Surg Pathol 2001;25:699-709.

119. Guillou L, Benhattar J, Gengler C, et al. Translocation-positive low-grade fibromyxoid sarcoma: clinicopathologic and molecular analysis of a series expanding the morphologic spectrum and suggesting a potential relationship with sclerosing epithelioid fibrosarcoma: a study from the French sarcoma group. Am J Surg Pathol 2007;31:1887-1402.

120. Rekhi B, Deshmukh M, Jambhekar NA. Low-grade fibromyxoid sarcoma: a clinicopathologic study of 18 cases, including histopathologic relationship with sclerosing epithelioid fibrosarcoma in a subset of cases. Ann Diagn Pathol 2011;15:303-311.

121. Doyle LA, Wang WL, Dal Cin P, et al. MUC4 is a sensitive and extremely useful marker for sclerosing epithelioid fibrosarcoma: association with FUS gene rearrangement. Am J Surg Pathol 2012;36:1444-1451.

Inflammatory Myofibroblastic Tumor

122. Coffin CM, Watterson J, Priest JR, Dehner LP. Extrapulmonary inflammatory myofibroblastic tumor (inflammatory pseudotumor). A clinicopathologic and immunohistochemical study of 84 cases. Am J Surg Pathol 1995;19:859-872.

123. Coffin CM, Dehner LP, Meis-Kindblom JM. Inflammatory myofibroblastic tumor, inflammatory fibrosarcoma, and related lesions: an historical review with differential diagnostic considerations. Semin Diagn Pathol 1998;15:102-110.

124. Coffin CM, Humphrey PA, Dehner LP. Extrapulmonary inflammatory myofibroblastic tumor: a clinical and pathological survey. Semin Diagn Pathol 1998;15:85-101.

125. Meis JM, Enzinger FM. Inflammatory fibrosarcoma of the mesentery and retroperitoneum. A tumor closely simulating inflammatory pseudotumor. Am J Surg Pathol 1991;15:1146-1156.

126. Meis-Kindblom JM, Kjellstrom C, Kindblom LG. Inflammatory fibrosarcoma: update, reappraisal, and perspective on its place in the spectrum of inflammatory myofibroblastic tumors. Semin Diagn Pathol 1998;15:133-143.

127. Coffin CM, Hornick JL, Fletcher CD. Inflammatory myofibroblastic tumor. Comparison of clinicopathologic, histologic, and immunohistochemical features including ALK-expression in atypical and aggressive cases. Am J Surg Pathol 2007;31:509-520.

128. Mariño-Enríquez A, Wang WL, Roy A, et al. Epithelioid inflammatory myofibroblastic sarcoma: an aggressive intra-abdominal variant of inflammatory myofibroblastic tumor with nuclear membrane or perinuclear ALK. Am J Surg Pathol 2011:35:135-144.

129. Griffin CA, Hawkins AL, Dvorak C, Henkle C, Ellingham T, Perlman EJ. Recurrent involvement of 2p23 in inflammatory myofibroblastic tumors. Cancer Res 1999;59:2776-2780.

130. Sukov WR, Cheville JC, Carlson AW, et al. Utility of ALK-1 protein expression and ALK rearrangements in distinguishing inflammatory myofibrolastic tumor from malignant spindle cell lesions of the urinary bladder. Mod Pathol 2007;20:592-603.

131. Lawrence B, Perez-Atayde A, Hibbard MK, et al. TPM3-ALK and TPM4-ALK oncogenes in inflammatory myofibroblastic tumors. Am J Pathol 2000;157:377-384.

132. Bridge JA, Kanamori M, Ma Z, et al. Fusion of the ALK gene to the clathrin heavy chain gene, CLTC, in inflammatory myofibroblastic tumor. Am J Pathol 2001;159:411-415.

133. Debelenko LV, Arthur DC, Pack SD, Helman LJ, Schrump DS, Tsokos M. Identification of CARS-ALK fusion in primary and metastatic lesions of an inflammatory myofibroblastic tumor. Lab Invest 2003;83:1255-1265.

134. Debiec-Rychter M, Marynen P, Hagemeijer A, Pauwels P. ALK-ATIC fusion in urinary bladder inflammatory myofibroblastic tumor. Genes Chomosomes Cancer 2003;38:187-190.

135. Ma Z, Hill DA, Collins MH, et al. Fusion of ALK to the Ran-binding protein 2 (RANBP2) gene in inflammatory myofibroblastic tumor. Genes Chromosomes Cancer 2003;37:98-105.

136. Panagopoulos I, Nilsson T, Domanski HA, et al. Fusion of the SEC31L1 and ALK genes in an inflammatory myofibroblastic tumor. Int J Cancer 2006;118:1181-1186.

137. Takeuchi K, Soda M, Togashi Y, et al. Pulmonary inflammatory myofibroblastic tumor expressing a novel fusion, PPFIBP1-ALK: reappraisal of anti-ALK immunohistochemistry as a tool of novel ALK fusion identification. Clin Cancer Res 2011;17:3341-3348.

138. Tothova Z, Wagner AJ. Anaplastic lymphoma kinase-directed therapy in inflammatory myofibroblastic tumors. Curr Opin Oncol 2012;24:409-413.

Inflammatory Myxohyaline Tumor of Distal Extremities/Acral Myxoinflammatory Fibroblastic Sarcoma

139. Meis-Kindblom JM, Kindblom LG. Acral myxoinflammatory fibroblastic sarcoma: a low-grade tumor of the hands and feet. Am J Surg Pathol 1998;22:911-924.

140. Montgomery EA, Devaney KO, Giordano TJ, Weiss SW. Inflammatory myxohyaline tumor of distal extremities with virocyte or Reed-Sternberg-like cells: a distinctive lesion with features simulating inflammatory conditions, Hodgkin's disease, and various sarcomas. Mod Pathol 1998;11:384-391.

141. Michal M. Inflammatory myxoid tumor of the soft parts with bizarre giant cells. Pathol Res Pract 1998;194:529-533.

142. Elco CP, Mariño-Enriquez A, Abraham JA, Dal Cin P, Hornick JL. Hybrid myxoinflammatory fibroblastic sarcoma/hemisiderotic fibrolipomatous tumor: report of a case providing further evidence for a pathogenetic link. Am J Surg Pathol 2010;34:1723-1727.

143. Lambert I, Debiec-Rychter M, Guelinckx P, Hagemeijer A, Sciot R. Acral myxoinflammatory fibroblastic sarcoma with unique clonal chromosomal changes. Virchows Arch 2001;438:509-512.

144. Mansoor A, Fidda N, Himoe E, Payne M, Lawce H, Magenis RE. Myxoinflammatory fibroblastic sarcoma with complex supernumerary ring chromosomes composed of chromosome 3 segments. Cancer Genet Cytogenet 2004;142:61-65.

145. Hallor KH, Sciot R, Staaf J, et al. Two genetic pathways, t(1;10) and amplification of 3p11-12, in myxoinflammatory fibroblastic sarcoma, hemosiderotic fibrolipomatous tumour, and morphologically similar lesions. J Pathol 2009;217:716-727.

146. Antonescu CR, Zhang L, Nielsen GP, Rosenberg AE, Dal Cin P, Fletcher CD. Consistent t(1;10) with rearrangements of TGFBR3 and MGEA5 in both myxoinflammatory fibroblastic sarcoma and hemosiderotic fibrolipomatous tumor. Genes Chromosom Cancer 2011;50:757-764.

147. Sakaki M, Hirokawa M, Wakatsuki S, et al. Acral myxoinflammatory fibroblastic sarcoma: a report of five cases and review of the literature. Virchows Arch 2003;442:25-30.

148. Tejwani A, Kobayashi W, Chen YL, et al. Management of acral myxoinflammatory fibroblastic sarcoma. Cancer 2010;116:5733-5739.

Infantile Fibrosarcoma (Congenital Fibrosarcoma)

149. Balsaver AM, Butler JJ, Martin RG. Congenital fibrosarcoma. Cancer 1967;20:1607-1616.

150. Chung EB, Enzinger FM. Infantile fibrosarcoma. Cancer 1976;38:729-739.

151. Soule EH, Pritchard DJ. Fibrosarcoma in infants and and children: a review of 110 cases. Cancer 1977;40:1711-1721.

152. Iwasaki H, Enjoji M. Infantile and adult fibrosarcomas of the soft tissues. Acta Pathol Jpn 1979;29:377-388.

153. Coffin CM, Jaszcz W, O'Shea PA, Dehner LP. So-called congenital-infantile fibrosarcoma: does it exist and what is it? Pediatr Pathol 1994;14:133-150.

154. Nonaka D, Sun CC. Congenital fibrosarcoma with metastasis in a fetus. Pediatr Develop Pathol 2004;7:187-191.

155. Salloum E, Caillaud JM, Flamant F, Landman J, Lemerle J. Poor prognosis infantile fibrosarcoma with pathologic features of malignant fibrous histiocytoma after local recurrence. Med Pediatr Oncol 1990;18:295-298.

156. Kodet R, Stejskal J, Pilat D, Kocourkova M, Smelhaus V, Eckschlager T. Congenital-infantile fibrosarcoma: a clinicopathological study of five patients entered on the Prague children's tumor registry. Pathol Res Pract 1996;192:845-853.

157. Sheng WQ, Hisaoka M, Okamoto S, et al. Congenital-infantile fibrosarcoma. A clinicopathologic study of 10 cases and molecular detection of the ETV6-NTRK3 fusion transcripts using paraffin-embedded tissues. Am J Clin Pathol 2001;115:348-355.

158. Dal Cin P, Brock P, Casteels-Van Daele M, De Wever I, Van Damme B, Van den Berghe H. Cytogenetic characterization of congenital or infantile fibrosarcoma. Eur J Pediatr 1991;150:579-581.

159. Sankary S, Dickman PS, Wiener E, et al. Consistent numerical chromosome aberrations in congenital fibrosarcoma. Cancer Genet Cytogenet 1993;65:152-156.

160. Knezevich SR, Mcfadden DE, Tao W, Lim JF, Sorensen PH. A novel ETV6-NTRK3 gene fusion in congenital fibrosarcoma. Nat Genet 1998;18:184-187.

161. Bourgeois JM, Knezevich SR, Mathers JA, Sorensen PH. Molecular detection of the ETV6-NTRK3 gene fusion differentiates congenital fibrosarcoma from other childhood spindle cell tumors. Am J Surg Pathol 2000;24:937-946.

162. Knezevich SR, Garnett MJ, Pysher TJ, Beckwith JB, Grundy PE, Sorensen PH. ETV6-NTRK3 gene fusions and trisomy 11 establish a histogenetic link between mesoblastic nephroma and congenital fibrosarcoma. Cancer Res 1998;58:5046-5048.

163. Rubin BP, Chen CJ, Morgan TW, et al. Congenital mesoblastic nephroma t(12;15) is associated with ETV6-NTRK3 gene fusion: cytogenetic and molecular relationship to congenital (infantile) fibrosarcoma. Am J Pathol 1998;153:1451-1458.

164. Argani P, Fritsch M, Kadkol SS, Schuster A, Beckwith JB, Perlman EJ. Detection of the ETV6-NTRK3 chimeric RNA of infantile fibrosarcoma/cellular congenital mesoblastic nephroma in paraffin-embedded tissue: application to challenging pediatric renal stromal tumors. Mod Pathol 2000;13:29-36.

165. Tognon C, Knezevich SR, Huntsman D, et al. Expression of the ETV6-NTRK3 gene fusion as a primary event in human secretory breast carcinoma. Cancer cell 2002;2:367-376.

166. Bernstein R, Zeltzer PM, Lin F, Carpenter PM. Trisomy 11 and other nonrandom trisomies in congenital fibrosarcoma. Cancer Genet Cytogenet 1994;78:82-86.

167. Cofer BR, Vescio PJ, Wiener ES. Infantile fibrosarcoma: complete excision is the appropriate treatment. Ann Surg Oncol 1996;3:159-161.

168. Kynaston JA, Malcolm AJ, Craft AW, et al. Chemotherapy in the management of infantile fibrosarcoma. Med Pediatr Oncol 1993;21:488-493.

Adult Fibrosarcoma and Myofibroblastic Sarcoma

169. Sheng WQ, Hashimoto H, Okamoto S, et al. Expression of COLIAI-PDGFB fusion transcripts in superficial adult fibrosarcoma suggests close relationship to dermatofibrosarcoma protuberans. J Pathol 2001;194:88-94.

170. Scott SM, Reiman HM, Pritchard DJ, Ilstrup DM. Soft tissue fibrosarcoma. A clincopathologic study of 132 cases. Cancer 1989;64:925-931.

171. Bahrami A, Folpe AL. Adult-type fibrosarcoma: A reevaluation of 163 putative cases diagnosed at a single instituition over a 48-year period. Am J Surg Pathol 2010;34:1504-1513.

172. Mentzel T, Dry S, Katenkamp D, Fletcher CD. Low-grade myofibroblastic sarcoma: analysis of 18 cases in the spectrum of myofibroblastic tumors. Am J Surg Pathol 1998;22:1228-1238.

173. Montgomery E, Goldblum JR, Fisher C. Myofibrosarcoma: a clinicopathologic study. Am J Surg Pathol 2001;25:219-228.

Myxofibrosarcoma

174. Angervall L, Kindblom LG, Merck C. Myxofibrosarcoma. A study of 30 cases. Acta Pathol Microbiol Scand A 1977;85A:127-140.

175. Weiss SW, Enzinger FM. Myxoid variant of malignant fibrous histiocytoma. Cancer 1977;39:1672-1685.

176. Mentzel T, Calonje E, Wadden C, et al. Myxofibrosarcoma. Clinicopathologic analysis of 75 cases with emphasis on the low-grade variant. Am J Surg Pathol 1996;20:391-405.

177. Fletcher CD, Gustafson P, Rydholm A, Willen H, Akerman M. Clinicopathologic re-evaluation of 100 malignant fibrous histiocytomas: prognostic relevance of subclassification. J Clin Oncol 2001;19:3045-3050.

178. Kindblom LG, Merck C, Angervall L. The ultrastructure of myxofibrosarcoma. A study of 11 cases. Virchows Arch A Pathol Anat Histol 1979;381:121-139.

179. Lagace R, Delage C, Seemayer TA. Myxoid variant of malignant fibrous histiocytoma: ultrastructural observations. Cancer 1979;43:526-534.

180. Antonescu CR, Baren A. Spectrum of low-grade fibrosarcomas: a comparative ultrastructural analysis of low-grade myxofibrosarcoma and fibromyxoid sarcoma. Ultrastruct Pathol 2004;28:321-332.

181. Antonescu CR, Erlandson RA, Huvos AG. Primary fibrosarcoma and malignant fibrous histiocytoma of bone—a comparative ultrastructural study: evidence of a spectrum of fibroblastic differentiation. Ultrastruct Pathol 2000;24:83-91.

182. Merck C, Angervall L, Kindblom LG, Oden A. Myxofibrosarcoma. A malignant soft tissue tumor of fibroblastic-histiocytic origin. A clinicopathologic and prognostic study of 110 cases using multivariate analysis. Acta Pathol Microbiol Immunol Scand Suppl 1983;282:1-40.

183. Huang HY, Lal P, Qin J, Brennan MF, Antonescu CR. Low-grade myxofibrosarcoma: a clinicopathologic analysis of 49 cases treated at a single institution with simultaneous assessment of the efficacy of 3-tier and 4-tier grading systems. Hum Pathol 2004;35:612-621.

184. Hisaoka M, Morimitsu Y, Hashimoto H, et al. Retroperitoneal liposarcoma with combined well-differentiated and myxoid malignant fibrous histiocytoma-like myxoid areas. Am J Surg Pathol 1999;23:1480-1492.

185. Antonescu CR, Elahi A, Humphrey M, et al. Specificity of TLS-CHOP rearrangement for classic myxoid/round cell liposarcoma: absence in predominantly myxoid well-differentiated liposarcomas. J Mol Diagn 2000;2:132-138.

186. Mansoor A, White CR, Jr. Myxofibrosarcoma presenting in the skin: clinicopathological features and differential diagnosis with cutaneous myxoid neoplasms. Am J Dermatopathol 2003;25:281-286.

187. Waters B, Panicek DM, Lefkowitz RA, et al. Low-grade myxofibrosarcoma: CT and MRI patterns in recurrent disease. AJR Am J Roentgenol 2007;188:W193-198.

188. Le Doussal V, Coindre JM, Leroux A, et al. Prognostic factors for patients with localized primary malignant fibrous histiocytoma: a multicenter study of 216 patients with multivariate analysis. Cancer 1996;77:1823-1830.

189. Mandahl N, Heim S, Kristoffersson U, et al. Telomeric association in a malignant fibrous histiocytoma. Hum Genet 1985;71:321-324.

190. Orndal C, Rydholm A, Willen H, Mitelman F, Mandahl N. Cytogenetic intratumor heterogeneity in soft tissue tumors. Cancer Genet Cytogenet 1994;78:127-137.

191. Willems SM, Debiec-Rychter M, Szuhai K, Hogendoorn PC, Sciot R. Local recurrence of myxofibrosarcoma is associated with increase in tumour grade and cytogenetic aberrations, suggesting a multistep tumour progression model. Mod Pathol 2006;19:407-416.

192. Barretina J, Taylor BS, Banerji S, et al. Subtype-specific genomic alterations define new targets for soft-tissue sarcoma therapy. Nat Genet 2010;42:715-721.

193. Willems SM, Mohseny AB, Balog C, et al. Cellular/intramuscular myxoma and grade I myxofibrosarcoma are characterized by distinct genetic alterations and specific composition of their extracellular matrix. J Cell Mol Med 2009;13:1291-1301.

194. Manoso MW, Pratt J, Healey JH, Boland PJ, Athanasian EA. Infiltrative MRI pattern and incomplete initial surgery compromise local control of myxofibrosarcoma. Clin Orthop Relat Res 2006;450:89-94.

195. Mutter RW, Singer S, Zhang Z, Brennan MF, Alektiar KM. The enigma of myxofibrosarcoma of the extremity. Cancer 2012;118:518-527.

Malignant Fibrous Histiocytoma/ Undifferentiated Pleomorphic Sarcoma

196. O'Brien JE, Stout AP. Malignant fibrous xanthomas. Cancer 1964;17:1445-1455.

197. Ozzello L, Stout AP, Murray MR. Cultural characteristics of malignant histiocytomas and fibrous xanthomas. Cancer 1963;16:331-344.

198. Fletcher CD, Gustafson P, Rydholm A, Willen H, Akerman M. Clinicopathologic re-evaluation of 100 malignant fibrous histiocytomas: prognostic relevance of subclassification. J Clin Oncol 2001;19:3045-3050.

199. Erlandson RA, Antonescu CR. The rise and fall of malignant fibrous histiocytoma. Ultrastruct Pathol 2004;28:283-289.

200. Dei Tos AP. Classification of pleomorphic sarcomas: where are we now? Histopathology 2006;48:51-62.

201. Fletcher CD. Pleomorphic malignant fibrous histiocytoma: fact or fiction? A critical reappraisal based on 159 tumors diagnosed as pleomorphic sarcoma. Am J Surg Pathol 1992;16:213-228.

202. Mitelman F, Johansson B, Mertens F. Mitelman Database of Chromosome Aberrations and Gene Fusions in Cancer. (http://cgap.nci.nih.gov/Chromosomes/Mitelman), 2012.

203. Gibault L, Pérot G, Chibon F, et al. New insights in sarcoma oncogenesis: a comprehensive analysis of a large series of 160 soft tissue sarcomas with complex genomics. J Pathol 2011;223:64-71.

204. Pérot G, Chibon F, Montero A, et al. Constant p53 pathway inactivation in a large series of soft tissue sarcomas with complex genetics. Am J Pathol 2010;177:2080-2090.

205. Deyrup AT, Haydon RC, Huo D, et al. Myoid differentiation and prognosis in adult pleomorphic sarcomas of the extremity: an analysis of 92 cases. Cancer 2003;98:805-813.

206. Massi D, Beltrami G, Capanna R, Franchi A. Histopathological re-classification of extremity pleomorphic soft tissue sarcoma has clinical relevance. Eur J Surg Oncol 2004;30:1131-1136.

Pleomorphic Hyalinizing Angiectatic Tumor

207. Smith ME, Fisher C, Weiss SW. Pleomorphic hyalinizing angiectatic tumor of soft parts. A low-grade neoplasm resembling neurilemoma. Am J Surg Pathol 1996;20:21-29

208. Groisman GM, Bejar J, Amar M, Ben-Izhak O. Pleomorphic hyalinizing angiectatic tumor of soft parts: immunohistochemical study including the expression of vascular endothelial growth factor. Arch Pathol Lab Med 2000;124:423-426.

209. Folpe AL, Weiss SW. Pleomorphic hyalinizing angiectatic tumor: analysis of 41 cases supporting evolution from a distinctive precursor lesion. Am J Surg Pathol 2004;28:1417-1425.

210. Mitsuhashi T, Barr RJ, Machtinger LA, Cassarino DS. Primary cutaneous myxofibrosarcoma mimicking pleomorphic hyalinizing angiectatic tumor (PHAT): a potential diagnostic pitfall. Am J Dermatopathol 2005:27:322-326.

211. Kazakov DV, Pavlovsky M, Mukensnabl P, Michal M. Pleomorphic hyalinizing angiectatic tumor with a sarcomatous component recurring as high-grade myxofibrosarcoma. Pathol Int 2007:57:281-284.

212. Illueca C, Machado I, Cruz J, et al. Pleomorphic hyalinizing angiectatic tumor: report of 3 new cases, 1 with sarcomatous myxofibrosarcoma component and another with unreported soft tissue palpebral location. Appl Immunohistochem Mol Morphol 2012;20:96-101.

Giant Cell Tumors of Soft Parts and Giant Cell Malignant Fibrous Histiocytoma

213. Folpe AL, Morris RJ, Weiss SW. Soft tissue giant cell tumor of low malignant potential: a proposal for the reclassification of malignant giant cell tumor of soft parts. Mod Pathol 1999;12:894-902.

214. Oliveira AM, Dei Tos AP, Fletcher CD, Nascimento AG. Primary giant cell tumor of soft tissues: a study of 22 cases. Am J Surg Pathol 2000;24:248-256.

215. O'Connell JX, Wehrli BM, Nielsen GP, Rosenberg AE. Giant cell tumors of soft tissue: a clinicopathologic study of 18 benign and malignant tumors. Am J Surg Pathol 2000;24:386-395.

216. Salm R, Sissons HA. Giant cell tumours of soft tissues. J Pathol 1972;107:27-39.

217. Guccion JG, Enzinger FM. Malignant giant cell tumor of soft parts. An analysis of 32 cases. Cancer 1972;29:1518-1529.

218. Angervall L, Hagmar B, Kindblom LG, Merck C. Malignant giant cell tumor of soft tissues: a clinicopathologic, cytologic, ultrastructural, angiographic and microangiographic study. Cancer 1981;47:736-747.

4 LIPOMATOUS TUMORS

LIPOMA AND VARIANTS

Benign lipomatous lesions (excluding atypical lipoma/atypical lipomatous tumors) are probably the most common soft tissue tumors. Most are composed of white fat (ordinary lipoma) with some variations, such as fibrolipoma with a fibrous element and lipoma with chondro-osseous metaplasia (chondrolipoma).

The term *lipomatosis* describes a heterogeneous group of clinical entities that are regional diffuse growths of adipose tissue; it is not known whether they are fat hyperplasias or true neoplasms. Only lipomatosis of the nerve is currently considered histologically distinctive. The other lipomatoses are summarized in Table 4-1.

Clinicopathologically distinctive variants with additional cellular components are considered separate entities. They include angiolipoma with clusters of capillaries, spindle cell/pleomorphic lipoma with a variably prominent spindle cell or myxoid component, chondroid lipoma composed of epithelioid cells with a vague resemblance to cartilage, and hemosiderotic fibrohistiocytic lipoma. Hibernoma is distinctive in its content of brown fat elements. Lipoblastoma is a histologically distinctive tumor featuring fetal-type fat and occurs exclusively in young children. Massive localized lymphedema is a tumor-like non-neoplastic processes that is clinically significant in its capability to simulate liposarcoma.

Myelolipoma, combining mature fat and bone marrow elements, usually occurs in the adrenal gland and angiomyolipoma in the kidney. These tumors infrequently occur in the retroperitoneum outside these parenchymal organs.

Table 4-1

MOST IMPORTANT CLINICAL LIPOMATOSIS SYNDROMES

Condition	Key Features
Diffuse lipomatosis	Lipomatous growth involving various tissue planes in an anatomic region, especially an extremity
Multiple symmetric lipomatosis (Madelung disease, Launois-Bensaude syndrome)	Prominent, symmetric fat collection involving the anterior neck, upper trunk, and arm; some cases are hereditary; also reported in association with alcoholism; connection with mitochondrial myopathy; debulking to prevent neurovascular and respiratory compromise when necessary
Pelvic lipomatosis	Diffuse deposition of fat between bladder, rectum, and large vessels; may cause urinary or colorectal obstruction; predilection to black males; associated with glandular metaplasia and adenocarcinoma of urinary bladder, also an association with achondroplasia
Encephalocraniocutaneous lipomatosis	Congenital malformation syndrome with facial and ipsilateral oculocerebral malformations, hydrocephalus, seizures, and mental retardation; multiple lipomas involving skin of face and scalp, and intracranial space (meninges, cranial fossae); lipomas may have fibrolipomatous features and are not principal cause of morbidity
Spinal epidural lipomatosis	May be associated with corticosteroid use or be idiopathic; spinal decompression may be needed
Steroid lipomatosis	Designation of lipomatous masses caused by excessive corticosteroid stimulation; may be endogenous (Cushing syndrome) or iatrogenic; a variety of sites can be involved; predilection to head and neck

Table 4-2

CLINICAL VARIANTS OF LIPOMA[a]

Condition	Description/Management of Lipomas
Nevus lipomatosus superficialis	Superficial lipoma involving the dermis; occurs in childhood and may be congenital; can form a solitary dermal nodule or linear streaks, often in the buttocks and proximal thigh
Lumbosacral lipoma	Lipoma involving subcutis and deeper structures at the midline; associated with spinal cord closure defects and usually attached to the spinal cord; manifests in early childhood; cord attachment may cause neurologic symptoms, especially related to autonomic nerve functions, especially those of the urinary bladder
Spermatic cord lipoma	Common lipomatous masses associated with spermatic cord and detected during herniography operations; it is uncertain whether these are reactive formations or true lipomas (adipocytic neoplasms)
Nerve sheath lipoma	May be external or internal to the nerve; some cases have overlapping features with lipomatosis of the nerve
Lipoma arborescens	Lipomatous mass involving synovial as multiple nodular protrusions; histologically composed of mature fat often associated with mild lymphoid infiltration

[a]Does not include variants of specific lipoma types.

Atypical lipoma/atypical lipomatous tumor and well-differentiated liposarcoma are clinically and genetically closely related entities and are discussed together in a separate chapter.

Ordinary Lipoma

Clinical Features. *Lipoma* is the most common soft tissue tumor and is estimated to comprise almost half of all of soft tissue tumors (1). Its incidence is difficult to determine with accuracy, because many lipomas never come to medical attention.

Soft tissue lipomas usually occur in adults over 40 years of age and appear to have a male predominance. They most commonly occur in the upper body, especially the back, shoulder, arm, forearm, and other extremity sites, especially the proximal ones. Familial occurrence has been reported (2). In addition, many visceral sites are affected, but lipomas in these sites are excluded from further discussion.

Most soft tissue lipomas are subcutaneous, circumscribed, mobile tumors, usually smaller than 5 cm (3). Some are intramuscular or located in intermuscular septa (4,5), and fewer are located in the retroperitoneum, where atypical lipomatous tumors/well-differentiated liposarcomas are more common and need to be always carefully excluded (6).

Numerous clinically distinctive lipoma variants exist. Those whose lipomatous components are histologically similar to ordinary lipoma include *nevus lipomatosus superficialis* (7,8), *lumbosacral lipoma* (9–11), *spermatic cord lipoma* (12), *nerve sheath lipoma* (13), and *lipoma arborescens of synovial tissues* (14,15). These are summarized in Table 4-2 and illustrated in figure 4-2.

Gross Findings. Grossly and histologically, lipomas resemble mature white adipose tissue. Although typically less than 5 cm, some are larger than 20 cm. Lipomas often form oval, flattened or discoid, well-circumscribed subcutaneous masses, often with larger longitudinal and lateral and smaller anteroposterior dimensions. On sectioning, the surface is typically golden yellow, especially in unfixed specimens, but it may be paler after fixation. Fibrolipomas are firmer and may have grayish streaks of fibrous tissue.

Microscopic Findings. Histologically, typical lipomas are surrounded by a thin collagenous pseudocapsule and composed of mature adipocytes closely resembling normal adipose tissue, except that lobulation is less distinct or absent (fig. 4-1). Some lipomas are mucoid (*myxoid lipoma*); this change is more common in spindle cell lipoma. Only minor adipocyte size variation is observed, and the lesion is usually free of diffuse lymphohistiocytic infiltration, although focal fat necrosis and calcification may be present, especially in larger lesions. Adipocyte nuclei are typically small and peripherally located, but

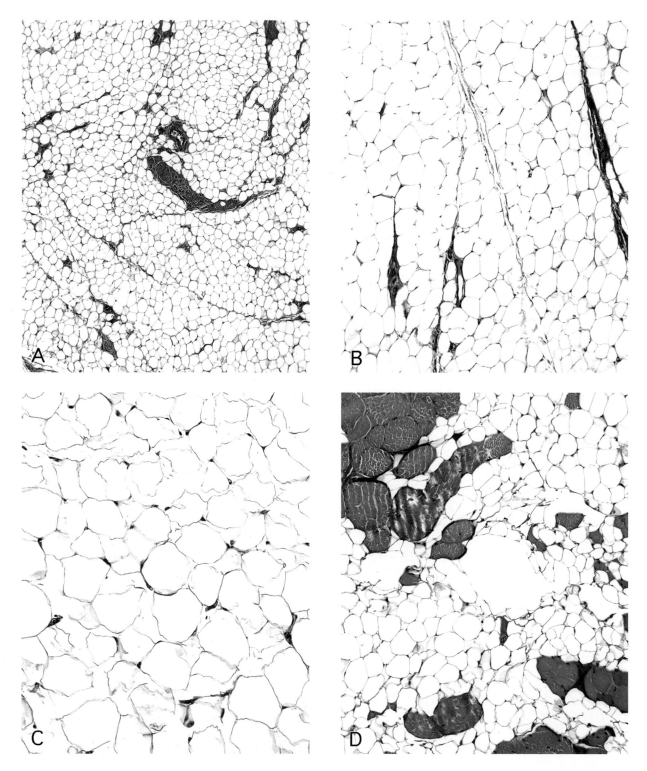

Figure 4-1

ORDINARY LIPOMA

A–D: The tumor is composed of mature adipose tissue that does not show distinct lobulation. Adipocytes are of approximately equal size, and significant nuclear atypia is absent. An infiltrative type of intramuscular lipoma dissects between skeletal muscle fibers.

because they are small, they are not seen in all cells in a given section plane.

Intramuscular lipoma can involve skeletal muscle in a checkerboard pattern of alternating fat and skeletal muscle cells (fig. 4-1), but may also be well demarcated, similar to a subcutaneous lipoma. Entrapped skeletal muscle giant cells (sarcoplasmic giant cells) should not be interpreted as atypical elements (fig. 4-1).

The variants with prominent, paucicellular fibrous septa are classified as *fibrolipomas*. Examples with myxoid stroma (*myxoid lipoma, myxolipoma*) should not be confused with myxoid liposarcoma. The lack of a prominent plexiform capillary pattern and lipoblasts separate them from the latter.

Genetics. Ordinary lipomas show clonal chromosomal aberrations in nearly 80 percent of cases, and such changes seem to be more common in lipomas of older patients and those of larger size or located in the extremities, as opposed to the trunk wall (17,18). Clonal chromosomal changes also support the idea that lipomas are clonal neoplasms and not fat hyperplasias.

Although malignant transformation of ordinary lipoma has not been believed to occur, lipomas show aberrations in the same chromosomal region as well-differentiated liposarcomas, 12q13-q15 (19), suggesting that there may be a biologic continuum. However, amplification of the 12q13-15 region, including the *MDM2* locus, is not observed in lipomas but only in atypical lipomatous tumors (20–22).

Differential Diagnosis. In some instances it is difficult to determine whether well-differentiated fat represents lipoma or normal fat. Lipoma of the hernia sac is more often reactive fat than a fatty neoplasm, but it is possible that a lipomatous tumor caused the hernia. Demarcation, pseudoencapsulation, and lack of well-defined lobulation, as seen in normal fat, are features of lipoma. Recently, fat herniations in the orbit that contained normal, displaced fat have been reported (16). Differentiating this condition from a lipoma requires clinico-radiologic correlation, although the presence of multinucleated cells slightly resembling pleomorphic lipoma might be a clue.

Large lipomas, especially the deep and intra-abdominal ones, should be sampled generously (at least 1 section per cm of tumor diameter) in order to comprehensively evaluate atypia, because atypia can be focal. Significant nuclear atypia in deep tumors indicates atypical lipoma/well-differentiated liposarcoma. The often focal atypia in atypical lipomatous tumors limits the value of small needle biopsies in this differential diagnosis.

Muscular dystrophy syndromes or muscle atrophy due to an adjacent tumor may be associated with substantial fatty replacement of skeletal muscle and even minor fat cell atypia, potentially simulating a lipomatous tumor. Also, intramuscular hemangioma can have a significant lipomatous component; in this tumor the presence of the hemangiomatous component traditionally outweighs the presence of fat (although historically the designation of infiltrative angiolipoma has been used of these fat-containing hemangiomas).

Optimal tissue processing and sectioning facilitates the interpretation of fatty tumors and especially the evaluation of atypia. In general, lipomas are best submitted for histology after (thin) slicing and overnight fixation.

Treatment and Prognosis. Simple excision is sufficient, but the infiltrative variant of intramuscular lipoma has significant potential to recur unless completely excised (4,5).

Lipoma with Metaplastic Cartilage and Bone

Rare lipomas contain foci of mature hyaline cartilage, metaplastic bone, or both (fig. 4-2). Such tumors have sometimes been designated as *chondrolipomas* or *osteolipomas* (23–26). Lipomas with metaplastic bone and cartilage occur in a wide age range from childhood to old age, and in locations such as hand, trunk wall, breast, pharynx, and neck. Such lipomas differ from chondroid lipoma, which does contain true hyaline cartilage.

Lipomatosis of the Nerve

Definition. *Lipomatosis of the nerve*, also known as *fibrolipomatous hamartoma of nerve* and *neural fibrolipoma*, is a rare tumor-like formation usually occurring in fingers and hands that contains a nerve splayed by fatty growth.

Clinical Features. This rare condition occurs mainly in children and young adults, equally in both sexes. In many cases, it is detected at birth. The median age in the Armed Forces Institute of Pathology (AFIP) case files is 25 years.

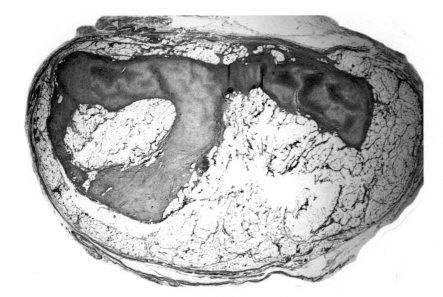

Figure 4-2

LIPOMA WITH CHONDRO-OSSEOUS METAPLASIA (CHONDROLIPOMA)

Cartilaginous foci and focal osseous metaplasia are seen. Paucicellular fibrous septa are also present.

Clinically, there is an ill-defined, often sausage-shaped, sometimes painful, tumor-like lesion usually developing on the volar aspects fingers and hands, most often around the median nerve (fig. 4-3). Other nerves of the hand may also be involved (ulnar nerve), and this tumor can also involve the foot. Some examples are associated with macrodactyly.

Gross and Microscopic Findings. Grossly the lesion represents a sausage or spindle-shaped fibrofatty mass involving a nerve, usually the median nerve (see fig. 4-1). Microscopically, the lesion contains branches of the nerve splayed by fibrofatty expansion of the epineurium. The nerve branches, usually seen as cross sections or sometimes longitudinally cut, vary from nearly normal to severely altered. They are often surrounded by epineurial fibrosis and contain endoneurial fibrosis (fig. 4-4, left). In some cases, onion bulb-like perineurial cell proliferation surrounds the axons, reminiscent of the histology of intraneural perineurioma (fig. 4-4, right). The fat is composed of evenly sized adipocytes with no nuclear atypia.

Differential Diagnosis. Lipomatosis of a nerve should be distinguished from atypical lipomatous tumors, which are composed of adipocytes of variable sizes and contain at least focal significant nuclear atypia.

Treatment and Prognosis. Because radical excision leads to nerve sacrifice and neural deficits, this condition, when involving major motor nerves, should generally be diagnosed by biopsy

and treated by nerve decompression when necessary (27,28). Lipomatosis of nerve may be associated with systemic lipomatosis, and nerves may also be involved by well-demarcated intraneural lipomas that do not separate the nerve bundles. These also cause nerve compression but can be removed without much morbidity (29).

Angiolipoma

Definition. *Angiolipoma* is a lipoma variant containing varying numbers of capillaries as clusters or peripheral streaks and often containing focal fibrin microthrombi. The terms "infiltrative angiolipoma" and "spinal angiolipoma" have been previously used for unrelated lesions: intramuscular hemangiomas combining vascular and mature lipomatous elements.

Clinical Features. Angiolipoma is a common tumor that presents as a small, circumscribed, often painful, superficial subcutaneous nodule, typically in young to middle-aged adults. There is a marked male predominance. The most frequent locations are chest wall and breast, forearm, arm, abdominal wall, thigh, and back. Occurrence in the distal extremities and head and neck region is rare. Multiple angiolipomas are seen in 10 percent of patients, sometimes on a familial basis.

Gross Findings. Angiolipomas are usually small, ovoid, circumscribed, pseudocapsulated lipomatous nodules typically measuring 1 to 2 cm in greatest diameter. They may appear firmer than ordinary lipomas and on sectioning may have a red tinge, reflecting the capillary content.

Figure 4-3

LIPOMATOSIS OF NERVE

A sausage-like mass is formed inside a nerve trunk.

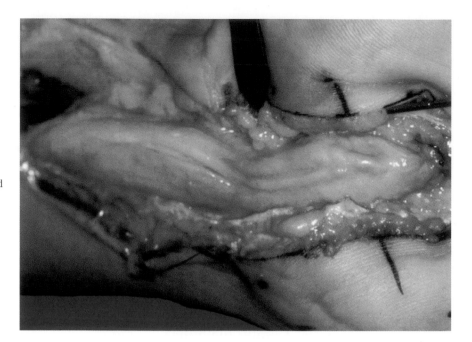

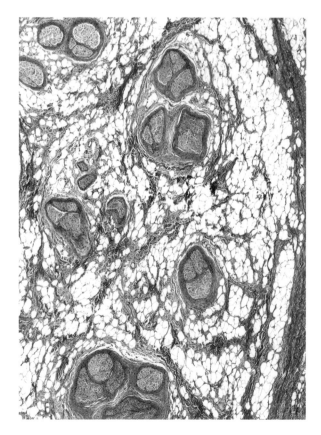
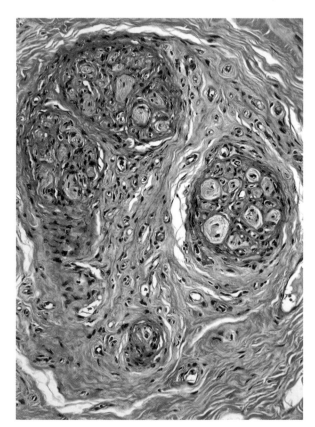

Figure 4-4

LIPOMATOSIS OF THE NERVE

Left: Histologically typical is a mature adipose tissue-dominated mass containing the splayed elements of a nerve trunk.
Right: The nerves may contain a perineurial cell proliferation remotely resembling intraneural perineurioma.

Microscopic Findings. Histologically, angiolipoma combines mature white fat with clusters and streaks of thick-walled capillaries, often radiating inward from the tumor periphery. The vessels may be congested, and some contain eosinophilic, feathery, fibrin-platelet microthrombi (fig. 4-5A,B). The number of vessels varies from few to numerous. Larger examples may contain regressive changes including fat necrosis and calcification.

Cellular angiolipoma is a variant with an extensive vascular component and focal to inconspicuous fatty element (34). This variant may grossly and histologically resemble a cellular capillary hemangioma, spindle cell hemangioma, or even Kaposi sarcoma (fig. 4-5C,D).

Genetics. No cytogenetic alterations were reported in a study of 20 angiolipomas, suggesting a genetic difference from ordinary lipomas (35).

Differential Diagnosis. Hemangiomas involving fat usually contain greater numbers of capillaries, and the vascular lumens are typically wider. Sharp demarcation, packeting of the vessels as lobules, slit like vascular spaces, lack of endothelial atypia, well-developed pericytes, and the presence of distinctive fibrin thrombi, help to separate cellular angiolipoma from hemangioendothelioma variants and malignant vascular tumors.

Treatment and Prognosis. Simple excision is curative, and there is no significant tendency for recurrence.

Spindle Cell Lipoma and Pleomorphic Lipoma

Definition. *Spindle cell lipoma* is a lipoma variant with a bland nonlipogenic, CD34-positive spindle cell component. *Pleomorphic lipoma* is a histologic variant with the additional content of floret-like or mildly pleomorphic multinucleated cells.

Clinical Features. Spindle cell and pleomorphic lipomas usually occur in middle-aged and older individuals; there is a strong male predominance (90 percent). The median age at the AFIP is 57 years, but many lesions have a long history, indicating an earlier onset. Over 80 percent of lesions occur in the subcutis of the (posterior) neck, back shoulder, scalp, face, and orofacial region. Only rare examples present elsewhere in the trunk wall (36–41). It is not clear whether lipomas in the distal extremities with a focal spindle cell component are fully comparable with spindle cell lipomas.

Spindle cell lipomas, although usually small (2 to 5 cm), may reach a size over 10 cm. Some patients have multiple lesions, and familial occurrence has been reported, mostly in older men (42).

Gross Findings. Spindle cell lipoma typically forms an oval or discoid, yellowish to grayish white mass depending on the extent of the fatty versus spindle cell component. The tumor is often firmer than an ordinary lipoma.

Microscopic Findings. Histologically, spindle cell lipoma is composed of mature fat and bland spindled mesenchymal cells that may be present as small clusters between the fat cells or dominate the tumor. The appearance varies from tumors that resemble ordinary lipomas but contain a focal spindle cell element to tumors that are mostly composed of spindle cells with only few fat cells (fig. 4-6). Only rare mitoses are detectable. Mast cells are a typical element often scattered between the spindle cells, and lymphocytes and plasma cells may occur, especially in pleomorphic lipomas. Coarse "rope-like" collagen bands are often seen between the cellular elements. Unusual features include nuclear palisading and perivascular hyalinization (fig. 4-6).

In the *myxoid variant* of spindle cell lipoma, the loose myxoid matrix may be dominant. Spindle cell lipomas with cleavage spaces resembling vascular slits have been designated *pseudoangiomatoid variant* (43). The rare *plexiform variant* consists of multiple, separate nodules, often set in fibrous matrix (44). Cytologically, the spindle cells are uniform, often have pointed ends, and may appear slightly hyperchromatic (fig. 4-7).

Pleomorphic lipoma is a variant of spindle cell lipoma. In addition to the above features, this tumor contains multinucleated floret-like giant cells, named so because its radially arranged nuclei appear like petals of flowers (fig. 4-7D). Some of these tumors have prominent nuclear atypia with hyperchromasia and even occasional atypical mitoses. In such instances the border between pleomorphic lipoma and atypical lipoma is arbitrary. The clinical features and behavior are similar to those of spindle cell lipoma.

Special Studies. Immunohistochemically, the spindle cells in both spindle cell and

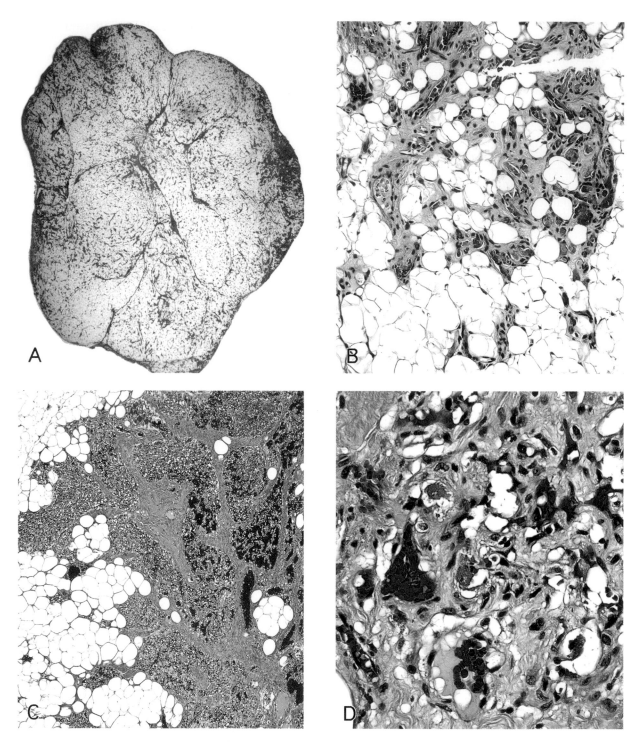

Figure 4-5

ANGIOLIPOMA

A: A sharply demarcated nodule contains capillaries as pericapsular foci or streaks streaming into the middle of nodule.

B: The fat cells are uniform in size with regular nuclei. The capillaries are often hyperemic and some contain fibrin thrombi.

C: Cellular angiolipoma forms a mass predominantly composed on lobules of capillaries. There is only a minor fatty component resulting in a hemangioma-like appearance.

D: Extensive fibrin thrombi are typical of cellular angiolipoma.

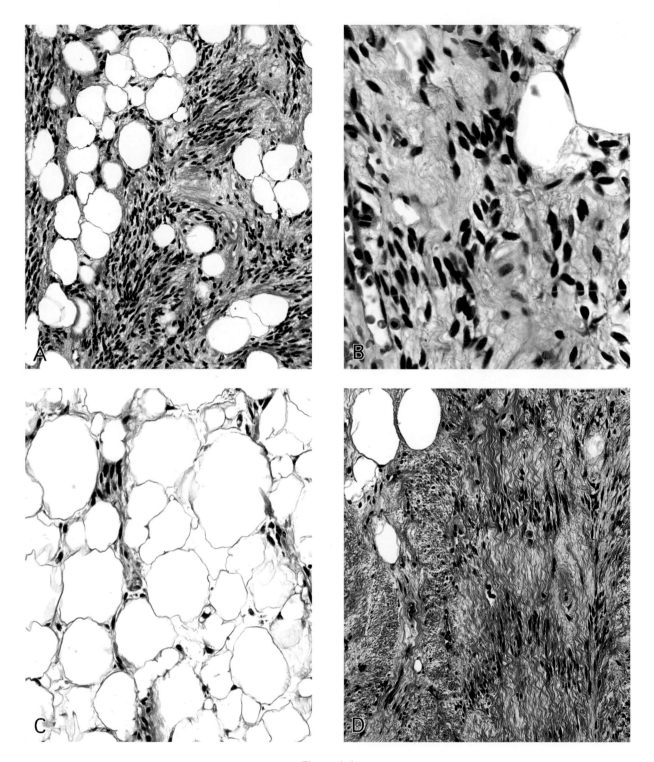

Figure 4-6

SPINDLE CELL LIPOMA

The tumor contains mature adipose tissue and a bland spindle cell component in varying proportions.
A,B: A prominent spindle cell component is present.
C: Fat-dominant spindle cell lipoma.
D: Nuclear palisading is an unusual feature of spindle cell lipoma.

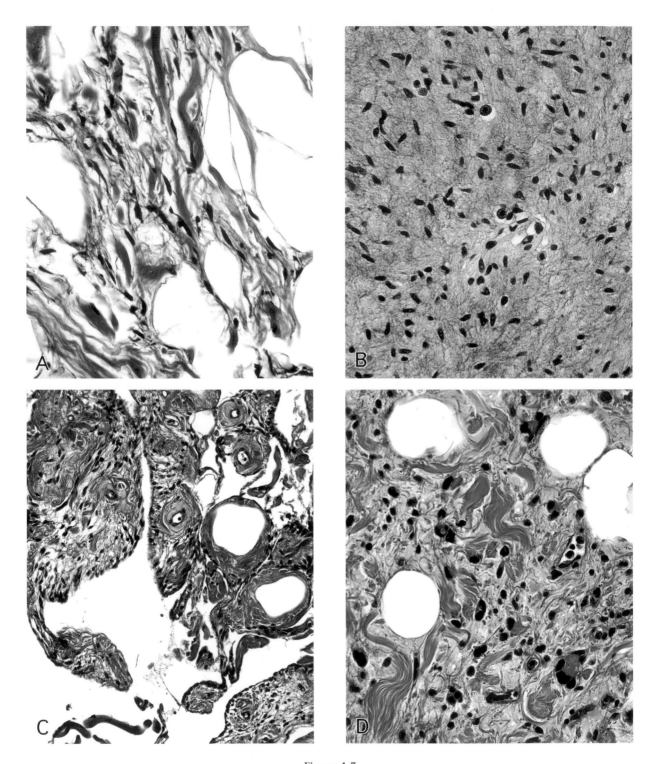

Figure 4-7

SPINDLE CELL LIPOMA

A: Lipoma cells.
B: Prominent myxoid matrix is seen in some cases.
C: A pseudoangiomatous pattern is created by stromal mucinous degeneration.
D: Pleomorphic lipoma is a spindle cell lipoma variant with multinucleated giant cells with a floret-like nuclear pattern.

pleomorphic lipomas are strongly positive for CD34 and negative for S-100 protein and smooth muscle actin (45,46). Loss of the retinoblastoma protein (RB1) by immunohistochemistry is another characteristic finding in these tumors (47). Some cases (10 to 20 percent) are desmin positive, a finding that should not lead to a misdiagnosis of a smooth muscle tumor (48).

Genetics. Chromosome 16q losses with partial monosomy are typical of spindle cell and pleomorphic lipomas and differ from the changes seen in other lipomas. The involved genes have not been specifically identified. Recurrent involvement of chromosome 13q has been reported (49–51), including loss of *RB1* locus. Spindle cell lipomas, however, characteristically lack the 12q13-15 alterations that are common in conventional and atypical lipomas (49–51).

Differential Diagnosis. The uniformity of the spindle cells, mature collagen fibers, and absence of lipoblasts separate spindle cell and pleomorphic lipomas from atypical lipomatous tumor/well-differentiated liposarcoma. Some tumors classified as spindle cell liposarcomas seem to be genetically similar to spindle cell lipomas and probably represent their progression forms (51a).

Treatment and Prognosis. Spindle cell and pleomorphic lipomas have a benign behavior and simple local excision is considered sufficient, although nondestructive recurrences may occur. However, spindle cell/pleomorphic lipoma may have a potential to evolve into more atypical forms (51a).

Chondroid Lipoma

Definition. *Chondroid lipoma* is a lipoma variant containing epithelioid cells with partial cytoplasmic clearing that resembles a cartilaginous neoplasm.

Clinical Features. Chondroid lipoma mainly occurs in young adults, with an 80 percent female predominance. The most common locations are shoulder, arm, and thigh (52,53). It has been also reported in oral cavity (54). The tumor can be subcutaneous or intramuscular. The size averages 3 to 4 cm, but examples exceeding 10 cm have occurred. The behavior is benign, but local recurrence is possible.

Gross Findings. Grossly, the tumor is typically well circumscribed, golden yellow, and slightly firmer than a lipoma. Often, lobulation and gray-white fibrous septa are visible.

Microscopic Findings. The tumor contains foci of intermingled white fat cells and distinctive chondroid lipoma cells in nests, sheets, or cords. Chondroid lipoma cells are small, often with multivacuolated, bubbly cytoplasm slightly resembling hibernoma cells. The cells may be in a lacunar space surrounded by a matrix varying from basophilic myxoid to fibrin-like or deeply eosinophilic, showing some resemblance to cartilage (fig. 4-8). Differentiated cartilage cells, however, are not present.

Chondroid lipoma cells typically have complex nuclear outlines, including curved and C-shaped forms. Mitotic figures are rare. Focal to extensive deeply eosinophilic fibrinous matrix, fat necrosis, and focal calcification may be present. Some tumors have a focal or widespread corded pattern resembling the appearance of extraskeletal myxoid chondrosarcoma.

Special Studies. Chondroid lipoma cells contain glycogen and are periodic acid–Schiff (PAS) positive. The myxoid matrix is Alcian blue positive at an acidic pH similar to the chondroid matrix. The tumor cells are variably positive for S-100 protein and CD68. Collagen IV immunoreactivity around tumor cells reflects the presence of basement membranes. Electron microscopic findings typically include prominent pinocytic vesicles and numerous cytoplasmic lipid vacuoles, interpreted to support white fat differentiation (52).

Genetics. Balanced translocation t(11;16)(q13;p12-13) has been described in three cases, suggesting that this aberration is characteristic of chondroid lipoma (55,56). The breakpoint in chromosome 11 is similar to that of hibernoma, while the breakpoint in chromosome 16 is different from that of myxoid liposarcoma.

Differential Diagnosis. Lipomas with sharply demarcated foci of cartilaginous differentiation are not chondroid lipomas, but are classified as lipomas with chondroid metaplasia (chondrolipoma). Mixed tumors with a fatty component should not be confused with chondroid lipoma. These often contain glandular epithelial differentiation and are immunohistochemically variably positive for epithelial-myoepithelial markers (keratins, actins, and glial fibrillary acidic protein [GFAP]).

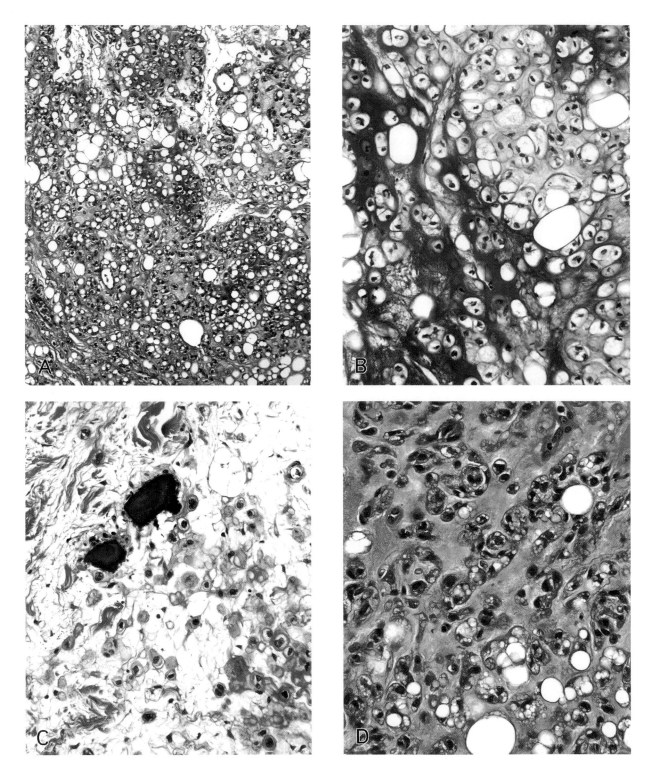

Figure 4-8

CHONDROID LIPOMA

A–C: A distinctive feature is the presence of multivacuolated cells resembling those in hibernoma and an eosinophilic fibrous matrix.

D: A prominent myxoid matrix that resembles extraskeletal myxoid chondrosarcoma is a rare finding.

234

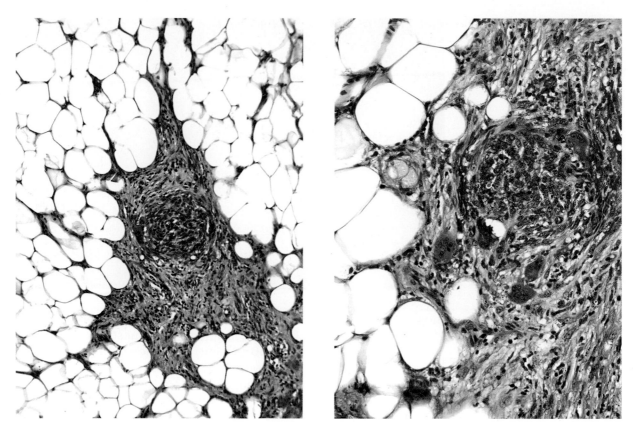

Figure 4-9

FIBROHISTIOCYTIC LIPOMA

Left, Right: Streaks of spindle cells are in a fibrous stroma with frequent hemosiderin deposits. Scattered osteoclast-like giant cells are also present.

Hemosiderotic Fibrohistiocytic Lipomatous Lesion/Tumor

Definition. *Hemosiderotic fibrohistiocytic lipomatous lesion/tumor* (HFLL) is a rare lipomatous neoplasm that contains hemosiderin and has a nonlipomatous "fibrohistiocytic"-like component.

Clinical Features. This tumor typically presents in middle-aged patients with a female predominance. Rare cases are reported in children. Most examples occur on the dorsal aspect of the foot or in the ankle, and a few in the hand and cheek (57,58).

Gross Findings. Grossly, this tumor resembles lipoma, but contains foci of yellow-brown hemosiderin pigment. The tumor size varies from 1 to over 10 cm.

Microscopic Findings. The tumor is characterized by fat cells with minimal size variation and no atypia, and quilt-like periseptal, periadipocytic, and perivascular foci of spindle cells, histiocytes, mast cells, and coarsely granulated iron pigment (fig. 4-9). The spindled cells resemble those of spindle cell lipoma and are CD34 positive. Calponin positivity has also been reported. The spindle cell component is negative for desmin, smooth muscle actin, and S-100 protein.

Genetics. A consistent t(1;10) translocation corresponding to *TGFBR3* and *MGEA5* gene rearrangements is a recurrent finding in HFLL, similar to inflammatory myxohyaline tumor of distal extremities, suggesting that these tumors are related (58a,58b).

Treatment and Prognosis. Local recurrence is common, but long-term follow-up has not identified further morbidity (57,58). Although a relationship with pleomorphic hyaline angioectatic tumor was proposed in one series (58), the two published series did not include any

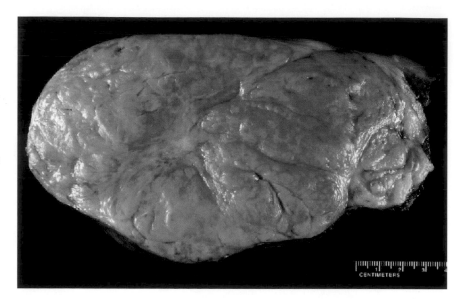

Figure 4-10

HIBERNOMA

The tumor is often distinctive as a brownish mass.

cases with transitional morphology, failing to support such an association.

Hibernoma

Definition. *Hibernoma* is a benign tumor of adipose tissue that contains multivacuolated fat cells mimicking the differentiation of brown fat.

Clinical Features. Hibernoma predominantly occurs in young adults: 61 percent are in the third and fourth decades of life. The youngest patients are teenaged children (5 percent) and 7 percent occur in those over 60 years of age. These tumors most commonly occur in the upper trunk (40 percent from neck to chest wall) (59–61). Tumors located in the neck and axillary region coincide with the normal location of brown fat. About 33 percent present in the deep thigh and inguinal region. Hibernoma can be subcutaneous or intramuscular. It is radiologically characterized by prominent tortuous "serpentine" feeder vessels (62).

Gross Findings. Hibernomas that contain brown fat cells among white fat cells are not grossly distinct from ordinary lipomas. Those tumors that have extensive brown fat differentiation are yellow brown to brown. Hibernomas usually measure between 3 and 10 cm and appear well demarcated (fig. 4-10).

Microscopic Findings. Histologically, hibernomas contain varying numbers of multivacuolated fat cells. In some cases these cells dominate, whereas in others they are only a minority among white fat cells. The cytoplasm of

hibernoma cells varies from eosinophilic to pale. The pale cell variant is the most common (more than 40 percent) and shows multivacuolated hibernoma cells with pale-staining cytoplasm. It has a predilection for the thigh. Rare variants contain a myxoid element or spindle cells resembling those in spindle cell lipoma (61,63).

Hibernomas are often lobulated by thin fibrous streaks or mildly dilated medium sized tortuous vessels that can be focally prominent (fig. 4-11).

Cytologically, hibernoma cells are multivacuolated, have small often centrally placed nuclei, and may have mildly prominent nucleoli (fig. 4-11D). Mitoses are exceptional.

Genetics. Rearrangement of 11q13, occurring in somewhat heterogeneous, sometimes complex translocations involving multiple chromosomes, appears to be the most common recurrent cytogenetic change. Breakpoints have been repeatedly found in 12q13-15 and 6p regions, sometimes involved in conventional lipomas (64–69).

Losses of the tumor suppressor genes *MEN1* and *AIP* are associated molecular genetic changes and have been considered major pathogenetic factors (70).

Differential Diagnosis. Myxoid liposarcoma and, rarely, well-differentiated liposarcoma may contain hibernoma-like multivacuolated cells. Attention should be paid to the diagnostic features of these liposarcoma types, especially the presence of prominent, delicate capillaries and uniform ovoid tumor cells in myxoid liposarcoma and atypical adipocytes with enlarged and

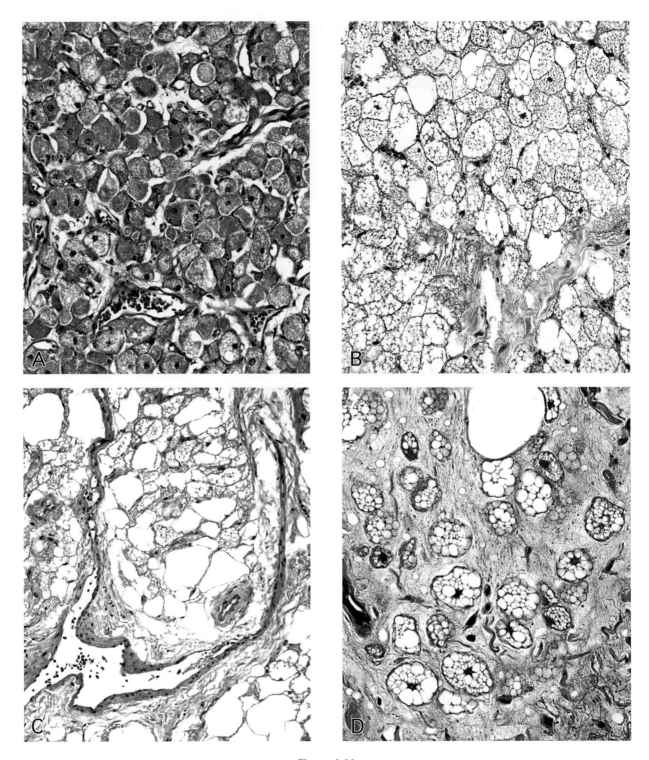

Figure 4-11

HIBERNOMA

A: Variants all have multivacuolated adipocytes with small, often central nuclei. This tumor is composed of eosinophilic cells.
B: An example with pale cells.
C: Prominent blood vessels characterize many hibernomas.
D: Hibernoma with prominent stromal myxoid change.

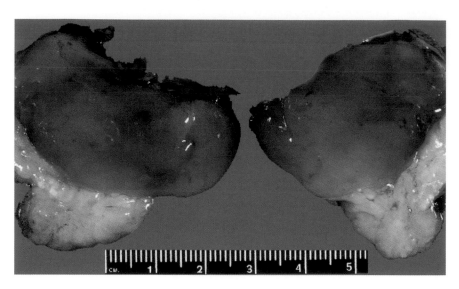

Figure 4-12

LIPOBLASTOMA

A demarcated fatty mass has a gelatinous, pinkish tan surface on sectioning.

hyperchromatic nuclei in atypical lipomatous tumor/well-differentiated liposarcoma.

Treatment and Prognosis. The behavior does not differ from that of ordinary lipoma. Recurrences are rare, so that simple excision is an acceptable option.

Lipoblastoma

Definition. *Lipoblastoma* is a benign early childhood lipomatous tumor consisting of lobulated, immature white fat cells with a prominent capillary pattern and often focal myxoid matrix. Larger tumors with grossly diffuse borders are designated *lipoblastomatosis*.

Clinical Features. Lipoblastoma is essentially restricted to children, and 75 percent of patients are under 3 years of age. Isolated, well-documented cases have been reported in young adults (71). There is a nearly 2 to 1 male predominance in most published series. The tumor typically presents in the extremities, trunk, head and neck, and sometimes in the retroperitoneum and mediastinum. Most examples are subcutaneous, but some tumors extend intramuscularly or are located in body cavities (72–76).

Gross Findings. Lipoblastoma is yellow or yellowish gray, often lobulated, and may show a lipoma-like or myxoid appearance on sectioning (fig. 4-12). Most examples are smaller than 5 cm, but a lipoblastoma over 20 cm has been reported in the retroperitoneum.

Microscopic Findings. Lipoblastoma and lipoblastomatosis are typically lobulated by connective tissue septa (fig. 4-13A). The lobules are composed of highly vascular nonatypical white fat cells and a variably myxoid stroma resembling embryonic fat (fig. 4-13B). Occasionally, a dominant spindle cell component may be present (fig. 4-13C). Foci of multivacuolated, hibernoma-like cells may also occur. In older children, lipoblastomas are typically composed of nearly mature fat with focal myxoid change resembling fibrolipoma (fig. 4-13D). Such maturation can also be observed in recurrences. Mitotic activity is inconspicuous.

Genetics. The genetic changes described in lipoblastoma typically include structural rearrangements, especially translocations and inversions involving chromosome 8q11-14 region. *PLAG1* gene rearrangement is the corresponding molecular event, and its demonstration by fluorescence in situ hybridization (FISH) may be of diagnostic value (77–81).

Differential Diagnosis. The lobular and more organized nature, lack of perivascular hypercellularity, and more commonly subcutaneous location of lipoblastoma aid in distinction from myxoid liposarcoma. In problematic cases, genetic analysis of the myxoid liposarcoma translocation and the presence of the *PLAG1* gene rearrangement are helpful. In addition to a prominent fatty component, lipofibromatosis contains cellular fibrous septa with a fibromatosis-like appearance.

Treatment and Prognosis. The tumor is benign, but may recur locally, especially if diffuse. The long-term prognosis is excellent and complete but conservative excision is sufficient.

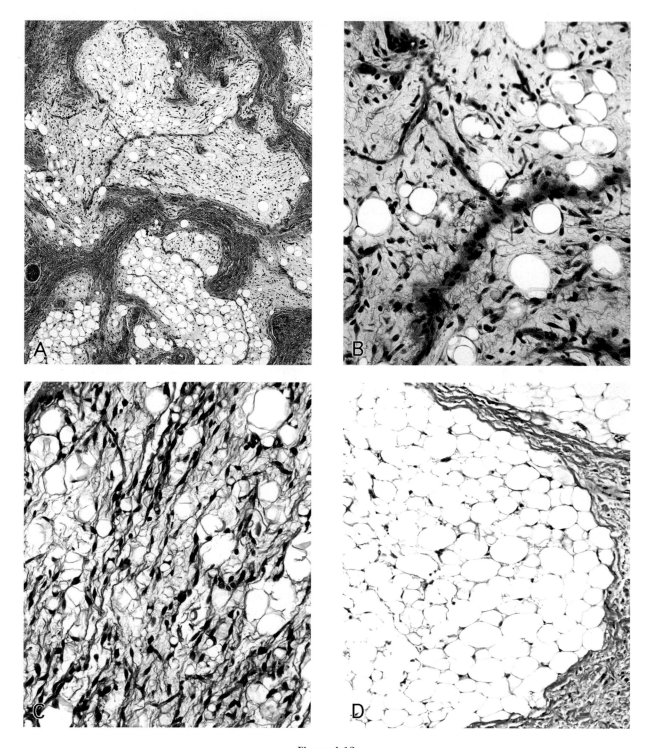

Figure 4-13

LIPOBLASTOMA

A: Multiple lobules are separated by variably developed fibrous septa.

B: Prominent capillaries and focally myxoid matrix are typical features.

C: A spindle cell component may be present in lipoblastoma.

D: In older children, lipoblastoma shows "maturation" with a greater resemblance to ordinary lipoma, but with distinct lobulation.

Massive Localized Lymphedema in the Obese

Definition. *Massive localized lymphedema* is the regional hypertrophy of a fat panniculus forming a large pendulant mass associated with localized lymphedema.

Clinical Features. This tumor-like condition usually occurs in middle-aged, seriously obese patients who weigh 150 to 200 kg, or more. The condition is more common in women. Clinically, a large, pendulant tumor-like panniculus forms on the medial proximal thigh, lower abdominal wall, or less commonly, scrotum or proximal arm. In some cases, the condition is precipitated by lymphadenectomy for carcinoma, varicose vein stripping, or trauma (82–85). Hypothyreosis is a contributing factor in some patients (83).

The tumor-like fat pannus commonly weighs 5 to 10 kg, and measures 20 to 30 cm longitudinally and up to 5 to 15 cm in depth. Bilateral lesions occur in some patients. These lesions are sometimes designated as pseudosarcomas. Regrowth is possible after excision, but there is no true neoplastic potential.

Gross Findings. The process involves the skin and subcutis, and overlying skin is usually included in the excision specimen. Grossly, the skin is thickened and indurated, with an orange peel appearance. The subcutaneous fat is greatly expanded. On sectioning, the adipose tissue appears edematous and punctuated by thickened and edematous fibrous septa.

Microscopic Findings. Histologically typical is marked fibrous thickening of the dermis with dilated lymphatics. The subcutaneous fat shows enhanced lobulation by thickened, edematous, paucicellular fibrous septa containing reactive fibroblasts and myofibroblasts (fig. 4-14). Fat is also edematous and may contain foci of fat necrosis and mild diffuse lymphohistiocytic infiltration. Occasional multinucleated fat cells are present, but there is no true adipocytic atypia. A zone of neovascular capillaries may border the fatty lobules, and dilated lymphatics may be present in the fat.

Differential Diagnosis. The most significant entity in the differential diagnosis is well-differentiated lipoma-like sarcoma, which is often a diagnostic consideration due to the large size of the lesion. Lymphedema is a superficial process that involves the skin (a major clue).

Furthermore, the fat shows distinct lobulation not observed in liposarcoma. Adipocytes are evenly sized and lack significant nuclear atypia, in contrast to well-differentiated liposarcoma.

LIPOSARCOMA

Liposarcoma is the most common soft tissue sarcoma, accounting for 20 percent of all sarcomas in adults. Liposarcomas occur anywhere in the body, but the most common sites are the thigh and retroperitoneum. Except for subcutaneous lipomas, there is little evidence that these lesions arise from mature tissue counterparts. In fact, many liposarcomas arise at sites devoid of adipose tissue.

The classification of malignant adipocytic tumors is now significantly based on their cytogenetic abnormalities. Four main categories have been defined: 1) *atypical lipomatous tumor/well-differentiated liposarcoma;* 2) *dedifferentiated liposarcoma;* 3) *myxoid/round cell liposarcoma;* and 4) *pleomorphic liposarcoma.* An additional histologic type, *spindle cell liposarcoma*, has been proposed but remains still somewhat controversial due to its less defined genetic abnormalities.

The anatomic distribution of liposarcoma appears to be closely related to the histologic type. The well-differentiated and dedifferentiated subtypes account for 46 percent and 18 percent of liposarcomas, respectively, and are more commonly found in the retroperitoneum. The myxoid/round cell and pleomorphic subtypes account for 28 percent and 8 percent of liposarcomas, respectively, and have a predilection for extremities, with more than two-thirds occurring in the thigh.

The extent of differentiation, as reflected by histologic grade, remains the most important determinant of clinical course and of ultimate prognosis for patients with liposarcoma after resection. Mortality rates for patients with liposarcoma range from 1 to 90 percent and recurrence rates from 5 to 83 percent depending on histologic subtype and location (86–89).

Atypical Lipomatous Tumor/ Well-Differentiated Liposarcoma

Definition. *Atypical lipomatous tumor/well-differentiated liposarcoma* (ALT/WDLS) is a locally aggressive but nonmetastasizing malignant fatty neoplasm composed mainly of a mature

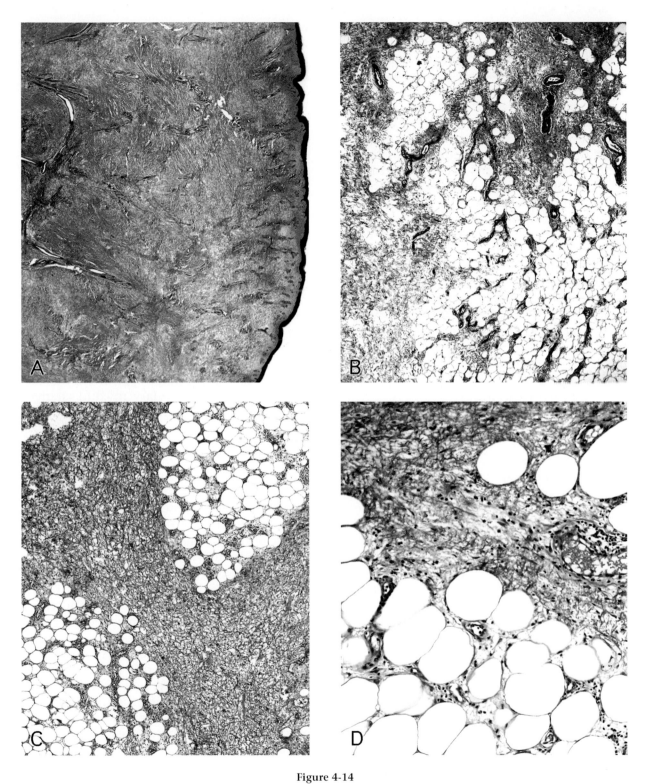

Figure 4-14

MASSIVE LOCALIZED LYMPHEDEMA IN THE OBESE

A: The skin is thickened by fibrosclerosis.

B–D: The subcutaneous fat retains lobulation, but the septa are edematous and expanded by paucicellular fibrosis. There is no adipocytic atypia.

adipocytic proliferation showing significant variation in the size and shape of the adipocytes and the presence of scattered atypical stromal cells and/or lipoblasts.

General Considerations. ALT/WDLS is a low-grade, nonmetastasizing tumor (unless it undergoes dedifferentiation) with a propensity for local recurrence. Due to its lack of metastatic potential, the designation of sarcoma is controversial, particularly for lesions arising at surgically amenable locations, such as the extremity and trunk. At these sites, wide excision is usually curative, and hence the use of term well-differentiated liposarcoma in these sites is being replaced with the term atypical lipomatous tumor. In the retroperitoneum, pelvis, and mediastinum, however, the well-differentiated liposarcoma designation is still preferred, as the mortality from this disease is significant, even in the absence of metastases. Atypical lipomatous tumor and well-differentiated liposarcoma are presently used interchangeably as synonyms, describing identical lesions both morphologically and karyotypically.

Clinical Features. These tumors account for 45 percent of all liposarcomas and represent the largest subgroup of malignant adipocytic neoplasms. They often arise in middle-aged adults, with a peak incidence in the sixth decade, and only rarely occur in the pediatric age group. There is no gender predilection. Most present in the deep soft tissue of the limbs, especially the thigh, followed by retroperitoneum, paratesticular/spermatic cord area, and mediastinum. Clinically, they present as a deep-seated, painless enlarging mass, with slow growth to attain very large sizes. In the retroperitoneal locations the tumors may exceed 20 cm before eliciting any symptomatology.

Gross Findings. ALT/WDLS is often composed of large, lobulated and well-circumscribed masses, surrounded by thin, translucent membranes, which appear easily shelled out (fig. 4-15). Only rarely is more infiltrative growth appreciated grossly. On cut surface, the tumors show variable yellow and white components (fig. 4-16). Fat necrosis may be noted in larger tumors.

Microscopic Findings. Microscopically, ALT/WDLS is divided into three morphologic types: lipoma-like, sclerosing and inflammatory. The presence of more than one morphologic pattern within the same lesion is common, particularly within retroperitoneal locations. Although the presence of lipoblasts is often believed to be the hallmark of any liposarcoma diagnosis, their absence does not exclude a diagnosis of ALT/WDLS. Large areas of mature adipose tissue or lipoma-like tissue associated with high variability in the adipocytic cell size and the presence of atypical stromal cells with hyperchromatic and multilobated nuclei are key diagnostic features for ALT/WDLS (fig. 4-17). The presence of fibrous septa dividing the tumor into solid compartments is also of diagnostic significance. The septa are typically composed of a delicate, silky fibrous stroma, have a variable thickness, and are often infiltrated by spindle or atypical stromal cells (fig. 4-18). The relative abundance of the fibrous component distinguishes the sclerosing variant from the predominantly fatty, lipoma-like ALT/WDLS.

In the retroperitoneum, the hyperchromatic atypical stromal cells are more numerous and more readily appreciated within the fibrous septa (fig. 4-19). Secondary myxoid changes may be noted and may represent diagnostic pitfalls, due to features that overlap with other myxoid sarcomas.

Inflammatory liposarcoma is a rare variant of ALT/WDLS that occurs more often within the retroperitoneum. The heavy inflammatory component is composed of lymphocytes and plasma cells and often obscures the adipocytic nature of the neoplasm, suggesting alternative diagnoses, such as Hodgkin lymphoma, Castleman disease, or inflammatory myofibroblastic tumor (fig. 4-20). By immunohistochemistry, the inflammatory infiltrate is composed of polyphenotypic lymphoplasmacytic aggregates in keeping with a reactive process.

Special Studies. Immunohistochemistry plays a limited role in the differential diagnosis of ALT/WDLS. Adipocytic cells stain with S-100 protein, while HMB-45 is consistently negative, which may be helpful to exclude a diagnosis of angiomyolipoma, occasionally entertained in the differential of retroperitoneal lesions. MDM2 and CDK4 immunoreactivity, potentially useful to distinguish between lipoma and ALT/WDLS, should be interpreted with caution due to the low cellularity and often only focal pattern of staining. In this distinction, FISH

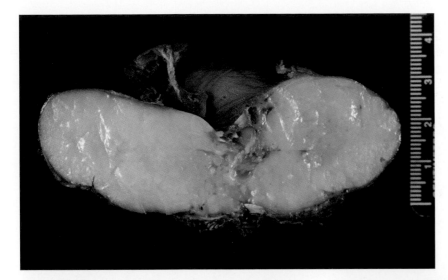

Figure 4-15

ATYPICAL LIPOMATOUS TUMOR/WELL-DIFFERENTIATED LIPOSARCOMA

A large, deep-seated tumor within the thigh shows a homogeneous, buttery yellow cut surface.

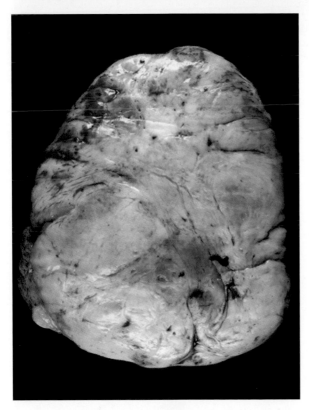

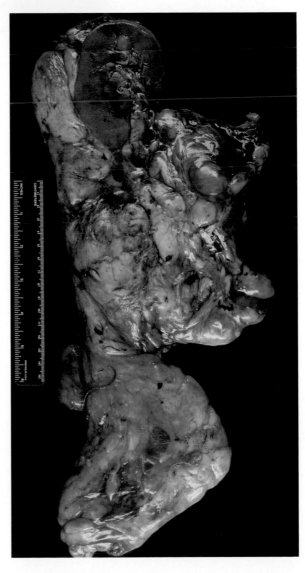

Figure 4-16

ATYPICAL LIPOMATOUS TUMOR/WELL-DIFFERENTIATED LIPOSARCOMA

Recurrent retroperitoneal well-differentiated liposarcoma as multiple discontiguous nodules within the retroperitoneum and abdomen, including a 30-cm mass (above) showing a yellow, lobulated cut surface. A 34-cm lesion is adherent to the kidney capsule (right).

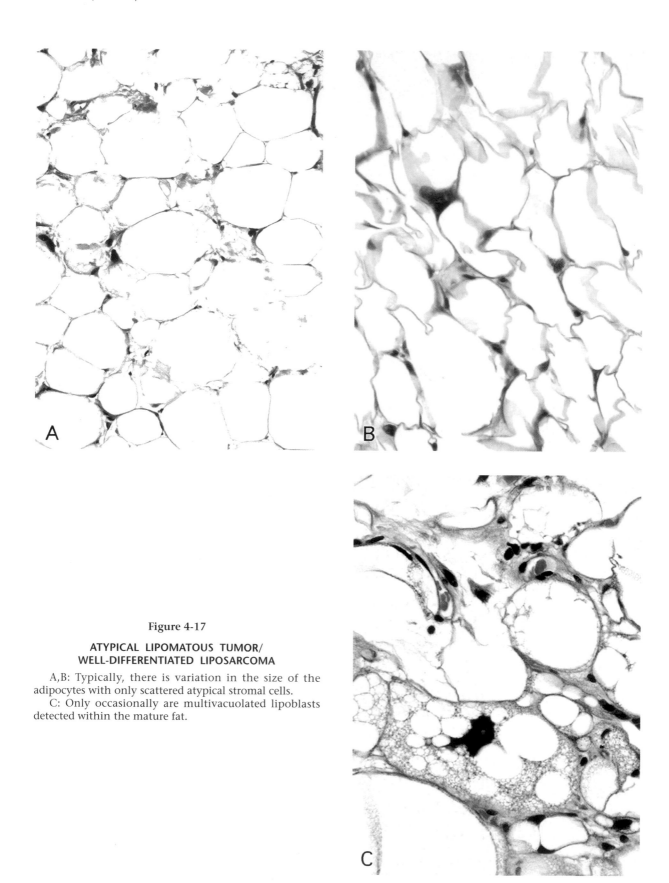

Figure 4-17

**ATYPICAL LIPOMATOUS TUMOR/
WELL-DIFFERENTIATED LIPOSARCOMA**

A,B: Typically, there is variation in the size of the adipocytes with only scattered atypical stromal cells.

C: Only occasionally are multivacuolated lipoblasts detected within the mature fat.

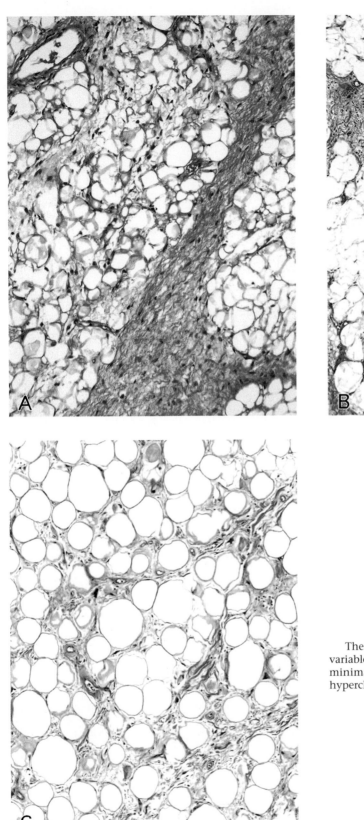

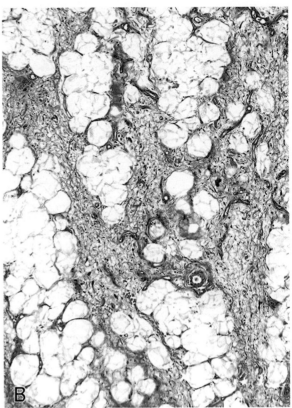

Figure 4-18

**ATYPICAL LIPOMATOUS TUMOR/
WELL-DIFFERENTIATED LIPOSARCOMA**

The sclerosing variant shows delicate fibrous septa of variable thickness infiltrated by either spindle cells with minimal cytologic atypia (A), or scattered atypical and hyperchromatic stromal cells (B,C).

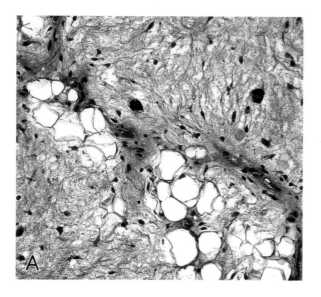

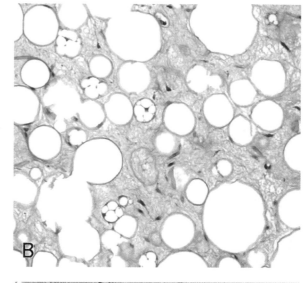

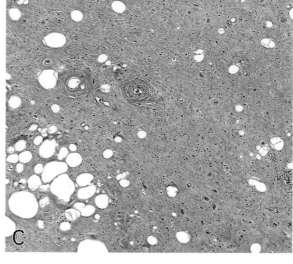

Figure 4-19

**ATYPICAL LIPOMATOUS TUMOR/
WELL-DIFFERENTIATED LIPOSARCOMA**

In the retroperitoneal location, the atypical stromal cells are usually more numerous and readily appreciated on the fibrous background.

A: The atypical cells often have multinucleated, lobulated nuclei with a floret-like appearance.

B: Multivacuolated lipoblasts are also detected.

C: In some cases the fibrous component appears more confluent, showing dense hyalinization of the collagenous stroma.

D: The tumors are often tightly adherent to the renal capsule, requiring nephrectomy.

E: Secondary myxoid changes are seen adjacent to or within the lipoma-like component.

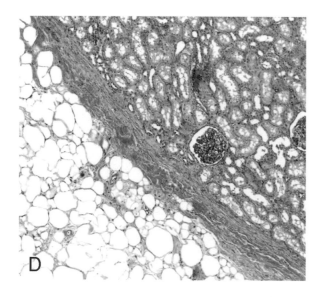

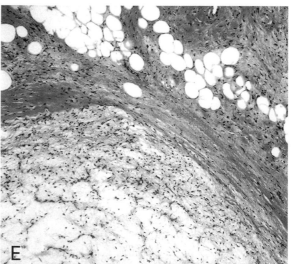

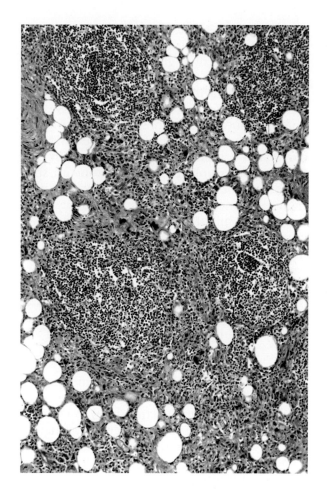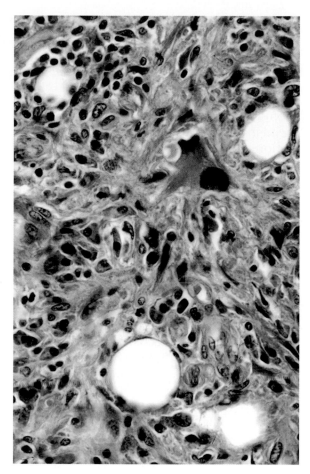

Figure 4-20

WELL-DIFFERENTIATED LIPOSARCOMA, INFLAMMATORY VARIANT

Left, Right: An abundant lymphocytic and plasmacytic infiltrate, arranged in tight aggregates as well as dispersed throughout the adipocytic component, may suggest an alternative lymphoproliferative diagnosis.

analysis for the presence of *MDM2* or *CDK4* gene amplification is preferred, being far more sensitive, and is the gold standard ancillary technique in challenging cases.

Genetics. The genetic hallmark of ALT/WDLS is the presence of supernumerary circular (ring) and giant rod chromosomes. These rings and giant markers contain amplification of the 12q14-15 region, which includes MDM2 and CDK4, and other co-amplified chromosomal regions. Most commonly, the supernumerary ring and marker chromosomes are the sole genetic abnormality; however, the telomeric associations may falsely give the impression of a more complex karyotype. FISH analysis is now widely applied on archival material to document the presence of the 12q14-15 amplicon, using fluorescent probes covering the *MDM2* or *CDK4* gene locus. This 12q14-15 amplification is not noted in lipomas, and its detection serves as a critical finding in confirming the diagnosis of ALT/WDLS.

Differential Diagnosis. The most common diagnostic challenge involves the distinction between ALT/WDLS and lipoma. This is particularly relevant in the extremity and trunk, where the ALT/WDLS can be composed of areas of mature adipose tissue, indistinguishable from lipoma, with only rare, scattered atypical cells. In nonretroperitoneal locations, the atypical cells should be large enough to be discerned at scanning magnification and the presence of even a single highly atypical and hyperchromatic stromal cell is sufficient for the diagnosis. The nuclei are often elongated, giving the fat cell a signet ring cell-like appearance, and multinucleation also occurs. Many cases also contain expanded septa with atypical cells. Furthermore, ALT/WDLS shows a higher variability in the adipocytic cell size and shape, in comparison with the even cell size in lipomas. The clinical presentation of a large, deep-seated tumor in the thigh also reinforces the high level of suspicion. A minimum of one section per centimeter of diameter of tumor or up to 10 sections should be routinely taken from lipomatous tumors removed from locations other than subcutaneous tissue.

The distinction of spindle cell lipoma from ALT/WDLS is based on the ropy collagen, uniform spindle cells, and subcutaneous location in the back, neck, or shoulder. Similarly, the presence of a subcutaneous fatty lesion within the shoulder and neck exhibiting numerous multinucleated, florette-type atypical cells favors a pleomorphic lipoma over an ALT/WDLS.

Secondary myxoid change is common in both lipomas and ALT/WDLS and its presence should not affect the diagnosis. However, myxoid features in an otherwise benign lipoma are often underrecognized and may suggest alternative diagnoses, including ALT/WDLS or myxoid liposarcoma. Particularly in acral locations, lipomas often exhibit secondary myxoid changes and may simulate an ALT/WDLS.

Occasionally myelolipoma may simulate an ALT/WLDS due to its heavy inflammatory infiltrate admixed with the mature adipose tissue component. Careful examination at high power reveals clusters of hematopoietic cells with scattered megakaryocytes that lead to the correct interpretation.

Fat necrosis can also be mistaken for an ALT/WLDS due to its lipid-filled macrophages, the multinucleated cells, and areas of fibrosis. Macrophages however, have small, centrally located, bland nuclei, which are not indented by lipoid vacuoles.

Angiomyolipoma with a prominent fatty component may be sometimes misinterpreted as ALT/WDLS, especially within the retroperitoneum, where the perivascular myoid cells may be confused with the atypical stromal cells. The prominent vascular component, with concentric arrangement of the smooth muscle cells is not a feature of ALT/WDLS, and while metaplastic smooth muscle may be found occasionally in ALT/WDLS, it does not have a perivascular distribution. Moreover, HMB-45 is positive in the myoid cells of angiomyolipoma while the cells of ALT/WDLS are negative.

Treatment and Prognosis. The most important prognostic factor for ALT/WDLS is the anatomic location. Lesions located within the extremity or easily amenable to wide excision are cured after complete surgical resection. In contrast, tumors arising in the retroperitoneum, spermatic cord, or mediastinum are associated with high recurrence rates and may eventually cause death as a result of uncontrolled local effects on critical adjacent organs. Additionally, the risk of dedifferentiation in subsequent recurrences varies from 20 percent in the retroperitoneum to less than 2 percent in the limbs (90). Overall mortality varies from 0 percent for patients with tumors of the extremities to over 80 percent for those occurring in the retroperitoneum (91).

Dedifferentiated Liposarcoma

Definition. *Dedifferentiated liposarcoma* is a well-differentiated liposarcoma that shows either an abrupt or more gradual transition to a nonlipogenic sarcoma. The process of dedifferentiation is often seen already in the primary tumor, but it some cases it only appears in a recurrence.

Clinical Features. Dedifferentiated liposarcomas typically present as large, deep-seated, painless masses, often detected incidentally or due to signs of obstruction of adjacent organs. The retroperitoneum is the most common anatomic location, outnumbering the extremity soft tissue by at least 3 to 1. Other locations include spermatic cord and trunk. Occurrence within a subcutaneous location is rare. There is no gender predilection and the peak incidence occurs in the seventh decade of life. Radiographically, these tumors show coexistence of both fatty and nonfatty solid components, which is helpful for the diagnosis.

Gross Findings. Grossly, dedifferentiated liposarcoma consists of large multinodular yellow masses (well-differentiated component) containing discrete, solid, often fleshy nonlipomatous areas (fig. 4-21). Morphologically, these regions have a heterogeneous appearances, ranging from low- to high-grade components.

Microscopic Findings. The most prevalent histology is a spindle and pleomorphic sarcoma, with a varying degree of myxoid stroma,

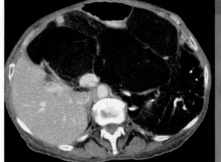
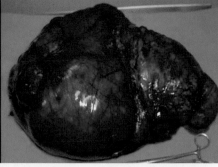
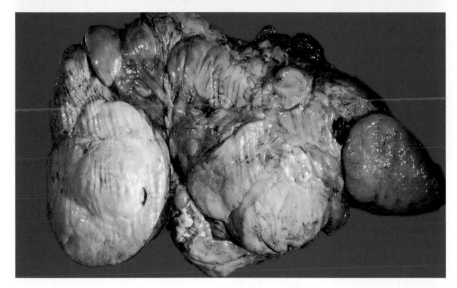

Figure 4-21

DEDIFFERENTIATED LIPOSARCOMA

Most dedifferentiated liposarcomas present as very large lesions within the retroperitoneum.

Top: CT scan and intraoperative gross photo of en-bloc resection of a voluminous retroperitoneal tumor.

Bottom: The tumors usually have a fish-flesh, gray-tan cut surface.

resembling myxofibrosarcoma or malignant fibrous histiocytoma (fig. 4-22). Although dedifferentiated liposarcoma was initially defined as a high-grade nonlipogenic component adjacent to a well-differentiated fatty lesion (92), the concept of low-grade dedifferentiation is now widely recognized (fig. 4-23A,B) (93,94). Low-grade dedifferentiation may exhibit a large variety of growth patterns, including bland spindle cell proliferations reminiscent of fibromatosis, solitary fibrous tumor/hemangiopericytoma low-grade fibrosarcoma, or gastrointestinal stromal tumor (fig. 4-23C–E). Recently, the concept of dedifferentiation was expanded even further to include "'homologous" lipogenic dedifferentiation, which closely resembles pleomorphic liposarcoma due to the presence of pleomorphic lipoblasts in the high-grade component (95).

Dedifferentiated liposarcoma undergoes heterologous differentiation in 5 to 10 percent of cases, with no apparent impact on clinical outcome. The most common lines of differentiation include osteochondrosarcoma/chondrosarcomatous (fig. 4-24, left) and myogenic (either leiomyosarcoma or rhabdomyosarcoma) elements. Other rare morphologic patterns include leiomyosarcoma-like elements and an undifferentiated/primitive component, resembling a small blue round cell tumor (fig. 4-24, right). A bland and peculiar "meningothelial-like" whorling pattern has been described in association with metaplastic ossification (fig. 4-25) (96,97).

Special Studies. The only reliable marker is the consistent nuclear reactivity of MDM2 and CDK4 reactivity (fig. 4-26A,B) (98). CD34 positivity is common. Otherwise, immunohistochemical studies are of limited value in distinguishing dedifferentiated liposarcoma from other spindle and pleomorphic sarcomas.

Genetics. Similar to ALT/WDLS, dedifferentiated liposarcomas exhibit the ring and marker giant chromosomes secondary to 12q14-15 region amplification (99,100). FISH analysis for detecting the *MDM2* or *CDK4* gene amplification

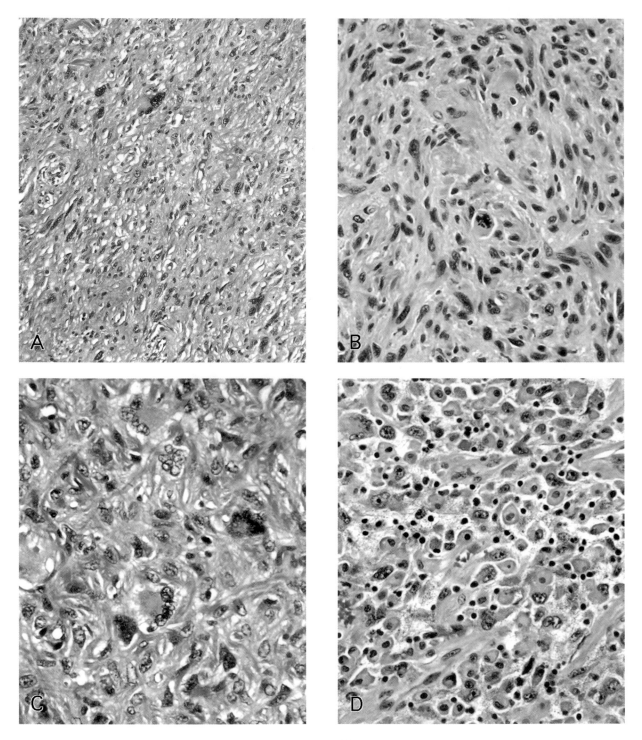

Figure 4-22

DEDIFFERENTIATED LIPOSARCOMA

A: Usually, dedifferentiated liposarcoma is a high-grade nonlipogenic spindle and pleomorphic sarcoma resembling malignant fibrous histiocytoma.

B: Mitotic figures are frequent.

C: Multinucleated, floret-type cells.

D: Occasionally, there is a more epithelioid, histiocytoid appearance.

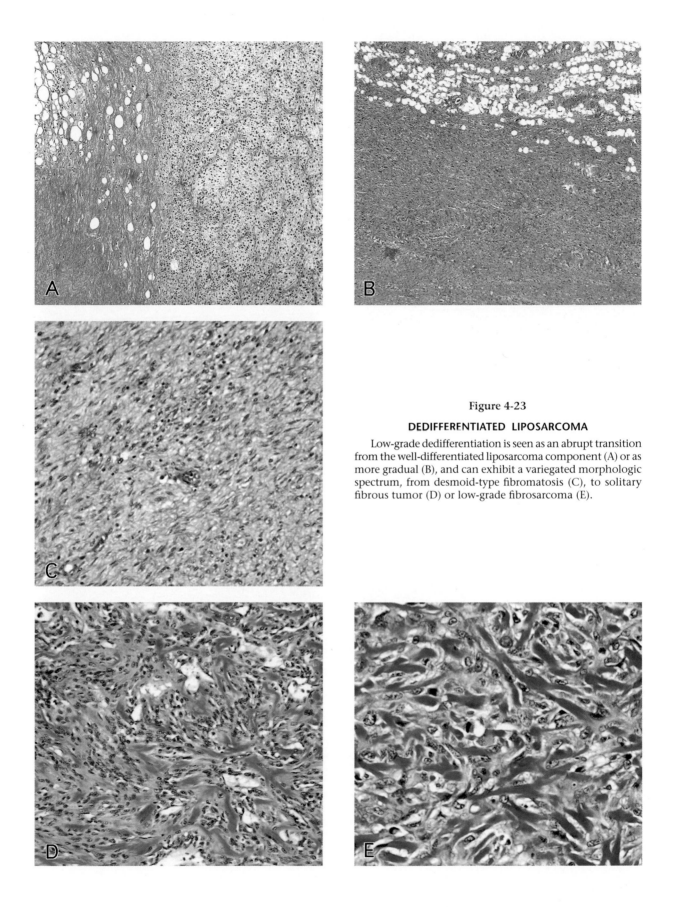

Figure 4-23

DEDIFFERENTIATED LIPOSARCOMA

Low-grade dedifferentiation is seen as an abrupt transition from the well-differentiated liposarcoma component (A) or as more gradual (B), and can exhibit a variegated morphologic spectrum, from desmoid-type fibromatosis (C), to solitary fibrous tumor (D) or low-grade fibrosarcoma (E).

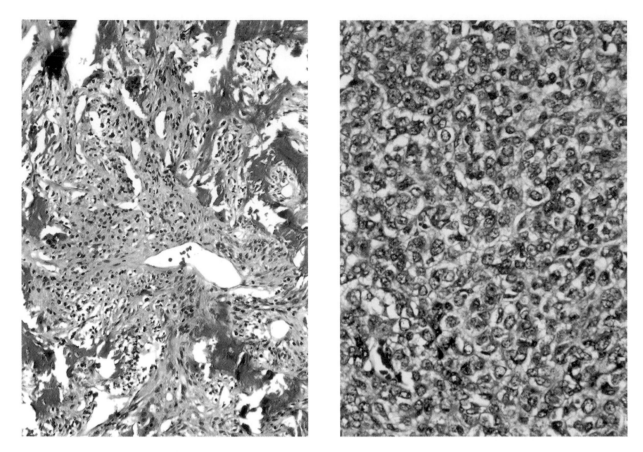

Figure 4-24

DEDIFFERENTIATED LIPOSARCOMA

Unusual microscopic features include divergent differentiation to a heterologous osteosarcoma component (left) or an undifferentiated small blue round cell tumor, reminiscent of Ewing sarcoma (right).

Figure 4-25

DEDIFFERENTIATED LIPOSARCOMA

Dedifferentiated liposarcoma variants, especially those in the retroperitoneum, contain meningothelial-like whorls.

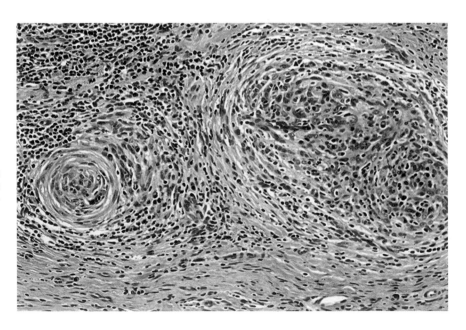

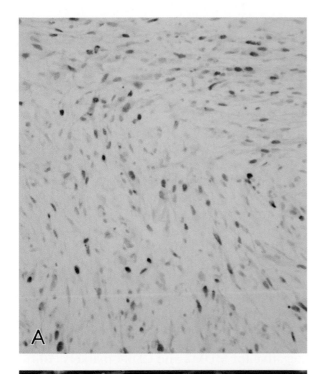

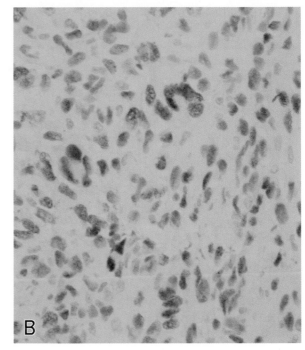

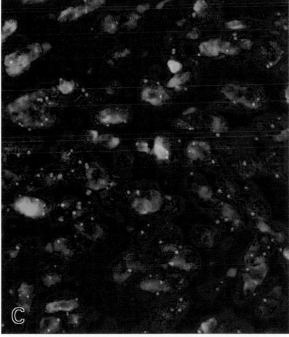

Figure 4-26

DEDIFFERENTIATED LIPOSARCOMA

Ancillary techniques are useful for detecting the consistent 12q14-15 genetic abnormalities. These are seen either at the protein level by nuclear immunoreactivity for MDM2 and CDK4 (A,B) or at the gene level by fluorescence in situ hybridization (FISH) for the detection of copy number abnormalities on interphase nuclei from archival material. A high level of *CDK4* gene amplification (C) (CDK4 = red signal; chromosome 12 centromeric probe = green signal) in a dedifferentiated liposarcoma.

may be applied on archival material in difficult diagnoses, such as lack of a well-differentiated liposarcoma component or limited material (fig. 4-26C).

Differential Diagnosis. Myxofibrosarcoma arising in the extremities or chest wall may exhibit an infiltrative growth pattern within the subcutaneous fat, and mimic a well-differentiated liposarcoma component. The extremity/ trunk presentation, however, and rather superficial location within the subcutis, are unusual for a diagnosis of dedifferentiated liposarcoma. In difficult cases, immunohistochemical studies for CDK4 and MDM2 overexpression or FISH analysis for *MDM2* gene amplification provide a more definitive classification.

In retroperitoneal tumors, the material available for review may show only a high-grade pleomorphic or myxoid sarcoma, reminiscent of a high-grade pleomorphic malignant fibrous histiocytoma or myxofibrosarcoma, without an obvious well-differentiated liposarcoma component. Careful and sometimes extensive sampling of these large tumors reveal the presence of a lipomatous component, which may have been initially overlooked. Alternatively, the status of CDK4 and MDM2 expression at the protein or gene level may be evaluated to confirm the diagnosis of dedifferentiated liposarcoma, even in the absence of a well-differentiated liposarcoma component. Most cases previously diagnosed as malignant fibrous histiocytoma or myxofibrosarcoma in the retroperitoneum are now considered dedifferentiated liposarcomas.

Treatment and Prognosis. Dedifferentiated liposarcomas have similar local effects to well-differentiated liposarcoma. Although they metastasize systemically (i.e., lungs), they have a significantly lower metastatic rate (10 to 15 percent) than would be predicted based on their high-grade morphology, large size, and a 5-year survival probability of 75 percent (87,101). In comparison, the probability of distant metastasis for all patients with larger than 5-cm, high-grade malignant fibrous histiocytoma of the extremity at 3 years is 59 percent (88).

For retroperitoneal tumors, the histologic subtype, incomplete resection, contiguous organ resection (excluding nephrectomy), and increasing patient age are strongly associated with death from tumor. Tumor burden and nephrectomy are not associated with disease-specific survival (88). Despite an aggressive surgical approach, over 80 percent of dedifferentiated liposarcomas recur locally.

Spindle Cell Liposarcoma

Definition. *Spindle cell liposarcoma* is a rare malignant lipogenic neoplasm occurring in the subcutaneous tissue of the shoulder girdle or upper limbs. It is composed of a deceptively bland spindle cell proliferation admixed with a limited adipocytic component.

General Considerations. The classification of spindle cell liposarcoma remains somewhat controversial and further work is needed to elucidate its place in the present classification of liposarcomas. Spindle cell liposarcoma has been initially regarded as a variant of ALT/WDLS, in which the bland spindle cell component predominates over the adipocytic areas (102). Spindle cell liposarcomas, however, do not share the same genetic abnormalities with ALT/WDLS and consistently lack the 12q14-15 amplification, suggesting a distinct pathologic entity.

Clinical Features. Spindle cell liposarcoma tends to occur in the subcutaneous tissue of the extremities, trunk, and head and neck region of adults.

Gross and Microscopic Findings. Grossly, the lesions are characterized by multinodularity. Microscopically, there is a bland spindle cell proliferation arranged in fascicles and whorls, set in a variably myxoid stroma (fig. 4-27).

Special Studies. The slightly atypical, spindled tumor cells often stain for CD34, but are negative for MDM2 and CDK4 markers (103).

Genetics. Spindle cell liposarcomas consistently lack the 12q14-15 amplicon by karyotype or *MDM2/CDK4* amplification by FISH. Instead, a partial or complete monosomy 7 has been reported as the sole anomaly or among a few additional simple numeric and structural abnormalities in two cases (104).

Differential Diagnosis. The differential diagnosis of spindle cell liposarcoma is broad and includes both benign lesions, such as spindle cell lipoma and diffuse neurofibroma, as well as low-grade sarcomas, such as dermatofibrosarcoma protuberans, sclerosing ALT/WDLS, low-grade myxofibrosarcoma, low-grade malignant peripheral nerve sheath tumor, and low-grade fibromyxoid sarcoma. The combination of an adipocytic component adjacent to a bland spindle cell proliferation usually helps in recognizing this tumor as a liposarcoma.

Treatment and Prognosis. Despite their bland morphologic appearance and superficial anatomic location, spindle cell liposarcomas are prone to multiple local recurrences (102).

Myxoid Liposarcoma

Definition. *Myxoid liposarcoma* is a tumor composed of uniform, round to oval, primitive nonlipogenic cells and a variable number of small signet ring cell lipoblasts in a prominent

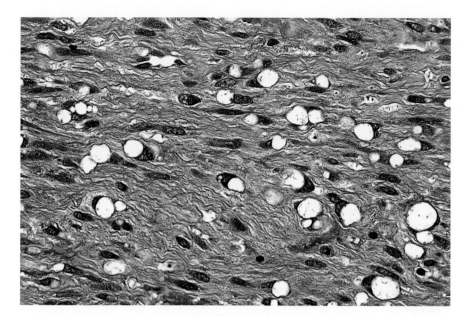

Figure 4-27

SPINDLE CELL LIPOSARCOMA

The tumor is composed of fairly uniform spindled cells with common fat vacuoles and a myxoid matrix.

myxoid stroma with a characteristic branching vascular pattern. Included in this category are lesions formerly known as *round cell liposarcoma.*

General Considerations. The gradual transition from myxoid to hypercellular/round cell areas provides strong support that myxoid and round cell liposarcomas represent a histologic continuum of myxoid liposarcoma. This concept is also supported by the presence of the identical translocation in both histologic types.

Clinical Features. Myxoid liposarcoma is the second most common subtype of liposarcoma, accounting for more than one third of liposarcomas and representing about 10 percent of all adult soft tissue sarcomas. The deep soft tissues of the extremities are usually involved by a large painless mass, and more than two thirds of cases arise within the musculature of the thigh (fig. 4-28). Myxoid liposarcoma rarely arises primarily in the retroperitoneum or subcutaneous tissue.

Myxoid liposarcoma is a disease of young adults, with the age at presentation on average a decade younger than with other histologic subtypes of liposarcoma. The peak incidence is in the fourth and fifth decades of life and, although rare, it is the most common form of liposarcoma in children and adolescents (105). There is no gender predilection (fig. 4-29).

Gross Findings. Grossly, myxoid liposarcomas are well-circumscribed, multinodular intramuscular tumors, showing a glistening, gelatinous cut surface in the myxoid areas (fig.

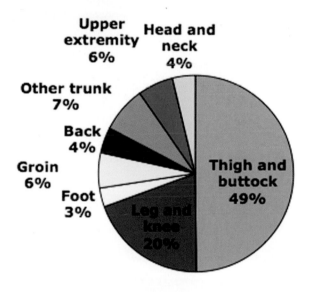

Figure 4-28

MYXOID LIPOSARCOMA

Anatomic distribution from data from the Armed Forces Institute of Pathology (AFIP).

4-30, top). In contrast, areas of the round cell component have instead a fleshy tan appearance (fig. 4-30, bottom). Gross evidence of tumor necrosis is uncommon.

Microscopic Findings. At low power, myxoid liposarcoma has a nodular growth pattern, with enhanced cellularity at the periphery of the lobules. There is a mixture of uniform round to oval nonlipogenic cells and small signet

Age and Sex Distribution of 1034 Patients with Myxoid Liposarcoma

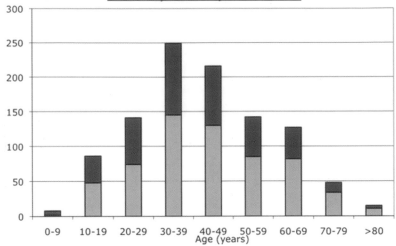

Figure 4-29

MYXOID LIPOSARCOMA

Age and sex distribution.

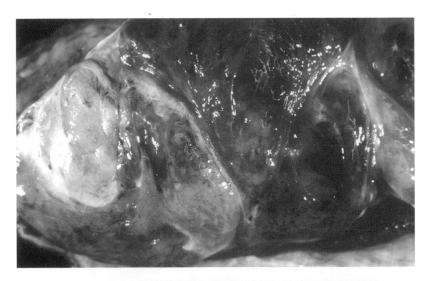

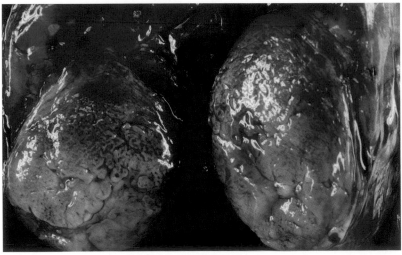

Figure 4-30

MYXOID LIPOSARCOMA

Top: A low-grade myxoid liposarcoma has a distinctive gelatinous appearance.

Bottom: In contrast, a high-grade tumor with a predominant round cell component shows a more fish-fleshy, tan cut surface.

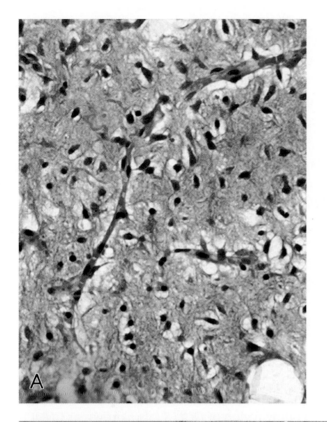

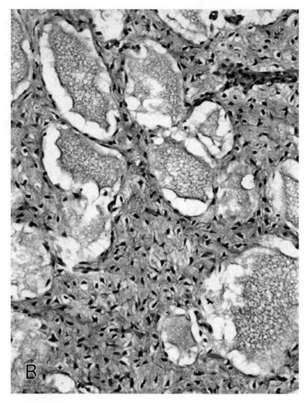

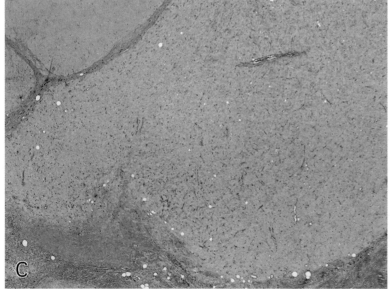

Figure 4-31

MYXOID LIPOSARCOMA

A: Low-grade myxoid liposarcoma has small, uniform round to oval cells embedded in a copious myxoid stroma with a rich capillary vascular network.

B: The mucopolysaccharides accumulate in small pools or microcysts, having a "pulmonary-edema" type appearance.

C: Remarkable tumor response to trabectedin (ET-743) in a myxoid liposarcoma of the buttock, microscopically showing more than 95 percent tumor fibrosis.

ring lipoblasts in a prominent myxoid stroma, rich with a delicate, arborizing "chicken-wire" capillary vasculature (fig. 4-31A). Frequently, the extracellular mucin forms large confluent pools, creating a microcystic lymphangioma-like or so-called pulmonary edema growth pattern (fig. 4-31B). Typically, myxoid liposarcoma lacks nuclear

pleomorphism, giant tumor cells, prominent areas of spindling, or significant mitotic activity. Post-treatment specimens can show extensive fibrosis and be unrecognizable (fig. 4-31C).

A subset of myxoid liposarcoma shows histologic progression to hypercellular or round cell morphology, which is associated with a

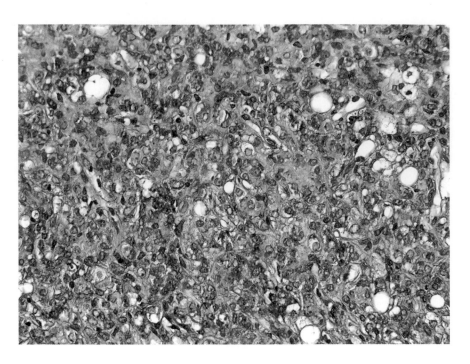

Figure 4-32

ROUND CELL LIPOSARCOMA

The round cell liposarcoma component consists of solid sheets of monotonous round cells, lacking cytologic atypia or spindling.

significantly poorer prognosis. The round cell areas are characterized by solid sheets of back-to-back primitive round cells with a high nuclear to cytoplasmic ratio, and no intervening myxoid stroma (fig. 4-32). The cytomorphology of the round cell component may resemble the small cells seen in the myxoid areas or may, less often, consist of larger rounded cells with variable amounts of eosinophilic cytoplasm. These two morphologic patterns show no difference in prognosis but have been responsible for some of the confusion regarding the definition of the round cell variant. The so-called areas of transition are defined as areas of increased cellularity, not reaching the level of the round cell component and still retaining a small amount of intercellular myxoid stroma.

Special Studies. In most cases, immunohistochemical studies are not needed for establishing a diagnosis of myxoid liposarcoma. In tumors with a predominantly round cell morphology, immunostains are performed to exclude other round cell malignancies, since S-100 protein is variably positive in the round cell component.

Genetics. Myxoid liposarcoma is characterized by the recurrent translocation t(12;16)(q13;p11) (106,107) that results in the *FUS-DDIT3* gene fusion, present in over 95 percent of cases (108–112). In the remaining cases, a variant t(12;22)(q13;q12) is present in which *DDIT3* fuses instead with

EWSR1, a gene highly related to *FUS* (111). In the most common fusion variants, a portion of the amino terminus of *FUS* is fused to the entire coding region of *DDIT3* (also known as *CHOP*). Three major recurrent fusion transcript types have been reported, in which exon 2 of *DDIT3* is fused in frame with either *FUS* exon 5 (type I, accounting for two thirds of cases), exon 7 (type II), or exon 8 (type III) (112–114). The monoclonal origin of the synchronous/metachronous multifocal myxoid liposarcoma has been confirmed by *FUS-DDIT3* genomic rearrangement structures in tumors from different sites (115). The presence of the *FUS-DDIT3* fusion is highly sensitive and specific for myxoid liposarcoma and is absent in other morphologic mimics, including predominantly myxoid well-differentiated/dedifferentiated liposarcoma of the retroperitoneum and myxofibrosarcoma (116). No convincing genetic evidence has been presented to date to support the concept of a mixed type liposarcoma composed of myxoid liposarcoma and dedifferentiated liposarcoma.

Activating *PIK3CA* mutations were recently demonstrated in 14 to 18 percent of cases, in either the helical (E542K and E545K) or kinase (H1047L and H1047R) domains (117,118). Mutations were more frequent in round cell liposarcoma and were associated with a shortened disease-specific survival period. Homozygous *PTEN* loss, an alternative mechanism for PI3K/Akt activation, was found in an additional subset of patients, mutually exclusive with *PIK3CA* mutations.

Differential Diagnosis. The differential diagnosis of myxoid liposarcoma involves tumors associated with an extensive myxoid stroma. Myxofibrosarcoma may have intracytoplasmic vacuoles reminiscent of lipoblasts and a prominent branching vasculature; however, most of the constituent cells of myxofibrosarcoma are spindled and display significantly more pronounced nuclear pleomorphism, with marked hyperchromasia and multilobated nuclei, even in low-grade tumors. Also, the conspicuous vessels show a distinctive curvilinear arrangement and are surrounded by pericytic cells, in contrast with the very delicate capillary-type network in myxoid liposarcoma. Most myxofibrosarcomas are superficial tumors with highly infiltrative growth in contrast to myxoid liposarcoma which is rather well circumscribed and typically confined to the skeletal muscle.

Extraskeletal myxoid chondrosarcoma shares the lobulated growth pattern and deep-seated location within the muscle. The tumor, however, is composed of round to epithelioid cells arranged in a distinctive reticular pattern or small nests. It typically lacks the conspicuous branching vascular network as well as lipoblasts of myxoid liposarcoma.

In retroperitoneal locations, often, well-differentiated liposarcoma has extensive myxoid changes, with significant overlap with myxoid liposarcoma. With extensive sampling, the presence of a lipoma-like or sclerosing component is revealed, with the hyperchromatic and often multilobated atypical stromal cells characteristic of well-differentiated liposarcoma. If in doubt, immunohistochemical stains for MDM2 and CDK4 are typically positive, while the FISH assay for *DDIT3* gene rearrangements is negative. Primary myxoid liposarcoma of the retroperitoneum is rare, and when it occurs, more often represents a soft tissue metastasis from an extremity primary.

Rarely, the material available for review is composed predominantly of a solid, nonmyxoid round cell component. In this setting, the differential diagnosis includes other small blue round cell tumors, including Ewing sarcoma. The lack of O13 membranous staining and S-100 protein reactivity suggests a round cell liposarcoma diagnosis, which can be confirmed by genetic testing for the *DDIT3* gene rearrangement.

Treatment and Prognosis. Myxoid liposarcoma is reported to be more radiosensitive than other soft tissue sarcomas, and higher rates of local control are achieved after combined surgery and radiation, suggesting a particular radiosensitivity that can be exploited to improve oncologic outcome in appropriate cases (119). Additionally, recent studies demonstrated that trabectedin (ecteinascidin 743 or ET-743), a chemotherapeutic agent derived from the sea, induces major antitumor effects in myxoid liposarcoma (120), apparently overcoming lipogenic cell differentiation block due to the tumor chromosomal translocation (121).

High histologic grade, often defined as a 5 percent or greater round cell component; presence of necrosis; and *TP53* and *CDKN2A* alterations are predictors of unfavorable outcome in localized myxoid liposarcoma (112,122–124). The prognostic significance of more limited hypercellularity (transitional areas) is less certain. The clinical outcome of for patients with multifocal myxoid liposarcoma is poor, regardless of its often bland or low-grade histologic appearance. The different isoforms of the *FUS-DDIT3* fusion transcripts are not associated with differences in histologic grade or clinical outcome (125).

One third of patients develop distant metastases; this is dependent on the histologic grade of the tumor. In contrast with other types of liposarcoma or myxoid sarcomas of the extremities, myxoid liposarcoma tends to metastasize to unusual locations in soft tissue (such as retroperitoneum, opposite extremity, axilla) or bone, with a predilection for the spine, even before spreading to the lungs (126). In a significant number of cases, patients present with synchronous or metachronous multifocal disease (115). This unusual clinical manifestation is due to hematogenous metastases to other sites by tumor cells seemingly incompetent to seed the lungs.

Pleomorphic Liposarcoma

Definition. *Pleomorphic liposarcoma* is a high-grade pleomorphic sarcoma that displays a varying degree of lipoblastic differentiation and contains pleomorphic lipoblasts.

Figure 4-33

PLEOMORPHIC LIPOSARCOMA

A large intramuscular pleomorphic liposarcoma of the thigh has a well-circumscribed, pseudo-encapsulated appearance. The cut surface has a multinodular, yellow-tan appearance with areas of hemorrhage and necrosis.

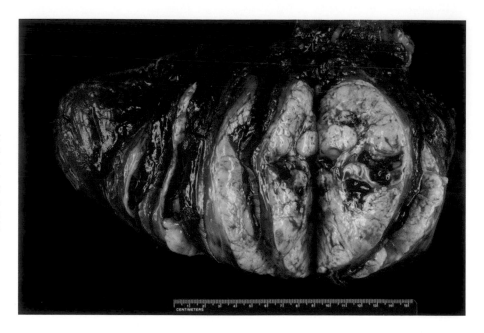

Clinical Features. Pleomorphic liposarcoma is the least common histologic subtype, accounting for less than 5 percent of all liposarcomas (127). Pleomorphic liposarcoma often occurs in the deep soft tissue of the extremities, with a predilection for the musculature of the thigh, whereas the retroperitoneum and trunk are only rarely affected (128). Most tumors occur in older individuals, with an equal sex distribution (129,130). The lesions are large at presentation and computerized tomography (CT) scans often do not demonstrate fat density.

Gross Findings. Pleomorphic liposarcoma has a tan, fleshy cut surface with variable areas of necrosis and myxoid/mucoid change. Yellow discoloration may be present (fig. 4-33).

Microscopic Findings. Microscopically, the tumors are highly cellular with overt nuclear pleomorphism, increased mitotic activity, and areas of necrosis. The diagnostic feature of pleomorphic liposarcoma is the presence of pleomorphic lipoblasts, which are typically arranged in solid sheets (fig. 4-34). The degree of lipoblastic differentiation is variable and may be extensive in some cases, but more often is focal and can be missed if not adequately sampled. Multinucleated giant cells and markedly bizarre and pleomorphic cells are common and may simulate a pleomorphic malignant fibrous histiocytoma (fig. 4-35A). Large areas of the tumor may show a myxoid stroma with an increased

vascular component that retains a degree of nuclear anaplasia (fig. 4-35B).

In some cases, pleomorphic liposarcoma has a round cell component, which may be misinterpreted as a true round cell/myxoid liposarcoma (fig. 4-35). The distinction is based on identifying clear nuclear pleomorphism and giant tumor cells, which are not features of a myxoid liposarcoma. The least common morphologic variant is the epithelioid type, composed of sheets of epithelioid-appearing cells with ample, variably eosinophilic cytoplasm. Often, the cell borders have a honeycomb-like pattern and little if any collagenous extracellular matrix (fig. 4-36).

Genetics. Pleomorphic liposarcoma displays a complex karyotype with numerous nonrecurrent chromosomal abnormalities, composed of gains or losses. At the molecular level they show frequent loss of retinoblastoma protein expression and high p53 mutation rates (approximately 60 percent) (131).

Differential Diagnosis. Since the diagnostic areas of lipoblastic differentiation may be quite focal, some pleomorphic liposarcomas composed predominantly of a myxoid and/or storiform-pleomorphic component may suggest an alternative diagnosis of malignant fibrous histiocytoma or myxofibrosarcoma, especially in limited needle biopsy material or if inadequately sampled. Immunohistochemical studies of the pleomorphic/myxoid components are usually

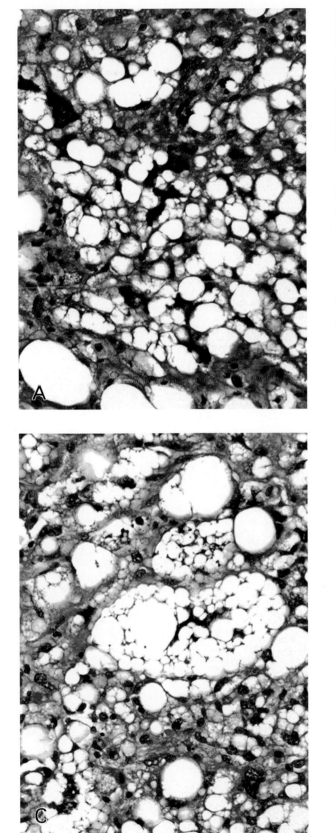

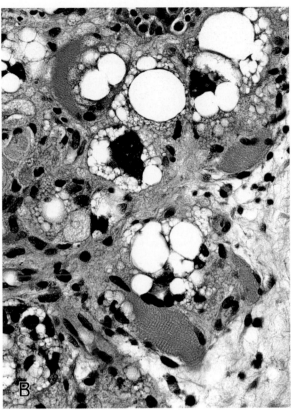

Figure 4-34

PLEOMORPHIC LIPOSARCOMA

The lipoblastic component is typically composed of solid sheets of lipoblasts (A), with marked cytologic atypia and hyperchromasia, involving skeletal muscle (B). The diagnostic hallmark is the pleomorphic lipoblast, with multivacuolated cytoplasm and marked indentations of the nucleus (B,C).

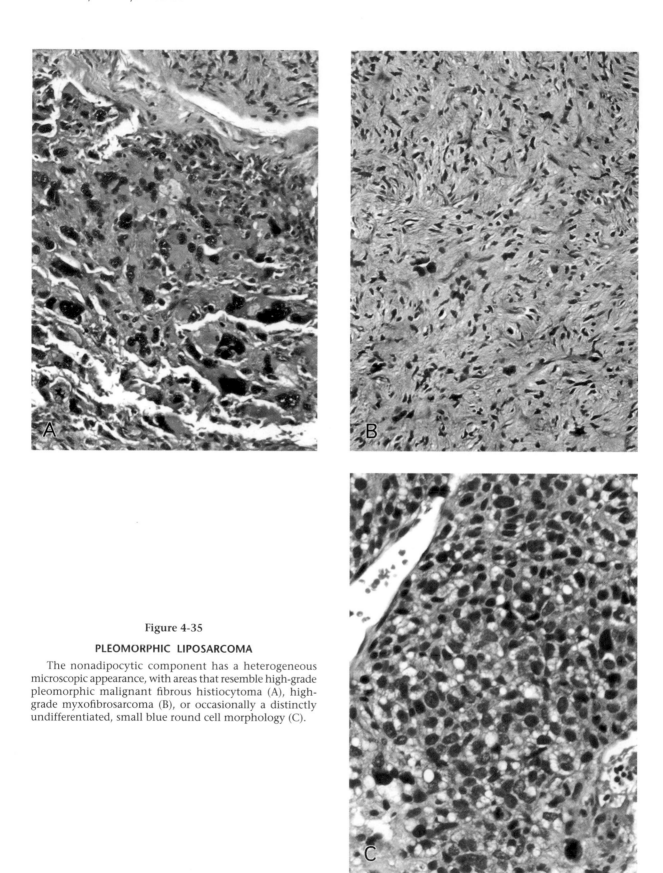

Figure 4-35

PLEOMORPHIC LIPOSARCOMA

The nonadipocytic component has a heterogeneous microscopic appearance, with areas that resemble high-grade pleomorphic malignant fibrous histiocytoma (A), high-grade myxofibrosarcoma (B), or occasionally a distinctly undifferentiated, small blue round cell morphology (C).

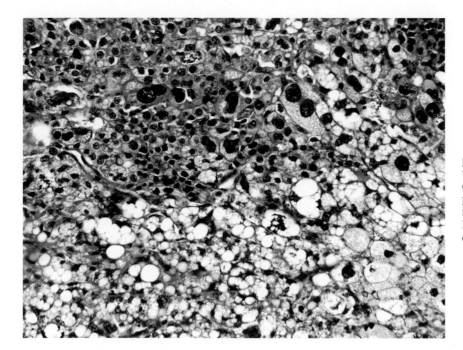

Figure 4-36

PLEOMORPHIC LIPOSARCOMA

The epithelioid variant of pleomorphic liposarcoma contains large cells with abundant cytoplasm. The epithelioid appearance potentially simulates renal or adrenocortical carcinoma. Lipomatous differentiation is diagnostic of this entity.

not useful for distinguishing between the two pathologic entities.

There has been occasional confusion between pleomorphic liposarcoma and ALT/WDLS based on the presence of scattered lipoblasts and pleomorphic atypical stromal cells seen in the latter. The main distinction is based on the large areas of lipoma-like or sclerosing components in ALT/WDLS. In the retroperitoneum, dedifferentiated liposarcoma with "homologous" lipogenic dedifferentiation may resemble pleomorphic liposarcoma, due to the presence of pleomorphic lipoblasts in the high-grade component (132). In most cases, however, careful examination reveals areas of sclerosing or lipoma-like morphology that excludes a diagnosis of pleomorphic liposarcoma. Similar to the other morphologic variants of dedifferentiated liposarcoma, these tumors are positive for MDM2 and CDK4, and have a high-level amplification of 12q14.3 by FISH. True pleomorphic liposarcomas rarely occur within the retroperitoneum, which is the preferred location for well-differentiated/dedifferentiated liposarcomas.

Occasionally, when the limited material available for review displays predominantly an epithelioid morphology (epithelioid variant of pleomorphic liposarcoma), an alternative consideration in the differential is metastatic carcinoma, possibly of adrenal or renal origin (133,134). Immunohistochemical studies have limited value in this setting, since the epithelioid variant of pleomorphic liposarcoma shows focal expression of epithelial markers in almost half of the cases (128,133).

Treatment and Prognosis. Compared to the other two subtypes of liposarcoma, pleomorphic liposarcoma has the most aggressive behavior, exhibiting a high propensity for systemic spread and a poor overall outcome. The 5-year disease-specific survival rate is 53 percent. Recurrent disease, unresectability, and microscopically positive margins are predictors of a poor prognosis. Systemic relapse (the strongest poor prognostic determinant) develops in about 35 percent of patients with localized pleomorphic liposarcoma (131). Surgical resection is currently the only potentially curative approach to these remarkably chemoresistant tumors; locally advanced and metastatic disease is generally noncurable.

REFERENCES

Ordinary Lipoma

1. Myhre-Jensen O. A consecutive 7-year series of 1331 benign soft tissue tumours. Clinicopathologic data. Comparison with sarcomas. Acta Orthop Scand 1981;52:287-293

2. Shanks JA, Paranchych W, Tuba J. Familial multiple lipomatosis. Can Med Assoc J 1957:77:881-884.

3. Rydholm A, Berg NO. Size, site and clinical incidence of lipoma. Factors in the differential diagnosis of lipoma and sarcoma. Acta Orthop Scand 1983;54:929-934.

4. Bjerregaard P, Hagen K, Daugaard S, Kofoed H. Intramuscular lipoma of the lower limb. Longterm follow-up after local resection. J Bone Joint Surg Br 1989;71:812-815.

5. Fletcher CD, Martin-Bates E. Intramuscular and intermuscular lipoma: neglected diagnoses. Histopathology 1988;12:275-287.

6. Macarenko RS, Erickson-Johnson M, Wang X, et al. Retroperitoneal lipomatous tumors without cytologic atypia: are they lipomas? A clinicopathologic and molecular study of 19 cases. Am J Surg Pathol 2006;33:1470-1476.

7. Mehregan AH, Tavafoghi V, Ghandchi A. Nevus lipomatosus cutaneus superficialis (Hoffmann-Zurhelle). J Cutan Pathol 1975;2:307-313.

8. Jones EW, Marks R, Pongsehirun D. Naevus superficialis lipomatosus. A clinicopathological report of twenty cases. Br J Dermatol 1975;93:121-133.

9. Lassman LP, James CC. Lumbosacral lipomas: critical survey of 26 cases submitted to laminectomy. J Neurol Neurosurg Psychiat 1967;30:174-181.

10. Kieck CF, De Villiers JC. Subcutaneous lumbosacral lipomas. S Afr Med J 1975;49:1563-1566.

11. Arai H, Sato K, Okuda O, et al. Surgical experience of 120 patients with lumbosacral lipomas. Acta Neurochir (Wein) 2001;143:857-864.

12. Carilli S, Alper A, Emre A. Inguinal cord lipomas. Hernia 2004;8:252-254.

13. Spinner RJ, Scheithauer BW, Amrami KK, Wenger DE, Hébert-Blouin MN. Adipose lesions of the nerve: the need for modified classification. J Neurosurg 2012;116:418-431.

14. Hallel T, Lew S, Bansal M. Villous lipomatous proliferation of the synovial membrane (lipoma arborescens). J Bone Joint Surg Am 1988;70A:264-270.

15. Yildiz C, Deveci MS, Ozcan A, Saracoglu HI, Erler K, Basbozkurt M. Lipoma arborescens (diffuse articular lipomatosis). J South Orthoped Assoc 2003;12:163-166.

16. Schmack I, Patel RM, Folpe AL, et al. Subconjunctival herniated orbital fat: a benign adipocytic lesion that may mimic pleomorphic lipoma and atypical lipomatous tumor. Am J Surg Pathol 2007;31:193-198.

17. Willen H, Akerman M, Dal Cin P, et al. Comparison of chromosomal patterns with clinical features in 165 lipomas: a report of the CHAMP study group. Cancer Genet Cytogenet 1998;102:46-49.

18. Sreekantaiah C, Leong SP, Karakousis CP, et al. Cytogenetic profile of 109 lipomas. Cancer Res 1991;51:422-433.

19. Mrózek K, Karakousis CP, Bloomfield CD. Chromosome 12 breakpoints are cytogenetically different in benign and malignant lipogenic tumors: localization of breakpoints in lipoma to 12q15 and in myxoid liposarcoma to 12q13.3 Cancer Res 1993;53:1670-1675.

20. Nilbert M, Rydholm A, Willén H, Mitelman F, Mandahl N. MDM2 gene amplification correlates with ring chromosomes in soft tissue tumors. Genes Chromosomes Cancer 1994;9:261-265.

21. Szymanska J, Virolainen M, Tarkkanen M, et al. Overrepresentation of 1q21-23 and 12q13-21 in lipoma-like liposarcomas but not in benign lipomas: a comparative genomic hybridization study. Cancer Genet Cytogenet 1997;99:14-18.

22. Sandberg AA. Updates on the cytognetics and molecular genetics of bone and soft tissue tumors: lipoma. Cancer Genet Cytogenet 2004; 150:93-115.

23. Marsh WL Jr, Lucas JG, Olsen J. Chondrolipoma of breast. Arch Pathol Lab Med 1989;113:369-371.

24. Nwaorgu OG, Akang EE, Ahmad BM, Nwachokor FN, Olu-Eddo AN. Pharyngeal lipoma with cartilaginous metaplasia (chondrolipoma): a case report and literature review. J Laryngol Otol 1997;111:656-658.

25. Hopkins JD, Rayan GM. Osteolipoma of the hand: a case report. J Okla State Med Assoc 1999; 92:535-537.

26. Rau T, Soeder S, Olk A, Aigner T. Parosteal lipoma of the thigh with cartilageneous and osseous differentiation: an osteochondrolipoma. Ann Diagn Pathol 2006;10:279-282,

Lipomatosis of the Nerve

27. Silverman TA, Enzinger FM. Fibrolipomatous hamartoma of nerve. A clinicopathologic analysis of 26 cases. Am J Surg Pathol 1985;9:7-14.

28. Brodwater BK, Major NM, Goldner RD, Layfield LJ. Macrodystrophia lipomatosa with associated fibrolipomatous hamartoma of the median nerve. Pediatr Surg Int 2000;16:216-218.

29. Spinner RJ, Scheithauer BW, Amrami KK, Wenger DE, Hébert-Blouin MN. Adipose lesions of nerve: the need for modified classification. J Neurosurg 2012;116:418-431.

Angiolipoma

30. Howard WR, Helwig EB. Angiolipoma. Arch Dermatol 1960;82:924-931.

31. Lin JJ, Lin F. Two entities in angiolipoma. A study of 459 cases of lipoma with review of literature on infiltrating angiolipoma. Cancer 1974;34:720-727.

32. Namba M, Kohda M, Mimura S, Nakagawa S, Ueki H. Angiolipoma in brothers. J Dermatol 1977;4:255-257.

33. Kazakov DV, Hes O, Hora M, Sima R, Michal M. Primary intranodal angiolipoma. Int J Surg Pathol 2005;13:99-101.

34. Hunt SJ, Santa Cruz DJ, Barr RJ. Cellular angiolipoma. Am J Surg Pathol 1990;14:75-81.

35. Sciot R, Akerman M, Dal Cin P, et al. Cytogenetic analysis of subcutaneous angiolipoma: further evidence supporting its difference from ordinary pure lipomas: a report of the CHAMP study group. Am J Surg Pathol 1997;21:441-444.

Spindle Cell Lipoma and Pleomorphic Lipoma

36. Enzinger FM, Harvey DA. Spindle cell lipoma. Cancer 1975;36:1852-1859.

37. Shmookler BM, Enzinger FM. Pleomorphic lipoma: a benign tumor simulating liposarcoma. A clinicopathologic analysis of 48 cases. Cancer 1981;47:126-133.

38. Angervall L, Dahl I, Kindblom LG, Säve-Soderbergh J. Spindle cell lipoma. Acta Pathol Microbiol Scand A 1976;84.477-487.

39. Fletcher CD, Martin-Bates E. Spindle cell lipoma: a clinicopathologic study with some original observations. Histopathology 1987;11:803-817.

40. Azzopardi JG, Iocco J, Salm R. Pleomorphic lipoma: a tumor simulating liposarcoma. Histopathology 1983;7:511-523.

41. Furlong MA, Fanburg-Smith JC, Childers EL. Lipoma of the oral and maxillofacial region: Site and and subclassification of 125 cases. Oral Surg Oral Med Oral Pathol Oral Radiol Endod 2004;98:441-450.

42. Fanburg-Smith JF, Devaney KO, Miettinen M, Weiss SW. Multiple spindle cell lipomas: a report of 7 familial and 11 nonfamilial cases. Am J Surg Pathol 1998;22:40-48.

43. Hawley IC, Krausz T, Evans DJ, Fletcher CD. Spindle cell lipoma—a pseudoangiomatous variant. Histopathology 1994;24:565-569.

44. Zelger BW, Zelger BG, Plörer A, Steiner H, Fritsch PO. Dermal spindle cell lipoma: plexiform and nodular variants. Histopathology 1995;27:533-540.

45. Templeton SF, Solomon AR Jr. Spindle cell lipoma is strongly CD34-positive. An immunohistochemical study. J Cutan Pathol 1996;23:546-550.

46. Suster S, Fisher C. Immunoreactivity for the human hematopoietic progenitor cell antigen (CD34) in lipomatous tumors. Am J Surg Pathol 1997;21:195-200.

47. Chen BJ, Mariño-Enriquez A, Fletcher CD, Hornick JL. Loss of retinoblastoma protein expression in spindle cell/pleomorphic lipomas and cytogenetically related tumors: an immunohistochemical study with diagnostic implications. Am J Surg Pathol 2012;36:1119-1128.

48. Tardio JC, Aramburu JA, Santonja C. Desmin expression in spindle cell lipomas: a potential diagnostic pitfall. Virchows Arch 2004;445:354-358.

49. Mandahl N, Mertens F, Willén H, Rydholm A, Brosjö O, Mitelman F. A new cytogenetic subgroup in lipomas: loss of chromosome 16 material in spindle cell and pleomorphic lipomas. J Cancer Res Clin Oncol 1994;120:707-711.

50. Dal Cin P, Sciot R, Polito P, et al. Lesions of 13q may occur independently of deletion of 16q in spindle cell/pleomorphic lipomas. Histopathology 1997;31:222-225.

51. Bartuma H, Nord KH, Macchia G, et al. Gene expression and single nucleotide polymorphism array analyses of spindle cell lipomas and conventional lipomas with 13q14 deletion. Genes Chromosom Cancer 2011;50:619-632.

51a. Mentzel T, Palmedo G, Kuhnen C. Well-differentiated spindle cell liposarcoma ('atypical spindle cell lipomatous tumor') does not belong to the spectrum of atypical lipomatous tumor but has a close relationship to spindle cell lipoma: clinicopathologic, immunohistochemical, and molecular analysis of six cases. Mod Pathol 2010;23:729-736.

Chondroid Lipoma

52. Meis JM, Enzinger FM. Chondroid lipoma. A unique tumor simulating liposarcoma and myxoid chondrosarcoma. Am J Surg Pathol 1993; 17:1103-1112.

53. Nielsen GP, O'Connell JX, Dickersin GR, Rosenberg AE. Chondroid lipoma, a tumor of white fat cells. A brief report of two cases with ultrastructural analysis. Am J Surg Pathol 1995;19:1272-1276.

54. Thomson TA, Horsman D, Bainbridge TC. Cytogenetic and cytologic features of chondroid lipoma of soft tissue. Mod Pathol 1999;12:88-91.

55. Gisselsson D, Domanski HA, Hoglund M, et al. Unique cytological features and chromosome aberrations in chondroid lipoma: a case report based on fine-needle aspiration cytology, histopathology, electron microscopy, chromosome banding, and molecular cytogenetics. Am J Surg Pathol 1999;23:1300-1304.

56. Ballaux F, Debiec-Rychter M, De Wever I, Sciot R. Chondroid lipoma is characterized by t(11;16)(q13;p12-13). Virchows Arch 2004;444:208-210.

Hemosiderotic Fibrohistiocytic Lipomatous Lesion/Tumor

57. Marshall-Taylor C, Fanburg-Smith JC. Hemosiderotic fibrohistiocytic lesion: ten cases of a previously undescribed fatty lesion of the foot/ankle. Mod Pathol 2000;13:1192-1199.

58. Browne TJ, Fletcher CD. Haemosiderotic fibrolipomatous tumour (so-called haemosiderotic fibrohistiocytic lipomatous tumour): analysis of 13 new cases in support of a distinct entity. Histopathology 2006;48:453-461.

58a. Hallor KH, Sciot R, Staaf J, et al. Two genetic pathways, t(1;10) and amplification of 3p11-12, in myxoinflammatory fibroblastic sarcoma, hemosiderotic fibrolipomatous tumour, and morphologically similar lesions. J Pathol 2009;217:716-727.

58b. Antonescu CR, Zhang L, Nielsen GP, Rosenberg AE, Dal Cin P, Fletcher CD. Consistent t(1;10) with rearrangements of TGFBR3 and MGEA5 in both myxoinflammatory fibroblastic sarcoma and hemosiderotic fibrolipomatous tumor. Genes Chromosomes Cancer 2011;50:757-764.

Hibernoma

59. Kindblom LG, Angervall L, Stener B, Wickbom I. Intramuscular and intermuscular lipomas and hibernomas. A clinical roentgenologic, histologic and prognostic study of 46 cases. Cancer 1974;33:754-762.

60. Gaffney EF, Hargreaves HK, Semple E, Vellios F. Hibernoma: distinctive light and electron microscopic features and relationship to brown adipose tissue. Hum Pathol 1983;14:677-687.

61. Furlong MA, Fanburg-Smith JC, Miettinen M. The morphologic spectrum of hibernoma: a clinicopathologic study of 170 cases. Am J Surg Pathol 2001;25:809-814.

62. Walker EA, Fenton ME, Salesky JS, Murphey MD. Magnetic resonance imaging of benign soft tissue neoplasms in adults. Radiol Clin North Am 2011;49:1197-2017.

63. Chirieac LR, Dekmezian RH, Ayala AG. Characterization of the myxoid variant of hibernoma. Ann Diagn Pathol 2006;10:104-106.

64. Dal Cin P, van Damme B, Hoogmartens M, Van Den Berghe H. Chromosome changes in a case of hibernoma. Genes Chromosomes Cancer 1992;5:178-180.

65. Meloni AM, Spanier SS, Bush CH, Stone JF, Sandberg AA. Involvement of 10q22 and 11q13 in hibernoma. Cancer Genet Cytogenet 1994;72:59-64.

66. Mertens F, Rydholm A, Brosjö O, Willén H, Mitelman F, Mandahl N. Hibernomas are characterized by rearrangements of chromosome bands 11q13-21. Int J Cancer 1994;58:503-505.

67. Mrozek K, Karakousis CP, Bloomfield CD. Band 11q13 is nonrandomly rearranged in hibernomas. Genes Chromosomes Cancer 1994;9:145-147.

68. Turaga KK, Silva-Lopez E, Sanger WG, et al. A (9;11)(q34;q13) translocation in a hibernoma. Cancer Genet Cytogenet 2006;170:163-166.

69. Maire G, Forus A, Foa C, et al. 11q13 alterations in two cases of hibernoma: large heterozygous deletions and rearrangement breakpoints near GARP in 11q13.5. Genes Chromosomes Cancer 2003;37:389-395.

70. Nord KH, Magnusson L, Isaksson M, et al. Concomitant deletions of tumopr suppressor genes MEN1 and AIP are essential for the pathogenesis of the brown fat tumor hibernoma. Proc Natl Acad Sci U S A 2010;107:221122-7.

Lipoblastoma

71. Sciot R, De Wever I, Debiec-Rychter M. Lipoblastoma in a 23-year-old male: distinction from atypical lipomatous tumor using cytogenetic and fluorescence in-situ hybridization analysis. Virchows Arch 2003;442:468-471.

72. Collins MH, Chatten J. Lipoblastoma/lipoblastomatosis: a clinicopathologic study of 25 tumors. Am J Surg Pathol 1997;21:1131-1137.

73. Chun YS, Kim WK, Park KW, Lee SC, Jung SE. Lipoblastoma. J Pediatr Surg 2001;36:905-907.

74. Miller GG, Yanchar NL, Magee JF, Blair GK. Lipoblastoma and liposarcoma in children: an analysis of 9 cases and review of the literature. Can J Surg 1998;41:455-458.

75. Hicks J, Dilley A, Patel D, Barrish J, Zhu SH, Brandt M. Lipoblastoma and lipoblastomatosis in infancy and childhood: histopathologic, ultrastructural, and cytogenetic features. Ultrastruct Pathol 2001;25:321-333.

76. Jung SM, Chang PY, Luo CC, Huang CS, Lau JY, Hsueh C. Lipoblastoma/lipoblastomatosis: a clinicopathologic study of 16 cases in Taiwan. Pediatr Surg Int 2005;21:809-812.

77. Dal Cin P, Sciot R, DeWever I, van Damme B, van den Berghe H. New discriminative chromosomal marker in adipose tissue tumors. The chromosome 8q11-q13 region in lipoblastoma. Cancer Genet Cytogenet 1994;78:232-235.

78. Astrom A, DíAmore ES, Sainati L, et al. Evidence of involvement of the PLAG1 gene in lipoblastomas. Int J Oncol 2000;16:1107-1110.

79. Hibbard MK, Kozakewich H, Dal Ci P, Sciot R, Tan X, Xiao S, Fletcher JA. PLAG1 fusion oncogenes in lipoblastoma. Cancer Res 2000;60:4869-4872.

80. Gisselsson D, Hibbard MK, Dal Cin P, et al. PLAG1 alterations in lipoblastoma: involvement in varied mesenchymal cell types and evidence for alternative oncogenic mechanisms. Am J Pathol 2001;159:955-962.

81. Morerio C, Rapelola A, Rosanda C, et al. PLAG1-HAS2 fusion in lipoblastoma with masked 8q intrachromosomal rearrangement. Cancer Genet Cytogenet 2005;156:183-184.

Massive Localized Lymphedema in the Obese

82. Farshid G, Weiss SW. Massive localized lymphedema in the morbidly obese: a histologically distinct reactive lesion simulating liposarcoma. Am J Surg Pathol 1998;22:1277-1283.

83. Wu D, Gibbs J, Cotral D, Intengan M, Brooks JJ. Massive localized lymphedema: additional locations and association with hypothyroidism. Hum Pathol 2000;31:1162-1168.

84. Oswald TM, Lineaweaver W. Limited segmental resection on symptomatic lower extremity lymhpodystrophic tissue in high-risk patients. South Med J 2003;96:689-691.

85. Goshtasby P, Dawson J, Agarwal N. Pseudosarcoma: massive localized lymphedema of the morbidly obese. Obes Surg 2006;16:88-93.

Liposarcoma

86. Linehan DC, Lewis JJ, Leung D, Brennan MF. Influence of biologic factors and anatomic site in completely resected liposarcoma. J Clin Oncol 2000;18:1637-1643.

87. McCormick D, Mentzel T, Beham A, Fletcher CD. Dedifferentiated liposarcoma. Clinicopathologic analysis of 32 cases suggesting a better prognostic subgroup among pleomorphic sarcomas. Am J Surg Pathol 1994;18:1213-1223.

88. Singer S, Antonescu CR, Riedel E, Brennan MF. Histologic subtype and margin of resection predict pattern of recurrence and survival for retroperitoneal liposarcoma. Ann Surg 2003;238:358-370; discussion 370-371.

89. Kooby DA, Antonescu CR, Brennan MF, Singer S. Atypical lipomatous tumor/well-differentiated liposarcoma of the extremity and trunk wall: importance of histological subtype with treatment recommendations. Ann Surg Oncol 2004;11:78-84.

Atypical Lipomatous Tumor/ Well-Differentiated Liposarcoma

90. Weiss SW, Rao VK. Well-differentiated liposarcoma (atypical lipoma) of deep soft tissue of the extremities, retroperitoneum, and miscellaneous sites. A follow-up study of 92 cases with analysis of the incidence of "dedifferentiation". Am J Surg Pathol 1992;16:1051-1058.

91. Lucas DR, Nascimento AG, Sanjay BK, Rock MG. Well-differentiated liposarcoma. The Mayo Clinic experience with 58 cases. Am J Clin Pathol 1994;102:677-683.

92. Evans HL. Liposarcoma: a study of 55 cases with a reassessment of its classification. Am J Surg Pathol 1979;3:507-523.

93. Elgar F, Goldblum JR. Well-differentiated liposarcoma of the retroperitoneum: a clinicopathologic analysis of 20 cases, with particular attention to the extent of low-grade dedifferentiation. Mod Pathol 1997;10:113-120.

94. Henricks WH, Chu YC, Goldblum JR, Weiss SW. Dedifferentiated liposarcoma: a clinicopathological analysis of 155 cases with a proposal for an expanded definition of dedifferentiation. Am J Surg Pathol 1997;21:271-281.

95. Marino-Enriquez A, Fletcher CD, Dal Cin P, Hornick JL. Dedifferentiated liposarcoma with "homologous" lipoblastic (pleomorphic liposarcoma-like) differentiation: clinicopathologic and molecular analysis of a series suggesting revised diagnostic criteria. Am J Surg Pathol 2010;34:1122-1131.

96. Nascimento AG, Kurtin PJ, Guillou L, Fletcher CD. Dedifferentiated liposarcoma: a report of nine cases with a peculiar neurallike whorling pattern associated with metaplastic bone formation. Am J Surg Pathol 1998;22:945-955.

97. Fanburg-Smith JC, Miettinen M. Liposarcoma with meningothelial-like whorls: a study of 17 cases of a distinctive histological pattern associated with dedifferentiated liposarcoma. Histopathology 1998;33:414-424.

98. Thway K, Flora R, Shah C, Olmos D, Fisher C. Diagnostic utility of p16, CDK4, and MDM2 as an immunohistochemical panel in distinguishing well-differentiated and dedifferentiated liposarcomas from other adipocytic tumors. Am J Surg Pathol 2012:36:470-477.

99. Fletcher CD, Akerman M, Dal Cin P, et al. Correlation between clinicopathological features and karyotype in lipomatous tumors. A report of 178 cases from the Chromosomes and Morphology (CHAMP) Collaborative Study Group. Am J Pathol 1996;148:623-630.

100. Gisselsson D, Hoglund M, Mertens F, et al. The structure and dynamics of ring chromosomes in human neoplastic and non-neoplastic cells. Human Genet 1999;104:315-325.

101. Huang HY, Brennan MF, Singer S, Antonescu CR. Distant metastasis in retroperitoneal dedifferentiated liposarcoma is rare and rapidly fatal: a clinicopathological study with emphasis on the low-grade myxofibrosarcoma-like pattern as an early sign of dedifferentiation. Mod Pathol 2005;18:976-984.

Spindle Cell Liposarcoma

102. Dei Tos AP, Mentzel T, Newman PL, Fletcher CD. Spindle cell liposarcoma, a hitherto unrecognized variant of liposarcoma. Analysis of six cases. Am J Surg Pathol 1994;18:913-921.

103. Mentzel T, Palmedo G, Kuhnen C. Well-differentiated spindle cell liposarcoma ('atypical spindle cell lipomatous tumor') does not belong to the spectrum of atypical lipomatous tumor but has a close relationship to spindle cell lipoma: clinicopathologic, immunohistochemical, and molecular analysis of six cases. Mod Pathol 2010;23:729-736.

104. Italiano A, Chambonniere ML, Attias R, Chibon F, Coindre JM, Pedeutour F. Monosomy 7 and absence of 12q amplification in two cases of spindle cell liposarcomas. Cancer Genet Cytogenet 2008;184:99-104.

Myxoid Liposarcoma

105. Huh WW, Yuen C, Munsell M, et al. Liposarcoma in children and young adults: a multi-institutional experience. Pediatric Blood Cancer 2011;57:1142-1146.

106. Turc-Carel C, Limon J, Dal Cin P, Rao U, Karakousis C, Sandberg AA. Cytogenetic studies of adipose tissue tumors. II. Recurrent reciprocal translocation t(12;16)(q13;p11) in myxoid liposarcomas. Cancer Genet Cytogenet 1986;23:291-299.

107. Sreekantaiah C, Karakousis CP, Leong SP, Sandberg AA. Cytogenetic findings in liposarcoma correlate with histopathologic subtypes. Cancer 1992;69:2484-2495.

108. Rabbitts TH, Forster A, Larson R, Nathan P. Fusion of the dominant negative transcription regulator CHOP with a novel gene FUS by translocation t(12;16) in malignant liposarcoma. Nat Genet 1993;4:175-180.

109. Crozat A, Aman P, Mandahl N, Ron D. Fusion of CHOP to a novel RNA-binding protein in human myxoid liposarcoma. Nature 1993;363:640-644.

110. Perez-Losada J, Pintado B, Gutierrez-Adan A, et al. The chimeric FUS/TLS-CHOP fusion protein specifically induces liposarcomas in transgenic mice. Oncogene 2000;19:2413-2422.

111. Panagopoulos I, Höglund M, Mertens F, Mandahl N, Mitelman F, Aman P. Fusion of the EWS and CHOP genes in myxoid liposarcoma. Oncogene 1996;12:489-494.

112. Antonescu CR, Tschernyavsky SJ, Decuseara R, et al. Prognostic impact of P53 status, TLS-CHOP fusion transcript structure, and histological grade in myxoid liposarcoma: a molecular and clinicopathologic study of 82 cases. Clin Cancer Res 2001;7:3977-3987.

113. Knight JC, Renwick PJ, Dal Cin P, Van den Berghe H, Fletcher CD. Translocation t(12;16)(q13;p11) in myxoid liposarcoma and round cell liposarcoma: molecular and cytogenetic analysis. Cancer Res 1995;55:24-27.

114. Panagopoulos I, Mandahl N, Ron D, et al. Characterization of the CHOP breakpoints and fusion transcripts in myxoid liposarcomas with the 12;16 translocation. Cancer Res 1994;54:6500-6503.

115. Antonescu CR, Elahi A, Healey JH, et al. Monoclonality of multifocal myxoid liposarcoma: confirmation by analysis of TLS-CHOP or EWS-CHOP rearrangements. Clin Cancer Res 2000;6:2788-2793.

116. Antonescu CR, Elahi A, Humphrey M, et al. Specificity of TLS-CHOP rearrangement for classic myxoid/round cell liposarcoma: absence in predominantly myxoid well-differentiated liposarcomas. J Mol Diagn 2000;2:132-138.

117. Barretina J, Taylor BS, Banerji S, et al. Subtype-specific genomic alterations define new targets for soft-tissue sarcoma therapy. Nat Genet 2010;42:715-721.

118. Demicco EG, Torres KE, Ghadimi MP, et al. Involvement of the PI3K/Akt pathway in myxoid/round cell liposarcoma. Mod Pathol 2012;25:212-221.

119. Chung PW, Deheshi BM, Ferguson PC, et al. Radiosensitivity translates into excellent local control in extremity myxoid liposarcoma: a comparison with other soft tissue sarcomas. Cancer 2009;115:3254-3261.

120. Grosso F, Jones RL, Demetri GD, et al. Efficacy of trabectedin (ecteinascidin-743) in advanced pretreated myxoid liposarcomas: a retrospective study. Lancet Oncol 2007;8:595-602.

121. Forni C, Minuzzo M, Virdis E, et al. Trabectedin (ET-743) promotes differentiation in myxoid liposarcoma tumors. Mol Cancer Ther 2009;8:449-457.

122. Moreau LC, Turcotte R, Ferguson P, et al. Myxoid\round cell liposarcoma (MRCLS) revisited: an analysis of 418 primarily managed cases. Ann Surg Oncol 2012;19:1081-1088.

123. Haniball J, Sumathi VP, Kindblom LG, et al. Prognostic factors and metastatic patterns in primary myxoid/round-cell liposarcoma. Sarcoma 2011;2011:538085.

124. Oda Y, Yamamoto H, Takahira T, et al. Frequent alteration of p16(INK4a)/p14(ARF) and p53 pathways in the round cell component of myxoid/round cell liposarcoma: p53 gene alterations and reduced p14(ARF) expression both correlate with poor prognosis. J Pathol 2005;207:410-421.

125. Bode-Lesniewska B, Frigerio S, Exner U, Abdou MT, Moch H, Zimmermann DR. Relevance of translocation type in myxoid liposarcoma and identification of a novel EWSR1-DDIT3 fusion. Genes Chromosomes Cancer 2007;46:961-971.

126. Schwab JH, Boland P, Guo T, et al. Skeletal metastases in myxoid liposarcoma: an unusual pattern of distant spread. Ann Surg Oncol 2007;14:1507-1514.

Pleomorphic Liposarcoma

127. Azumi N, Curtis J, Kempson RL, Hendrickson MR. Atypical and malignant neoplasms showing lipomatous differentiation. A study of 111 cases. Am J Surg Pathol 1987;11:161-183.

128. Hornick JL, Bosenberg MW, Mentzel T, McMenamin ME, Oliveira AM, Fletcher CD. Pleomorphic liposarcoma: clinicopathologic analysis of 57 cases. Am J Surg Pathol 2004;28:1257-1267.

129. Downes KA, Goldblum JR, Montgomery EA, Fisher C. Pleomorphic liposarcoma: a clinicopathologic analysis of 19 cases. Mod Pathol 2001;14:179-184.

130. Gebhard S, Coindre JM, Michels JJ, et al. Pleomorphic liposarcoma: clinicopathologic, immunohistochemical, and follow-up analysis of 63 cases: a study from the French Federation of Cancer Centers Sarcoma Group. Am J Surg Pathol 2002;26:601-616.

131. Ghadimi MP, Liu P, Peng T, et al. Pleomorphic liposarcoma: clinical observations and molecular variables. Cancer 2011;117:5359-5369.

132. Marino-Enriquez A, Fletcher CD, Dal Cin P, Hornick JL. Dedifferentiated liposarcoma with "homologous" lipoblastic (pleomorphic liposarcoma-like) differentiation: clinicopathologic and molecular analysis of a series suggesting revised diagnostic criteria. Am J Surg Pathol 2010;34:1122-1131.

133. Miettinen M, Enzinger FM. Epithelioid variant of pleomorphic liposarcoma: a study of 12 cases of a distinctive variant of high-grade liposarcoma. Mod Pathol 1999;12:722-728.

134. Huang HY, Antonescu CR. Epithelioid variant of pleomorphic liposarcoma: a comparative immunohistochemical and ultrastructural analysis of six cases with emphasis on overlapping features with epithelial malignancies. Ultrastruct Pathol 2002;26:299-308.

5 SMOOTH MUSCLE TUMORS

This chapter includes benign and malignant tumors with primary smooth muscle differentiation: leiomyomas and leiomyosarcomas. In addition, two related entities, myopericytoma, related to angioleiomyoma, and glomus tumor with smooth muscle differentiation although a separate clinicopathologic entity, are also discussed.

ANGIOLEIOMYOMA

Definition. *Angioleiomyoma* is a benign, well-differentiated, nodular smooth muscle tumor involving the walls of small veins. Alternative terminology includes *angiomyoma* and *vascular leiomyoma*.

Clinical Features. Angioleiomyoma is a fairly common tumor. It occurs in all ages but is more common in middle age. Based on Armed Forces Institute of Pathology (AFIP) civilian cases, there is a 2 to 1 male predominance in upper extremity tumors but an even sex distribution in lower extremity tumors.

Angioleiomyoma appears as a solitary, small (usually smaller than 1 cm) subcutaneous nodule, which is often painful. There is a predilection to the distal half of the extremities. Occurrence in the trunk wall and head and neck is rare. Angioleiomyomas also occur in the oral cavity and orofacial region. Simple excision is curative (1–3).

Gross and Microscopic Findings. Angioleiomyoma typically forms an ovoid, well-circumscribed rubbery nodule with a homogeneous yellow-white surface on sectioning. Histologically, it is composed of well-differentiated smooth muscle cells that arise from the walls of small veins (fig. 5-1). The vascular lumens may be very narrow (*solid variant*), gaping (*venous variant*), or cavernous blood filled-spaces (*cavernous variant*); the solid variant is most common (1). Unusual histologic features include calcification, lipomatous metaplasia, and focal nuclear atypia (fig. 5-1D).

Special Studies. Immunohistochemically, angioleiomyoma cells are positive for α-smooth muscle actin and calponin, and usually but not always, for desmin and heavy caldesmon. The lesional cells are negative for S-100 protein.

Differential Diagnosis. Smooth muscle tumors with both atypia and mitotic activity should be approached with caution. Complete excision and follow-up are necessary. Angioleiomyomas with lipomatous metaplasia are not related to angiomyolipoma and are negative for HMB-45 (4).

Angioleiomyoma-like tumors with a less differentiated smooth muscle component are designated myopericytoma. These tumors are discussed in a separate chapter. There is conceptual overlap between angioleiomyoma and myopericytoma, and the designation is arbitrary in some cases (5).

MYOPERICYTOMA

Definition. *Myopericytoma* is a mesenchymal tumor with features intermediate between angioleiomyoma and glomus tumor.

Clinical Features. Myopericytoma occurs in a wide age range, from the second decade to old age, but there is a predilection to young and middle-aged adults and a 2 to 1 male predominance. The most common locations are leg and knee, and forearm and hand. Most cases have been reported in the extremities, more commonly distally. Rare examples have been reported in the head and neck and trunk wall. The tumor usually forms a small, subcutaneous, often longstanding nodule that may be painful. Local excision is sufficient, but recurrence is possible (6–9).

Gross and Microscopic Findings. Myopericytoma typically forms a well-demarcated subcutaneous nodule measuring 1 to 2 cm. The tumor has a prominent vascular pattern, often containing round vascular profiles with patent lumens (fig. 5-2). Surrounding the vessels are spindled or epithelioid (glomus tumor-like) cells, often in a concentric pattern. Mitotic activity and atypia are limited.

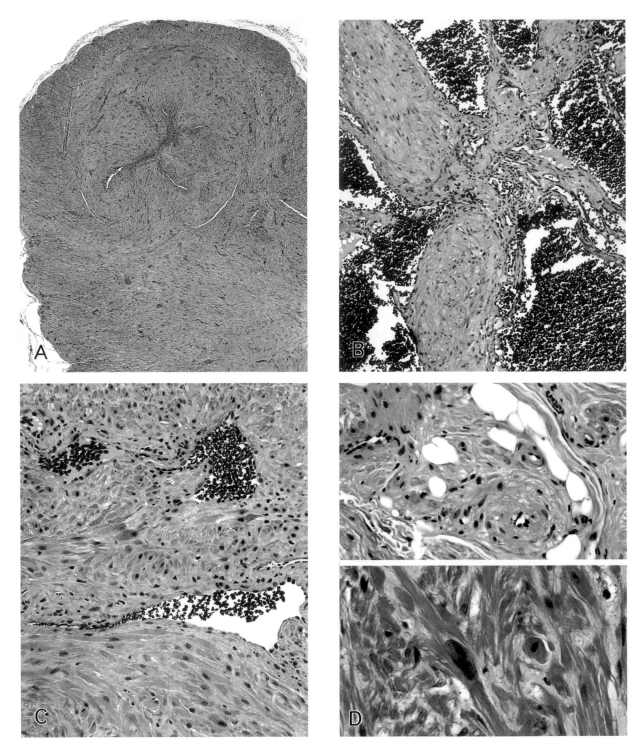

Figure 5-1

VARIANTS OF ANGIOLEIOMYOMA

A: Solid variant with narrow vascular lumens.
B: Cavernous variant with large blood-filled spaces separated by thick bands of smooth muscle.
C: An example with mildly dilated venous channels. Well-differentiated smooth muscle cells have eosinophilic cytoplasm.
D: Lipomatous metaplasia and focal nuclear atypia in angioleiomyoma.

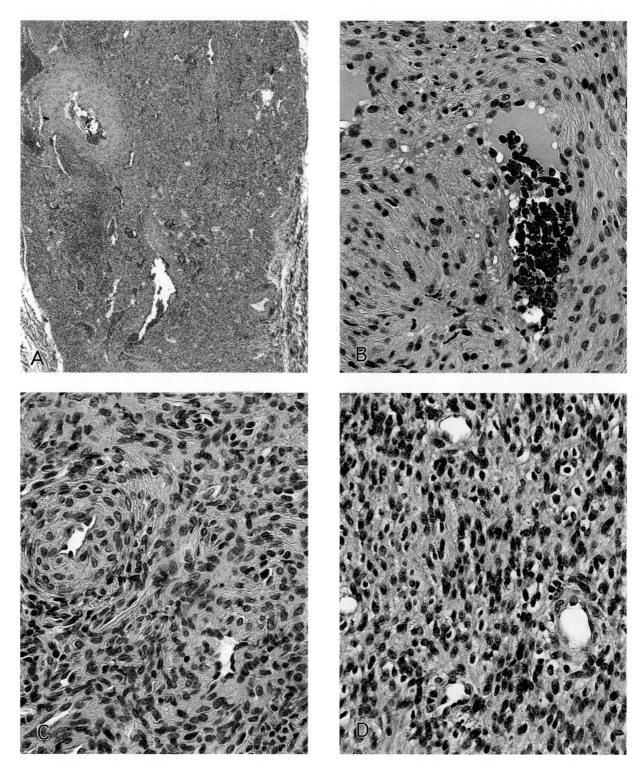

Figure 5-2

MYOPERICYTOMA

A: A sharply demarcated subcutaneous mass has prominent blood vessels with muscular walls.

B–D: The oval, fairly uniform tumor cells involve the vessel walls. The cells do not show features typical of smooth muscle cells.

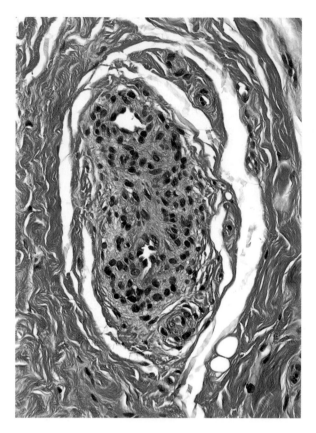

Figure 5-3

GLOMUS BODY

A glomus body, a normal anatomic counterpart of the glomus tumor, is seen in peripheral soft tissues, such as fingers and hand, and the coccygeal region. It is composed of epithelioid cells occupying walls of small vessels.

Special Studies. Immunohistochemically, myopericytomas are variably positive for α-smooth muscle actin and CD34, but are negative for desmin, keratins, and S-100 protein. Caldesmon positivity is detectable in some cases.

Differential Diagnosis. Myopericytoma, angioleiomyoma, and glomus tumor form a continuum, and in some cases the designation is arbitrary.

Treatment and Prognosis. Typical cases are managed with simple excision since recurrences are rare. The rare histologically malignant examples are managed as soft tissue sarcomas. Specific experience concerning these is currently limited.

GLOMUS TUMOR

Definition. *Glomus tumor* is a generally benign mesenchymal tumor composed of oval to epithelioid, smooth muscle-related cells analogous to cells forming the glomus bodies that regulate peripheral blood flow.

General Comments. Glomus bodies, the normal tissue counterpart of glomus tumor, occur in peripheral soft tissues, especially fingers, and also in the sacrococcygeal region; they are sometimes found incidentally in surgical specimens from those sites (10–12). Pathologic lesions such as retrorectal cystic hamartomas also contain glomus bodies (13). The glomus body consists of uniform epithelioid cells embedded in the smooth muscle walls of vessels (fig. 5-3).

Glomus tumors are usually benign, but there is a small group of atypical and potentially malignant ones. The truly malignant (metastasizing) glomus tumors are rare and the criteria for prediction of tumor behavior remain incomplete.

Clinical Features. Glomus tumors occur in a wide age range, although they are more common in young adults. They usually arise in the subcutaneous soft tissue, most commonly in the distal extremities. The nail bed is a typical location, and nail bed tumors have a female predominance (5). Glomus tumor occurs less frequently in the proximal extremities and trunk wall, and rarely in the head and neck region.

Most glomus tumors are small. The subungual examples typically measure only a few millimeters, whereas most others are 1 to 2 cm in diameter. These tumors are often painful (14).

Multiple clustered glomus tumors, designated as *glomuvenous malformations*, are rare. Clinically, they form cobblestone-like pink to purplish blue cutaneous and subcutaneous lesions, especially in the distal extremities. These are often present at birth, expand during childhood, are usually evident by the age of 20 years, and like ordinary glomus tumors, are often painful (15).

The affected individuals with familial glomuvenous malformations have loss of function germline mutations in the *glomulin* gene, located at 1p21-22. Studies of lesional tissue have shown a second nonsense mutation in the *glomulin* gene leading to complete inactivation of this gene and loss of glomulin protein, according the principle of classic tumor suppressor genes (16,17).

Gross Findings. Glomus tumors typically form circumscribed, subcutaneous, rarely intramuscular, ovoid or round nodules that are sometimes surrounded by collagenous capsule-like fibrous bands. On sectioning, the tumor is solid, or cystic and hemorrhagic (*glomangioma*).

Microscopic Findings. Histologically, glomus tumor typically forms a circumscribed nodule composed of clusters or solid sheets of glomus cells. The cellular nests are set in a myxoid or collagenous matrix as cords or perivascular clusters (fig. 5-4A,B). The solid examples contain uniform, round or slightly polygonal, epithelioid-like cells with sharp cellular borders and pale to bright eosinophilic, even oncocytic, cytoplasm. The nuclei are small and uniform, and are often surrounded by a paler halo zone (fig. 5-4C,D).

In some tumors, glomus cells line cavernously dilated vascular spaces and are designated glomangiomas (fig. 5-5A,B). An intravascular component may be present but has no adverse significance in conventional glomus tumors (fig. 5-5C). Tumors combining the features of glomus tumor and angioleiomyoma are designated *glomangiomyoma* and those diffusely infiltrating skeletal muscle as *glomangiomatosis* (fig. 5-5D).

Atypical and Malignant Glomus Tumors. Glomus tumors with a multinodular invasive pattern are associated with a potential for local recurrence but none for metastasis (18). Focal nuclear atypia and isolated mitotic figures may be present in a conventional glomus tumor and these features are not associated with a significant risk for metastasis, but a combination of atypia and mitotic activity may indicate metastatic potential (fig. 5-6). Metastasizing glomus tumors are rare and therefore information on predictive features is scant. Nevertheless, factors associated with a significant risk of metastasis include the presence of atypical mitoses (strongest association), tumor location deep to fascia, tumor size over 2 cm, and mitotic rate of more than 5 mitoses per 50 high-power fields (19,20). In rare cases, glomus tumors not fulfilling any of these criteria have also metastasized.

Special Studies. Glomus tumor cells are immunohistochemically positive for smooth muscle actin, and 20 to 30 percent are focally or extensively positive for CD34. Laminin- and collagen IV-positive basement membranes are typically detectable around the tumor cells. Expression of heavy caldesmon and calponin is variable. Only rarely are glomus tumors positive for desmin (especially glomangiomyomas), and they are negative for keratins and S-100 protein

(21), although small positive nerve twigs may be present. Electron microscopy shows smooth muscle-like features in the glomus cells: prominent cytoplasmic actin bundles, attachment plaques, pinocytic vesicles, and pericellular basement membrane (22).

Differential Diagnosis. Glomus tumors may resemble certain skin adnexal tumors, especially the more solid variants of hidradenoma (eccrine acrospiroma). The presence of ductular structures, clear cytoplasmic cells, and keratin expression helps to identify the latter. Superficial variants of the Ewing family tumors are distinguished by their much higher cellularity and scant cytoplasm. Metastatic melanoma typically shows greater atypia and is positive for S-100 protein and usually for other melanocytic markers.

Hemangiopericytoma/solitary fibrous tumor is composed of less differentiated ovoid to spindled cells with scant, generally noneosinophilic cytoplasm. This tumor almost uniformly lacks markers for smooth muscle cells, in contrast to glomus tumor.

Especially terminologically, glomus tumors may be confused with variants of paraganglioma sometimes called glomus tumors (especially glomus jugulare tumors). However, these paragangliomas have variably organoid patterns and are positive for the neuroendocrine markers chromogranin A and synaptophysin.

Treatment and Prognosis. Conventional glomus tumors are adequately managed by simple excision. Examples with atypical or malignant features should be excised with negative margins and the patients followed.

ESTROGEN RECEPTOR–POSITIVE SMOOTH MUSCLE TUMORS IN WOMEN

Clinical Features. *Leiomyoma in abdominal soft tissues* is a newly discovered category of tumors that occurs exclusively in women, typically in early middle age, and shows a histologic spectrum similar to that of uterine leiomyoma (23,24). They are considered extrauterine examples of uterine-type, estrogen receptor- and progesterone receptor-positive leiomyoma. The most common sites are various pelvic locations and the retroperitoneum. In our experience, however, similar tumors also occur elsewhere in the abdominal cavity, attached to intestines,

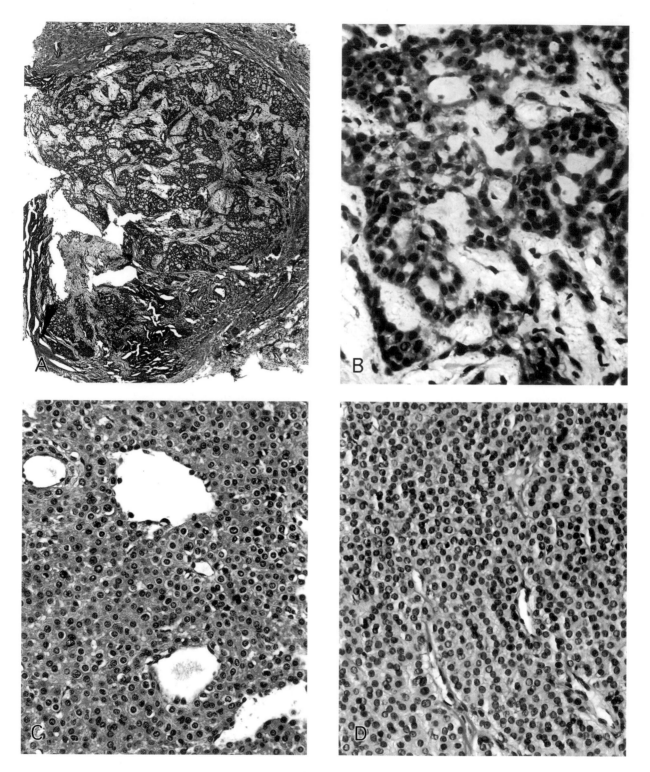

Figure 5-4

GLOMUS TUMOR

A: A small glomus tumor forms a circumscribed mass.
B: The tumor cells are organized to form interconnecting trabeculae in a fibromyxoid matrix.
C,D: These tumors are composed of solid sheets of uniform epithelioid cells. A perinuclear halo is formed in C.

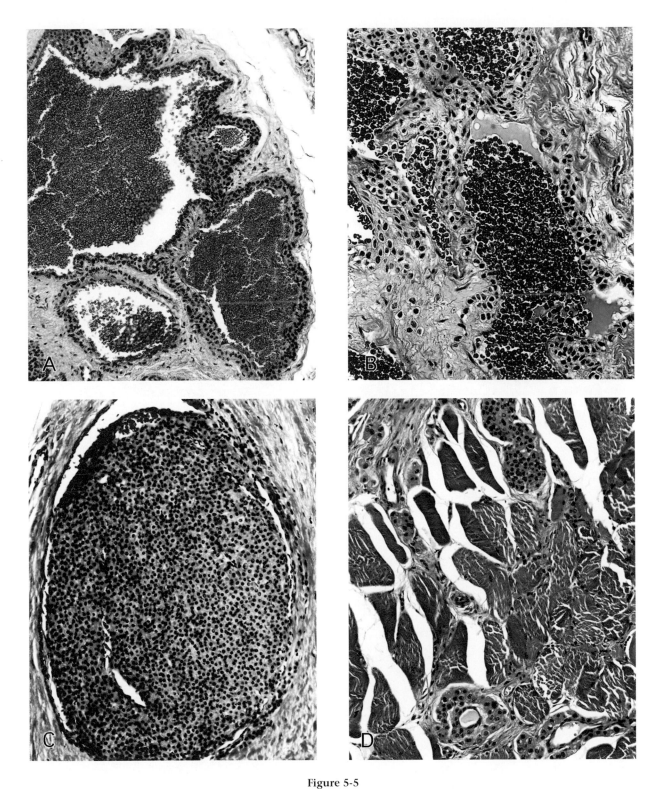

Figure 5-5

GLOMUS TUMORS

A,B: Two glomus tumors (glomangiomas) are composed of dilated vascular spaces lined by glomus cells.

C: An intravascular element of glomus tumor.

D: Multiple intramuscular nests of glomus tumor (glomangiomatosis).

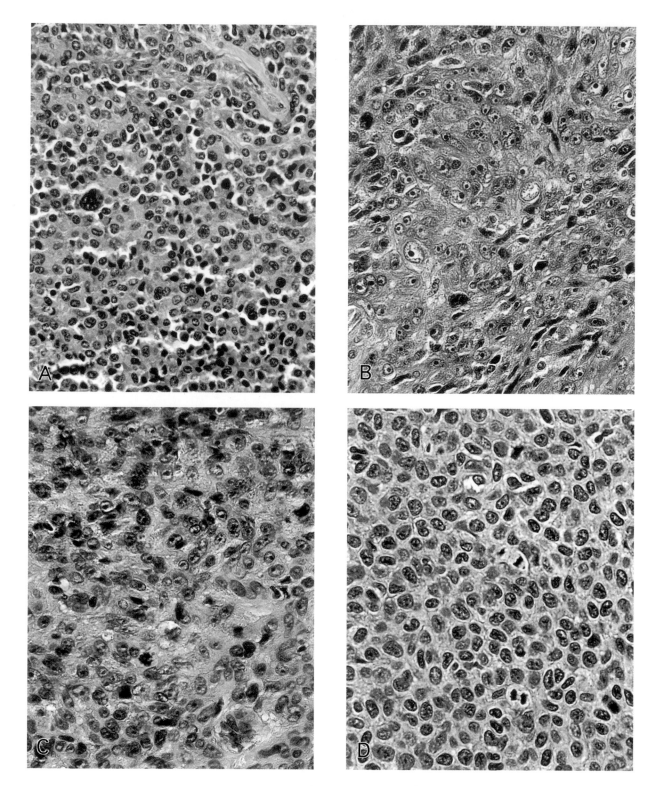

Figure 5-6

GLOMUS TUMOR

A,B: Cytologic and nuclear atypia in a glomus tumor.
C,D: Highly cellular glomus tumors with mitotic activity.

omentum, abdominal wall, and inguinal region (25). In the latter location, leiomyomas may originate from the round ligament.

Abdominal leiomyomas vary from nodules smaller than 1 cm to larger masses; the latter is especially true for retroperitoneal leiomyomas. The prognosis of patients with these tumors is excellent, as long as the mitotic activity is low (3 mitoses or less per 50 high-power fields) (23–25). There are no data on tumor behavior for examples with higher mitotic rates, which would still qualify as benign in the uterus. Such tumors with nonatypical features but higher mitotic rates have to be considered of uncertain biologic potential until more experience is obtained.

Gross Findings. Abdominal, especially retroperitoneal, leiomyomas vary from small 1- to 3-cm nodules to large tumors of over 15 cm that weigh more than 1 kg. They are firm, gray-white masses, often with a whorled appearance, and cysts may be present on sectioning. Similar tumors in the omentum and around intestines are typically smaller.

Microscopic Findings. Histologically, the tumors are generally paucicellular to moderately cellular, similar to uterine leiomyomas. Myxoid change, hyalinization, and microtrabecular patterns are part of their spectrum (fig. 5-7). Examples with fat infiltration are called *lipoleiomyomas*.

Special Studies. Similar to uterine leiomyomas, abdominal leiomyomas are immunohistochemically positive for smooth muscle actin, desmin, heavy caldesmon, and estrogen and progesterone receptors (fig. 5-8). Highly cellular examples with mitotic activity have to be classified as having uncertain malignant potential or as leiomyosarcomas, even if they are hormone receptor positive.

EPSTEIN-BARR VIRUS–ASSOCIATED SMOOTH MUSCLE TUMORS

Definition. *Epstein-Barr virus* (EBV)–associated smooth muscle tumors are mesenchymal tumors with smooth muscle differentiation that contain nuclear EBV-associated RNA (EBV early RNA [EBER] positive) and occur in immunosuppressed patients. Although previously considered leiomyosarcomas, they are presently classified as smooth muscle tumors to reflect their generally favorable outcome.

Clinical Features. EBV-associated smooth muscle tumors most commonly occur in children and young adults with acquired immunodeficiency syndrome (AIDS) (26–30), or in rare cases, with a congenital immunodeficiency syndrome (31). These tumors are less common in older adults and are then usually associated with immunosuppression following solid organ transplantation or, occasionally, corticosteroid treatment (32–34).

The patient mean age in series of AIDS-associated cases was 25 years and 39 years in a series of mixed background cases (30,34). Only one third of these tumors occur in peripheral soft tissues and two thirds in visceral organs, such as central nervous system, lung, and liver. Tumor multiplicity is common and seems to reflect independent multiple primaries rather than metastatic disease, based on molecular fingerprinting (34).

Gross and Microscopic Findings. EBV-associated smooth muscle tumors form 1- to 7-cm solid masses. Histologically, they vary from well-differentiated smooth muscle tumors similar to ordinary smooth muscle tumors to less differentiated ones. Occasional cases have myopericytoma-like histologic features (35). The tumors are often composed of uniform oval cells without much pleomorphism and with a less-differentiated appearance than typical smooth muscle cells (fig. 5-9). Numerous tumor-infiltrating T lymphocytes are common. Most cases have a mitotic rate of 2 or less mitoses per 10 high-power fields.

Special Studies. Although these tumors are generally uniformly α-smooth muscle actin positive, they are variably (50 to 80 percent) positive for desmin (30,33). Nuclear positivity for EBER in the context of a smooth muscle tumor is diagnostic (fig. 5-10); ordinary leiomyosarcomas are not EBER positive (36).

Treatment and Prognosis. Surgical excision is the main treatment, but surgically incurable multiple tumors may respond to a decrease of immunosuppression. EBV-associated smooth muscle tumors are unpredictable, and their behavior does not correlate with traditional criteria for smooth muscle tumors. Despite tumor multiplicity and signs of histologic malignancy, only rare patients die as a result of EBV-related smooth muscle tumors, and the immunosuppressive condition and infections play a major role in patient outcome (30,34).

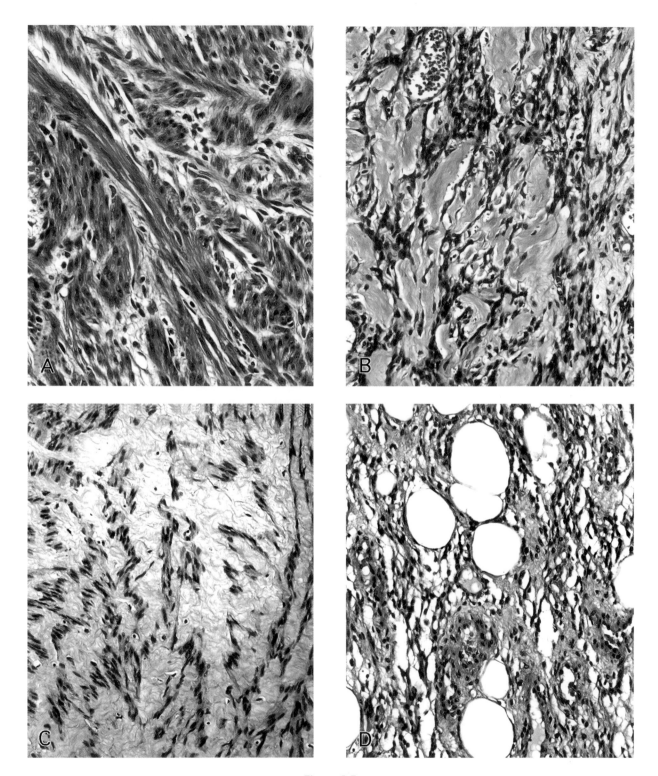

Figure 5-7

ABDOMINAL SOFT TISSUE LEIOMYOMA

A–C: Estrogen receptor-positive soft tissue leiomyomas in women show features similar to uterine leiomyomas, including fascicular, trabecular, and hyalinizing patterns.

D: Cases with a fatty component are designated lipoleiomyomas.

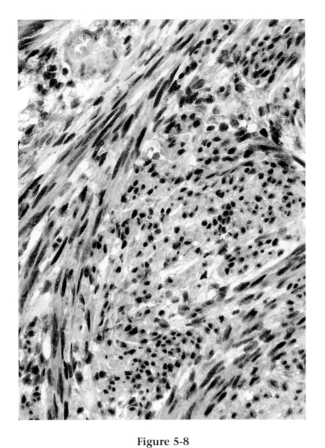

Figure 5-8

ABDOMINAL SOFT TISSUE LEIOMYOMA

Typical of abdominal leiomyomas in women is immuno-histochemical nuclear positivity for estrogen receptor.

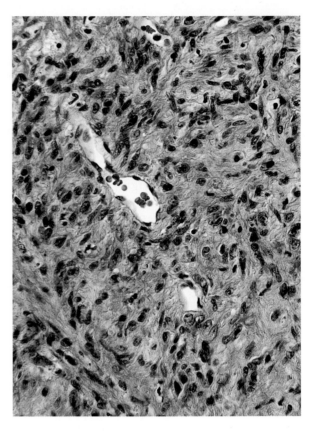

Figure 5-9

EPSTEIN-BARR VIRUS–ASSOCIATED SMOOTH MUSCLE TUMOR

The tumor is composed of fairly uniform oval cells.

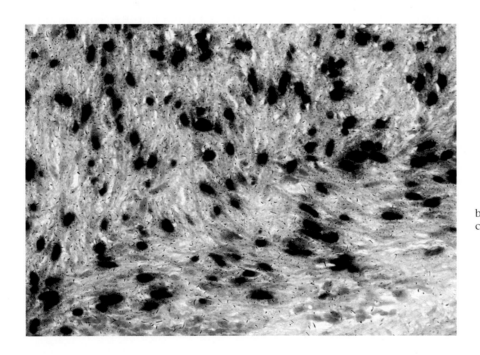

Figure 5-10

EPSTEIN-BARR VIRUS–ASSOCIATED SMOOTH MUSCLE TUMOR

The nuclei are EBER positive by in situ hybridization (blue chromogen).

LEIOMYOSARCOMA

Definition. *Leiomyosarcoma* is a malignant soft tissue tumor primarily or entirely composed of cells with smooth muscle differentiation. In general, smooth muscle tumors in soft tissues with nuclear atypia and any mitotic activity are considered leiomyosarcomas. Some tumors may contain differentiated smooth muscle and undifferentiated elements (*dedifferentiated leiomyosarcoma*).

General Considerations. This text covers leiomyosarcomas occurring in the extremities, trunk wall, and body cavities, including those of vascular origin. Estrogen receptor–dependent soft tissue leiomyosarcomas in the abdominal cavity or abdominal wall are considered separately below. EBV-associated smooth muscle tumors are now considered a separate group (see previous section). Cutaneous and visceral leiomyosarcomas are excluded and are discussed in other Fascicles.

Clinical Features. A Swedish study estimated the incidence of peripheral tumors (extremity and trunk wall leiomyosarcomas excluding cutaneous ones) as 1.3 per million people (37). Leiomyosarcoma is primarily a tumor of older adults, although it infrequently occurs in children, especially in connection with rare germline mutation syndromes affecting the *retinoblastoma* (38) and *TP53 (p53)* genes (39). While peripheral soft tissue leiomyosarcoma has a male predominance, retroperitoneal occurrence is more common in women (40).

There are a wide variety of soft tissue locations in the extremities, trunk wall, and body cavities. Thigh and buttocks are among the most common sites for peripheral leiomyosarcoma (41–46). A significant proportion of leiomyosarcomas are believed to arise from vascular smooth muscle, especially of veins (46–48). Venous origin is more commonly detected in retroperitoneal examples. Such tumors usually arise from the inferior vena cava, and less commonly from other veins, such as renal, iliac, or genital veins. Origin from peripheral veins is also possible, but less frequently detected. Most commonly recognized peripheral venous leiomyosarcomas are those arising from the saphenous vein.

Although the peripheral leiomyosarcomas present as mass lesions similar to many other sarcomas, the vascular ones entail specific clinical complications related to vascular luminal compromise. Those of the inferior vena cava involving the intrahepatic or perihepatic portions especially tend to compromise hepatic circulation and may thereby be fatal without metastatic spread (49–53).

Leiomyosarcomas most commonly metastasize into the lungs, liver, and bones. Cutaneous and soft tissue metastases also occur. The possibility of metastatic origin from deep soft tissue (such as retroperitoneum) must always be considered in the diagnosis of a peripheral soft tissue leiomyosarcoma when facing a small, circumscribed lesion and especially when multiple lesions are present (41).

Leiomyosarcomas of visceral origin usually involve the uterus and rarely the gastrointestinal tract. In the latter, most tumors previously classified as leiomyosarcomas are now considered gastrointestinal stromal tumors.

Gross Findings. Most leiomyosarcomas form circumscribed, solitary masses. Smaller tumors are often solid, homogeneous masses with a pale gray to yellowish, sometimes trabeculated surface on sectioning. Larger tumors typically contain extensive central necrosis and a variably thick peripheral rim of viable tissue. Some leiomyosarcomas are intimately associated with blood vessels (especially veins), and are considered of vascular origin (*vascular leiomyosarcomas*).

Microscopic Findings. Typical leiomyosarcoma is composed of spindled cells, but focal pleomorphism is a usual finding. The spindled cells often form intersecting fascicles (fig. 5-11A,B). In some cases, microscopic examination reveals a close connection/origin from a vein (fig. 5-11C). The spindle cell nuclei are typically blunt-ended (cigar-shaped) and display variable atypia, including prominent hyperchromasia. Cytoplasm varies from pale staining to deeply eosinophilic, and some cases contain rhythmic densities of eosinophilic cytoplasm, designated as contraction bands (54). Mitotic activity varies from rare mitoses to high counts of over 20 per 10 high-power fields, and atypical mitotic figures are common. Coagulative necrosis is a common finding in higher-grade tumors.

In some cases, the majority of tumor is undifferentiated, with only focal remnants of differentiated leiomyosarcoma (*dedifferentiated leiomyosarcoma*) (fig. 5-11D) (55). A collagenous or sometimes myxoid stromal element is variably

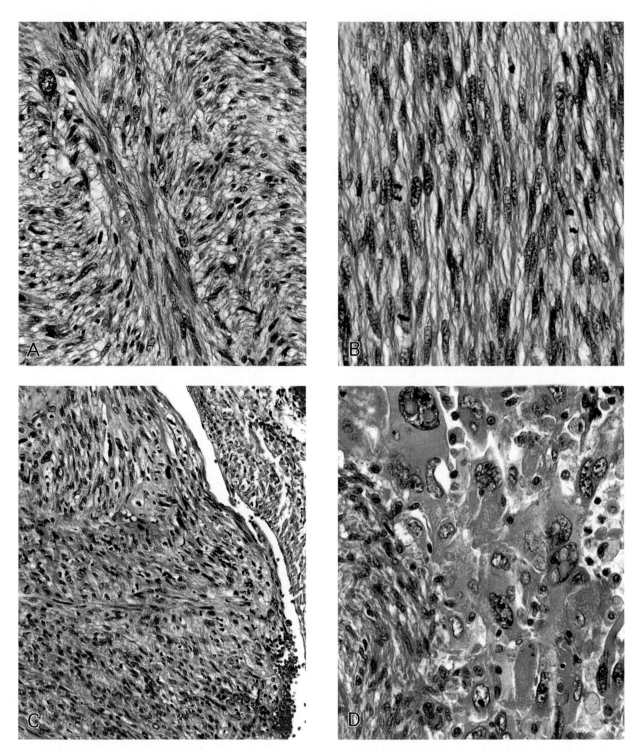

Figure 5-11

LEIOMYOSARCOMA

A,B: Typical leiomyosarcoma is composed of intersecting fascicles of spindle cells with blunt-ended nuclei. Focal nuclear pleomorphism is a common finding.

C: Some leiomyosarcomas are intimately associated with an originating vein.

D: Severe pleomorphism may be present, here seen sharply demarcated as the differentiated component.

present. Unusual variants with prominent lymphoid infiltration have been designated as *inflammatory leiomyosarcoma.*

Special Studies. Leiomyosarcoma cells typically stain yellow with trichrome stains such as van Gieson. Immunohistochemically, they are almost definitionally positive for α-smooth muscle actin. Most are positive for desmin and heavy caldesmon, although such staining can be focal, especially in poorly differentiated examples (57–60). Keratin and EMA positivity (usually focal) is detectable in up to one third of leiomyosarcomas, which should be considered in differential diagnosis of carcinomas (61,62). CD34 positivity (usually focal) is observed in one third, but these tumors are typically negative for S-100 protein.

By electron microscopy, leiomyosarcomas are distinctive in their content of bundled cytoplasmic actin filaments (dense bodies), and similar juxtamembranous structures are designated attachment plaques. Pinocytic vesicles may be present at the cell membrane. In the better differentiated variants, the cells are variably surrounded by basement membrane material.

No diagnostic genetic testing is routinely available for leiomyosarcoma, which has a complex genomic profile with unbalanced karyotypes (63).

Differential Diagnosis. The most significant entities in the differential diagnosis are those related to malignancy and benign smooth muscle tumors. Also, leiomyosarcoma has to be separated from tumors of other lineages, such as myofibroblastic and undifferentiated sarcomas. Separation of leiomyosarcoma from gastrointestinal stromal tumor is a common problem among abdominal smooth muscle tumors.

Well-differentiated smooth muscle tumors of the abdominal cavity, abdominal wall, and genital region in women are often hormonally influenced, estrogen receptor–positive tumors. Without significant nuclear atypia, these are usually benign, especially if the mitotic count is low (fewer than 10 per 50 high-power fields).

Small biopsies of well-differentiated smooth muscle tumors of soft tissue have to be approached with caution. Because some leiomyosarcomas have low mitotic rates and only focal marked atypia, it is wise to designate them in needle core biopsies as "well-differentiated smooth muscle tumors" and mention that malignancy cannot be (totally) excluded. Tumors that either contain significant atypia but no mitoses, or abundant mitoses with limited atypia, may be designated "smooth muscle tumors of uncertain malignant potential (STUMP)."

Sarcomas that are smooth muscle actin positive but lack the eosinophilic cytoplasm and other morphologic features of differentiated smooth muscle cells are better designated as myofibroblastic or undifferentiated sarcomas. These tumors are usually heavy caldesmon and desmin negative, but focal positivity for the latter may occur.

Inflammatory myofibroblastic tumor usually occurs in children and young adults. It typically shows a heterogeneous admixture of large myofibroblastic tumor cells marked by elongated nuclei with prominent nucleoli, amphophilic cytoplasm, and lymphoplasmacytic infiltration. Immunohistochemically, these tumors are usually positive for ALK, but they may be variably positive for α-smooth muscle actin and desmin.

Some dedifferentiated liposarcomas contain areas of smooth muscle differentiation. Although these may be difficult to separate from leiomyosarcoma in a small sample, a liposarcomatous component and a tumor component with nuclear MDM2 positivity are diagnostic of dedifferentiated liposarcoma.

Gastrointestinal stromal tumors (GISTs) are often grossly distinctive from leiomyosarcomas. They often form hemorrhagic masses that are most often characterized as pink-tan on sectioning, in contrast to the generally pale yellowish appearance of leiomyosarcoma tissue. GISTs generally lack the cytoplasmic eosinophilia seen in leiomyosarcoma, showing more amphophilic or pale cytoplasm. GISTs less commonly show significant nuclear pleomorphism. Immunohistochemically, they are distinctive by being generally positive for KIT (CD117) and anoctamin-1 (DOG1). Although GISTs may show smooth muscle traits in their variable expression of α-smooth muscle actin and heavy caldesmon, they are usually negative for desmin, or at most, show only sporadic positive cells.

Schwann cell tumors, especially cellular schwannoma, can resemble leiomyosarcoma by its spindle cell appearance. However, these tumors may contain nuclear palisading and foci of xanthoma cells. Immunohistochemically, schwannomas are negative for smooth muscle actin and desmin, and positive for S-100 protein in contrast to leiomyosarcoma. Malignant peripheral nerve sheath tumors, however, may be negative for S-100 protein and contain focal desmin. Their occurrence in nerve trunks and association with preexisting neurofibroma are diagnostic.

Treatment and Prognosis. Complete excision and follow-up is the main mode treatment whenever feasible. No specific targeted treatment is currently available for leiomyosarcoma. Although leiomyosarcoma limited to the dermis (cutaneous leiomyosarcoma) almost never metastasizes, tumors with subcutaneous involvement metastasize in 20 to 33 percent of cases (45). In retroperitoneal leiomyosarcomas a mitotic rate of less than 10 per 10 high-power fields seems to be associated with longer survival rates (40).

REFERENCES

Angioleiomyoma

1. Hachisuga T, Hashimoto H, Enjoji M. Angioleiomyoma. A clinicopathologic reappraisal of 562 cases. Cancer 1984;54:126-130.
2. Katenkamp D, Kohmehl H, Lengbein L. [Angiomyoma. A pathologo-anatomic analysis of 229 cases]. Zentralbl Allg Pathol 1988;134:423-433. [German]
3. Brooks JK, Nikitakis NG, Goodman NJ, Levy BA. Clinicopathologic characterization of oral angioleiomyomas. Oral Surg Oral Med Oral Pathol Oral Radiol Endod 2002;94:221-227.
4. Beer TW. Cutaneous angiomyolipomas are HMB45 negative, not associated with tuberous sclerosis, and should be considered as angioleiomyomas with fat. Am J Dermatopathol 2005;27:418-421.
5. Matsuyama A, Hisaoka M, Hashimoto H. Angioleiomyoma: a clinicopathologic and immunohistochemical reappraisal with special reference to the correlation with myopericytoma. Hum Pathol 2007;38:645-651.

Myopericytoma

6. Granter SR, Badizadegan K, Fletcher CD. Myofibromatosis in adults, glomangiopericytoma, and myopericytoma: a spectrum of tumors with perivascular myoid differentiation. Am J Surg Pathol 1998;22:513-525.
7. Mentzel T, Dei Tos AP, Sapi Z, Kutzner H. Myopericytoma of the skin and soft tissues: clinicopathologic and immunohistochemical study of 54 cases. Am J Surg Pathol 2006;30:104-113.
8. Matsuyama A, Hisaoka M, Hashimoto H. Angioleiomyoma; a clinicopathologic and immunohistochemical reappraisal with special reference to the correlation with myopericytoma. Hum Pathol 2007;38:645-651.
9. McMenamin ME, Fletcher CD. Malignant myopericytoma: expanding the spectrum of tumours with myopericytic differentiation. Histopathology 2002;41:450-460.

Glomus Tumor

10. Albrecht S, Zbieranowski I. Incidental glomus coccygeum. When a normal structure looks like a tumor. Am J Surg Pathol 1990;14:922-924.
11. Gatalica Z, Wang L, Lucio ET, Miettinen M. Glomus coccygeum in surgical pathology specimens: small troublemaker. Arch Pathol Lab Med 1999;123:905-908.
12. Santos LD, Chow C, Kennerson AR. Glomus coccygeum may mimick glomus tumour. Pathology 2002;34:339-343.
13. McDermott NC, Newman J. Tailgut cyst (retrorectal cystic hamartoma) with prominent glomus bodies. Histopathology 1991;18:265-266.
14. Tsuneyoshi M, Enjoji M. Glomus tumor. A clinicopathologic and electron microscopic study. Cancer 1982;50:1601-1607.
15. Boon LM, Mulliken JB, Enjolras O, Vikkula M. Glomuvenous malformation (glomangioma) and venous malformation: distinct clinicopathologic and genetic entities. Arch Dermatol 2004;140:971-976.
16. Brouillard P, Boon LM, Mulliken JM, et al. Mutations in a novel factor "glomulin" are responsible for glomuvenous malformations ("glomangiomas"). Am J Hum Genet 2002;70:866-874

17. Brouillard P, Ghassibe M, Penington A, et al. Four common glomulin mutations cause two thirds of glomuvenous malformations ("familial glomangiomas"): evidence for a founder effect. J Med Genet 2005;42:e13.

18. Gould EW, Manivel JC, Albores-Saavedra J, Monforte H. Locally infiltrative glomus tumors and glomangiosarcomas. A clinical, ultrastructural, and immunohistochemical study. Cancer 1990;65:310-318.

19. Khoury T, Balos L, McGrath B, Wong MK, Cheney RT, Tan D. Malignant glomus tumor: a case report and review of the literature, focusing on its clinicopathologic features and immunohistochemical profile. Am J Dermatopathol 2005;27:428-431.

20. Folpe AL, Fanburg-Smith JC, Miettinen M, Weiss SW. Atypical and malignant glomus tumors: analysis of 52 cases with a proposal for the reclassification of glomus tumors. Am J Surg Pathol 2001;25:1-12.

21. Porter PL, Bigler SA, McNutt M, Gown AM. The immunophenotype of hemangiperipcytomas and glomus tumors, with special reference to muscle protein expression: an immunohistochemical study and review of the literature. Mod Pathol 1991;4:46-52.

22. Murad TM, von Haam E, Murthy MS. Ultrastructure of hemangiopericytoma and a glomus tumor. Cancer 1968;22:1239-1249.

Estrogen Receptor–Positive Smooth Muscle Tumors in Women

23. Billings SD, Folpe AL, Weiss SW. Do leiomyomas of deep soft tissue exist? An analysis of highly differentiated smooth muscle tumors of deep soft tissue supporting two distinct subtypes. Am J Surg Pathol 2001;25:1134-1142.

24. Paal E, Miettinen M. Retroperitoneal leiomyomas: a clinicopathologic and immunohistochemical study of 56 cases with a comparison to retroperitoneal leiomyosarcomas. Am J Surg Pathol 2001;25:1355-1363.

25. Patil DT, Laskin WB, Fetsch JF, Miettinen M. Inguinal smooth muscle tumors in women-a dichotomous group consisting of Müllerian-type leiomyomas and soft tissue leiomyosarcomas: an analysis of 55 cases. Am J Surg Pathol 2011;35:315-324.

Epstein-Barr Virus–Associated Smooth Muscle Tumors

26. McClain KL, Leach CT, Jenson HB, et al. Association of Epstein-Barr virus with leiomyosarcomas in children with AIDS. N Engl J Med 1995;332:12-18.

27. Ross JS, Del Rosario A, Bui HX, Sonbati H, Solis O. Primary hepatic leiomyosarcoma in a child with the acquired immunodeficiency syndrome. Hum Pathol 1992;23:69-72.

28. Orlow SJ, Kamino H, Lawrence RL. Multiple subcutaneous leiomyosarcomas in an adolescent with AIDS. Am J Pediatr Hematol Oncol 1992;14:265-268.

29. van Hoeven KH, Factor SM, Kress Y, Woodruff JM. Visceral myogenic tumors. A manifestation of HIV infection in children. Am J Surg Pathol 1993;17:1176-1181.

30. Purgina B, Rao UN, Miettinen M, Pantanowitz L. AIDS-related EBV-associated smooth muscle tumors: review of 64 published cases. Patholog Res Int 2011;2011:561548.

31. Tulbah A, Al-Dayel F, Fawaz I, Rosai J. Epstein-Barr virus-associated leiomyosarcoma of the thyroid in a child with congenital immunodeficiency: a case report. Am J Surg Pathol 1998;23:473-476.

32. Timmons CF, Dawson DB, Richards CS, Andrews WS, Katz JA. Epstein-Barr virus-associated leiomyosarcomas in liver transplantation recipients. Origin from either donor or recipient tissue. Cancer 1995;76:1481-1489.

33. Somers GR, Tesoriero AA, Hartland E, et al. Multiple leiomyosarcomas of both donor and recipient origin arising in heart-lung transplant patient. Am J Surg Pathol 1998;22:1423-1428.

34. Deyrup AT, Lee VK, Hill CE, et al. Epstein-Barr virus-associated smooth muscle tumors are distinctive mesenchymal tumors reflecting multiple infection events: a clinicopathologic and molecular analysis of 29 tumors from 19 patients. Am J Surg Pathol 2006;30:75-82.

35. Lau PP, Wong OK, Lui PC, et al. Myopericytoma in patients with AIDS: a new class of Epstein-Barr virus-associated tumor. Am J Surg Pathol. 2009;33:1666-1672.

36. Hill MA, Araya JC, Eckert MW, Gillespie AT, Hunt JD, Levine EA. Tumor specific Epstein-Barr virus infection is not associated with leiomyosarcoma in human immunodeficiency virus negative individuals. Cancer 1997;80:204-210.

Leiomyosarcoma

37. Gustafson P, Willen H, Baldetrop B, Ferno M, Akerman M, Rydholm A. Soft tissue leiomyosarcoma. A population-based epidemiologic and prognostic study of 48 patients, including cellular DNA content. Cancer 1992;70:114-119.

38. Kleinerman R, Tucker MA, Abramson DH, Seddon JM, Terone RE, Faumeni JF Jr. Risk of soft tissue sarcomas by individual subtype in survivors of hereditary retinoblastoma. J Natl Cancer Inst 2007;99:24-31.

39. Ognjanovic S, Olivier M, Bergemann TL, Hainaut P. Sacomas in TP53 germline mutation carriers: a review of the IARC TP53 database. Cancer 2012;118:1387-1396.

40. Rajani B, Smith TA, Reith JD, Goldblum JR. Retroperitoneal leiomyosarcomas unassociated with the gastrointestinal tract: a clinicopathologic analysis of 17 cases. Mod Pathol 1999;12:21-28.

41. Dahl I, Angervall L. Cutaneous and subcutaneous leiomyosarcoma. A clinicopathologic study of 47 patients. Pathol Eur 1974;9:307-315.

42. Fields JP, Helwig EB. Leiomyosarcoma of the skin and subcutaneous tissue. Cancer 1981;47:156-169.

43. Hashimoto H, Daimaru Y, Tsuneyoshi M, Enjoji M. Leiomyosarcoma of the external soft tissues. A clinicopathologic, immunohistochemical and electron microscopic study. Cancer 1986;57:2077-2088.

44. Jensen ML, Jensen OM, Michalski W, Nielsen OS, Keller J. Intradermal and subcutaneous leiomyosarcoma: a clinicopathological and immunohistochemical study of 41 cases. J Cutan Pathol 1996;23:458-463.

45. Svarvar C, Böhling T, Berlin O, et al. Clinical course of nonvisceral soft tissue leiomyosarcoma in 225 patients from the Scandinavian Sarcoma Group. Cancer 2007;109:282-291.

46. Farshid G, Pradham M, Goldblum J, Weiss SW. Leiomyosarcoma of somatic soft tissues: a tumor of vascular origin with multivariate analysis of outcome in 42 cases. Am J Surg Pathol 2002;26:14-24.

47. Varela-Duran J, Oliva H, Rosai J. Vascular leiomyosarcoma: the malignant counterpart of vascular leiomyoma. Cancer 1979;44:1684-1691.

48. Berlin O, Stener B, Kindblom LG, Angervall L. Leiomyosarcoma of venous origin in the extremities. A correlated clinical, roentgenologic, and morphologic study with diagnostic surgical implications. Cancer 1984;54:2147-2159.

49. Mingoli A, Cavallaro A, Sapienza P, Di Marzo L, Feldhaus RJ, Cavallari N. International registry of inferior vena cava leiomyosarcoma: analysis of a world series on 218 patients. Anticancer Res 1996;16:3201-3205.

50. Hines OJ, Nelson S, Quinones-Baldrich WJ, Eilber FR. Leiomyosarcoma of the inferior vena cava: prognosis and comparison with leiomyosarcoma of other anatomic sites. Cancer 1999;85:1077-1083.

51. Hollenbeck ST, Grobmyer SR, Kent KC, Brennan MF. Surgical treatment and outcomes in patients with primary inferior vena cava leiomyosarcoma. J Am Coll Surg 2003;197:575-579.

52. Ito H, Hornick JL, Bertagnolli MM, et al. Leiomyosarcoma of the inferior vena cava: survival after aggressive management. Ann Surg Oncol 2007;14:3534-3541.

53. Laskin WB, Fanburg-Smith JC, Burke AP, Krazewska E, Fetsch JF, Miettinen M. Leiomyosarcoma of the inferior vena cava: a clinicopathologic study of 40 cases. Am J Surg Pathol 2010;34:873-881.

54 Venance SL, Burns KL, Veinot JP, Walley VM. Contraction bands in visceral and vascular smooth muscle. Hum Pathol 1996;27:1035-1041.

55. Nicolas MM, Tamboli P, Gomez JA, Czerniak B. Pleomorphic and dedifferentiated leiomyosarcoma: clinicopathologic and immunohistochemical study of 41 cases. Hum Pathol 2010;41:663-671.

56. Merchant W, Calonje E, Fletcher CD. Inflammatory leiomyosarcoma: a morphologic subgroup within the heterogeneous family of so-called malignant fibrous histiocytoma. Histopathology 1995;27:525-532.

57. Schürch W, Skalli O, Seemayer TA, Gabbiani G. Intermediate filament proteins and actin isoforms as markers for soft tissue tumor differentiation and origin. I. Smooth muscle tumors. Am J Pathol 1987;128:91-103.

58. Azumi N, Ben-Ezra J, Battifora H. Immunophenotypic diagnosis of leiomyosarcomas and rhabdomyosarcomas with monoclonal antibodies to muscle-specific actin and desmin in formalin-fixed tissue. Mod Pathol 1988;1:469-474.

59. Watanabe K, Kusakabe T, Hoshi N, Saito A, Suzuki T. h-caldesmon in leiomyosarcoma and tumors with smooth muscle cell-like differentiation: its specific expression in the smooth muscle cell tumor. Hum Pathol 1999;30:392-396.

60. Miettinen MM, Sarlomo-Rikala M, Kovatich AJ, Lasota J. Calponin and h-caldesmon in soft tissue tumors: consistent h-caldesmon immunoreactivity in gastrointestinal stromal tumors indicates traits of smooth muscle differentiation. Mod Pathol 1999;12:756-762.

61. Miettinen M. Immunoreactivity for cytokeratin and epithelial membrane antigen in leiomyosarcoma. Arch Pathol Lab Med 1988;112:637-640.

62. Iwata J, Fletcher CD. Immunohistochemical detection of cytokeratin and epithelial membrane antigen in leiomyosarcoma: a systematic study of 100 cases. Pathol Int 2000;50:7-14.

63. Sandberg AA. Updates on the cytogenetics and molecular genetics of bone and soft tissue tumors: leiomyosarcoma. Cancer Genet Cytogenet 2005;161:1-19.

6 TUMORS WITH SKELETAL MUSCLE DIFFERENTIATION

This chapter includes a spectrum of benign and malignant tumors with skeletal muscle differentiation. Malignant skeletal muscle differentiation (rhabdomyosarcomatous differentiation) occurs in many other diagnostic entities as well, and a thorough morphologic examination and an adequate immunohistochemical panel are used to rule them out. In adult patients especially, rhabdomyosarcomatous differentiation is much more common in nonrhabdomyosarcomatous tumors, such as malignant mixed mullerian tumor in women, dedifferentiated liposarcoma, and a variety of carcinomas.

RHABDOMYOMATOUS MESENCHYMAL HAMARTOMA

Definition. *Rhabdomyomatous mesenchymal hamartoma (striated muscle hamartoma)* is an extremely rare benign tumor of the face and neck in newborns, characterized by an intradermal or subcutaneous collection of mature skeletal muscle, myxoid stroma, and other mesenchymal tissues.

Clinical Features. Rhabdomyomatous mesenchymal hamartoma usually presents as a small papule or pedunculated lesion, most often involving the head and neck region (1–5). Rare cases occur in the digits and genital region (6,7). Almost all reported cases have occurred in males, sometimes in association with other congenital anomalies (8,9).

Gross Findings. Rhabdomyomatous mesenchymal hamartomas appear as small papular or polypoid lesions of the skin. They are sometimes umbilicated (1–5).

Microscopic Findings. Histologically, rhabdomyomatous hamartoma consists of an intradermal and subcutaneous collection of mature-appearing skeletal muscle cells, arranged singly and in small groups. These are arrayed in a collagenized and variably myxoid stroma, with admixed mature adipose tissue, dermal adnexal structures, nerves, and blood vessels. Ossification or calcification may be present (fig. 6-1) (1–5). Rhabdomyomatous mesenchymal hamartoma does not require ancillary studies for diagnosis.

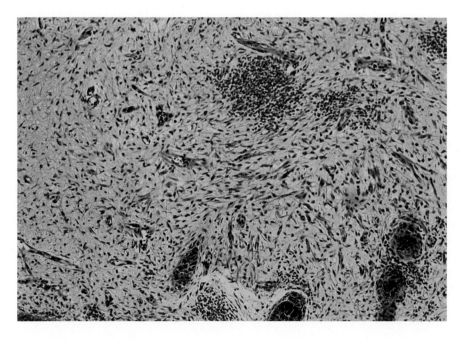

Figure 6-1

RHABDOMYOSARCOMATOUS MESENCHYMAL HAMARTOMA

Rhabdomyomatous mesenchymal hamartoma contains a bland spindle cell proliferation with skeletal muscle differentiation (this lesion was also verified as desmin positive). (Courtesy of Dr. D. M. Parham, Los Angeles, CA.)

Genetics. A specific genetic abnormality has not been reported. The rare occurrence of this tumor in girls suggests that it is not an X-linked disorder, as has been suggested (6).

Differential Diagnosis. Neuromuscular choristoma (benign triton tumor) arises in association with a peripheral nerve and consists of an admixture of nerves and muscle, without fat. Nevus lipomatosus superficialis lacks skeletal muscle. Fibrous hamartoma of infancy is a triphasic tumor, consisting of primitive mesenchyme, fat, and mature fibrous tissue, without skeletal muscle. Embryonal rhabdomyosarcoma is very rare in the skin and is a much more cellular tumor consisting of mitotically active immature skeletal muscle and rhabdomyoblasts.

Treatment and Prognosis. Rhabdomyomatous mesenchymal hamartoma is adequately treated with local excision and does not recur.

RHABDOMYOMA

Definition. *Rhabdomyomas* are rare benign mesenchymal tumors showing skeletal muscle differentiation. They are classified into the cardiac (not covered here) and extracardiac types. Extracardiac rhabdomyomas are subclassified as fetal and adult type, with genital rhabdomyoma representing a differentiated (adult-type) rhabdomyoma of the genital tract.

Clinical Features. *Fetal Rhabdomyoma.* Fetal rhabdomyomas typically occur as a solitary mass in the subcutaneous tissue of the head and neck region of young boys (under 5 years of age) (10–16). *Predominantly myxoid fetal rhabdomyoma* most often occurs in the preauricular and postauricular regions of infants; less myxoid, more cellular tumors *(intermediate-type fetal rhabdomyoma)* occur more often in adults and tend to involve the orbit, tongue, nasopharynx, and soft palate. Some cases of fetal rhabdomyoma are associated with the basal cell nevus syndrome (13).

Adult Rhabdomyoma. Adult rhabdomyomas usually occur in the head and neck of older males (median, 60 years of age), most often in the pharynx, oral cavity, tongue base, and larynx (12,16–21). Multiple lesions occur in up to 20 percent of cases.

Genital Rhabdomyoma. Genital rhabdomyoma most often presents as a polypoid lesion of the cervix or vagina in middle-aged women (range,

30 to 48 years) (22–24). Rare cases have been reported to occur in men in the paratesticular region or epididymis (25–28).

Gross Findings. Rhabdomyomas of all types are typically small (3 to 5 cm) and well-circumscribed. Fetal rhabdomyomas appear more myxoid than do their adult counterparts.

Microscopic Findings. *Fetal Rhabdomyoma.* Fetal rhabdomyomas are well delineated but not encapsulated. The myxoid type of fetal rhabdomyoma shows an abundant myxoid matrix, within which are bland spindle cells and rare immature skeletal muscle fibers (10–16). Mitoses, pleomorphism, and necrosis are absent. More mature skeletal muscle cells are present at the periphery of the lesion.

Intermediate-type fetal rhabdomyomas consist of numerous differentiated skeletal muscle fibers with little myxoid matrix. Ganglion-like rhabdomyoblasts, mature-appearing skeletal muscle cells with easily identified cross striations, and vacuolated cells are typically found. Mild pleomorphism may be present, but necrosis and mitotic figures are absent (fig. 6-2) (10–16).

Adult Rhabdomyoma. Adult rhabdomyomas are well-circumscribed but unencapsulated, often lobulated tumors that are composed of large polygonal or round cells with abundant eosinophilic cytoplasm, a large nucleus, and a prominent nucleolus (12,16–21). "Spider cells," consisting of large cells with predominantly clear cytoplasm and thin strands of eosinophilic cytoplasm extending from the nucleus to the cytoplasmic membrane, are often found. Cross striations and intracytoplasmic crystalline material may be present. Mitoses are rare to absent (fig. 6-3).

Genital Rhabdomyoma. Genital rhabdomyomas are composed of haphazardly arranged, round or strap-like rhabdomyoblasts with copious eosinophilic cytoplasm and cross striations, resembling intermediate fetal rhabdomyomas (22–24). In general, however, genital rhabdomyomas show a greater degree of stromal fibrosis and less cellular variability than do fetal rhabdomyomas.

Special Studies. Rhabdomyomas have a mature skeletal muscle phenotype, with expression of desmin, skeletal muscle actin isoforms, and myoglobin (12). Few cases have been studied for myogenin or MyoD1 expression, and it is unclear whether the expression of these markers

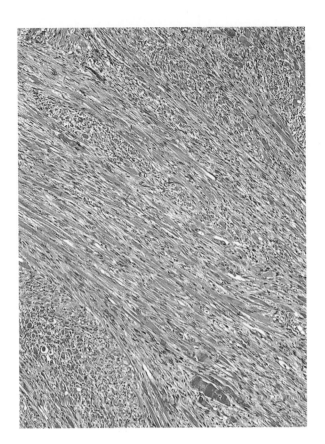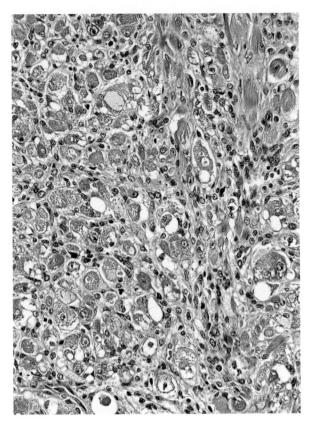

Figure 6-2

INTERMEDIATE-TYPE FETAL RHABDOMYOMA

Left: The tumor consists of a moderately cellular proliferation of fairly well-differentiated skeletal muscle cells in various stages of maturation.

Right: Nuclear atypia and mitotic activity are absent, in contrast to embryonal rhabdomyosarcoma.

is of value in the distinction of rhabdomyoma from differentiated forms of rhabdomyosarcoma (22).

Genetics. A specific genetic event has not been reported in rhabdomyomas of any type.

Differential Diagnosis. Embryonal rhabdomyosarcoma is the most important differential diagnostic consideration for fetal rhabdomyoma. Unlike fetal rhabdomyomas, embryonal rhabdomyosarcomas are poorly circumscribed, mitotically active, contain hyperchromatic cells, and typically show a reversed pattern of zonation, with the least mature cells present at the periphery of the lesion. A submucosal cambium layer may be present in embryonal rhabdomyosarcoma.

Adult rhabdomyomas may be confused with granular cell tumors, hibernomas, paragangliomas, and reticulohistiocytomas, as well as with rhabdomyosarcomas. Unlike rhabdomyomas, such tumors lack cross striations and do not express skeletal muscle markers. Rhabdomyosarcomas are much more infiltrative lesions that display prominent pleomorphism, mitotic activity, and often necrosis, and which usually occur in younger patients.

Treatment and Prognosis. Rhabdomyomas of all types have a low risk for local recurrence, but no risk for aggressive behavior or metastasis. Complete excision with negative margins is recommended.

RHABDOMYOSARCOMA

Rhabdomyosarcomas are highly malignant soft tissue sarcomas recapitulating various stages in the embryonic differentiation of skeletal (striated) muscle. Rhabdomyosarcomas are classified as *embryonal, alveolar,* and *pleomorphic subtypes.*

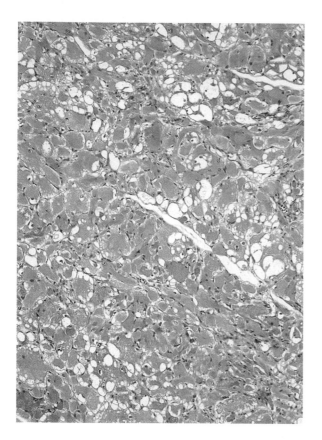 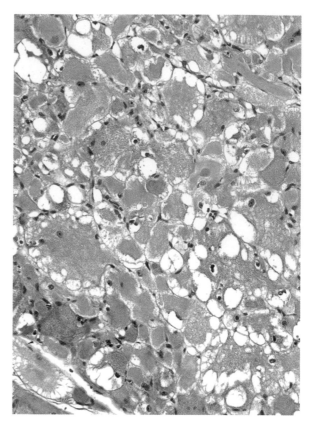

Figure 6-3

ADULT RHABDOMYOMA

Left: The well-circumscribed mass has large polygonal cells with abundant eosinophilic cytoplasm, a large nucleus, and a prominent nucleolus.

Right: Large eosinophilic cells and "spider cells" are seen.

Embryonal rhabdomyosarcoma is in turn divided into *conventional, botryoid, spindle cell,* and *anaplastic variants*. Alveolar rhabdomyosarcoma occurs in both *classic* and *solid variants*. The recently described *sclerosing variant of rhabdomyosarcoma* may represent a variant of embryonal rhabdomyosarcoma or a distinct entity, and is described separately.

Embryonal Rhabdomyosarcoma

Clinical Features. *Embryonal rhabdomyosarcoma* is the most frequent sarcoma of childhood, with an incidence of roughly 3 per million children under 15 years of age in the United States (29–31). It represents 70 to 75 percent of all rhabdomyosarcomas. Children between 5 and 15 years are most often affected (45 percent), with up to 35 percent of cases occurring in children under 5 years of age (30,32–34).

It is not widely appreciated that embryonal rhabdomyosarcoma is also the most common subtype of rhabdomyosarcoma in adults (35). The tumors are slightly more common in males than in females (1.2 to 1.0).

Approximately 50 percent of cases occur in the head and neck region, including tumors located in the orbit, eyelid, oropharynx, parotid gland, auditory canal, middle ear, pterygoid fossa, nose, paranasal sinuses, tongue, and cheek (32,33,36). The genitourinary system is the next most common location, comprising approximately 30 percent of cases, most often with involvement of the urinary bladder, vagina, prostate gland, and paratesticular soft tissues. Fewer than 9 percent of embryonal rhabdomyosarcomas arise in the skeletal musculature of the extremities. Involvement of visceral organs, retroperitoneum, pelvis, and perineum is rare. The well-differentiated spindle cell variant typically occurs in scrotal soft tissues and the head and neck (37,38), with the botryoid variant predominating in the wall of hollow organs or beneath mucosal linings (32,34,39,40). The symptoms of embryonal rhabdomyosarcoma are generally nonspecific and relate to mass effects and obstruction in the involved organ.

Gross Findings. Embryonal rhabdomyosarcomas are poorly circumscribed, fleshy, partially hemorrhagic or necrotic masses of widely variable size (1 to 32 cm). The well-differentiated spindle cell variant may be more firm and fibrous, whereas the botryoid variant typically has a gelatinous, polypoid appearance resembling a "bunch of grapes."

Microscopic Findings. Embryonal rhabdomyosarcomas are characterized by primitive mesenchymal cells showing varying degrees of rhabdomyoblastic differentiation. In most cases a spectrum of differentiation is present: primitive small round blue cells, undifferentiated spindled cells, ganglion-like rhabdomyoblasts, and strap cells with brightly eosinophilic cytoplasm and cross striations, sometimes showing a characteristic "broken arrow" appearance (32,34,39,40).

The tumors may be extremely poorly differentiated, resembling an undifferentiated sarcoma (fig. 6-4), or very well differentiated, simulating rhabdomyoma (fig. 6-5). Mitotic activity is invariably present and necrosis is frequent. Myxoid stromal change is frequently present. The botryoid variant, occurring in a submucosal location, typically grows in a polypoid fashion and has a zone of increased cellularity immediately below the mucosa (cambium zone) (fig. 6-6). Extensively myxoid embryonal rhabdomyosarcomas may show minimal cytologic atypia. The spindle cell variant is characterized by well-differentiated, bland-appearing spindled cells arranged in a fascicular or storiform pattern, reminiscent of a smooth muscle tumor or a fibrous histiocytoma (fig. 6-7) (37,38).

Embryonal rhabdomyosarcoma showing "anaplasia" is characterized by enlarged, markedly atypical cells with hyperchromatic nuclei that are three times larger than the nuclei of the surrounding cells (41). Atypical mitotic figures are commonly present. Generally, the anaplasia must be multifocal or diffuse before the tumor is designated as anaplastic. The significance of anaplasia in embryonal rhabdomyosarcoma is still unclear. Some embryonal rhabdomyosarcomas have epithelioid changes (*epithelioid rhabdomyosarcoma*) (42).

Special Studies. Embryonal rhabdomyosarcomas are typically diffusely immunoreactive for desmin with variable expression of myogenin and MyoD1 (11,40,43–46). Antibodies to pan-muscle actins (HHF-35) are less often positive than are those to desmin, and smooth muscle actin isoforms are expressed in some cases, a potential diagnostic pitfall, particularly in well-differentiated spindle cell variants (45,47,48). Expression of myoglobin is much less frequent, particularly in poorly differentiated tumors. Occasional embryonal rhabdomyosarcomas express unexpected markers such as cytokeratin and S-100 protein, potentially resulting in misdiagnoses, particularly in the head and neck region (49).

Genetics. At the cytogenetic level, embryonal rhabdomyosarcoma is characterized by complex structural and numerical abnormalities, including trisomies of chromosomes 2, 8, and 13 (50–53). Molecular analyses commonly show allelic loss at chromosome 11p15, a site containing a number of putative tumor suppressor genes, including *IGF2*, *H19*, and *CDKN1C*. Embryonal rhabdomyosarcomas lack a specific translocation, unlike alveolar rhabdomyosarcoma.

Differential Diagnosis. Conventional embryonal rhabdomyosarcoma may show a spectrum of differentiation, and may therefore be confused with other primitive round blue cell tumors when poorly differentiated, or with rhabdomyomas and leiomyomas when well differentiated. Positivity for desmin, myogenin, and MyoD1 is critical in the distinction of embryonal rhabdomyosarcoma from other round cell tumors.

Malignant peripheral nerve sheath tumors with rhabdomyoblastic differentiation (malignant triton tumor) may closely resemble embryonal rhabdomyosarcoma, but typically occur in much older patients with a long history of neurofibromatosis (NF)1, and may arise from a preexisting neurofibroma. Infantile fibrosarcoma occurs in slightly younger patients than does embryonal rhabdomyosarcoma, lacks expression on myogenic markers, and often contains the specific translocation, t(12;15) (*ETV6-NTRK3*).

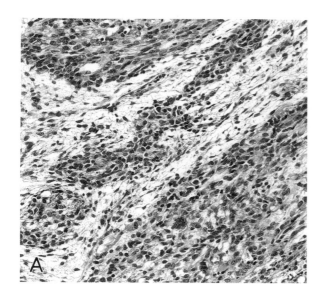

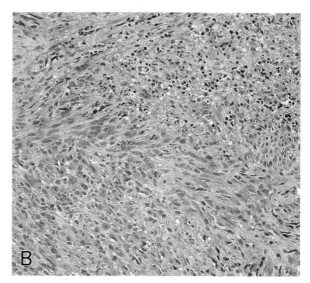

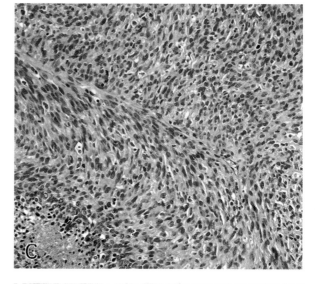

Figure 6-4

POORLY DIFFERENTIATED
EMBRYONAL RHABDOMYOSARCOMA

A: The tumor contains an admixture of primitive round cells and differentiating rhabdomyoblasts.

B: Poorly differentiated embryonal rhabdomyosarcoma, spindle cell type, with focal rhabdomyoblastic differentiation.

C: Fibrosarcoma-like poorly differentiated embryonal rhabdomyosarcoma.

D: Poorly differentiated embryonal rhabdomyosarcoma with rhabdoid features.

E: Small clusters of differentiating rhabdomyoblasts in an otherwise poorly differentiated embryonal rhabdomyosarcoma.

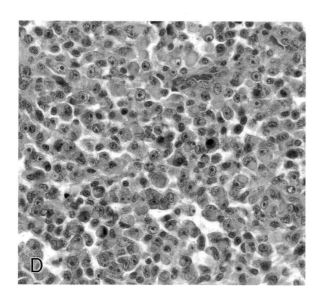

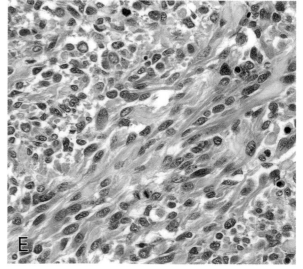

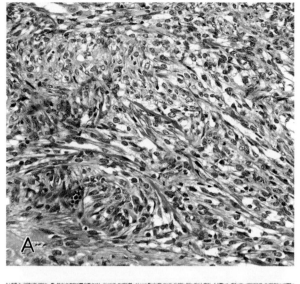

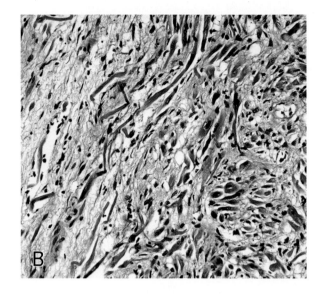

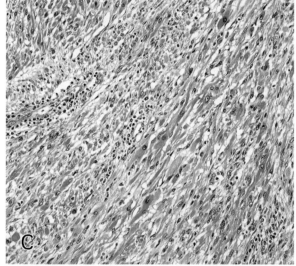

Figure 6-5

EMBRYONAL RHABDOMYOSARCOMA

A: The tumor contains numerous strap-like rhabdomyoblasts.

B: Strap-like rhabdomyoblasts show acute angle bending ("broken arrow sign").

C: Ganglion-like rhabdomyoblasts in embryonal rhabdomyosarcoma.

D: Embryonal rhabdomyosarcoma composed largely of differentiating strap-like rhabdomyoblasts.

E: Well-differentiated embryonal rhabdomyosarcoma mimicking fetal rhabdomyoma. Elsewhere this tumor showed mitotic activity and more primitive-appearing cells.

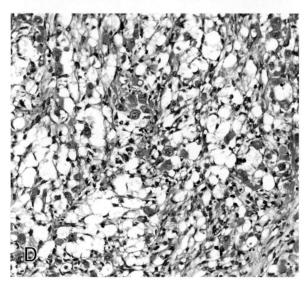

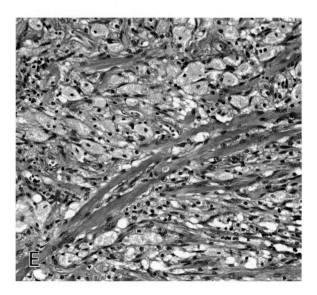

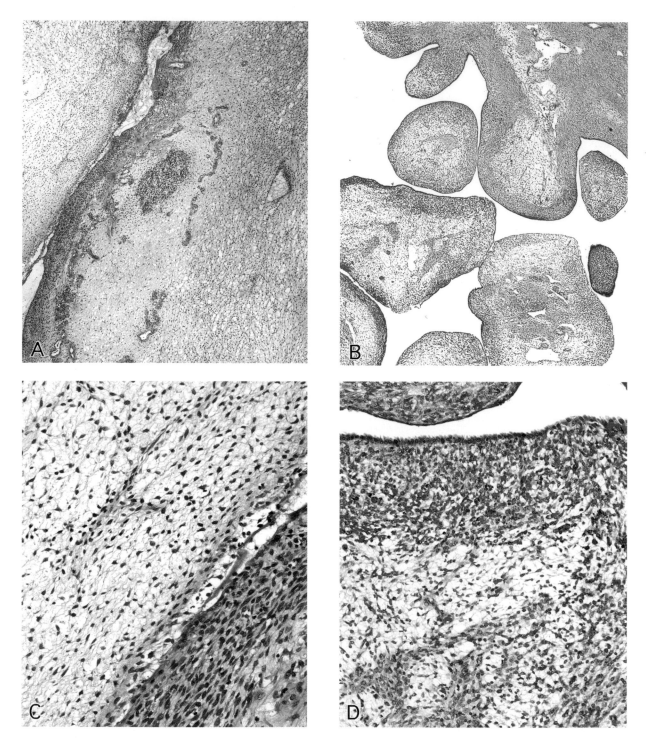

Figure 6-6

BOTRYOID RHABDOMYOSARCOMA

A: The tumor grows as multiple "grape-like" myxoid nodules within the endometrial cavity of a young girl.

B: The submucosal "cambium cell layer" and subjacent hypocellular myxoid zone in botryoid rhabdomyosarcoma.

C: Extensively myxoid botryoid rhabdomyosarcoma of the vagina.

D: Higher-power view shows that the malignant cells present in the myxoid zones are deceptively bland in appearance.

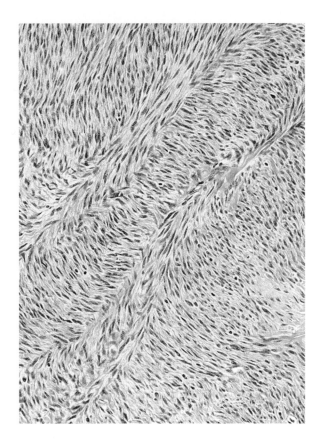 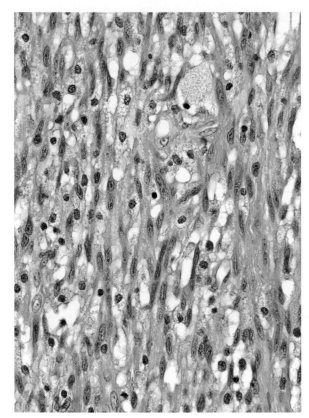

Figure 6-7

WELL-DIFFERENTIATED SPINDLE CELL RHABDOMYOSARCOMA

Left: This tumor mimics low-grade fibrosarcoma.

Right: Well-differentiated spindle cell rhabdomyosarcoma, composed of deceptively bland spindled cells, resembles smooth muscle.

Extremely well-differentiated embryonal rhabdomyosarcoma differs from rhabdomyomas by the presence of infiltrative growth, mitotic activity, and greater cytologic atypia. Positivity for myogenin and MyoD1 is valuable in the distinction of well-differentiated spindle cell rhabdomyosarcoma from smooth muscle tumors and fibrous histiocytomas.

Many types of tumors may contain rhabdomyosarcomatous differentiation, especially in adults: carcinosarcomas, dedifferentiated liposarcoma, and certain carcinomas, such as Merkel cell carcinoma. These alternative diagnoses have to be ruled out before (embryonal) rhabdomyosarcoma is diagnosed in an adult patient.

Treatment and Prognosis. With the widespread use of multiagent chemotherapy, adjuvant radiotherapy, and modern surgical techniques, the disease-free survival rate has improved from 20 percent to about 70 percent (32,36,54). The prognosis is heavily dependent on three factors: histologic subtype, tumor location, and stage (Intergroup Rhabdomyosarcoma Study clinical group). The prognosis for patients with botryoid and well-differentiated spindle cell variants is generally excellent, whereas tumors showing diffuse anaplasia confer a worse prognosis (41). The prognosis for patients with tumors located in the orbit is excellent (92 percent 5-year survival rate), followed by tumors of the head/neck and genitourinary tract, exclusive of the bladder and prostate gland (80 percent 5-year survival rate). Less favorable tumor locations include the bladder/prostate gland, parameningeal locations, and other soft tissue locations. Other adverse prognostic features include adult age, large tumor size, and unresectability (55). Common sites of metastasis are the lungs, lymph nodes, liver, and brain.

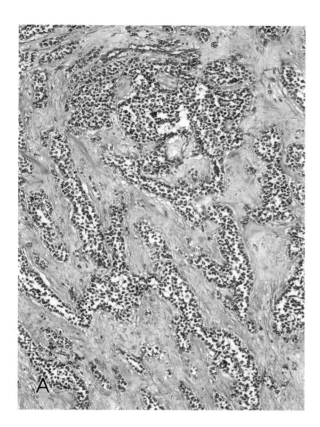 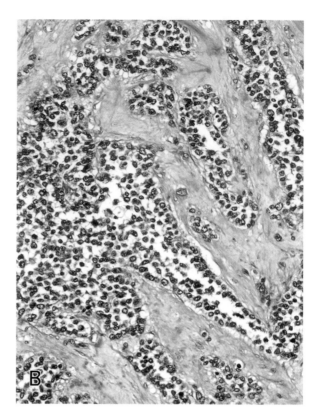

Figure 6-8

ALVEOLAR RHABDOMYOSARCOMA

A: There is a pseudoalveolar proliferation of discohesive, primitive round cells surrounded by highly vascular fibrous septa.

B: Nests of discohesive, hyperchromatic round cells have moderate nuclear variability and scattered small differentiating rhabdomyoblasts.

Alveolar Rhabdomyosarcoma

Clinical Features. *Alveolar rhabdomyosarcomas* account for 20 to 25 percent of all rhabdomyosarcomas. They occur in older patients than do embryonal rhabdomyosarcomas, with a median age of 7 to 9 years (33,40,56,57). Many alveolar rhabdomyosarcomas also occur in adolescents and young adults. Most tumors arise in the soft tissues of the extremities, including the hands and feet (57). They are less common than embryonal rhabdomyosarcoma in the head and neck, where they most often involve the nose and paranasal sinuses.

Alveolar rhabdomyosarcoma in any location typically presents as a rapidly growing painless mass, with other symptoms dependent on tumor location. Alveolar rhabdomyosarcomas frequently present as metastases, including to lymph nodes and bone marrow, from unknown primary tumors (36).

Gross Findings. Alveolar rhabdomyosarcomas are typically 2 to 8 cm at the time of diagnosis. They are fleshy, hemorrhagic or necrotic masses with a variable amount of fibrous tissue (57).

Microscopic Findings. In its classic form, alveolar rhabdomyosarcoma is a highly malignant-appearing, diffusely infiltrative tumor composed of nests of discohesive, primitive-appearing round cells surrounded by highly vascular fibrous bands, creating a distinctive pseudoalveolar pattern (fig. 6-8) (32,39,57). Multinucleated eosinophilic tumor giant cells are occasionally identified within these nests, as are scattered ganglion-like rhabdomyoblasts. Strap cells are seldom present. The solid form of alveolar rhabdomyosarcoma lacks the prominent nested pattern and cellular discohesion seen in classic alveolar rhabdomyosarcoma, although small areas of nested growth are usually present if searched for carefully (fig. 6-9) (32,40,58,59).

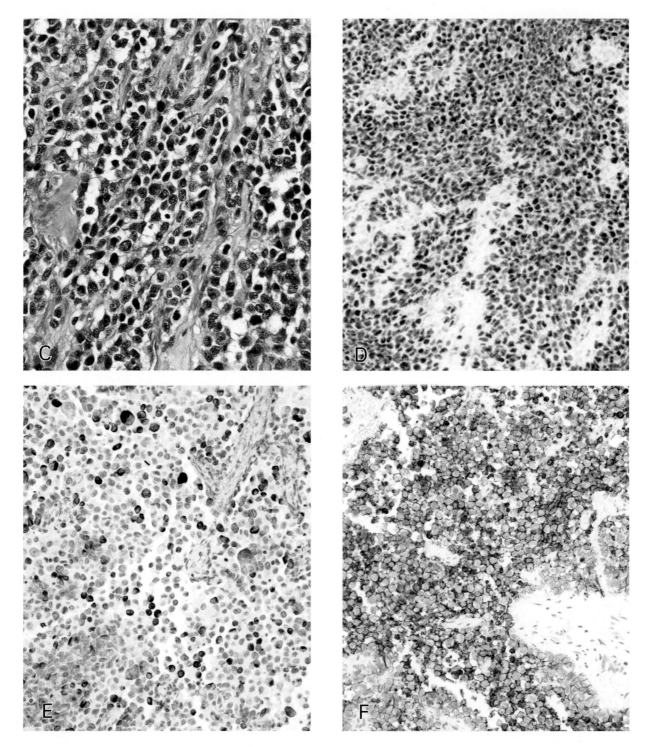

Figure 6-8, continued

C: The cells of alveolar rhabdomyosarcoma tend to show greater nuclear variability and enlargement compared with other small blue round cell tumors.

D: Diffuse myogenin expression is characteristic of alveolar rhabdomyosarcoma.

E,F: Anomalous expression of cytokeratins (E) and neuroendocrine markers, such as CD56 (F), is seen in a significant percentage of alveolar rhabdomyosarcomas, potentially resulting in a misdiagnosis as neuroendocrine carcinoma, particularly in head/neck locations.

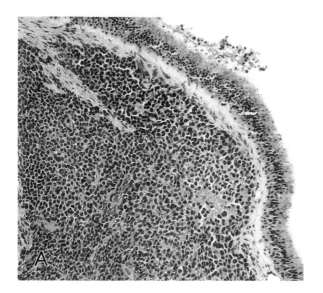

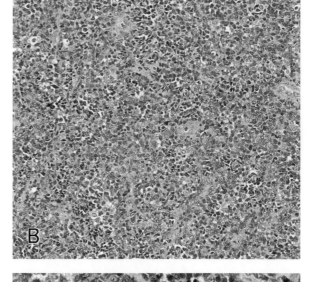

Figure 6-9

ALVEOLAR RHABDOMYOSARCOMA

A: The solid variant of alveolar rhabdomyosarcoma arises in the nasal cavity.

B: Although fibrous septa are present in most solid variants of alveolar rhabdomyosarcoma, they are poorly developed, and the characteristic pseudoalveolar pattern may be difficult to appreciate.

C: This solid variant consists of a sheet-like proliferation of primitive round cells. Only scattered cells show a small amount of brightly eosinophilic cytoplasm, indicative of rhabdomyoblastic differentiation.

D: Multinucleated tumor giant cells may be a clue to the diagnosis of solid alveolar rhabdomyosarcomas.

E: Clear cell change in the solid variant of alveolar rhabdomyosarcoma.

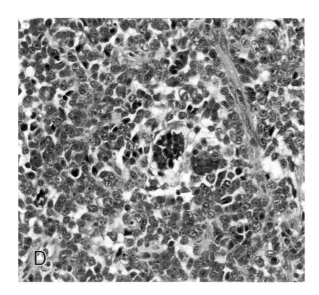

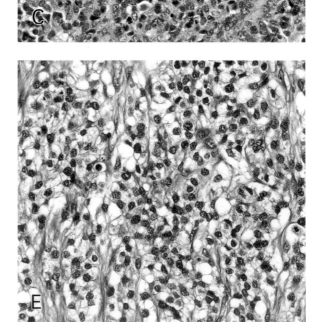

Clear cell change may be prominent. Foci identical to embryonal rhabdomyosarcoma may occasionally be found; such *mixed alveolar/embryonal rhabdomyosarcomas* appear to behave as alveolar rhabdomyosarcoma, with a poor prognosis (32).

Special Studies. Alveolar rhabdomyosarcomas express desmin, myogenin, and MyoD1, similar to embryonal rhabdomyosarcomas (11, 37,38,43,46,48,60–72). Myogenin expression is often much stronger than is MyoD1, which may occasionally aid in the subclassification of a given tumor as alveolar rhabdomyosarcoma (64). As in embryonal rhabdomyosarcoma, cytokeratin, S-100 protein, CD56, and synaptophysin are occasionally expressed, with the potential for the misclassification of alveolar rhabdomyosarcoma as a small cell carcinoma or melanoma (73). CD99 may be expressed by some alveolar rhabdomyosarcomas, as may TLE1 (74,75).

Genetics. Alveolar rhabdomyosarcomas are characterized in approximately 75 percent of cases by t(2; 13)(q35; q14)(*PAX3-FOXO1A*) and in approximately 10 percent of cases by t(1; 13)(p36; q14)(*PAX7-FOXO1A*) (52,53). Although approximately 15 percent of alveolar rhabdomyosarcomas have traditionally been considered to be "fusion-negative," the noncanonical translocations t(2; 2)(p23; q35)(*PAX3-NCOA1*) or t(2; 8)(q35; q13)(*PAX3-NCOA2*) have recently been identified in some cases (76–80). To date, all of these molecular genetic events are specific for alveolar rhabdomyosarcoma. They are detected by karyotyping, reverse transcriptase polymerase chain reaction (RT-PCR), or fluorescence in situ hybridization (FISH).

Differential Diagnosis. Alveolar rhabdomyosarcoma differs from embryonal rhabdomyosarcoma by an older patient age, a distinctive pseudoalveolar pattern, a lack of strap cells, and strong myogenin rather than MyoD1 expression. Identification of an alveolar rhabdomyosarcoma-associated fusion gene may be necessary for the distinction of alveolar rhabdomyosarcoma from the most primitive forms of embryonal rhabdomyosarcoma. Immunohistochemistry for myogenic markers, in particular, myogenin and MyoD1, is critical in the distinction of alveolar rhabdomyosarcoma from other small round cell tumors, such as Ewing sarcoma, lymphoblastic lymphoma, small cell carcinoma, and melanoma. Desmoplastic round cell tumor may display a nested pattern reminiscent of alveolar rhabdomyosarcoma and frequently expresses desmin, but lacks expression of myogenin or MyoD1, and contains a diagnostic t(11;22) (*EWS-WT1*) gene fusion. Despite its similar name, alveolar soft part sarcoma is a wholly dissimilar-appearing tumor, composed of large eosinophilic cells with prominent nucleoli.

Treatment and Prognosis. The prognosis for patients with alveolar rhabdomyosarcoma is considerably worse than for those with embryonal rhabdomyosarcoma, irrespective of other clinical or pathologic features, with many tumors presenting at a high clinical stage. The 5-year survival rate is only approximately 50 percent (81,82). Some data suggest an improved prognosis for patients with metastatic disease if their tumor contains a *PAX7-FOXO1A* fusion gene, rather than a *PAX3-FOXO1A* fusion gene, although fusion subtype does not appear to be a prognostic factor for patients with localized disease (76).

Pleomorphic Rhabdomyosarcoma

Clinical Features. *Pleomorphic rhabdomyosarcoma* is the rarest subtype of rhabdomyosarcoma, occurring essentially only in adults over 45 years of age (median age, 55 years) (67,83–87). The precise incidence of pleomorphic rhabdomyosarcoma is difficult to discern, as many tumors previously reported as such likely represent undifferentiated pleomorphic sarcomas. Pleomorphic rhabdomyosarcoma usually occurs in the deep soft tissues of the extremities, in particular, the thigh, but have been reported in a wide variety of anatomic locations (67,83–87).

Gross Findings. Most pleomorphic rhabdomyosarcomas present as large (over 10 cm) soft tissue masses, often with grossly visible necrosis.

Microscopic Findings. Pleomorphic rhabdomyosarcoma consists of a sheet-like to fascicular proliferation of large, deeply eosinophilic, round to spindled cells with anaplastic-appearing nuclei, frequent mitotic figures, and geographic necrosis (fig. 6-10). Cross striations are typically difficult to identify (67,83–87).

Special Studies. Markers of skeletal muscle differentiation, including myoglobin, MyoD1, myogenin, and desmin, are expressed. Expression

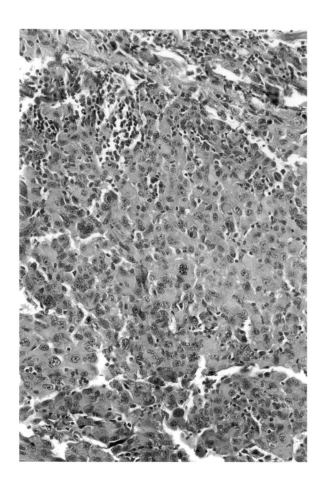 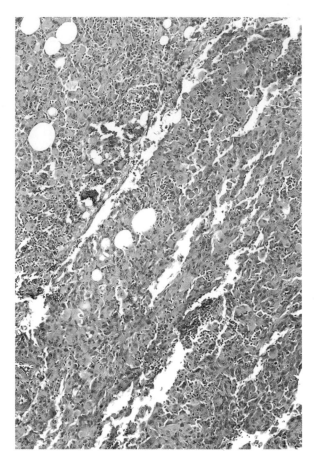

Figure 6-10

PLEOMORPHIC RHABDOMYOSARCOMA

Left: The tumor consists of a sheet-like proliferation of large polygonal cells with abundant eosinophilic cytoplasm.

Right: Higher-power view shows marked nuclear pleomorphism, abundant eosinophilic cytoplasm, tumor giant cells, and mitotic figures.

of myogenin and MyoD1 may be limited, and some authors have accepted as pleomorphic rhabdomyosarcomas tumors lacking expression of these markers (85). Distinguishing such tumors from other pleomorphic sarcomas showing (anomalous) desmin expression may be extremely difficult, if not arbitrary (88).

Genetics. Pleomorphic rhabdomyosarcomas lack a specific genetic alteration, showing instead only highly abnormal karyotypes with numerous numerical and structural aberrations (83,84,89).

Differential Diagnosis. The differential diagnosis includes a variety of pleomorphic sarcomas, including undifferentiated pleomorphic sarcoma (malignant fibrous histiocytoma), pleomorphic liposarcoma, and pleomorphic leiomyosarcoma.

In general, the cells of pleomorphic rhabdomyosarcoma show much more striking cytoplasmic eosinophilia than do these other tumors. The presence of pleomorphic lipoblasts is definitional of pleomorphic liposarcoma. Pleomorphic leiomyosarcomas do not express MyoD1 and myogenin. In children, rhabdomyosarcomas showing striking pleomorphism likely represent embryonal rhabdomyosarcomas with anaplasia rather than pleomorphic liposarcomas and should be treated as such.

Treatment and Prognosis. The prognosis of patients with pleomorphic rhabdomyosarcoma is dismal, with over 70 percent of patients dead of disease in less than 5 years (67,83–87). The lung is the most common site of metastasis.

Sclerosing Rhabdomyosarcoma

Clinical Features. *Sclerosing rhabdomyosarcoma* is a rare, recently described rhabdomyosarcoma variant. Fewer than 30 cases have been described (60,61,63, 90). Initially felt to be a rhabdomyosarcoma of adults, cases of sclerosing rhabdomyosarcoma have now been described in children as young as 3 months of age (60). Approximately 30 percent of these tumors arise in the head and neck, with the rest occurring in a variety of somatic soft tissue locations.

Gross Findings. Sclerosing rhabdomyosarcoma presents as a slowly enlarging, nonspecific soft tissue mass, usually 3 to 8 cm in size.

Microscopic Findings. These are highly infiltrative lesions that produce an abundant hyaline matrix that varies from eosinophilic to basophilic, resembling either primitive osteoid or chondroid (although calcification and lacunae are absent). This stroma often comprises most of the tumor mass and divides the neoplastic cells into lobules and small nests, similar to those seen in primitive chondroid tumors, and single-file arrays reminiscent of those seen in sclerosing osteosarcoma or sclerosing epithelioid fibrosarcoma (fig. 6-11) (60,61,63,90). The tumor may also form pseudovascular spaces, raising the possibility of angiosarcoma (63).

The cells of sclerosing rhabdomyosarcoma are primitive appearing, with a minute amount of eosinophilic cytoplasm, irregular nuclear contours with coarse chromatin, and small, occasionally multiple nucleoli. Although a microalveolar pattern is often present, the distinctive large alveolar pattern characteristic of alveolar rhabdomyosarcoma is not seen. Occasional cases form anastomosing cords, reminiscent of an angiosarcoma. Strap-like rhabdomyoblasts, as seen in embryonal rhabdomyosarcoma, are found focally in a minority of cases.

Special Studies. Sclerosing rhabdomyosarcoma often shows only limited desmin expression, sometimes with a "dot-like" pattern, but is strongly positive for MyoD1. Myogenin expression may be confined to only a few tumor cells or absent entirely (60,61,63,90). Smooth muscle actin expression may be present. Occasional sclerosing rhabdomyosarcomas express CD99; S-100 protein and cytokeratin are not expressed.

Genetics. Very few cases of sclerosing rhabdomyosarcoma have been evaluated by genetic methods. Alveolar rhabdomyosarcoma-associated fusion genes have not been identified in any tested cases (60,61,63,90). Loss of 10q22 and the Y chromosome, amplification of the 12q13-15 region with amplification of *MDM2* and *HMGA2* but not *CDK4*, and trisomy 18 have been reported, as have numerical abnormalities similar to those seen in embryonal rhabdomyosarcoma (90–92). These studies have not clearly established whether sclerosing rhabdomyosarcoma represents a distinct entity or a variant of one of the better established rhabdomyosarcoma subtypes.

Differential Diagnosis. The differential diagnosis includes osteosarcoma, extraskeletal myxoid chondrosarcoma, mesenchymal chondrosarcoma, sclerosing epithelioid fibrosarcoma, and angiosarcoma. Sclerosing osteosarcoma shows matrix calcification, osteoclastic giant cells, pleomorphic epithelioid to plasmacytoid cells, and, frequently, other patterns of osteosarcoma. Extraskeletal myxoid chondrosarcoma consists of bland eosinophilic cells arranged in cords and chains, without the densely hyalinized matrix and highly malignant small round cells seen in sclerosing rhabdomyosarcoma. Mesenchymal chondrosarcoma typically shows an admixture of primitive round cell areas and nodules of well-differentiated cartilage, and often displays a prominent hemangiopericytoma-like branching vasculature. Sclerosing epithelioid fibrosarcoma often contains areas resembling low-grade fibromyxoid sarcoma and lacks expression of myogenic markers. Angiosarcoma lacks pseudoalveolar structures and rhabdomyoblasts and expresses endothelial markers such as CD31 rather than myogenic markers.

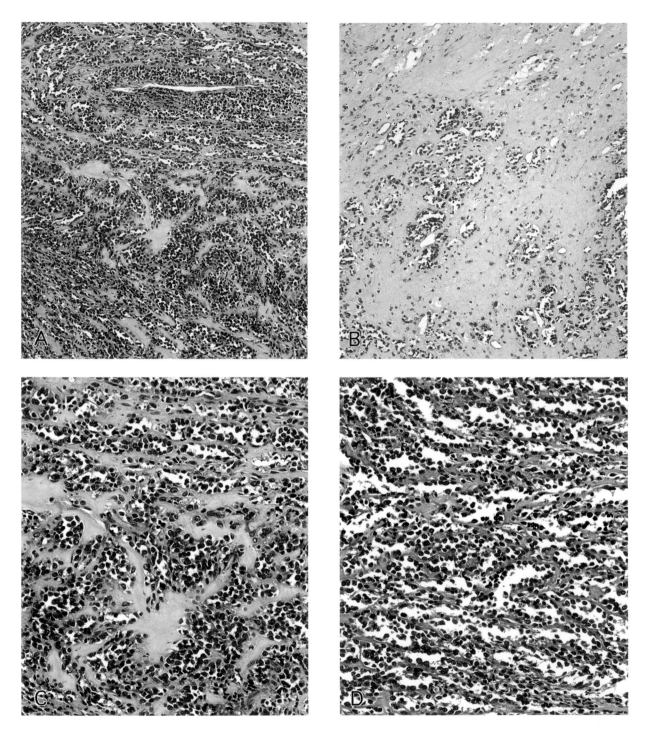

Figure 6-11

SCLEROSING RHABDOMYOSARCOMA

A: A cord-like to microalveolar proliferation of primitive round cells is in a hyalinized, eosinophilic, osteoid-like background.

B: Microalveolar nests of undifferentiated, hyperchromatic round cells are embedded in an abundant osteochondroid-like matrix.

C: Although the microalveolar pattern of sclerosing rhabdomyosarcoma may suggest the diagnosis of alveolar rhabdomyosarcoma, alveolar rhabdomyosarcoma-associated gene fusion events are not found.

D: Some cases of sclerosing rhabdomyosarcoma show a pseudovascular pattern, mimicking angiosarcoma.

REFERENCES

Rhabdomyomatous Mesenchymal Hamartoma

1. Ashfaq R, Timmons CF. Rhabdomyomatous mesenchymal hamartoma of skin. Pediatr Pathol 1992;12:731-775.
2. White G. Congenital rhabdomyomatous mesenchymal hamartoma. Am J Dermatopathol 1990;12:539-40.
3. Sahn EE, Garen PD, Pai GS, Levkoff AH, Hagerty RC, Maize JC. Multiple rhabdomyomatous mesenchymal hamartomas of skin. Am J Dermatopathol 1990;12:485-491.
4. Katsumata M, Keong CH, Satoh T. Rhabdomyomatous mesenchymal hamartoma of skin. J Dermatol 1990;17:384-387.
5. Mills AE. Rhabdomyomatous mesenchymal hamartoma of skin. Am J Dermatopathol 1989;11:58-63.
6. Han SH, Song HJ, Hong WK, Lee HS, Choi GS, Shin JH. Rhabdomyomatous mesenchymal hamartoma of the vagina. Pediatr Dermatol 2009;26:753-755.
7. Brinster NK, Farmer ER. Rhabdomyomatous mesenchymal hamartoma presenting on a digit. J Cutan Pathol 2009;36:61-63.
8. Read RW, Burnstine M, Rowland JM, Zamir E, Rao NA. Rhabdomyomatous mesenchymal hamartoma of the eyelid: report of a case and literature review. Ophthalmology 2001;108:798-804.
9. Rosenberg AS, Kirk J, Morgan MB. Rhabdomyomatous mesenchymal hamartoma: an unusual dermal entity with a report of two cases and a review of the literature. J Cutan Pathol 2002;29:238-243.

Rhabdomyoma

10. Dehner LP, Enzinger FM, Font RL. Fetal rhabdomyoma. An analysis of nine cases. Cancer 1972;30:160-166.
11. Seidal T, Kindblom LG, Angervall L. Myoglobin, desmin and vimentin in ultrastructurally proven rhabdomyomas and rhabdomyosarcomas. An immunohistochemical study utilizing a series of monoclonal and polyclonal antibodies. Appl Pathol 1987;5:201-219.
12. Eusebi V, Ceccarelli C, Daniele E, Collina G, Viale G, Mancini AM. Extracardiac rhabdomyoma: an immunocytochemical study and review of the literature. Appl Pathol 1988;6:197-207.
13. DiSanto S, Abt AB, Boal DK, Krummel TM. Fetal rhabdomyoma and nevoid basal cell carcinoma syndrome. Pediatr Pathol 1992;12:441-447.
14. Crotty PL, Nakhleh RE, Dehner LP. Juvenile rhabdomyoma. An intermediate form of skeletal muscle tumor in children. Arch Pathol Lab Med 1993;117:43-47.

15. Kapadia SB, Meis JM, Frisman DM, Ellis GL, Heffner DK. Fetal rhabdomyoma of the head and neck: a clinicopathologic and immunophenotypic study of 24 cases. Hum Pathol 1993;24:754-765.
16. Hansen T, Katenkamp D. Rhabdomyoma of the head and neck: morphology and differential diagnosis. Virchows Arch 2005;447:849-854.
17. Di Sant'Agnese PA, Knowles DM 2nd. Extracardiac rhabdomyoma: a clinicopathologic study and review of the literature. Cancer 1980;46:780-789.
18. Balatsouras DG, Eliopoulos PN, Economou CN. Adult-type rhabdomyoma of the submandibular region. J Otolaryngol 1993;22:14-17.
19. Kapadia SB, Meis JM, Frisman DM, Ellis GL, Heffner DK, Hyams VJ. Adult rhabdomyoma of the head and neck: a clinicopathologic and immunophenotypic study. Hum Pathol 1993;24:608-617.
20. Box JC, Newman CL, Anastasiades KD, Lucas GW, Latouff OM. Adult rhabdomyoma: presentation as a cervicomediastinal mass (case report and review of the literature). Am Surg 1995;61:271-276.
21. Sanchez Jimenez J, Dean Ferrer A, Alamillos Granados F, et al. Adult rhabdomyoma in the masticatory area. New case presentation and review of the literature. Med Oral 2001;6:64-68.
22. Lu DY, Chang S, Cook H, et al. Genital rhabdomyoma of the urethra in an infant girl. Hum Pathol 2012;43:597-600.
23. Hanski W, Hagel-Lewicka E, Daniszewski K. Rhabdomyomas of female genital tract. Report on two cases. Zentralbl Pathol 1991;137:439-442.
24. Konrad EA, Meister P, Hubner G. Extracardiac rhabdomyoma: report of different types with light microscopic and ultrastructural studies. Cancer 1982;49:898-907.
25. Davies B, Noh P, Smaldone MC, Ranganathan S, Docimo SG. Paratesticular rhabdomyoma in a young adult: case study and review of the literature. J Pediatr Surg 2007;42:E5-7.
26. Cooper CL, Sindler P, Varol C, McCarthy SW, Karim RZ, Scolyer RA. Paratesticular rhabdomyoma. Pathology 2007;39:367-369.
27. Sencan A, Mir E, Sencan AB, Ortac R. Intrascrotal paratesticular rhabdomyoma: a case report. Acta Paediatr 2000;89:1020-1022.
28. Maheshkumar P, Berney DM. Spermatic cord rhabdomyoma. Urology 2000;56:331.
29. Toro JR, Travis LB, Wu HJ, Zhu K, Fletcher CD, Devesa SS. Incidence patterns of soft tissue sarcomas, regardless of primary site, in the surveillance, epidemiology and end results program, 1978-2001: an analysis of 26,758 cases. Int J Cancer 2006;119:2922-2930.

30. Perez EA, Kassira N, Cheung MC, Koniaris LG, Neville HL, Sola JE. Rhabdomyosarcoma in children: a SEER population based study. J Surg Res 2011;170:e243-251.

31. Gurney JG, Davis S, Severson RK, Fang JY, Ross JA, Robison LL. Trends in cancer incidence among children in the U.S. Cancer 1996;78:532-541.

32. Qualman SJ, Coffin CM, Newton WA, et al. Intergroup Rhabdomyosarcoma Study: update for pathologists. Pediatr Dev Pathol 1998;1:550-561.

33. Newton WA Jr, Gehan EA, Webber BL, et al. Classification of rhabdomyosarcomas and related sarcomas. Pathologic aspects and proposal for a new classification—an Intergroup Rhabdomyosarcoma Study. Cancer 1995;76:1073-1085.

34. Newton WA Jr, Soule EH, Hamoudi AB, et al. Histopathology of childhood sarcomas, Intergroup Rhabdomyosarcoma Studies I and II: clinicopathologic correlation. J Clin Oncol 1988;6:67-75.

35. Hawkins WG, Hoos A, Antonescu CR, et al. Clinicopathologic analysis of patients with adult rhabdomyosarcoma. Cancer 2001;91:794-803.

36. Ruymann FB, Grovas AC. Progress in the diagnosis and treatment of rhabdomyosarcoma and related soft tissue sarcomas. Cancer Invest 2000;18:223-241.

37. Rubin BP, Hasserjian RP, Singer S, Janecka I, Fletcher JA, Fletcher CD. Spindle cell rhabdomyosarcoma (so-called) in adults: report of two cases with emphasis on differential diagnosis. Am J Surg Pathol 1998;22:459-464.

38. Cavazzana AO, Schmidt D, Ninfo V, et al. Spindle cell rhabdomyosarcoma. A prognostically favorable variant of rhabdomyosarcoma. Am J Surg Pathol 1992;16:229-235.

39. Parham DM. Pathologic classification of rhabdomyosarcomas and correlations with molecular studies. Mod Pathol 2001;14:506-14.

40. Tsokos M. The diagnosis and classification of childhood rhabdomyosarcoma. Semin Diagnostic Pathol 1994;11:26-38.

41. Qualman S, Lynch J, Bridge J, et al. Prevalence and clinical impact of anaplasia in childhood rhabdomyosarcoma: a report from the Soft Tissue Sarcoma Committee of the Children's Oncology Group. Cancer 2008;113:3242-3247.

42. Jo VY, Marino-Enriquez A, Fletcher CD. Epithelioid rhabdomyosarcoma: clinicopathologic analysis of 16 cases of a morphologically distinct variant of rhabdomyosarcoma. Am J Surg Pathol 2011;35:1523-1530.

43. Engel ME, Mouton SC, Emms M. Paediatric rhabdomyosarcoma: MyoD1 demonstration in routinely processed tissue sections using wet heat pretreatment (pressure cooking) for antigen retrieval. J Clin Pathol 1997;50:37-39.

44. Wang NP, Marx J, McNutt MA, Rutledge JC, Gown AM. Expression of myogenic regulatory proteins (myogenin and MyoD1) in small blue round cell tumors of childhood. Am J Pathol 1995;147:1799-1810.

45. Rangdaeng S, Truong LD. Comparative immunohistochemical staining for desmin and muscle-specific actin. A study of 576 cases. Am J Clin Pathol 1991;96:32-45.

46. Carter RL, Jameson CF, Philp ER, Pinkerton CR. Comparative phenotypes in rhabdomyosarcomas and developing skeletal muscle. Histopathology 1990;17:301-309.

47. Skalli O, Gabbiani G, Babai F, Seemayer TA, Pizzolato G, Schurch W. Intermediate filament proteins and actin isoforms as markers for soft tissue tumor differentiation and origin. II. Rhabdomyosarcomas. Am J Pathol 1988;130:515-31.

48. Jones H, Steart PV, Du Boulay CE, Roche WR. Alpha-smooth muscle actin as a marker for soft tissue tumours: a comparison with desmin. J Pathol 1990;162:29-33.

49. Coindre JM, de Mascarel A, Trojani M, de Mascarel I, Pages A. Immunohistochemical study of rhabdomyosarcoma. Unexpected staining with S100 protein and cytokeratin. J Pathol 1988;155:127-132.

50. Bridge JA, Liu J, Qualman SJ, et al. Genomic gains and losses are similar in genetic and histologic subsets of rhabdomyosarcoma, whereas amplification predominates in embryonal with anaplasia and alveolar subtypes. Genes Chromosomes Cancer 2002;33:310-321.

51. Wang C. Childhood rhabdomyosarcoma: recent advances and prospective views. J Dent Res 2012;91:341-350.

52. Pazzaglia L, Chiechi A, Conti A, et al. Genetic and molecular alterations in rhabdomyosarcoma: mRNA overexpression of MCL1 and MAP2K4 genes. Histol Histopathol 2009;24:61-67.

53. Gallego Melcon S, Sanchez de Toledo Codina J. Molecular biology of rhabdomyosarcoma. Clin Transl Oncol 2007;9:415-419.

54. Raney RB, Maurer HM, Anderson JR, et al. The Intergroup Rhabdomyosarcoma Study Group (IRSG): major lessons from the IRS-I through IRS-IV studies as background for the current irs-v treatment protocols. Sarcoma 2001;5:9-15.

55. Raney RB, Walterhouse DO, Meza JL, et al. Results of the Intergroup Rhabdomyosarcoma Study Group D9602 protocol, using vincristine and dactinomycin with or without cyclophosphamide and radiation therapy, for newly diagnosed patients with low-risk embryonal rhabdomyosarcoma: a report from the Soft Tissue Sarcoma Committee of the Children's Oncology Group. J Clin Oncol 2011;29:1312-1318.

56. Caillaud JM, Gerard-Marchant R, Marsden HB, et al. Histopathological classification of childhood rhabdomyosarcoma: a report from the International Society of Pediatric Oncology pathology panel. Med Pediatr Oncol 1989;17:391-400.

57. Enzinger FM, Shiraki M. Alveolar rhabdomyosarcoma. An analysis of 110 cases. Cancer 1969;24: 18-31.
58. Parham DM, Shapiro DN, Downing JR, Webber BL, Douglass EC. Solid alveolar rhabdomyosarcomas with the t(2;13). Report of two cases with diagnostic implications. Am J Surg Pathol 1994;18:474-478.
59. Tsokos M, Webber BL, Parham DM, et al. Rhabdomyosarcoma. A new classification scheme related to prognosis. Arch Pathol Lab Med 1992;116:847-855.
60. Chiles MC, Parham DM, Qualman SJ, et al. Sclerosing rhabdomyosarcomas in children and adolescents: a clinicopathologic review of 13 cases from the Intergroup Rhabdomyosarcoma Study Group and Children's Oncology Group. Pediatr Dev Pathol 2004;7:583-594.
61. Folpe AL, McKenney JK, Bridge JA, Weiss SW. Sclerosing rhabdomyosarcoma in adults: report of four cases of a hyalinizing, matrix-rich variant of rhabdomyosarcoma that may be confused with osteosarcoma, chondrosarcoma, or angiosarcoma. Am J Surg Pathol 2002;26:1175-1183.
62. Cessna MH, Zhou H, Perkins SL, et al. Are myogenin and myoD1 expression specific for rhabdomyosarcoma? A study of 150 cases, with emphasis on spindle cell mimics. Am J Surg Pathol 2001;25:1150-1157.
63. Mentzel T, Katenkamp D. Sclerosing, pseudovascular rhabdomyosarcoma in adults. Clinicopathological and immunohistochemical analysis of three cases. Virchows Arch 2000;436:305-111.
64. Dias P, Chen B, Dilday B, et al. Strong immunostaining for myogenin in rhabdomyosarcoma is significantly associated with tumors of the alveolar subclass. Am J Pathol 2000;156:399-408.
65. Cui S, Hano H, Harada T, Takai S, Masui F, Ushigome S. Evaluation of new monoclonal anti-MyoD1 and anti-myogenin antibodies for the diagnosis of rhabdomyosarcoma. Pathol Int1999;49:62-68.
66. Coffin CM, Rulon J, Smith L, Bruggers C, White FV. Pathologic features of rhabdomyosarcoma before and after treatment: a clinicopathologic and immunohistochemical analysis. Mod Pathol 1997;10:1175-1187.
67. Hollowood K, Fletcher CD. Rhabdomyosarcoma in adults. Semin Diagn Pathol 1994;11:47-57.
68. Seidal T, Angervall L, Kindblom LG. Expression of muscle-specific actins and myosin in light microscopically undifferentiated small and dark cell malignancies of soft tissues. APMIS 1990;98:1105-1112.
69. Fisher C. The value of electronmicroscopy and immunohistochemistry in the diagnosis of soft tissue sarcomas: a study of 200 cases. Histopathology 1990;16:441-454.
70. Dias P, Parham DM, Shapiro DN, Webber BL, Houghton PJ. Myogenic regulatory protein (MyoD1) expression in childhood solid tumors: diagnostic utility in rhabdomyosarcoma. Am J Pathol 1990;137:1283-1291.
71. Miettinen M, Rapola J. Immunohistochemical spectrum of rhabdomyosarcoma and rhabdomyosarcoma-like tumors. Expression of cytokeratin and the 68-kD neurofilament protein. Am J Surg Pathol 1989;13:120-132.
72. Brooks JJ. Immunohistochemistry of soft tissue tumors. Myoglobin as a tumor marker for rhabdomyosarcoma. Cancer 1982;50:1757-1763.
73. Bahrami A, Gown AM, Baird GS, Hicks MJ, Folpe AL. Aberrant expression of epithelial and neuroendocrine markers in alveolar rhabdomyosarcoma: a potentially serious diagnostic pitfall. Mod Pathol 2008;21:795-806.
74. Stevenson A, Chatten J, Bertoni F, Miettinen M. CD99 (p30/32MIC2) neuroectodermal/Ewing's sarcoma antigen as an immunohistochemical marker. Review of more than 600 tumors and the literature experience. Appl Immunohistochemistry 1994;2:231-240.
75. Kosemehmetoglu K, Vrana JA, Folpe AL. TLE1 expression is not specific for synovial sarcoma: a whole section study of 163 soft tissue and bone neoplasms. Mod Pathol 2009;22:872-878.
76. Sorensen PH, Lynch JC, Qualman SJ, et al. PAX3-FKHR and PAX7-FKHR gene fusions are prognostic indicators in alveolar rhabdomyosarcoma: a report from the Children's Oncology Group. J Clin Oncol 2002;20:2672-2679.
77. Parham DM, Qualman SJ, Teot L, et al. Correlation between histology and PAX/FKHR fusion status in alveolar rhabdomyosarcoma: a report from the Children's Oncology Group. Am J Surg Pathol 2007;31:895-901.
78. Kikuchi K, Rubin BP, Keller C. Developmental origins of fusion-negative rhabdomyosarcomas. Curr Top Dev Biol 2011;96:33-56.
79. Anderson JR, Barr FG, Hawkins DS, Parham DM, Skapek SX, Triche TJ. Fusion-negative alveolar rhabdomyosarcoma: modification of risk stratification is premature. J Clin Oncol 2010;28:e587-8; author reply e9-90.
80. Sumegi J, Streblow R, Frayer RW, et al. Recurrent t(2;2) and t(2;8) translocations in rhabdomyosarcoma without the canonical PAX-FOXO1 fuse PAX3 to members of the nuclear receptor transcriptional coactivator family. Genes Chromosomes Cancer 2010;49:224-236.
81. Raney RB, Anderson JR, Brown KL, et al. Treatment results for patients with localized, completely resected (group I) alveolar rhabdomyosarcoma on Intergroup Rhabdomyosarcoma Study Group (IRSG) protocols III and IV, 1984-1997: a report from the Children's Oncology Group. Pediatr Blood Cancer 2010;55:612-616.

82. Wharam MD, Meza J, Anderson J, et al. Failure pattern and factors predictive of local failure in rhabdomyosarcoma: a report of group III patients on the third Intergroup Rhabdomyosarcoma Study. J Clin Oncol 2004;22:1902-1908.

83. Stock N, Chibon F, Binh MB, et al. Adult-type rhabdomyosarcoma: analysis of 57 cases with clinicopathologic description, identification of 3 morphologic patterns and prognosis. Am J Surg Pathol 2009;33:1850-1859.

84. Guillou L, Aurias A. Soft tissue sarcomas with complex genomic profiles. Virchows Arch 2010; 456:201-217.

85. Furlong MA, Mentzel T, Fanburg-Smith JC. Pleomorphic rhabdomyosarcoma in adults: a clinicopathologic study of 38 cases with emphasis on morphologic variants and recent skeletal muscle-specific markers. Mod Pathol 2001;14:595-603.

86. Gaffney EF, Dervan PA, Fletcher CD. Pleomorphic rhabdomyosarcoma in adulthood. Analysis of 11 cases with definition of diagnostic criteria. Am J Surg Pathol 1993;17:601-609.

87. Seidal T, Kindblom LG, Angervall L. Rhabdomyosarcoma in middle-aged and elderly individuals. APMIS. 1989;97:236-248.

88. Deyrup AT, Haydon RC, Huo D, et al. Myoid differentiation and prognosis in adult pleomorphic sarcomas of the extremity: an analysis of 92 cases. Cancer 2003;98:805-813.

89. Mertens F, Fletcher CD, Dal Cin P, De Wever I, Mandahl N, Mitelman F, et al. Cytogenetic analysis of 46 pleomorphic soft tissue sarcomas and correlation with morphologic and clinical features: a report of the CHAMP Study Group. Chromosomes and MorPhology. Genes Chromosomes Cancer. 1998;22:16-25.

90. Croes R, Debiec-Rychter M, Cokelaere K, De Vos R, Hagemeijer A, Sciot R. Adult sclerosing rhabdomyosarcoma: cytogenetic link with embryonal rhabdomyosarcoma. Virchows Arch 2005;446:64-67.

91. Kuhnen C, Herter P, Leuschner I, et al. Sclerosing pseudovascular rhabdomyosarcoma-immunohistochemical, ultrastructural, and genetic findings indicating a distinct subtype of rhabdomyosarcoma. Virchows Arch 2006;449:572-578.

92. Bouron-Dal Soglio D, Rougemont AL, Absi R, et al. SNP genotyping of a sclerosing rhabdomyosarcoma: reveals highly aneuploid profile and a specific MDM2/HMGA2 amplification. Hum Pathol 2009;40:1347-1352.

7 VASCULAR TUMORS

This chapter includes reactive, benign, and malignant vascular proliferations. The classification of hemangiomas is complex. The approach here is to describe all well-defined hemangioma entities and discuss other hemangiomas composed of certain vessel types (capillary, cavernous, and venous hemangiomas). Some hemangiomatous lesions contain many types of vessels, including lymphatic vessels, and then the designation mixed angioma is in order.

The classification of many vascular lesions as vascular malformations as opposed to hemangioma is a major trend in pediatric surgery (and pathology). This issue is further discussed in the general comments for hemangiomas.

Hemangioendotheliomas are a group of vascular tumors with variable biologic potential, including lesions with metastatic capability (especially, epithelioid hemangioendothelioma).

Angiosarcoma and Kaposi sarcoma are malignant vascular endothelial tumors. Each of these forms a morphologically distinct group that can be divided in several clinicopathologic subgroups.

PAPILLARY ENDOTHELIAL HYPERPLASIA

Definition. *Papillary endothelial hyperplasia* is a benign papillary endothelial proliferation associated with vascular thrombosis in reactive conditions, hemangioma, or vascular malformation. It is also termed *Masson tumor* or *Masson vegetant intravascular hemangioendothelioma*.

Clinical Features. The lesion occurs in all ages, with median age at 40 years, slightly more commonly in women. It appears as a subcutaneous or, rarely, cutaneous, often purplish protuberance, most commonly in the fingers and hand. Other common sites include head and neck and trunk wall. Hemorrhoids frequently contain a papillary endothelial hyperplasia component within the thrombosed veins. These "secondary" lesions associated with vascular tumors or malformations may have a broader anatomic distribution. The nodule size is generally less than 2 cm, but some examples have been larger, especially when associated with hemangiomas (1–4).

Gross and Microscopic Findings. Grossly, the lesion is a hemorrhagic, well-circumscribed nodule. Histologically, there is a sharply circumscribed, usually intravascular nodule often partially filled with thrombosis. Areas of the lesion contain intravascular papillary projections with hyalinized stroma lined by hyperplastic endothelia (fig. 7-1). Stromal hemosiderin may be present. The endothelial cells may appear slightly hyperchromatic but lack significant nuclear enlargement, pleomorphism, and mitotic activity.

Differential Diagnosis. The presence of numerous vascular channels unassociated with papillary endothelial hyperplasia signals hemangioma or vascular malformation. Papillary endothelial hyperplasia differs from angiosarcoma in that the former is typically intravascular and associated with thrombosis. The endothelial cells in papillary endothelial hyperplasia are not multilayered and they lack areas of solid cellular proliferation, nuclear atypia, and significant mitotic activity seen in angiosarcoma.

HEMANGIOMAS

Hemangiomas are a heterogeneous group of benign vascular lesions containing differentiated blood vessels. Clinicopathologic entities recognized within this group are summarized in Table 7-1. Other hemangiomas not belonging in any of these specific categories are characterized descriptively using several sets of parameters, which include type of vessels involved, location, and whether the lesion is considered a hemangioma or vascular malformation.

According to vessel type, hemangiomas are descriptively classified as *capillary, cavernous,* or *venous*. When lymphatic vessels are present along with blood vessels, then the designation *mixed angioma* is applicable. By location, hemangiomas are classified as *cutaneous, intramuscular, synovial,* and so forth.

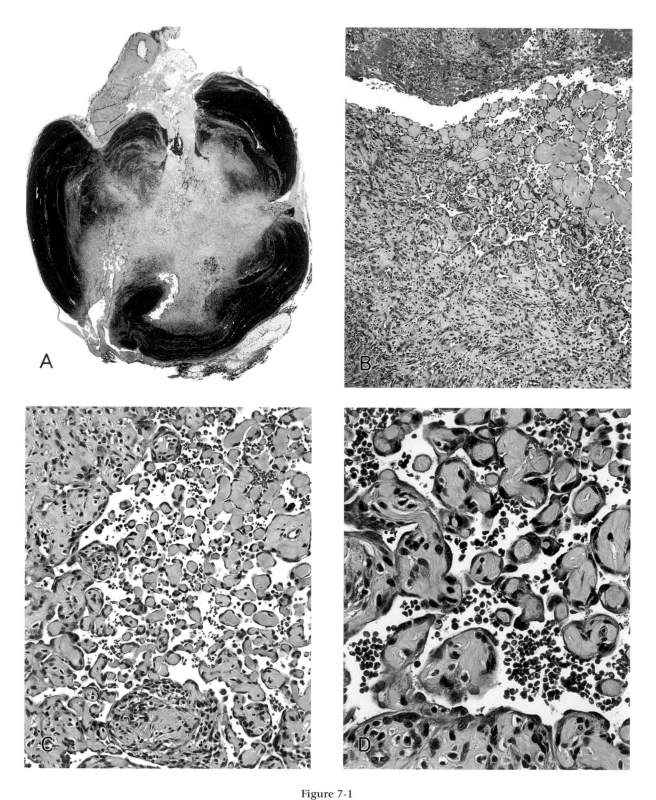

Figure 7-1

PAPILLARY ENDOTHELIAL HYPERPLASIA

A: At low magnification, papillary endothelial hyperplasia forms a well-circumscribed, intravascular, blood-filled lesion.
B–D: Papillary endothelial hyperplasia has a placental-like, villiform appearance, with limited endothelial atypia.

Table 7-1

CLASSIFICATION OF HEMANGIOMAS

By Vessel Type
   Capillary hemangioma
   Cavernous hemangioma
   Microvenular hemangioma
   Venous hemangioma

By Location
   Intramuscular hemangioma
   Synovial hemangioma

Distinct Clinicopathologic Entities
   Arteriovenous hemangioma
   Epithelioid hemangioma
   Glomeruloid hemangioma
   Hobnail hemangioma
   Lobular capillary hemangioma
   Spindle cell hemangioma
   Tufted angioma
   Verrucous hemangioma

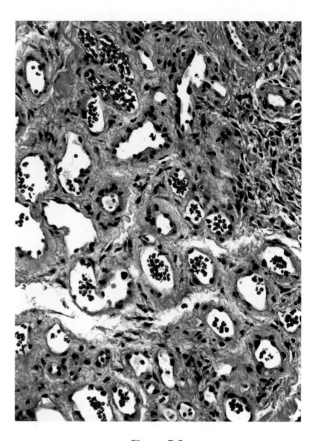

Figure 7-2

CAPILLARY HEMANGIOMA

A capillary hemangioma (cherry angioma) is a superficial angioma composed of a cluster of capillaries.

The treatment is generally local excision, with the exception of juvenile hemangiomas, which can regress spontaneously.

Many vascular lesions previously categorized as hemangiomas are now considered vascular malformations, especially in children, for the lesions composed of large caliber vessels, and vascular tumors with multiple components. Also, many childhood lymphangiomas are alternatively designated as lymphatic malformations.

Capillary Hemangioma

Hemangiomas composed of capillary type vessels and not falling into any of the other categories listed in Table 7-1 are designated as *capillary hemangiomas*. This is a clinicopathologically heterogeneous group. Many cutaneous hemangiomas belong to this group, among them small nodular formations designated as *cherry angiomas* (fig. 7-2). A subgroup of intramuscular hemangiomas is also composed of capillary hemangiomas (fig. 7-3). Typical of all these is the presence of well-differentiated capillary type vessels containing a single endothelial cell layer surrounded by pericytes.

Cavernous Hemangioma

Hemangiomas entirely or predominantly composed of dilated vascular spaces are designated as *cavernous hemangiomas*. These hemangiomas often form well-demarcated soft tissue nodules. Microscopically, they are composed of dilated, cavernous vascular spaces lined by a single layer of nonatypical endothelial cells. Pericytes are often less prominent, and in the walls of the cavernous spaces there is a nearly acellular fibrous matrix (fig. 7-4).

Venous Hemangioma

Hemangiomas composed of large vein-like vessels with discontinuous smooth muscle walls lined by a single endothelial cell layer are designated *venous hemangiomas* (fig. 7-5). Many contain additional vascular elements and are better characterized as *mixed angiomas*. Most of these are now designated as *vascular malformations* (*venous malformations*). Venous and cavernous hemangiomas are partly overlapping groups.

Based on the Armed Forces Institute of Pathology (AFIP) data, venous angiomas are most common in young adults but occur in all ages, with a male predominance. Half of these lesions

311

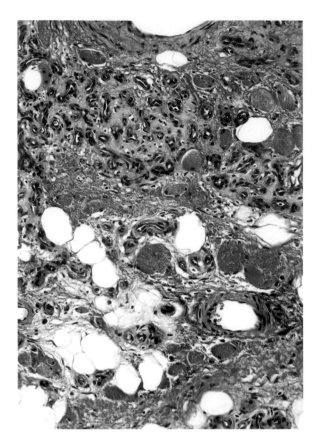 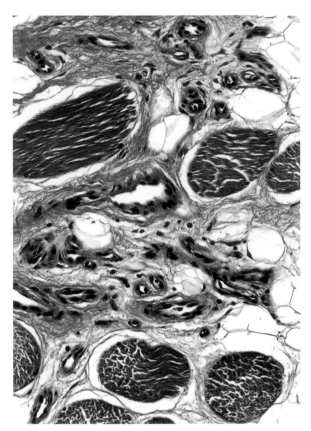

Figure 7-3

CAPILLARY HEMANGIOMA

Left, Right: Intramuscular capillary hemangioma infiltrates between skeletal muscle fibers and is composed of capillary-type vessels with nonatypical endothelial cells.

are located in the extremities and the other half in the trunk wall, head and neck, and body cavities (mediastinum and retroperitoneum).

Microvenular Hemangioma

Microvenular hemangioma is a rarely reported cutaneous hemangioma usually diagnosed in young to middle-aged adults. It appears as a small reddish patch, nodule, or plaque, especially in the forearms and elsewhere in the extremities or trunk wall (5,6). Occurrence of multiple eruptive lesions has been reported (7). This hemangioma is composed of venule-like vascular channels embedded in a collagenous matrix. The vessels have narrow lumens that often run parallel to the skin surface (fig. 7-6). The vessels contain a single endothelial layer without nuclear atypia and have well-defined pericytes.

Intramuscular Hemangioma

Intramuscular capillary hemangiomas are composed of small, uniform capillary vessels forming an infiltrative mass within the skeletal muscle (see fig. 7-3). The lesion may be associated with fatty metaplasia. Intramuscular angiomas of mixed type vessels, including venous elements, are often designated as vascular malformations.

Cutaneous Arteriovenous Hemangioma

Cutaneous arteriovenous hemangioma is composed of tightly organized lobules of blood vessels with dilated lumens and muscular walls (fig. 7-7). An overlying component including thin-walled capillaries may also be present. This lesion is also called *cirsoid aneurysm*.

Cutaneous arteriovenous hemangioma usually occurs in middle-aged and older adults,

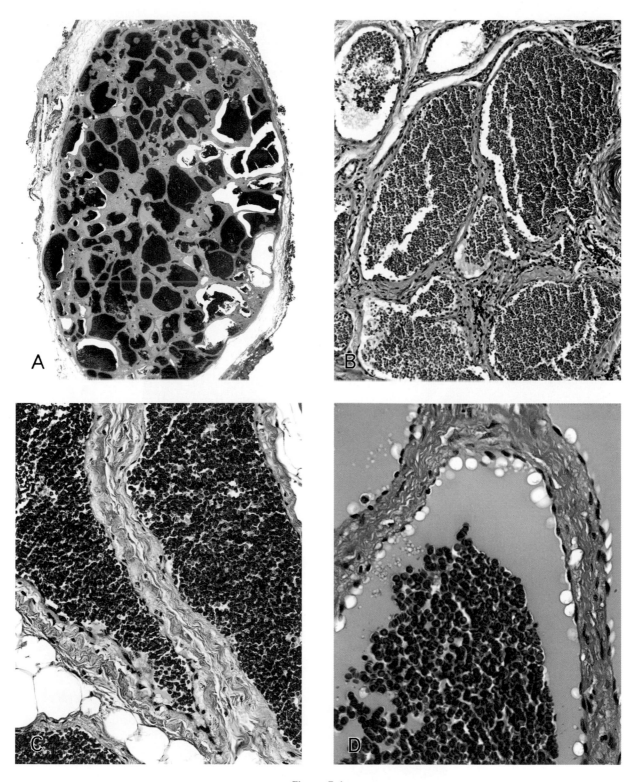

Figure 7-4

CAVERNOUS HEMANGIOMA

A,B: A sharply demarcated mass consists of cavernously dilated vessels.
C, D: The endothelial cells form a monolayer, and the septa are nearly acellular.

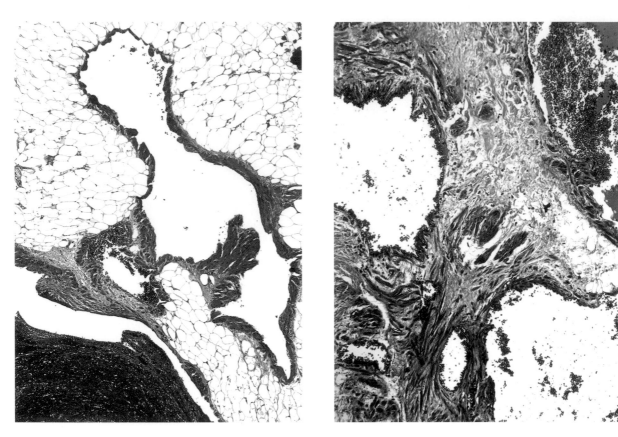

Figure 7-5

VENOUS HEMANGIOMA

Left, Right: Vein-like vessels have incompletely developed smooth muscle layers.

Figure 7-6

**MICROVENULAR
HEMANGIOMA**

Parallel, mildly dilated venule-like vessels are in a dense collagenous stroma.

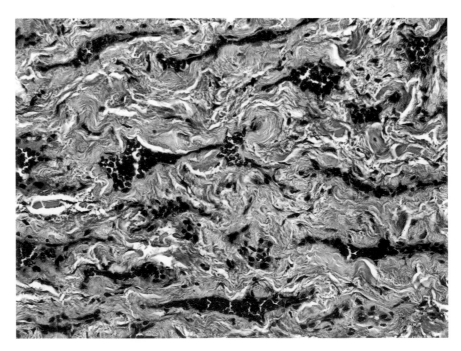

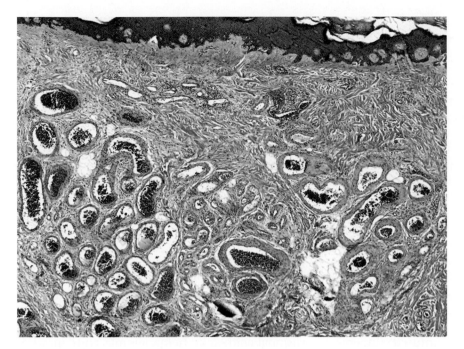

Figure 7-7

CUTANEOUS ARTERIOVENOUS HEMANGIOMA

The tumor consists of a cluster of large caliber vessels with smooth muscle walls.

and there is a male predominance. The tumor is typically located in the orofacial region and the extremities. This hemangioma is not associated with arteriovenous shunting, which occurs in some large vessel-type hemangiomas or vascular malformations (8–10). It forms an asymptomatic, less than 1 cm, red, raised nodule of plaque. Simple excision is curative.

Epithelioid Hemangioma

Definition. *Epithelioid hemangioma* is a benign vascular tumefaction that presents as a dermal, subcutaneous, or rarely, deep-seated process. All examples feature a prominent population of plump epithelioid endothelial cells, which form well-developed, but often immature-appearing, vessels with an accompanying myopericytic component without significant endothelial atypia. An inflammatory infiltrate rich in lymphocytes and eosinophils is usually present.

Angiolymphoid hyperplasia with eosinophilia is the most widely used synonym (11–15). Other terms used in the literature include: *nodular angioblastic hyperplasia with eosinophilia and lymphofolliculosis* (16), *subcutaneous angioblastic lymphoid hyperplasia with eosinophilia* (17), *atypical* or *pseudopyogenic granuloma* (18–21), *inflammatory angiomatous nodule* (21), and *intravenous atypical vascular proliferation* (28). Kimura disease and histiocytoid hemangioma are not acceptable

synonyms. Kimura disease differs both clinically and histomorphologically from epithelioid hemangioma (22–27). Histiocytoid hemangioma is best avoided as a diagnostic term because it encompasses unrelated entities, ranging from reactive to low-grade malignant (13,14,26,28).

General Considerations. This discussion primarily deals with the subcutaneous variant of epithelioid hemangioma, which is the type usually seen in soft tissue pathology. It is controversial whether subcutaneous epithelioid hemangioma is a reactive tumefaction or true neoplasm (14,26,29). Features that raise the possibility of a reactive process include the following: 1) a predilection for superficial soft tissue sites that overly bone and have minimal soft tissue padding; 2) a tendency for the process to be symmetrically distributed around a small arterial segment with evidence of damage; 3) the existence of cases that have some morphologic overlap with traumatic pseudoaneurysm (especially of the superficial temporal artery) (30); 4) a compelling history of trauma in some instances; 5) a pronounced inflammatory reaction; and 6) histologic evidence of lesional maturation over time (29). However, there are cases that have the characteristics of a benign neoplasm. These often have greater cellularity, less maturation, subjectively more atypia, and less discrete growth, sometimes with infiltration of regional structures. Epithelioid hemangiomas primary to bone (31–33) and a variety of deep soft tissue sites (12,14,29) are also documented, but it is unclear whether all of these lesions have similar behavior and share a common pathogenesis with the more superficial lesions discussed in this section (31,34–36).

Clinical Features. Subcutaneous epithelioid hemangiomas occur over a wide age range, but the peak incidence is in the third through fifth decades (13,29). A slight female predominance has been noted in the literature. Patients usually present with a mass of 1 year or less in duration; rare lesions are present for more than 15 years.

The most common site of involvement is the head, with a predilection for the forehead, and preauricular and temporal scalp, in the distribution of the superficial temporal artery (13,29). Next in frequency is the distal portion of the extremities, especially the digits. The penis is an uncommon site, but noteworthy as lesions in this location have often been confused with epithelioid hemangioendotheliomas (13,29,37,38). The process is usually uninodular but occasionally multinodular (13,27,29,37,39).

Gross Findings. Gross examination usually reveals a well-demarcated nodular mass, 0.5 to 2.0 cm in size (22,27,33). Only rarely do lesions exceed 5 cm. Careful inspection may reveal an intimate association with a small artery. Some examples have the hemorrhagic appearance of a hemangioma; others may be confused with a lymph node because of circumscription and a prominent peripheral lymphoid reaction.

Microscopic Findings. Subcutaneous epithelioid hemangiomas usually form well-demarcated masses with a prominent proliferation of capillaries, often lined by epithelioid endothelial cells. The process is commonly organized around a small, frequently damaged arterial segment (fig. 7-8) (12,13,27,29,37). The arterial lumen and wall may contain epithelioid endothelial cells (fig. 7-9), and small immature vessels lined by similar cells often radiate outward from the arterial wall. At low magnification, the process is often symmetric, and there is evidence of vessel maturation from the center to the periphery of the lesion.

Some epithelioid endothelial cells contain cytoplasmic vacuoles (fig. 7-8A,B). These vessels often have an immature appearance and may lack patent lumens, but they are well-formed and have single cell layering of the endothelia and an intact myopericytic layer (37). Peripherally located vessels tend to have well-defined lumens and are often lined by hobnail or attenuated endothelial cells. An inflammatory milieu rich in lymphocytes and eosinophils is present in most cases, and some examples are bordered by a lymphoid reaction, occasionally with follicle formation.

The epithelioid endothelial cells characteristically have abundant amphophilic or eosinophilic cytoplasm and a large, eccentrically placed nucleus with an open chromatin pattern, delicate nuclear membrane, and prominent central nucleolus. The cytologic features associated with malignancy, including significantly coarsened chromatin, chromatin clumping along the nuclear membrane, sharp angulations of the nuclear membrane, and significant variation in the number, size, and location of nucleoli, are absent. Atypical mitotic figures are also absent. Occasional epithelioid hemangiomas contain solid, sheet-like foci of epithelioid endothelial cells (37). Although these lesions may appear worrisome, their cytomorphologic features and zonal maturation pattern indicate a benign nature.

Dermal epithelioid hemangiomas also feature a proliferation of small vessels lined by epithelioid endothelial cells set in an inflammatory milieu rich in lymphocytes and eosinophils (fig. 7-10) (13,18,19,21,39). These superficial lesions, however, lack an associated arterial segment, and the proliferating vessels tend to be more mature, with well-canalized lumens. Also, the endothelial cells are often less plump, with a more hobnail-like appearance, and are often less well-marginated than subcutaneous lesions. We tentatively regard "cutaneous epithelioid angiomatous nodule" as an exuberant variant of dermal epithelioid hemangioma (40).

Special Studies. Remnants of the arterial segment, often seen in association with subcutaneous epithelioid hemangioma, are highlighted with the Movat pentachrome stain. The arterial elastic lamina is also highlighted with the Verhoeff elastic stain.

The epithelioid endothelial cells are immunoreactive for CD31 and factor VIIIrAg (12,13,27,37,38). Immunoreactivity for CD34 is also frequently present, although sometimes to a lesser degree. Keratin expression is uncommon, but it is occasionally detected in a few

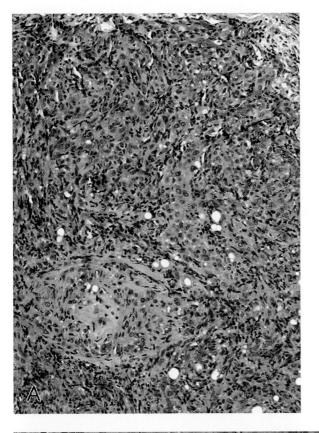

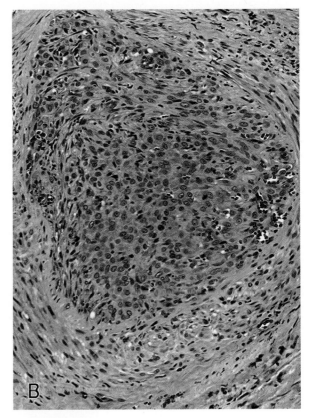

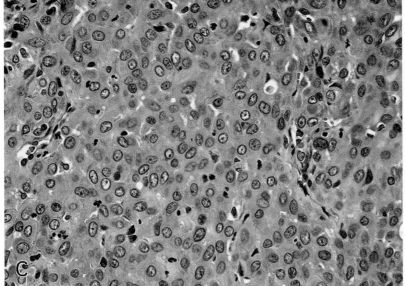

Figure 7-8

EPITHELIOID HEMANGIOMA

A: Epithelioid hemangioma associated with a small artery.

B: The process forms a florid intraluminal proliferation.

C: High-power examination shows that the cells have uniform nuclear morphology with an open chromatin pattern, distinct central nucleolus, and abundant amphophilic cytoplasm.

endothelial cells (37). Both well-developed and immature-appearing vessels are characteristically bordered by a distinct cuff of α-smooth muscle actin–positive myopericytes (fig. 7-9C) (37). These latter cells become more abundant toward the periphery of the lesion.

Differential Diagnosis. Kimura disease differs both clinically and histologically from epithelioid hemangioma (22–26). It has a greater predilection for young males, it is more frequently bilateral, it more commonly affects the parotid region, and it characteristically

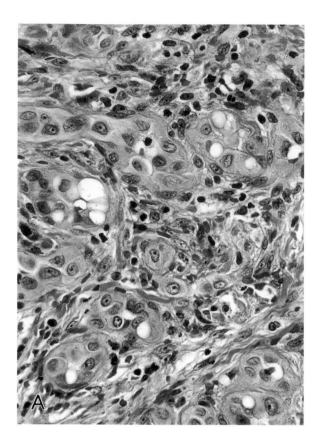

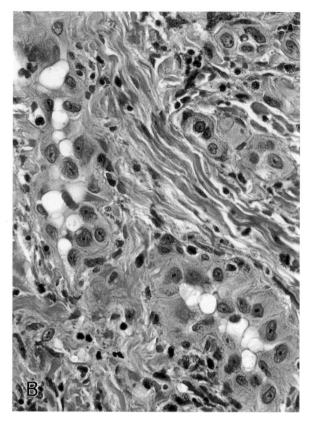

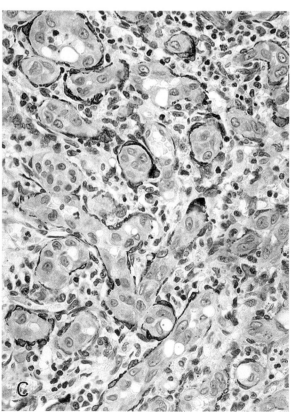

Figure 7-9

EPITHELIOID HEMANGIOMA

A,B: The immature (but well-formed) vessels encountered in subcutaneous epithelioid hemangioma are lined by a fairly uniform population of epithelioid endothelial cells with an open chromatin pattern and distinct central nucleolus. Some cells contain luminally oriented cytoplasmic vacuoles. There is a lymphoeosinophilic inflammatory infiltrate in the background.

C: A smooth muscle actin immunostain highlights the well-developed myopericytic layer associated with the immature vessels.

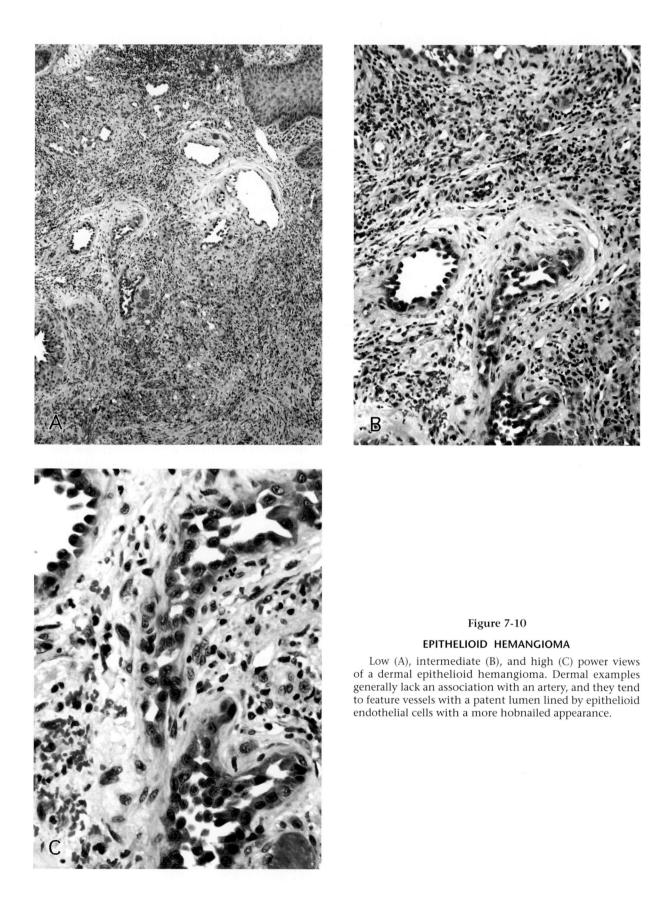

Figure 7-10

EPITHELIOID HEMANGIOMA

Low (A), intermediate (B), and high (C) power views of a dermal epithelioid hemangioma. Dermal examples generally lack an association with an artery, and they tend to feature vessels with a patent lumen lined by epithelioid endothelial cells with a more hobnailed appearance.

produces a larger mass than epithelioid hemangioma. Regional lymphadenopathy and peripheral eosinophilia are also more frequently associated with Kimura disease. Histologically, Kimura disease forms a poorly demarcated, extensively fibrotic mass with a prominent lymphocytic-eosinophilic inflammatory infiltrate. Whereas eosinophilic microabscesses are a frequent finding in Kimura disease, they are not a feature of epithelioid hemangioma. Additionally, the vessels in Kimura disease lack both epithelioid endothelial cells and an "immature" appearance. This unusual fibroinflammatory process is thought to represent an aberrant immunologic host response to an unidentified antigenic stimulus.

Epithelioid hemangioendothelioma contains single, short cords, clusters, and randomly arranged groups of atypical epithelioid endothelial cells, frequently embedded in a myxohyaline matrix (41–46). The majority of the neoplastic cells do not form well-developed vascular spaces or channels. As a result, one of the few clues to the vascular nature of this process is the presence of rudimentary intracytoplasmic lumens, sometimes containing red blood cells. Another clue is the occasional involvement and destruction of preexisting small to medium-sized veins. The much more primitive vascular architecture, infiltrative and destructive growth pattern, scarcity of α-smooth muscle actin-positive myopericytes, more pronounced cytologic atypia, and peculiar myxohyaline milieu help distinguish this entity from epithelioid hemangioma.

Epithelioid angiosarcoma contains plump epithelioid endothelial cells with eosinophilic or amphophilic cytoplasm and enlarged, highly atypical nuclei with prominent nucleoli (45–47). This process typically contains abundant mitoses, including atypical forms, and has an irregular, infiltrative and destructive growth pattern.

Epithelioid endothelial cells are also identified in a wide variety of vascular lesions, including reactive vascular proliferations secondary to infections (e.g., bacillary angiomatosis), other benign vascular lesions, borderline tumors (e.g., Dabska tumor, retiform hemangioendothelioma), low-grade malignant tumors (e.g., epithelioid hemangioendothelioma), and high-grade malignancies (e.g., both conventional and epithelioid angiosarcomas). As a result, accurate classification requires careful consideration of all pertinent clinical and histopathologic findings.

Superficial (traumatic) pseudoaneurysms have an anatomic distribution and clinical appearance that overlap with subcutaneous epithelioid hemangioma (30). These lesions usually affect the temporal artery or one of its branches. There is mural disruption of the affected vessel, often accompanied by organizing thrombus; granulation tissue with numerous capillaries near the defect; proteoglycans deposition; and active fibrointimal proliferation. Some endothelial cells have a hobnail or mildly epithelioid morphology. If there is a notably accentuated small vessel proliferation and the endothelial population has well-developed epithelioid morphology, we classify the lesion as an epithelioid hemangioma and note the accompanying arterial trauma.

Treatment and Prognosis. Complete local excision with follow-up is optimal management. Local recurrence has been documented in up to one third of patients (13,25). Most recurrences are cured by re-excision, but rarely, recurrences are locally aggressive. Occasional recurrences may appear separated from the presentation site, but they characteristically occur along the distribution of the initially affected vessel. There is one report of regional lymph node seeding that had no adverse outcome after 5 years of follow-up (17). There are no reports of distant metastases.

Glomeruloid Hemangioma

Definition. *Glomeruloid hemangioma* is a benign, probably reactive, vascular proliferation often linked to POEMS (polyneuropathy, organomegaly, endocrinopathy, M protein, skin changes) syndrome and multicentric Castleman disease (48–53) and characterized by dilated, thin-walled vessels with intraluminal aggregates of capillaries that assume a glomeruloid/papillary architecture. The intraluminal capillaries are lined by plump endothelial cells, and there are associated pericytes and stromal cells. Eosinophilic globules are usually identified within some of the plump endothelial and stromal cells. Similar lesions have been reported as *papillary hemangiomas*.

General Considerations. This distinctive vascular proliferation may be an early manifestation of POEMS syndrome, so in some cases, it may take several years of follow-up before patients fulfill the minimum diagnostic criteria for this disorder (49,54). It is also well documented that some patients with glomeruloid hemangiomas have no evidence, even after long-term follow-up, of POEMS syndrome or multicentric Castleman disease (51,55–58).

Clinical Features. POEMS syndrome usually affects patients between the ages of 30 to 80 years, with median ages ranging from 46 to 51 years in the largest series (59). Males are affected more often than females by a margin of 3 or more to 2. The major elements of this syndrome are polyneuropathy, organomegaly (hepatomegaly, splenomegaly), endocrinopathy (hypogonadism), presence of M protein, and skin changes. Additional important features not represented in the acronym are Castleman disease of lymph nodes (60), sclerotic bone lesions, papilledema, pleural and peritoneal effusions, and peripheral edema. The polyneuropathy and the M protein are considered major criteria for diagnosis and the other mentioned features are minor criteria. Both major criteria and at least one minor criterion are needed, at a minimum, for a diagnosis of POEMS syndrome (59). The M protein is almost invariably gamma light chain (59,61,62). It has been estimated that 10 to 30 percent of patients with POEMS syndrome have multicentric Castleman disease (59,61).

Most glomeruloid hemangiomas occur between the ages of 40 and 79 years. They present as reddish or purplish, well-circumscribed, sessile, papulonodular or pedunculated lesions, or as bluish compressible subcutaneous masses (50,53,54,56,63). Some examples, on close inspection, have a multilobulated, cerebriform appearance (48,53). Involvement of the trunk and proximal portions of the extremities has been stressed in the literature, but the face, neck, and other sites may also be affected, especially in nonsyndromic cases.

Gross Findings. Surgical specimens usually consist of a piece of skin and subcutis with a reddish blue papulonodular lesion ranging from 2 to 20 mm.

Microscopic Findings. The lower dermis or subcutis typically contains ectatic, thin-walled vascular spaces. These vessels have attenuated endothelial cells and their lumen is occupied by variably sized conglomerates of capillary channels lined by plump endothelial cells with abundant pale cytoplasm, with or without clear vacuoles; some cells have variably sized, pale-staining eosinophilic globules (fig. 7-11). The capillaries have an associated pericytic population, and there are scattered interposed plump stromal cells with lightly eosinophilic cytoplasm that also frequently contains cytoplasmic globules. Nuclear atypia is absent, and mitotic figures are rare. Similar vascular lesions are encountered in deep soft tissue sites and within organs (64,65). Although occasionally suggested, it is doubtful whether POEMS syndrome-associated and sporadic glomeruloid hemangiomas can be histologically distinguished (51,66,67).

Special Studies. The eosinophilic globules of glomeruloid hemangioma are periodic acid–Schiff (PAS) positive, diastase resistant, and generally have only weak peripheral immunoreactivity for immunoglobulins, which may be due to nonspecific antigen adsorption (51). The endothelial cells are immunoreactive for factor VIIIrAg and CD31 (49,51,57,66,67). The (myo)pericytes are smooth muscle actin positive. There is no immunoreactivity for human herpesvirus (HHV)-8 (48,56) or D2-40 (67).

Differential Diagnosis. Intravascular lobular capillary hemangioma, acquired tufted hemangioma, and Dabska tumor are all histologically distinctive although variably share the intravascular pattern of glomeruloid hemangioma. Cutaneous angiosarcomas are characterized by infiltrative and often destructive growth. There is both cytologic atypia and mitotic activity, and the endothelial cells lining vascular spaces often have disorganized growth with cell piling and detachment.

Treatment and Prognosis. Glomeruloid hemangioma is a benign, presumably reactive, process. Therefore, resection is generally not required. Some lesions recur after simple excision, and new independent lesions may develop over time. The importance of recognizing this entity is to avoid misdiagnosis as a potentially malignant vascular tumor and to alert clinicians of the possible association with POEMS syndrome and multicentric Castleman disease.

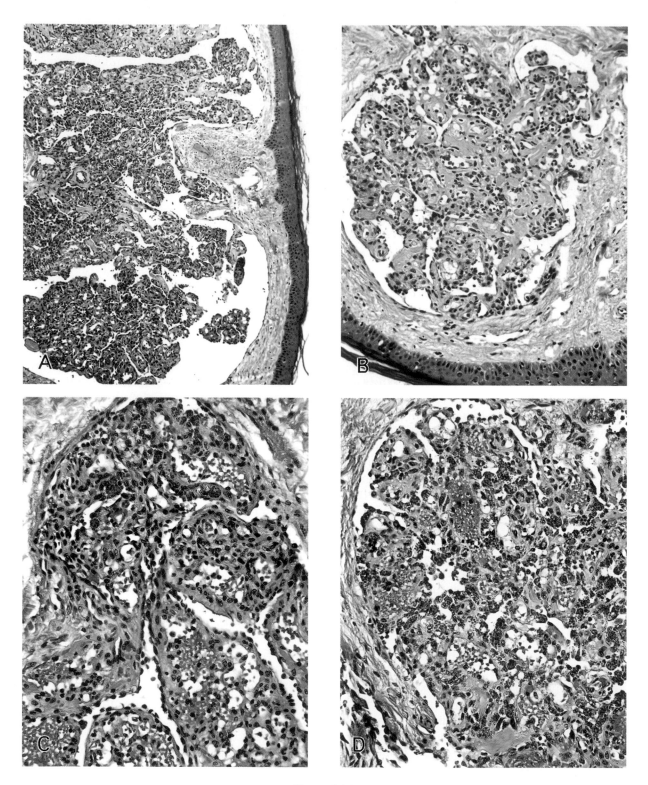

Figure 7-11

GLOMERULOID HEMANGIOMA

A,B: The intraluminal growth pattern is distinctive.
C,D: Scattered cells with multiple eosinophilic cytoplasmic globules are seen.

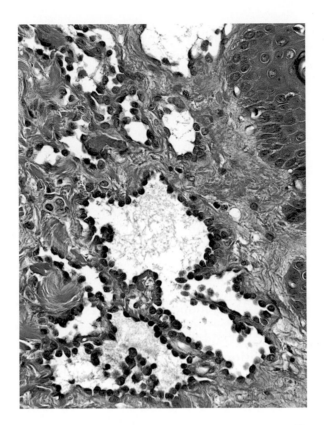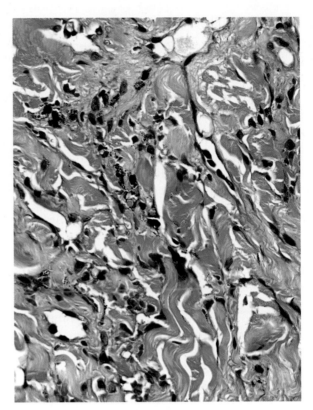

Figure 7-12

HOBNAIL HEMANGIOMA

Left: The vascular spaces are lined by inward protruding, hobnail-like endothelial cells.
Right: A deeper component contains vessels with narrow lumens and stromal hemosiderin deposition.

Hobnail Hemangioma

Definition. *Hobnail hemangioma* is a superficial, dermal hemangioma containing vessels with inward protuberant "hobnail-like" endothelial cells (68). A deeper dermal component may contain hemosiderin. It is synonymous to *targetoid hemosiderotic hemangioma*.

Clinical Features. Hobnail hemangioma often presents as a rounded erythematous macule containing a darker, mildly elevated central zone, thus the alternative name targetoid hemosiderotic hemangioma. It occurs from childhood to old age but is most common in young adults, with a male predominance. The most common locations are the skin of thigh and buttocks. In the upper extremity, there is a predilection to proximal sites. The back is the most common site in the trunk wall, whereas occurrence in the head and neck is rare. The lesions are typically small, usually less than 1 cm.

Microscopic Findings. Histologically, hobnail hemangiomas are distinctive for their dilated, irregularly shaped vascular channels lined by variably luminally protruding, cobblestone-like hobnail endothelial cells, which lack multilayering and significant nuclear atypia (fig. 7-12, left). A deeper dermal component of this hemangioma has slit-like capillaries and interstitial hemosiderin (fig. 7-12, right). Hobnail hemangioma differs from retiform hemangioendothelioma by its lack of complex, anastomosing vascular channels showing a higher cellularity and mild nuclear atypia.

Immunohistochemically typical is expression of lymphatic vascular phenotypic markers, VEGFR3, and podoplanin (69,70).

Treatment and Prognosis. Hobnail hemangioma has a uniformly benign behavior with no tendency for recurrence and simple excision is adequate (69–72).

Juvenile Capillary Hemangioma

Definition. *Juvenile capillary hemangioma* is a hemangioma variant typically occurring in infants and often composed of fairly primitive, pericyte-rich capillaries with variable lumen formation. Immunohistochemical positivity for glucose transporter type 1 (GLUT-1) is a feature unique to this hemangioma.

Clinical Features. Juvenile hemangiomas are common and occur in 10 percent of infants, with a predilection to female sex and Caucasian race. They can be congenital, especially in premature babies, or appear during the first year of life as a rapidly growing mass. Gradual involution is typical. Sites of occurrence vary, but the head and neck region is a common site. Involvement of the skin is most common, but the lesions often extend into the subcutis and may also involve deeper structures such as parotid gland, orbital soft tissue, and lacrimal glands. Large hemangiomas are associated with high-output cardiac failure.

Gross and Microscopic Findings. Grossly, juvenile capillary hemangiomas often form elevated, bright red, nodular cutaneous lesions, and therefore, are referred to as *strawberry nevi*. Histologically, these hemangiomas are typically lobulated (fig. 7-13A). They entrap surrounding elements such as skin adnexa, subcutaneous fat, and salivary gland tissue. The degree of vasoformation varies from inconspicuous to prominent lumen formation (fig. 7-13B–D). Endothelial mitotic activity is often present. A prominent pericytic, actin-positive component typically accompanies the endothelial cells. Infantile hemangiomas contain numerous mast cells and infiltrating histiomonocytic cells (73–76).

Special Studies. Immunohistochemically, the endothelial cells of juvenile capillary hemangiomas are uniquely positive for GLUT-1, similar to the capillaries of placental villi (fig. 7-14) (77,78). The capillaries contain prominent smooth muscle actin-positive pericytes, a feature that helps to identify the vascular differentiation typical of benign angiomas (79).

Differential Diagnosis. Rapidly involuting congenital hemangioma, noninvoluting congenital hemangioma (80), and congenital nonprogressive hemangioma (81) are uncommon congenital hemangiomas that mainly occur in the head and neck, have no gender bias, are large (often larger than 5 cm), and sometimes are associated with mild hemangioma-related platelet trapping without disseminated intravascular coagulation (Kasabach-Merritt syndrome).

Histologically these lesions do not have a unifying morphology, but show a spectrum of changes. Many are lobulated, and some resemble lobular capillary hemangioma, tufted angioma, or Kaposiform hemangioendothelioma. These hemangiomas are presently better recognized as clinical rather than distinct histopathologic entities. They seem to differ from juvenile capillary hemangioma by their lack of GLUT-1 expression.

Treatment and Prognosis. Surgical treatment can often be delayed in view of the spontaneous involution of the lesion. Medical treatment options include corticosteroids and interferon-alpha-2, which induce tumor regression.

Lobular Capillary Hemangioma

Definition. *Lobular capillary hemangioma* is a hemangioma variant composed of lobules of capillaries, often containing a central feeder vessel. *Pyogenic granuloma* (especially when occurring in skin mucosal sites, and intravascularly) is a synonym.

Clinical Features. This hemangioma variant occurs in all ages, but has a predilection to children and young adults. There is a male predominance. Most present as a polypoid mass on the skin or at mucosal sites, but some occur in the subcutis or rarely in deeper sites as palpable nondescript nodules (82–88). A few occur as an intravenous mass, also designated as *intravascular pyogenic granuloma* (89,90).

Gross Findings. Cutaneous and mucosal lesions form purplish, polypoid, dome-shaped nodules that may be secondarily ulcerated. They vary from a few millimeters to 1 cm or, occasionally, larger. Subcutaneous examples vary from yellowish to reddish nodules.

Microscopic Findings. The cutaneous and mucosal examples are often surrounded by a peripheral epithelial collar. The lesions, in general, are composed of variably lobulated capillaries, with the lobules often containing larger "feeder" vessels. The capillaries are lined by monolayered endothelium that may occasionally show mild atypia (fig. 7-15). Mitotic activity is common and is not an alarming finding. Intravascular examples involve lumens of small veins (fig. 7-16).

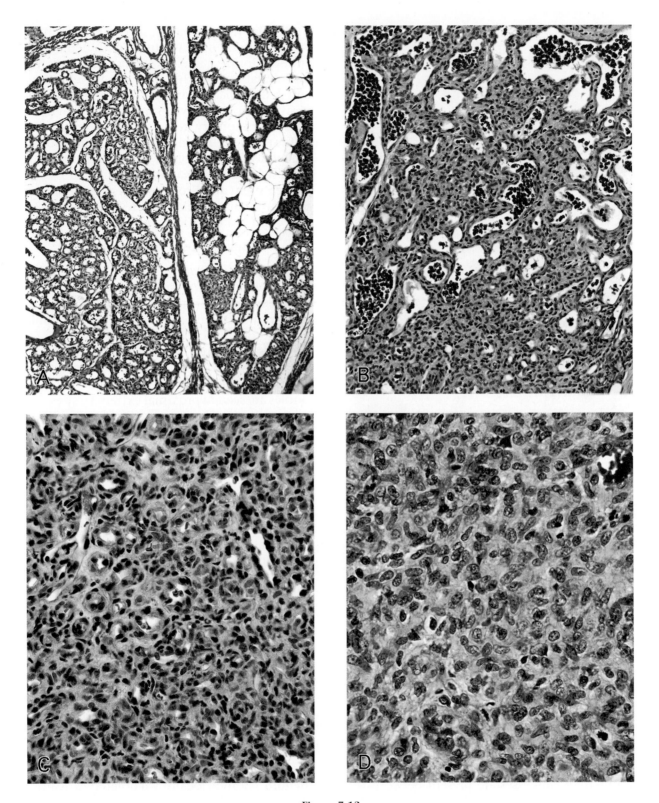

Figure 7-13

JUVENILE CAPILLARY HEMANGIOMA

This tumor is often lobulated (A) and shows densely packed capillaries with variable lumen formation (B–D).

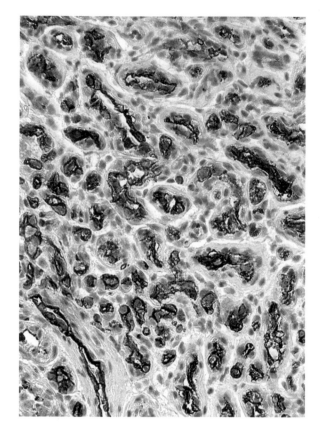

Figure 7-14

JUVENILE CAPILLARY HEMANGIOMA

The capillary endothelial cells are typically GLUT-1 positive.

Special Studies. The capillaries involved in lobular capillary hemangioma are typically well-developed and contain a component of monolayered endothelial cells positive for endothelial markers (CD31, ERG), and a prominent pericytic component positive for smooth muscle actin. The lesional endothelial cells are negative for HHV-8.

Differential Diagnosis. Infection-associated reactive vascular proliferations, especially bacillary angiomatosis, may resemble lobular capillary hemangioma, although they are typically less conspicuously lobulated. These reactive vascular proliferations are suspected if neutrophilic microabscesses are present between the capillaries. The diagnosis of bacillary angiomatosis is confirmed by demonstrating numerous bacilli with the Warthin-Starry stain.

Cellular variants of lobular capillary hemangioma should not be confused with hemangioendothelioma or angiosarcoma. The tendency for lobulation and the presence of well-differentiated capillaries with a smooth muscle actin-positive pericytic layer support the diagnosis of lobular capillary hemangioma. The lack of a solid spindle cell component and immunohistochemical expression of HHV-8 separate this hemangioma from Kaposi sarcoma.

Treatment and Prognosis. In general, simple excision is curative, although lesions may persist or recur if not completely excised.

Spindle Cell Hemangioma

Definition. *Spindle cell hemangioma* is a distinctive hemangioma variant mostly seen in the distal extremities. It resembles cavernous hemangioma but contains cellular septa with spindle cells and often vacuolated endothelial cells.

Clinical Features. Spindle cell hemangioma has a predilection for distal sites, mostly the hands and feet and adjacent tissues. Rare examples are seen in proximal extremity sites and head and neck. There is a predilection to young adults, without gender preference.

Clinical associations include early onset varicose veins and Klippel-Trenaunay syndrome (91–95). Patients with Maffucci syndrome often develop multiple spindle cell hemangiomas, which can form innumerable confluent masses extensively involving an extremity (fig. 7-17). These patients also develop osseous chondrosarcomas (96,97).

Gross Findings. Spindle cell hemangioma typically forms a solitary, circumscribed, subcutaneous purplish nodule measuring 1 to 2 cm. There may be multiple concurrent lesions, especially in connection with Maffucci syndrome.

Microscopic Findings. Spindle cell hemangioma consists of a circumscribed mass composed of dilated vascular channels and an interstitial bland spindle cell component without atypia or much mitotic activity. In some cases, the vascular lumens contain spherical hyalinized or sometimes calcified bodies, referred to as phleboliths ("vein stones"). The lining endothelium is often focally vacuolated, a feature helpful in identifying this lesion (fig. 7-18). More solid spindle cell growth can occupy a portion of the tumor.

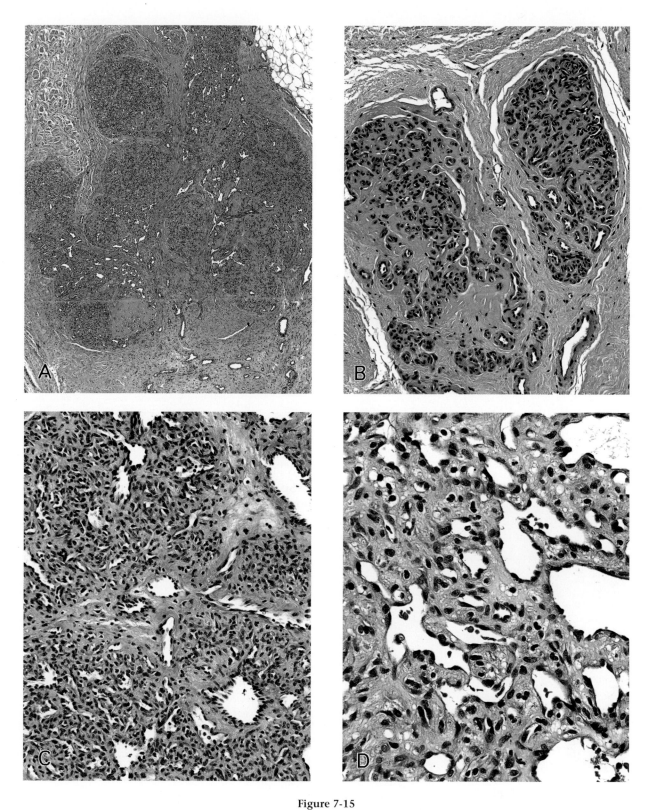

Figure 7-15

LOBULAR CAPILLARY HEMANGIOMA

The capillary units are organized as lobules (A,B), and these lobules contain larger caliber "feeder" vessels (C,D).

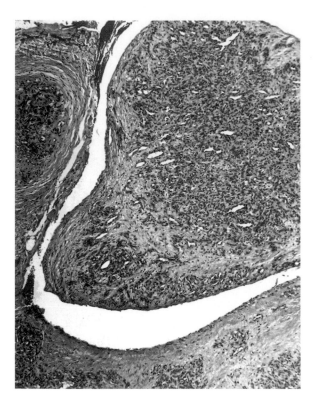 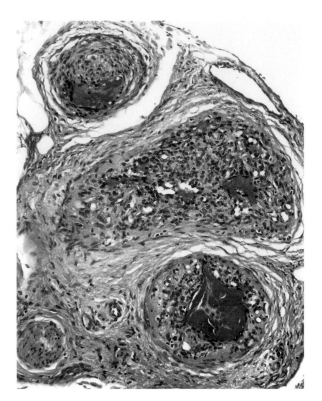

Figure 7-16

INTRAVASCULAR LOBULAR CAPILLARY HEMANGIOMA

Left, Right: Clusters of capillary vessels are located inside a small vein.

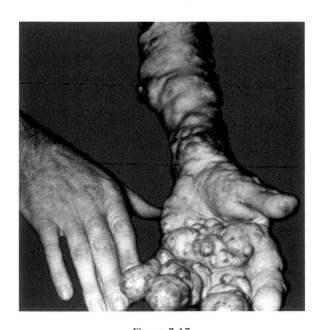

Figure 7-17

SPINDLE CELL HEMANGIOMAS

Extensive spindle cell hemangiomas involve the left hand of a patient with Maffucci syndrome.

Special Studies. Only the endothelial component is positive for CD31, ERG, and other endothelial markers, whereas the spindle cells are positive for smooth muscle actin.

Genetics. *IDHI* and *IDH2* somatic mosaic mutations have been reported in both sporadic and Maffucci syndrome-associated spindle cell hemangiomas. They seem to be specific to spindle cell hemangiomas among vascular tumors (97a,b).

Differential Diagnosis. The bland endothelial cytology and lesional circumscription distinguish this tumor from angiosarcoma and Kaposi sarcoma. In contrast with the latter two, there is no immunopositivity for HHV-8 antigens.

Treatment and Prognosis. Spindle cell hemangiomas often recur and multiple locoregional recurrences develop over time. They have, however, no metastatic potential.

Tufted Angioma

Definition. *Tufted angioma* is a superficial hemangioma variant composed of rounded

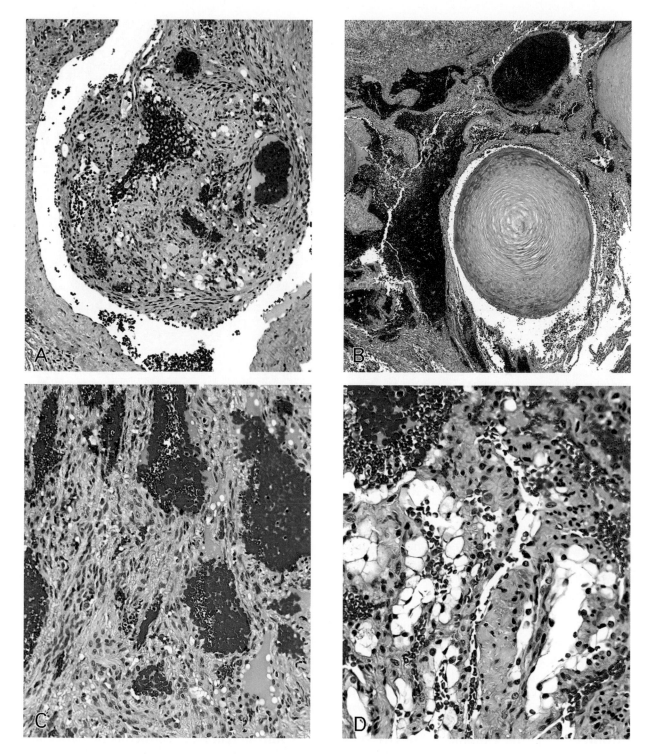

Figure 7-18

SPINDLE CELL HEMANGIOMA

A: Spindle cell hemangioma often forms an intravascular growth in a lumen of a vein.
B: Some lumens contain round fibrous bodies, often referred to as phleboliths.
C: Between the vascular lumens are cellular septa containing bland spindle cells.
D: Endothelial cell vacuolization is a common finding.

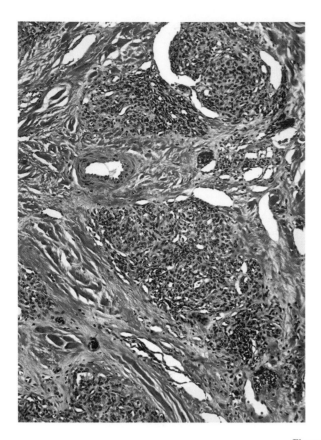 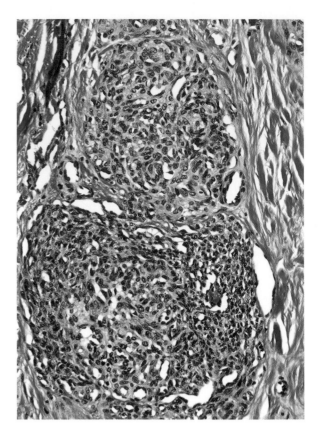

Figure 7-19

TUFTED ANGIOMA

Left: Tufted angioma consists of multiple rounded clusters of capillaries with prominent pericytes.
Right: The vessels typically have narrow or indistinguishable lumens.

nodules of capillaries, often with prominent pericytes. It is also called *acquired tufted angioma, progressive capillary hemangioma,* and *angioblastoma of Nakagawa.*

Clinical Features. This rare capillary hemangioma usually develops in early childhood; some lesions are congenital. It often forms a progressively enlarging cutaneous macule over years that persists into adulthood. The most common sites are head and neck and upper trunk wall, but cases have also been reported in the extremities and genital region. The lesion is associated with platelet trapping and severe thrombocytopenia (Kasabach-Merritt syndrome), or chronic coagulopathy (98–103).

Microscopic Findings. Histologically, the lesion is composed of clustered rounded lobules (described as a "cannon ball pattern") or band-like infiltrates of tightly packed capillaries with small lumens and prominent pericytes (fig.

7-19). Some of the nodules are intravascular, which results in their sharp demarcation. There is a single endothelial cell layer with no atypia. A pericytic smooth muscle actin-positive element is prominent and may give the lesion a spindled appearance. The endothelial cells are GLUT-1 negative.

Verrucous Hemangioma

Definition. *Verrucous hemangioma* is a cutaneous/subcutaneous hemangioma with a superficial component associated with verrucous epidermal change, especially in longstanding lesions.

Clinical Features. Verrucous hemangioma usually occurs in early childhood and is present at birth in half of the cases. There is no gender predilection, and most cases involve the lower extremities, especially the foot and ankle. The lesion may enlarge over time to form a large patch or a linear or irregular cluster of purple nodules that over years evolve into a verrucous formation. The superficial location is associated with bleeding after minor trauma.

Gross and Microscopic Findings. The lesions vary from solitary purplish nodules to a large plaque-like lesion several centimeters in diameter. Longstanding lesions are covered by a papillomatous and acanthous (verrucous) epidermis. The vascular component contains dilated, blood-filled capillaries. Cavernous, thick-walled, blood-filled vascular spaces may extend from just below the epidermis into the deep dermis and sometimes into the subcutis, in contrast with angiokeratoma. The endothelial lining forms an inconspicuous monolayer without atypia (fig. 7-20). The lesional endothelia may be focally positive for GLUT-1.

Treatment and Prognosis. This is a benign hemangioma variant. Complete surgical excision is advocated as these hemangiomas persist and recur following dermal shave, incomplete surgical excision, or topical treatments (104–108).

LYMPHANGIOMA (LYMPHATIC MALFORMATION)

Definition. *Lymphangioma* is a benign vascular lesion composed of lymphatic-like vascular channels. Childhood lymphangiomas, especially those involving head and neck, are largely synonymous to *lymphatic malformations*.

General Considerations. Similar to the dilemma of hemangioma versus vascular malformation, it is not known by scientific evidence whether lymphatic vascular lesions are true neoplasms or developmental anomalies (malformations). Nevertheless, the clinical literature currently prefers the designation lymphatic malformation, especially for cystic and cavernous lesions in children.

Clinical Features. Children are usually affected, and some have some form already during fetal life. Fewer lymphangiomas, especially cutaneous ones, are also seen in adults. There is no gender predilection. The most common locations are head and neck and abdominal cavity; occurrence in the extremities is less common. In the head and neck, lymphangioma most commonly involves the neck and orbit (109–112).

The *cystic lymphangiomas* in the neck (*cystic hygromas*) occur from infancy on and have an increased incidence in patients with Turner syndrome and various trisomies (113). Cystic lymphangiomas appear as fluctuant, ill-defined masses. Intra-abdominal or intrathoracic lymphangiomas form spongy or microcystic masses, and these lesions can be extensive. Soft tissue lymphangiomas in the body cavities often involve multiple contiguous organs and some are thereby designated as *lymphangiomatosis*.

Cutaneous lymphangiomas often form limited focal lesions referred to as *lymphangioma circumscriptum*. They extend superficially close to epidermis, and/or deeper with subcutaneous involvement.

Gross Findings. Larger lymphangiomas are often grossly distinctive, forming spongy masses that collapse after surgery. Neck lymphangiomas in young children are often extensively cystic (cystic lymphangioma) and contain serous or milky fluid.

Microscopic Findings. Deep soft tissue lymphangiomas are composed of dilated lymphatic channels often filled with clear or proteinaceous fluid; sometimes they contain lymphocytes (fig 7-21A). The lymphatic vessels in cystic lymphangioma vary from dilated, thin-walled vessels to thick fibrous bands. Lymphoid aggregates or small lymph nodes are often seen in the septa (fig. 7-21B).

Abdominal lymphangiomas are typically composed of cystically dilated lymphatics. The vessel walls often contain discontinuous smooth muscle (fig. 7-21C). In some cases, the lymphangiomatous nature is obscured by an extensive reactive myofibroblastic proliferation (114).

Cutaneous lymphangioma circumscriptum is composed of scattered, small-caliber lymphatic vessels lined by attenuated, monolayered lymphatic endothelial cells (fig. 7-21D). Clusters of lymphocytes may be present around or inside the lumens.

Special Studies. The vessels of lymphangioma are immunohistochemically distinctive in the expression of four vascular markers: podoplanin (D2-40) and PROX1 are the most practical but not totally specific; Lyve-1 and vascular endothelial growth factor receptor3 are also lymphatic vessel specific, but availability of good antibodies limits their diagnostic application (115,116). Lymphangioma vessels are CD31 positive but often demonstrate weaker CD34 positivity than blood vessels.

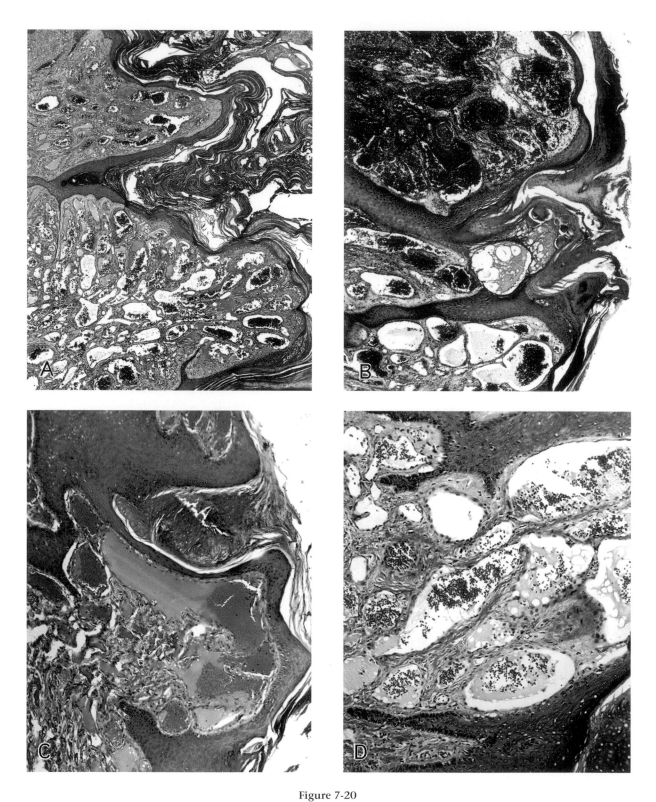

Figure 7-20

VERRUCOUS HEMANGIOMA

A,B: The hemangioma is overlaid by a verrucous, hyperplastic epidermis.

C,D: Capillary vessels are present below the epidermis, but by definition, they extend into deep dermis.

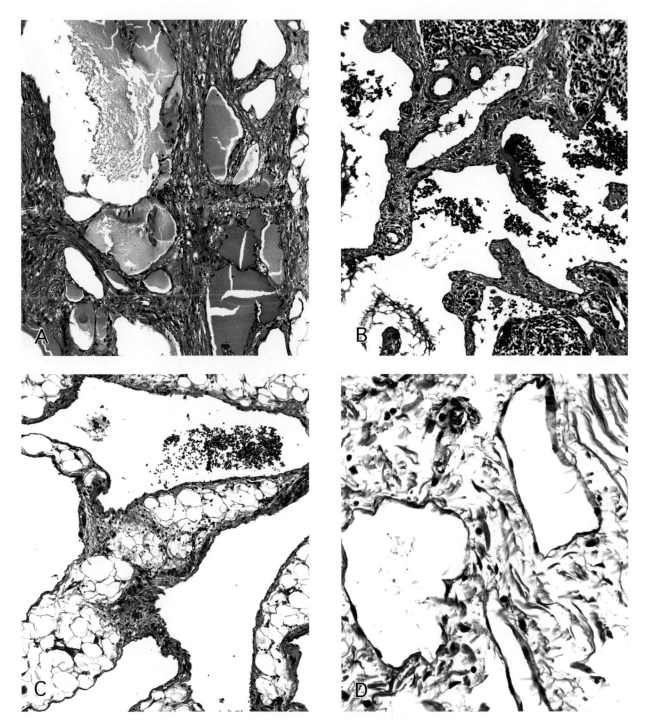

Figure 7-21

LYMPHANGIOMA

A: Soft tissue lymphangioma is composed of multiple vascular channels containing proteinaceous fluid.

B: Cystic lymphangioma contains thick collagenous septa, and lymphoid aggregates are present between the cystically dilated lymphatic channels.

C: An abdominal lymphangioma with dilated lymphatic vascular channels.

D: Cutaneous lymphangioma circumscriptum shows the delicate nature of apparently discontinuous endothelia typical of lymphangiomas.

Differential Diagnosis. Many vascular tumors contain both lymphatic and blood vessels and are therefore named angioma. In some cases, lesions in serosal cavities may be confused with a cystic mesothelial proliferation. Lymphedema appears as dilated lymphatics and stromal edema, without an increase in the number of lymphatic vessels, as seen in lymphangioma. Cystic mesothelial lesions should not be confused with lymphangiomas. Immunohistochemical positivity for keratin and calretinin identifies a mesothelial cyst, whereas podoplanin in present in both mesothelia and lymphatic endothelia.

Treatment and Prognosis. Large to massive lymphangiomas may cause local and potentially fatal complications, such as airway or cardiopulmonary compromise. Benign lymphangiomas may persist or recur, but there is no tendency to malignant transformation. Surgical excision in a function-preserving manner is the main approach when feasible, and surgical staging is significant, as a suprahyoid location and bilaterality of cervical lymphangiomas are associated with more complicated surgery. Additional modalities include sclerotherapy and advanced targeted therapies, as discussed below with lymphangiomatosis (117).

LYMPHANGIOMATOSIS

Definition. *Lymphangiomatosis* is a clinical term referring to extensive lymphangioma formation. The term is used variably in the literature to refer to a large organ-based or multiorgan lymphangioma or a more widespread process involving discontiguous organ systems. Due to the rarity of this condition, most information is in case reports (118–120).

Clinical Features. Lymphangiomatosis is typically diagnosed in early childhood, usually by the age of 10 years. There is a significant male predominance. The clinical manifestations include a diffuse soft tissue mass (most often in the lower extremity), regional bone involvement sometimes with massive osteolysis (Gorham disease, vanishing bone disease), and thoracic involvement with chylothorax. Splenic, hepatic, and other visceral lesions are common.

Microscopic Findings. Lymphangiomatosis in the extremities often involves both soft tissue

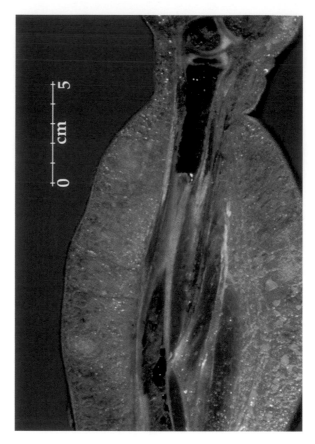

Figure 7-22

LYMPHANGIOMATOSIS

Massive soft tissue and bone involvement of the thigh.

and bone (fig. 7-22). Reported lymphangiomatosis is histologically heterogeneous and varies from lymphangioma-like to lymphangioendothelioma-like (119,120). These pathologic features are discussed above with the corresponding histopathologic entities.

Treatment and Prognosis. The treatment is often problematic. Surgery may include local resections, and in extreme cases, amputations for massive extremity lesions. Low-dose radiotherapy has been used in thoracic involvement. Modern drug treatment options include interferon alpha 2b, antibody-based or other antiangiogenic therapy (bevacizumab, thalidomide), and MTOR inhibitors (sirolimus). The prognosis varies and is better in extremity-based lesions. Extensive thoracic involvement is associated with significant mortality (118).

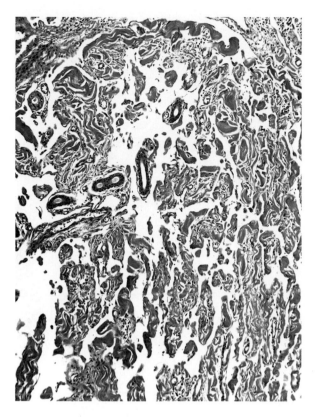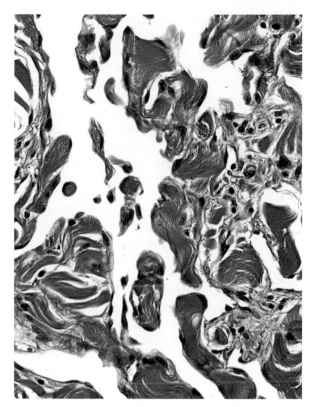

Figure 7-23

LYMPHANGIOENDOTHELIOMA

Left, Right: Anastomosing lymphatic-like vessels are lined by slightly prominent endothelial cells with limited atypia. These vessels permeate normal tissues leaving islands of skin adnexa inside the lesion.

LYMPHANGIOENDOTHELIOMA (ACQUIRED PROGRESSIVE LYMPHANGIOMA)

Definition. *Lymphangioendothelioma* is a benign, superficial lymphatic vascular tumor composed of anastomosing lymphatic channels.

Clinical Features. Lymphangioendothelioma is a cutaneous or subcutaneous tumor. It occurs in a wide age range, from early childhood to old age, with no gender predilection. The lesion clinically forms a discolored, reddish to purplish macule or plaque or an elevated lump that may enlarge over years, sometimes exceeding 10 cm in diameter, reflecting the original name *acquired progressive lymphangioma*. Most lesions measure 2 cm or less. Multiple/multifocal lesions have been reported in some patients (121–126).

The most commonly involved cutaneous sites are upper extremity, especially shoulder and forearm, head and neck, and lower extremity and trunk. Associated malignancies (hepa-toma, pulmonary small cell cancer) precede the skin lesion by 0.5 to 2.0 years.

A clinical syndrome of multifocal lymphangioendotheliomas (*lymphangioendotheliomatosis*) with thrombocytopenia has been reported in children (125). These patients had innumerable congenital cutaneous and multiple gastrointestinal lesions with severe gastrointestinal bleeding. The histologic features differ from those of adult lymphangioendothelioma and seem to resemble those of papillary intralymphatic angioendothelioma.

Gross and Microscopic Findings. Grossly, lymphangioendothelioma often appears as porous, reflecting the abundant content of lymphatic, vascular lumens. Histologically the lesions involve the dermis, and the larger examples usually extend into the subcutis. A key feature is a permeative, anastomosing network of lymphatic vascular channels (fig. 7-23). These channels tend to run horizontally and are more open in the upper dermis and more slit-like or closed in the lower dermis. The lining cells form a single layer of attenuated lymphatic endothelial cells without mitotic activity, although the cellularity is greater than seen in a typical lymphangioma. A focal hobnail appearance and papillary intraluminal proliferation resembling papillary endothelial hyperplasia are common, and some vascular channels contain focal smooth muscle elements. The vascular channels may contain erythrocytes. Scattered lymphoid cells are often present around the vascular channels, and hemosiderin deposition is infrequent. The lining endothelial cells are positive for the panendothelial markers CD31, CD34, ERG, and FVIIIRAg, and lymphatic endothelial markers podoplanin and PROX1.

Differential Diagnosis. The presence of perivascular inflammation and multiplicity of lesions should prompt consideration of lymphangioma-like variants of Kaposi sarcoma. Immunohistochemical HHV-8 positivity is the best discriminatory marker for Kaposi sarcoma. Benign lymphangioendothelioma lacks the endothelial multilayering, nuclear atypia, and frequent mitotic activity typically seen in angiosarcoma.

Lymphangiomatosis can be histologically similar to benign lymphangioendothelioma. It differs from it by the greater extent of the lesion and prominent subcutaneous and intramuscular involvement; visceral cases are also classified as lymphangiomatosis. Some examples of lymphangiomatosis are histologically similar to lymphangioma, with a simple vascular configuration and lack of papillary elements (127,128).

Treatment and Prognosis. Lymphangioendothelioma may persist or recur after an incomplete excision, but there is no metastatic potential. Although postoperative follow-up in the published series has been of short duration, a long history of a stable lesion supports a benign process. Complete, function-preserving excision and follow-up are generally optimal.

RETIFORM HEMANGIOENDOTHELIOMA

Definition. *Retiform hemangioendothelioma* is a hemangioendothelioma variant usually occurring in the skin that contains vascular spaces in a rete testis-like pattern and prominent, partly inward protruding endothelial cells. Originally considered low-grade angiosarcoma, this tumor

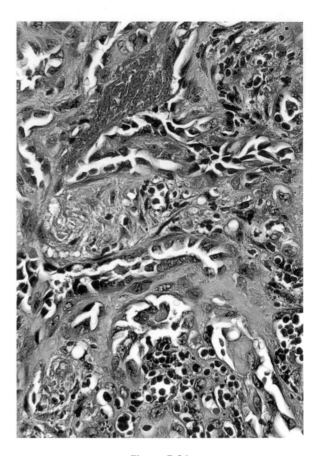

Figure 7-24

RETIFORM HEMANGIOENDOTHELIOMA

The vascular spaces are organized in a pattern resembling rete testis. Endothelial cells are inward protruding and somewhat prominent, but atypia is mild.

is currently included among borderline malignant vascular tumors.

Clinical Features. Retiform hemangioendothelioma often occurs in peripheral cutaneous locations, especially the hands and feet. It has a predilection to young adults with no gender preference. A solitary nodule is the typical manifestation, but multiple synchronous tumors have also been reported (129–131).

Gross and Microscopic Findings. Retiform hemangioendothelioma is usually small, measuring 1 to 2 cm. It is typically centered in the dermis, but often extends into the subcutis. It is composed of gaping, clustered vessels configurationally resembling rete testis structures (fig. 7-24). The endothelium is tall, with inward protruding cytoplasmic hobnail cells, which are more proliferative than those in hobnail

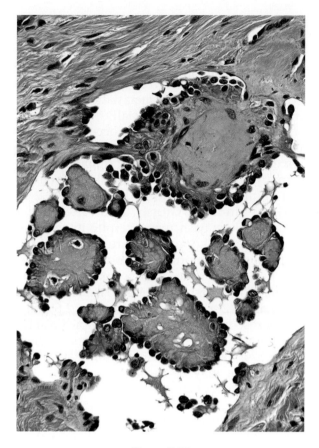

Figure 7-25

PAPILLARY INTRALYMPHATIC ANGIOENDOTHELIOMA

Intravascular papillary units are lined by mildly proliferative endothelial cells in a rosette-like pattern.

hemangioma. Focal solid areas are present in some tumors. Endothelial atypia and mitotic activity are scant. The endothelial cells are typically positive for podoplanin and PROX1 transcription factor, indicating a lymphatic endothelial-like phenotype (132).

Differential Diagnosis. The lesions are more extensive and endothelial cells are more prominent and proliferative than in hobnail hemangioma. Those lesions that contain intraluminal papillary proliferations overlap with papillary intralymphatic lymphangioendothelioma (133).

Treatment and Prognosis. Complete function-preserving excision is appropriate since this tumor has some potential to recur or persist. There is no distant metastatic potential, however, although regional lymph node involvement has been reported (129).

PAPILLARY INTRALYMPHATIC ANGIOENDOTHELIOMA

Definition. *Papillary intralymphatic angioendothelioma* is a lymphatic vessel-related vascular tumor with distinctive intraluminal proliferations containing endothelial cells in pseudo-rosette formations, surrounding fibrous cores. The tumor is also known as *Dabska tumor* and *Dabska hemangioendothelioma*.

Clinical Features. Most cases occur in children and young adults. The lesions usually form 1- to 3-cm subcutaneous soft tissue masses in a wide variety of anatomic regions. The spleen may also be involved (134–136).

Gross Findings. Grossly, the mass is pale tan to yellowish and appears poorly circumscribed. Dilated vascular lumens may give the cut surface a microcystic appearance.

Microscopic Findings. Histologically, the tumor is composed of anastomosing, dilated vascular channels. These often have papillary intravascular proliferations with radially arranged endothelial cells surrounding a fibrous core in a "match-stick" pattern (fig. 7-25). Lymphangioma-like components, with vascular lumens containing proteinaceous fluid and lymphocytes, are often present. Occurrence with lymphangioma has been reported (137).

Special Studies. Consistent positivity for podoplanin (D2-40), PROX1, and vascular endothelial growth factor receptor 3 is associated with a lymphatic vascular phenotype. The hyaline cores of the intravascular pseudorosette formations contain laminin- and collagen IV-positive basement membrane material.

Treatment and Prognosis. Complete excision with follow-up is the optimal treatment. Current series indicate a favorable outcome, although lymph node metastases occur rarely.

KAPOSIFORM HEMANGIOENDOTHELIOMA

Definition. *Kaposiform hemangioendothelioma* is a rare hemangioma variant with a multinodular pattern composed of vascular channels with prominent spindled pericytes.

Clinical Features. This tumor most commonly presents in the abdominal cavity and retroperitoneum of infants, but it has also been reported in peripheral soft tissue. Occurrence is essentially restricted to the pediatric age group. Large intra-abdominal lesions are commonly associated with platelet consumption coagulopathy (Kasabach-Merritt syndrome), which may be fatal. Otherwise, this tumor is benign (138–142).

Microscopic Findings. Histologically, the tumor is composed of multinodular, congealed aggregates of primitive vascular channels. These are lined by nonatypical but somewhat proliferative endothelial cells with some mitotic activity. These vascular channels are surrounded by prominent spindle-shaped pericytes, which give the lesion an overall spindle cell appearance (fig. 7-26). Erythrocyte extravasation and gross lesional hemorrhage are common features, especially in the larger abdominal lesions.

Special Studies. The endothelial component is positive for panendothelial cell markers (CD31, CD34, ERG) and for the lymphatic endothelial markers podoplanin (D2-40) and PROX1. Immunohistochemistry for α-smooth muscle actin highlights the prominent pericytic component (143).

Differential Diagnosis. The multinodular vascular proliferation in kaposiform hemangioendothelioma resembles tufted angioma, which is generally composed of separate multiple dermal or subcutaneous nodules forming a "cannon ball" pattern. Although the clinical context and the overall solid mass formation differ from Kaposi sarcoma, problems with this differential diagnosis can be solved with an immunostain for HHV-8 antigens, which are detected in Kaposi sarcoma only.

Treatment and Prognosis. This tumor is benign, but complications of associated platelet consumption into the lesional vessels can cause fatal bleeding diathesis.

EPITHELIOID HEMANGIOENDOTHELIOMA

Definition. *Epithelioid hemangioendothelioma* (EHE) is a low-grade malignant vascular neoplasm composed of cords of epithelioid endothelial cells set in a prominent myxoid or hyaline extracellular matrix with variable primitive luminal formation. This tumor typically involves the walls of veins. Genetically the tumor is characterized by a *WWTR1-CAMTA1* gene fusion translocation.

Clinical Features. EHE occurs in adults of all ages and rarely in children. There is a moderate female predominance. In soft tissue locations, EHE typically presents in the deep soft tissues of the extremities, forming ill-defined nodular masses, but some lesions are cutaneous. The tumor also occurs in viscera, especially liver, as well as lung and bone. Clinicopathologic correlation is required to determine whether a bone lesion is primary or metastatic. Occurrence in visceral locations, especially if multifocal, should prompt a search for an occult soft tissue primary tumor or a past history thereof, as some visceral lesions are metastatic from soft tissue primary tumors (144–148). Pleural involvement can mimic malignant mesothelioma (149).

Gross Findings. Grossly, EHE varies, but is often a pale grayish mass, despite its vascular nature (fig. 7-27). Some EHEs are grossly notable by forming a hemorrhagic venous thrombosis. The tumor size varies from a small, superficial dermal nodule less than 1 cm to a deep soft tissue mass of 2 to 10 cm (median size, 2.5 cm)

Microscopic Findings. Microscopically, EHE often involves the walls and lumens of small veins, and focal to extensive hyalinization and calcification may be present (fig. 7-28). The tumor consists of clusters, cords, or sometimes more solid sheets of epithelioid to slightly spindled cells in a myxoid or collagenous matrix (fig. 7-29). The tumor cells have pale eosinophilic cytoplasm and small nuclei with delicate nucleoli, but variants with greater nuclear atypia occur. The tumor cells often have intracytoplasmic vacuoles representing primitive vascular lumens, which may contain erythrocytes. The mitotic rate is typically low (less than 2 mitoses per 10 high-power fields).

Special Studies. The lesional cells are immunohistochemically positive for the endothelial cell markers CD31 (often membrane accentuation) and ERG (nuclear labeling). Focal von Willebrand factor expression (granular cytoplasmic pattern) is common and may highlight primitive vascular lumens. Approximately half of cases are positive for CD34. Keratins are often present (AE1/AE3 cocktail and CK7 in 30 percent of cases but CK18 in nearly all cases). Epithelial membrane antigen is rarely expressed, and usually shows weak luminal staining in the intracytoplasmic vacuoles, at the most (150).

Genetics. EHE is characterized by a t(1;3)(p36;q25) reciprocal chromosomal translocation involving a fusion of the promoter of the *WWTR1* gene with the carboxyl terminus of

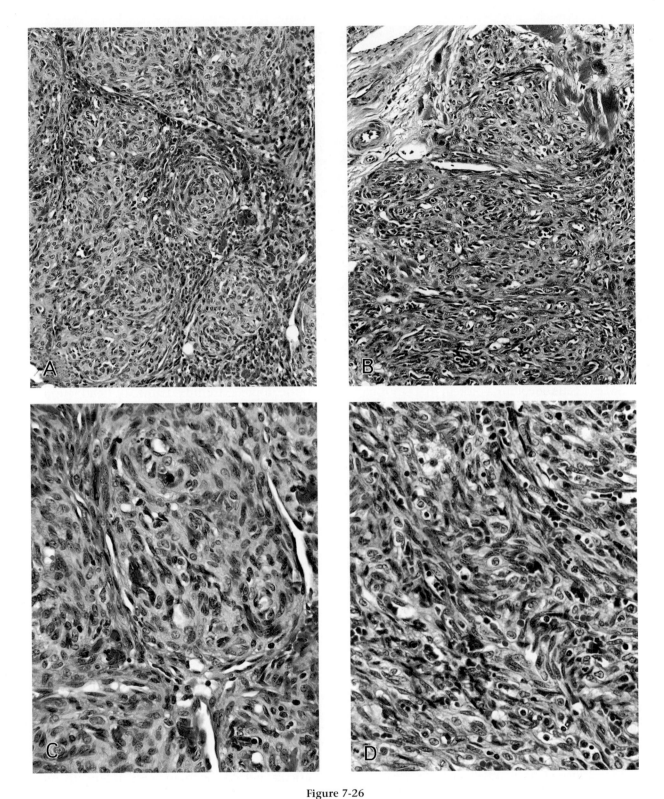

Figure 7-26

KAPOSIFORM HEMANGIOENDOTHELIOMA

A,B: The tumor contains rounded, merging clusters of capillaries with prominent spindle cell pericytes.
C,D: At high magnification, both endothelial cells and pericytes have a spindle cell appearance.

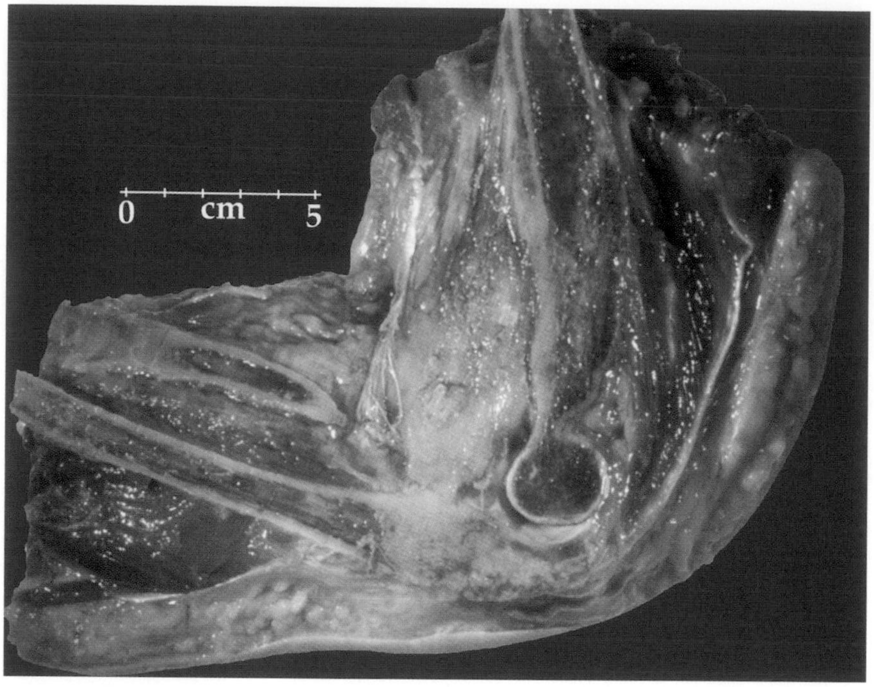

Figure 7-27

EPITHELIOID HEMANGIOENDOTHELIOMA

Grossly, this epithelioid hemangioendothelioma forms a pale mass in the deep soft tissues of the distal inner arm.

CAMTA1 gene encoding a protein that is normally expressed only in the brain. Available data indicate that this translocation is specific for EHE and is a potentially useful tumor marker (151–153).

Treatment and Prognosis. Complete excision should be performed whenever possible. The tumor has an unpredictable behavior, and up to 30 percent of patients develop metastases in regional lymph nodes, liver, bone, or lung, often long after the primary surgery.

Low cellularity and small tumor size, lack of striking atypia, and low mitotic rate correlate with better outcome, whereas nuclear atypia does not seem to have prognostic significance (154).

EPITHELIOID SARCOMA-LIKE HEMANGIOENDOTHELIOMA

Definition. *Epithelioid sarcoma-like hemangioendothelioma* is a spindle cell and epithelioid mesenchymal neoplasm that generally involves superficial soft tissues. It shows immunohistochemical reactivity for endothelial markers (CD31, ERG) and keratins AE1/AE3. This tumor has also been reported under the name *pseudomyogenic hemangioendothelioma*.

Clinical Features. The tumor has a predilection to young adults with 4 to 1 male predominance. It most commonly occurs in the lower extremity, with a minority of cases appearing in the upper extremity, trunk, or head. Tumors vary from cutaneous to subcutaneous and deep intramuscular, and usually measure 1 to 4 cm, although some superficial examples are smaller and occasional tumors larger than 5 cm. Regionally multifocal occurrence is common, and bones may also be involved (155,156).

Gross Findings. The tumor forms a gray-white nodule or ill-defined mass, which sometimes contains gross necrosis. Tumors involving skin may be ulcerated.

Microscopic Findings. Histologically, the tumor consists of cellular sheets or irregular fascicles of spindled cells, many of which have epithelioid features in their abundant, eosinophilic cytoplasm, and some cases have a distinctly epithelioid component. Despite endothelial differentiation, there is no vasoformation or hemorrhage, but focal cytoplasmic vacuolization may be present. The epithelioid cells may resemble epithelioid sarcoma cells or rhabdomyoblasts, as reflected in the alternative designations for this tumor (fig. 7-30). Focal mild pleomorphism may be present. The nuclei are vesicular with delicate nucleoli and mostly only mild atypia, although some cases show greater nuclear atypia, including focal pleomorphism. Mitotic figures are infrequent and usually fewer than 2 mitoses per 10 high-power fields. A

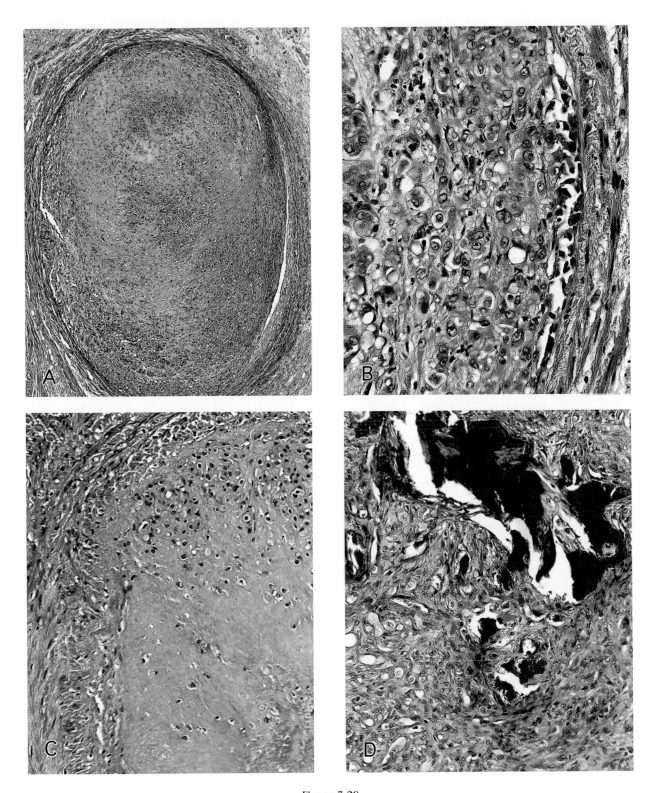

Figure 7-28

EPITHELIOID HEMANGIOENDOTHELIOMA

Epithelioid hemangioendothelioma often involves the wall and intraluminal space of veins (A). Focal cytoplasmic vacuolization (B), hyaline change (C), and focal calcification (D) are seen.

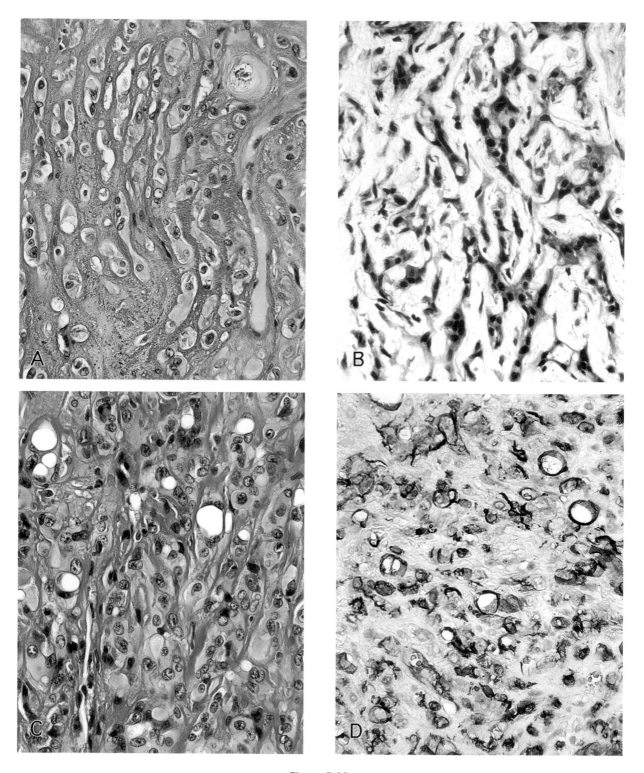

Figure 7-29

EPITHELIOID HEMANGIOENDOTHELIOMA

A–C: Corded histologic patterns are typical, and extracellular matrix varies from hyalinizing to myxoid.

D: The neoplastic cells are CD31 positive, and this marker also highlights the endothelial cell vacuolization as primitive lumen formation.

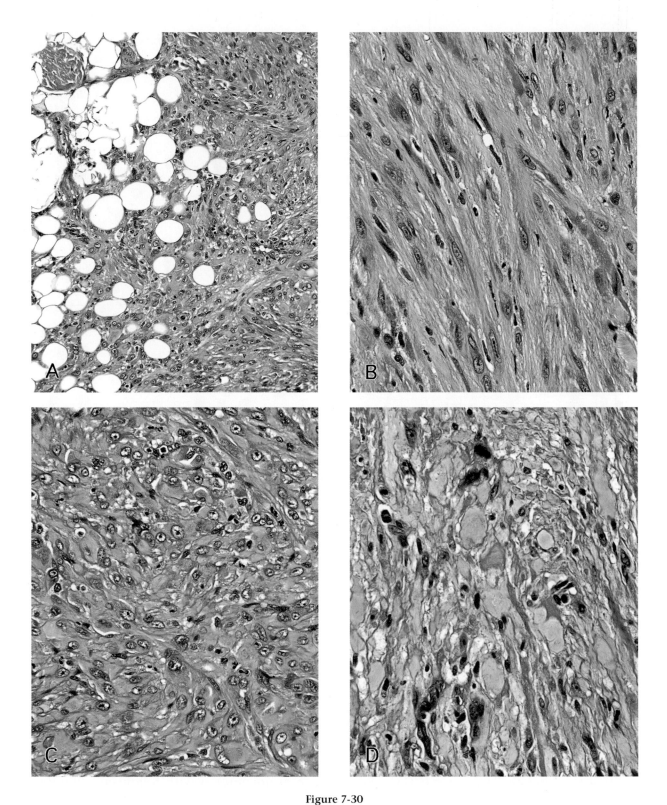

Figure 7-30

EPITHELIOID SARCOMA-LIKE HEMANGIOENDOTHELIOMA

The tumor contains spindle and epithelioid cells (A,C), some of which have prominently eosinophilic cytoplasm resembling epithelioid sarcoma cells or rhabdomyoblasts (B,D).

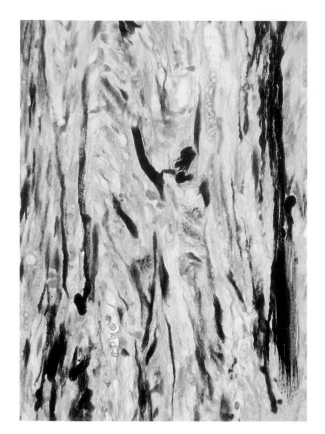
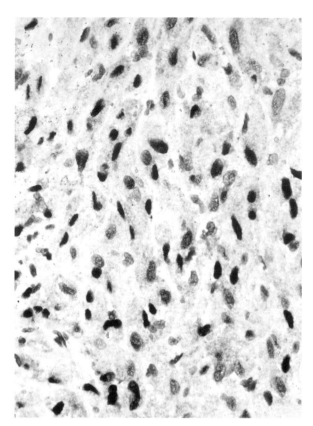

Figure 7-31

EPITHELIOID SARCOMA-LIKE HEMANGIOENDOTHELIOMA

Immunohistochemically, epithelioid sarcoma-like hemangioendothelioma is positive for keratin cocktail AE1/AE3 (left) and ETS-related gene (ERG) (right).

desmoplastic or myxoid stromal component and interstitial neutrophilic infiltration may be present and vascular invasion has been reported.

Special Studies. The tumor cells are variably positive for CD31 but consistently positive for panendothelial markers ERG and Fli-1. These tumors are also positive for AE1/AE3 keratin cocktail (fig. 7-31), for smooth muscle actin in some cases, and rarely for epithelial membrane antigen. They are negative for CD34, desmin, and S-100 protein. In contrast with epithelioid sarcoma, the tumor cells retain INI1/SMARCB1 protein expression.

Differential Diagnosis. The immunohistochemical combination of keratin AE1/AE3 positivity and endothelial markers (CD31, ERG) is unique for this tumor and helps to separate it from carcinomas. The tumor should be differentiated from skin adnexal and metastatic carcinomas and epithelioid sarcoma (the latter

is negative for INI1). Epithelioid hemangioendothelioma typically shows a microtrabecular pattern with focal vacuolization and primitive luminal formation. Epithelioid angiosarcomas show significant nuclear atypia with prominent nucleoli and frequent mitotic figures.

Treatment and Prognosis. Available follow-up data indicate an indolent course of disease. Complete excision and follow-up are generally optimal in solitary tumors and may be curative even in multifocal cases. In some cases, multifocal involvement of skeletal muscle and bone has been treated with radical surgery (amputation), or with oncologic modalities (radiation, chemotherapy). Local recurrences occur but appear uncommon with follow-up of limited duration. Lymph node and distant metastases seem rare, but nevertheless, the long-term prognosis remains uncertain due to limited long-term follow-up studies (155,156).

Table 7-2

CLINICOPATHOLOGIC VARIANTS OF ANGIOSARCOMA

Site/Circumstances	Age	Estimated Frequency	Characteristics
Scalp and face, cutaneous	Elderly	40%	Often multifocal, difficult to control surgically
Trunk and extremities, cutaneous (nonradiation associated)	Usually elderly	5%	Circumscribed, often smaller tumors
Postradiation, breast and chest wall, less often other sites	Middle age to elderly	25%	Purple skin nodules developing on radiated skin; can also involve subcutis and deeper tissues
Lymphedema associated	Varies	<5%	Develops in extremities involved by congenital or acquired lymphedema; can involve skin and deeper soft tissues
Deep soft tissue	Varies	10%	May clinically simulate hematoma or deep vascular thrombosis
Breast parenchyma	Young women	<5%	Deep, often hemorrhagic mass; can be remarkably well-differentiated, but is typically highly permeative in fat and breast parenchyma; described in detail in Fascicle of breast tumors
Body cavities	Varies	<5%	Diffuse growth on serosal surfaces that can stimulate malignant mesothelioma
In germ cell tumors	Young	<1%	Second most common somatic sarcoma, especially in mediastinal and testicular germ cell tumors
Visceral and miscellaneous sites	Varies	10-20%	Heart, liver, spleen (most common visceral sites), gastrointestinal tract, genitourinary system; described in other Fascicles

ANGIOSARCOMA

Definition. *Angiosarcoma* is a malignant vascular neoplasm essentially composed of cells with an endothelial phenotype and showing varying degrees of vasoformation. It is typically positive for panendothelial markers such as CD31 and ERG.

General Considerations. Angiosarcoma is a rare mesenchymal malignancy comprising no more than 1 to 2 percent of all sarcomas (157). Earlier reports on tumors defined without immunohistochemistry have included other malignancies with pseudoangiomatoid patterns as angiosarcomas. Also, a number of distinctive hemangioma types have been delineated that historically have sometimes been included among angiosarcomas, so that the true incidence of angiosarcoma is much lower than historical accounts suggest. Because of its common multifocality and the difficulty defining the tumor size, angiosarcoma is exempted from sarcoma staging systems.

Clinical Features. Several distinctive clinicopathologic variants related to tumor site and clinical circumstances are recognized, and these are summarized in Table 7-2. The most common is the *cutaneous angiosarcoma* of scalp and upper face in the elderly. This sarcoma forms single or multiple plaque-like or vague nodular formations that may involve large contiguous areas with multiple satellite plaques, and frequently also involves the subcutis (157–162). Cutaneous angiosarcoma in the extremities and trunk wall is much more uncommon, and is occasionally also seen in children (163,164). Xeroderma pigmentosum is one of the predisposing condition in early-onset cutaneous angiosarcoma (165).

Postradiation angiosarcoma in the breast and chest wall following breast cancer surgery and radiation is the second most common type. Radiation-associated angiosarcomas frequently have a latency of 2 to 5 years after radiation, shorter than for postradiation sarcomas in general. This may be a result of their earlier detection as superficial tumors. These angiosarcomas often form multiple cutaneous, subcutaneous, or sometimes deeper masses of varying sizes. Radiation-associated angiosarcomas also occur in other sites, especially in the lower abdominal wall following radiation for urogenital or gynecological cancer (166–170). Some atypical vascular lesions following radiation may be precursor lesions, although studies have not found a particularly high risk for angiosarcoma during limited follow-up of the presumed precursor lesions (171–174).

Lymphedema-associated angiosarcoma is presently rare. It was a notable complication of historically performed radical mastectomies combined with radical lymph node dissections. It also occurs in patients with longstanding congenital lymphedema (Milroy disease) and, rarely, in association with filarial lymphedema (175–178).

Angiosarcoma in deep soft tissues is rare. These tumors are often larger and frequently form hematomas or occlude large vessels and therefore are potentially confused with reactive processes (179,180). A rare form involves pleura or peritoneum in a diffuse manner, clinically simulating malignant mesothelioma (181–186).

A very small number of reports have described the development of angiosarcoma around a foreign body, such as shrapnel or implanted surgical device (187,188). Angiosarcoma can also develop as a rare complication of other tumors, most notably (malignant) peripheral nerve sheath tumors (188–190) and as a somatic development in germ cell tumors (191).

Gross Findings. Cutaneous angiosarcoma typically forms purplish plaques or nodules that are often ill-defined. Larger tumors often contain discontinuous multiple foci. On sectioning, angiosarcomas are typically purplish, often hemorrhagic, masses (fig. 7-32). Larger tumors, especially in the deep soft tissues, often contain necrosis and central cavitation and therefore grossly and clinically simulate a hematoma.

Microscopic Findings. Rare, purely well-differentiated angiosarcomas, which especially occur in the skin and breast parenchyma, consist of anastomosing, vasoformative units composed of mildly to moderately atypical endothelial cells (fig. 7-33). These tumors are highly permeative, especially in the subcutaneous fat. They frequently feature focal endothelial multilayering and some mitotic activity. In some cutaneous angiosarcomas, extensive lymphoid infiltration masks the endothelial malignancy.

Most angiosarcomas are high grade and composed of vasoformative and solid areas (fig. 7-34). The tumor cells vary from spindled to

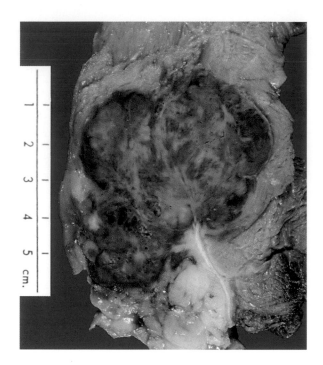

Figure 7-32

ANGIOSARCOMA

Grossly, a deep soft tissue angiosarcoma forms a hemorrhagic intramuscular mass.

ovoid and epithelioid. Tumors predominantly composed of epithelioid cells are referred to as *epithelioid angiosarcoma*. In rare instances, angiosarcomas (especially in small biopsies) are composed of entirely solid sheets or poorly differentiated round to ovoid cells. These tumors can histologically mimic lymphoma, and their identification as angiosarcoma should be based on immunohistochemical demonstration of the endothelial phenotype.

Special Studies. Immunohistochemical verification is highly desirable and usually necessary. The best panendothelial markers for this purpose are CD31 (PECAM1), ERG transcription factor, VEGFR2, and CD34 (fig. 7-35). CD31 labels nearly all angiosarcomas with a membrane and cytoplasmic pattern. However, it also detects histocytes, plasma cells, and megacaryocytes, which should be taken into account in the differential diagnosis (192,193). ERG labels nuclei in most angiosarcomas (over 95 percent) (fig. 7-35). This marker also labels extramedullary myeloid tumors and a subset of prostate carcinomas, including poorly differentiated

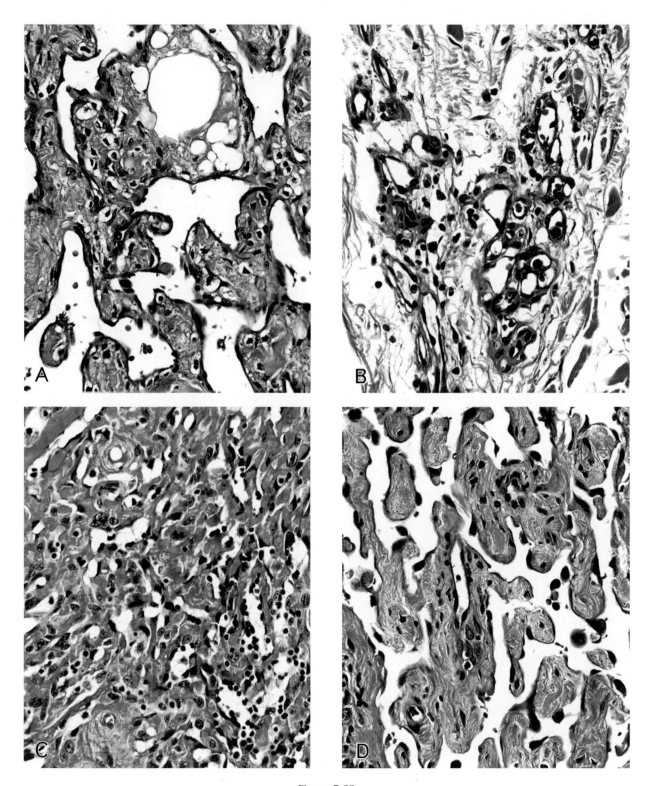

Figure 7-33

ANGIOSARCOMAS

A–D: Well-differentiated angiosarcomas show blood vessels with anastomosing or clustered nonanastomosing patterns and distinct endothelial atypia.

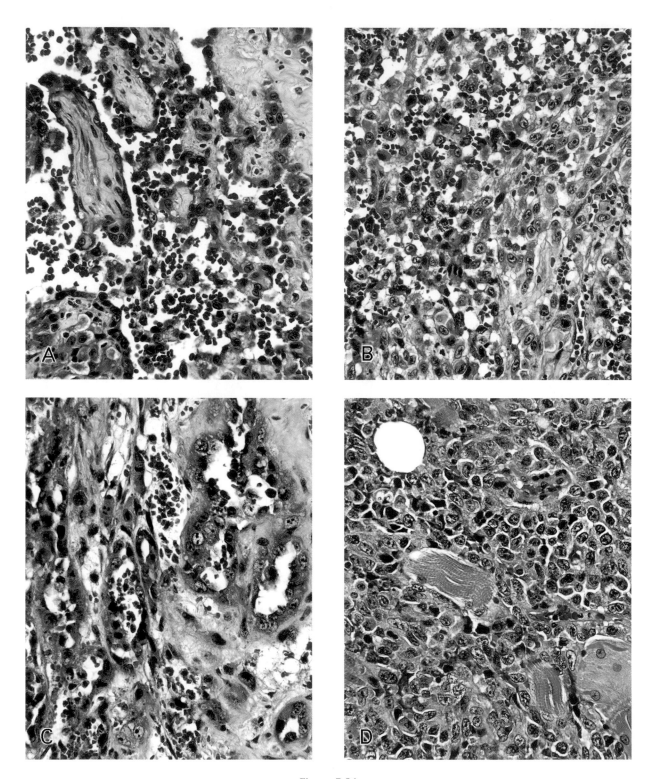

Figure 7-34

ANGIOSARCOMA

A–C. Variably epithelioid patterns are commonly seen in both cutaneous and soft tissue angiosarcomas.

D: Some angiosarcomas also contain solid nonvasoformative areas that are difficult to recognize as angiosarcoma in the absence of a differentiated component or confirmatory immunohistochemistry.

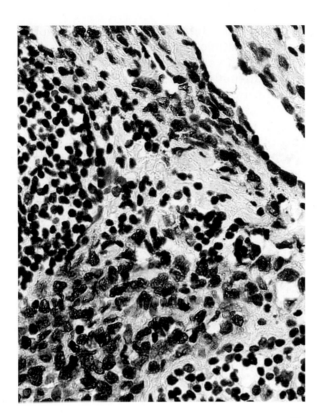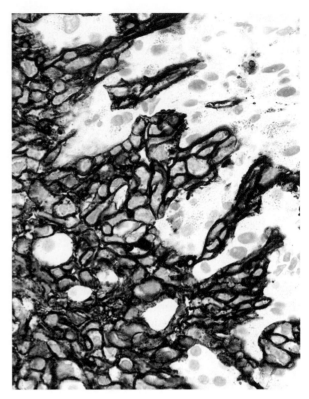

Figure 7-35

ANGIOSARCOMA

Left: Nuclear positivity for ERG transcription factor is seen in a cutaneous angiosarcoma with a prominent lymphoid response.

Right: Strong membranous CD31 immunoreactivity is shown here in an epithelioid angiosarcoma involving liver.

variants (194). CD34 positivity is variable and expressed in only 50 to 60 percent angiosarcomas. Von Willebrand factor (factor VIII-related antigen) is usually detectable in well-differentiated endothelial cells. It is often only focally, if at all, detectable in true angiosarcomas. In addition, podoplanin (D2-40) (195,196) and PROX1 transcription factor are usually detectable in cutaneous angiosarcomas and less commonly in other clinicopathologic variants. Neither marker is specific for endothelial phenotype, as many carcinomas and other malignancies are also positive. HHV-8 antigens are not detectable in angiosarcomas, an important differential diagnostic parameter in their separation from Kaposi sarcoma.

The absence of α-smooth muscle actin-positive pericytes is a clue indicating an immature vascular phenotype. It is useful in the differential diagnosis of cellular hemangioma and angiosarcoma.

Genetics. High level *MYC* gene amplification has been often detected in radiation- and lymph-edema-associated, but not sporadic, angiosarcomas (197a,b). FISH studies seem to be useful for distinguishing postradiation angiosarcoma from other atypical vascular proliferations, as the latter lack MYC amplification (197c,d).

Differential Diagnosis. Angiosarcomas have to be differentiated from a variety of hemangiomas. In general, angiosarcomas lack the well-organized vascular channels composed of both endothelial cells and pericytes. The latter component is highlighted with an α-smooth muscle actin immunostain, and its presence supports hemangioma as opposed to angiosarcoma. Specific hemangioma types that have to be separated from angiosarcoma include spindle cell hemangioma, anastomosing hemangioma, microvenular hemangioma, and Kaposiform hemangioendothelioma. Angiosarcomas typically lack the lobular organization seen in many hemangiomas, such as lobular capillary hemangioma.

Various carcinomas and malignant melanoma resemble angiosarcoma when showing hemorrhagic or pseudovascular histologic patterns. They are separated from angiosarcoma by the immunohistochemical lack of endothelial markers CD31 and ERG, and the presence of epithelial and melanocytic markers. Angiosarcomas may contain keratins, however, although they are only rarely extensively positive for AE/AE3 keratin cocktail, and usually lack epithelial membrane antigen expression (197).

Treatment and Prognosis. Smaller cutaneous and subcutaneous angiosarcomas are successfully treated with surgical excision, although locoregional recurrences and metastases may occur. Larger tumors involving scalp and face are difficult to eradicate even by large excisions, and these tumors typically show positive surgical margins. Tumor differentiation may not correlate with prognosis. Some success has been had with taxane-based chemotherapy (paclitaxel). Treatment with tyrosine kinase inhibitors with specificity toward VEGFR2 is a new, targeted therapy approach. In general, the prognosis of patients with angiosarcoma is poor, and metastases often develop in lung, bones, body cavities, and distant soft tissue and cutaneous sites.

KAPOSI SARCOMA

Definition. *Kaposi sarcoma* is a malignant spindle cell vascular endothelial tumor primarily involving the skin and strongly associated with human HHV-8 and immunosuppression.

Clinical Features. Kaposi sarcoma occurs in four clinicopathologic forms: 1) classic (chronic) with predilection for Mediterranean and Ashkenazi Jewish populations; 2) epidemic, associated with the acquired immunodeficiency syndrome (AIDS); 3) endemic in Africa, non-AIDS associated; and 4) other, mainly iatrogenic immunosuppression associated. The histologic features of the different forms are essentially identical. All these forms are associated with HHV-8 infection of the endothelial cells, a gamma herpesvirus that is greatly promoted by immunosuppression (198–202).

Classic Kaposi sarcoma typically presents in adults over 60 years, with a strong (10 to 1) male predominance. The AIDS-associated form, including the rapidly lethal disseminated form, occurs in all ages but is now less common with the antiretroviral therapies. In the classic form, single or multiple, purple to reddish skin lesions develop predominantly in the distal parts of the lower extremities, sometimes in the hands and occasionally in other acral sites.

AIDS-associated tumors involve a wide variety of sites in addition to skin, especially oral and gastrointestinal mucosae, and lymph nodes. Advanced disease can involve multiple internal organs, such as lung, intestine, abdominal cavity, bone, and rarely, deep soft tissues (203).

Endemic Kaposi sarcoma is one of the most common cancer types in sub-Saharan equatorial Africa. It occurs in both children and adults, and varies from indolent cutaneous disease to massive nodal and internal organ involvement.

Non-AIDS immunosuppression-associated Kaposi sarcoma mainly occurs in solid organ transplant patients who receive immunosuppressive drugs. It probably is reactivated HHV-8 infection triggered by immunosuppression, in view of its more common occurrence in patient populations with a higher incidence of HHV-8 infection (204,205).

Gross and Microscopic Findings. The skin lesions develop through several stages: patch, plaque-like, and nodular. The early lesion is a macular patch with no visible tumor formation (206,207). It may be difficult to diagnose, even histologically, because it merely consists of dilated, irregularly shaped vascular channels, perivascular lymphocytes, and plasma cells, resembling a reactive inflammatory process, lymphangioma, or hemangioma (fig. 7-36). Small clusters of atypical spindle cells, intravascular protrusion of spindle cells (promontory sign), and focal lymphoplasmacytic infiltration are signs that should prompt immunohistochemical testing for HHV-8 for confirmation. The plaque lesion is intermediate to the patch and nodular lesion, and has a richer spindle cell component that gradually evolves into a nodule.

The grossly purplish nodular, often elevated cutaneous lesion is the classic manifestation of Kaposi sarcoma. It may grossly resemble lobular capillary hemangioma. Histologically, however, the lesion is composed of irregular fascicles of mildly atypical cells forming cleft-like spaces often containing erythrocytes (fig. 7-37A,B). Cytoplasmic pink periodic acid–Schiff (PAS)-positive hyaline globules are formed by degenerating erythrocytes

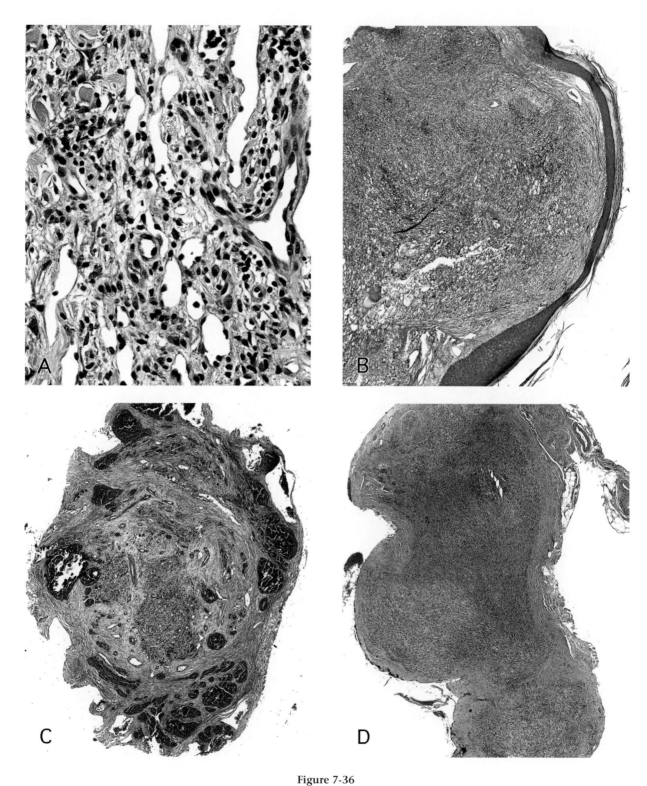

Figure 7-36

KAPOSI SARCOMA

A: The patch stage of Kaposi sarcoma shows lymphangioma-like features, but a subtle spindle cell population and interstitial lymphoplasmacytoid infiltration are present.

B–D: Examples of nodular Kaposi sarcomas. Some histologically simulate hemangiomas (C).

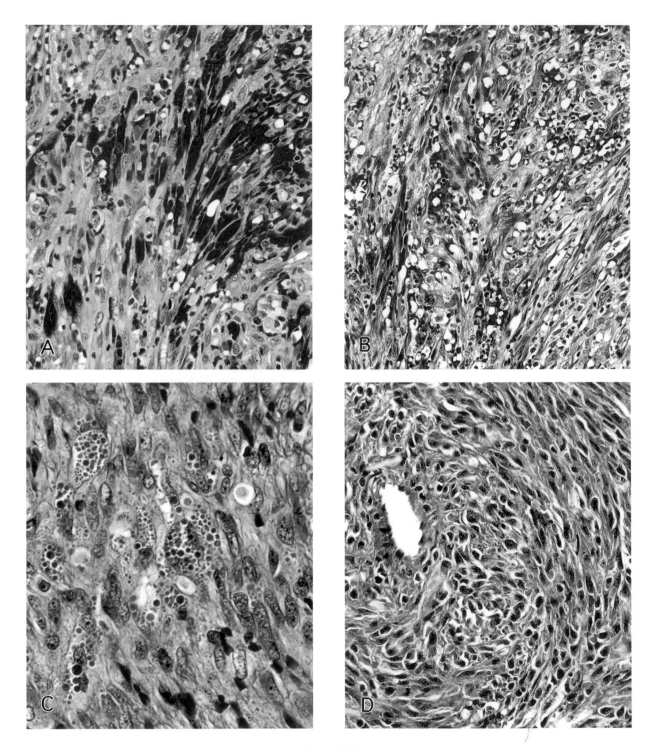

Figure 7-37

KAPOSI SARCOMA

A,B: Nodular Kaposi sarcoma contains an atypical spindle cell proliferation that has mildly vasoformative and fascicular features.

C: Cytoplasmic hyaline globules are typical although not totally diagnostic for Kaposi sarcoma.

D: Some forms of aggressive Kaposi sarcoma form solid sheets of sarcomatoid spindle cells, simulating other soft tissue sarcomas.

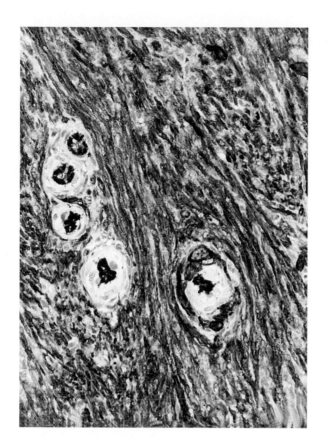 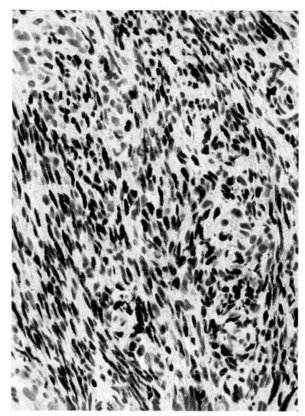

Figure 7-38

KAPOSI SARCOMA

The cytoplasm is positive for CD34 (left) and the nucleus is positive for human herpesvirus 8 (HHV-8) (right).

and are seen in most lesions (fig. 7-37C) (208). A solid spindle cell sarcomatous appearance may be seen in advanced tumors (fig. 7-37D).

Special Studies. Nuclear positivity for HHV-8 latent nuclear antigen-1 (LNA-1) is detectable in almost all cases (fig. 7-38). The neoplastic spindle cells have an endothelial phenotype and are positive for panendothelial markers CD31, CD34, and ERG and for the lymphatic endothelial markers podoplanin (D240), VEGFR3, and PROX1. The tumor cells are negative for S-100 protein, actins, desmin, keratins, and epithelial membrane antigen, which helps to separate Kaposi sarcoma from smooth muscle, myofibroblastic, and epithelial neoplasms (209–212).

Differential Diagnosis. Benign cutaneous lesions that may simulate Kaposi sarcoma include acral angiodermatitis, lobular capillary hemangioma/pyogenic granuloma, and various other hemangiomas. These typically contain more developed capillary vessels, whose endothelia

lack HHV-8 immunoreactivity. Spindle cell vascular transformation of lymph nodes occurring in association with metastatic carcinomas and other benign angiomatous proliferations involving lymph nodes should not be confused with Kaposi sarcoma; these lesions are negative for HHV-8 (213,214).

Advanced Kaposi sarcoma with extensive organ involvement may histologically resemble other sarcomas, especially angiosarcoma or leiomyosarcoma, or gastrointestinal stromal tumor. Immunohistochemistry for endothelial markers and HHV-8 is decisive.

Treatment and Prognosis. Chronic Kaposi sarcoma is usually clinically indolent, although the tumors are typically multifocal and recur locally. Local excision and radiation therapy in some cases usually keep the tumor under satisfactory control. Reversal of immunosuppression is a major contributor in the treatment of immunosuppression-associated Kaposi sarcoma.

REFERENCES

Papillary Endothelial Hyperplasia

1. Kuo TT, Sayers CP, Rosai J. Masson's "vegetant intravascular hemangioendothelioma:" a lesion often mistaken for angiosarcoma: study of seventeen cases located in the skin and soft tissues. Cancer 1976;38:1227-1236.
2. Clearkin KP, Enzinger FM. Intravascular papillary endothelial hyperplasia. Arch Pathol Lab Med 1976;100:441-444.
3. Hashimoto H, Daimaru Y, Enjoji M. Intravascular papillary endothelial hyperplasia. A clinicopathologic study of 91 cases. Am J Dermatopathol 1983;5:539-546.
4. Amérigo J, Berry CL. Intravascular papillary endothelial hyperplasia in the skin and subcutaneous tissue. Virchows Arch A Pathol Anat Histol 1980;387;81-90.

Microvenular Hemangioma

5. Hunt SJ, Santa Cruz DJ, Barr RJ. Microvenular hemangioma. J Cutan Pathol 1991;18:235-240.
6. Aloi F, Tomasini C, Pippione M. Microvenular hemangioma. Am J Dermatopathol 1993;15:534-538.
7. Xu XL, Xu CR, Chen H, et al. Eruptive microvenular hemangiomas in 4 Chinese patients: clinicopathologic correlation and review of literature. Am J Dermatopathol 2010;32:837-840.

Cutaneous Arteriovenous Hemangioma

8. Girard C, Graham J, Johnson WC. Arteriovenous hemangioma (artriovenous shunt). A clinicopathological and histochemical study. J Cutan Pathol 1974;1:73-87.
9. Carapeto FJ, Garcia-Perez A, Winkelmann RK. Acral arteriovenous tumor. Acta Dermatovener 1977;157:155-158.
10. Connelly MG, Winkelmann RK. Acral arteriovenous tumor. A clinicopathologic review. Am J Surg Pathol 1985;9:15-21.

Epithelioid Hemangioma

11. Castro C, Winkelmann RK. Angiolymphoid hyperplasia with eosinophilia in the skin. Cancer 1974;34:1696-1705.
12. Morton K, Robertson AJ, Hadden W. Angiolymphoid hyperplasia with eosinophilia: report of a case arising from the radial artery. Histopathology 1987;11:963-969.
13. Olsen TG, Helwig EB. Angiolymphoid hyperplasia with eosinophilia. A clinicopathologic study of 116 patients. J Am Acad Derrmatol 1985:12;781-796.
14. Rosai J. Angiolymphoid hyperplasia with eosinophilia of the skin. Its nosological position in the spectrum of histiocytoid hemangioma. Am J Dermatol 1982;4:175-184.
15. Wells GC, Whimster IW. Subcutaneous angiolymphoid hyperplasia with eosinophilia. Br J Dermatol 1969;81:1-15.
16. Bendl BJ, Asano K, Lewis RJ. Nodular angioblastic hyperplasia with eosinophilia and lymphofolliculosis. Cutis 1977;19:327-329.
17. Reed RJ, Terazakis N. Subcutaneous angioblastic lymphoid hyperplasia with eosinophilia (Kimura's disease). Cancer 1972;29:489-497.
18. Eady RA, Jones EW. Pseudopyogenic granuloma: enzyme histochemical and ultrastructural study. Hum Pathol 1977;8:653-668.
19. Kandii E. Dermal angiolymphoid hyperplasia with eosinophilia versus pseudopyogenic granuloma. Br J Dermatol 1970;83:405-408.
20. Peterson WC Jr, Fusaro RM, Goltz RW. Atypical pyogenic granuloma; a case of benign hemangioendotheliosis. Arch Dermatol 1964;90:197-201.
21. Jones EW, Bleehen SS. Inflammatory angiomatous nodules with abnormal blood vessels occurring about the ears and scalp (pseudo or atypical pyogenic granuloma). Br J Dermatol 1969;81:804-816.
22. Allen PW, Ramakrishna B, MacCormac LB. The histiocytoid hemangiomas and other controversies. Pathol Annu 1992;27(Part 2):51-87.
23. Googe PB, Harris NL, Mihm MC Jr. Kimura's disease and angiolymphoid hyperplasia with eosinophilia: two distinct histopathological entities. J Cutan Pathol 1987;14:263-271.
24. Kung IT, Gibson JB, Bannatyne PM. Kimura's disease: a clinicopathological study of 21 cases and its distinction from angiolymphoid hyperplasia with eosinophilia. Pathology 1984;16:39-44.
25. Kuo TT, Shih LY, Chan HL. Kimura's disease. Involvement of regional lymph nodes and distinction from angiolymphoid hyperplasia with eosinophilia. Am J Surg Pathol 1988;12:843-854.
26. Tsang WY, Chan JK. The family of epithelioid vascular tumors. Histol Histopathol 1993;8:187-212
27. Urabe A, Tsuneyoshi M, Enjoji M. Epithelioid hemangioma versus Kimura's disease. A comparative clinicopathologic study. Am J Surg Pathol 1987;11:758-766.
28. Rosai J, Gold J, Landy R. The histiocytoid hemangiomas. A unifying concept embracing several previously described entities of the skin, soft tissue, large vessels, bone, and heart. Hum Pathol 1979;10:707-730.

29. Fetsch JF, Weiss SW. Observations concerning the pathogenesis of epithelioid hemangioma (angiolymphoid hyperplasia). Mod Pathol 1991;4:449-455.

30. Burke AP, Jarvelainen H, Kolodgie FD, Goel A, Wight TN, Virmani R. Superficial pseudoaneurysms: clinicopathologic aspects and involvement of extracellular matrix proteoglycans. Mod Pathol 2004;17:482-488.

31. Floris G, Deraedt K, Samson I, Brys P, Sciot R. Epithelioid hemangioma of bone: a potentially metastasizing tumor? Int J Surg Pathol 2006;14:9-15.

32. Nielsen GP, Srivastava A, Kattapuram S, et al. Epithelioid hemangioma of bone revisited: a study of 50 cases. Am J Surg Pathol 2009;33:270-277.

33. O'Connell JX, Kattapuram SV, Mankin HJ, Bhan AK, Rosenberg AE. Epithelioid hemangioma of bone. A tumor often mistaken for low-grade angiosarcoma or malignant hemangioendothelioma. Am J Surg Pathol 1993;17:610-617.

34. Evans HL, Raymond AK, Ayala AG. Vascular tumors of bone: a study of 17 cases other than ordinary hemangioma, with an evaluation of the relationship of hemangioendothelioma of bone to epithelioid hemangioma, epithelioid hemangioendothelioma, and high-grade angiosarcoma. Hum Pathol 2003;34:680-689.

35. Evans HL. Expert commentary 1. Int J Surg Pathol 2006;14:16.

36. Rosenberg AE. Expert commentary 2. Int J Surg Pathol 2006;14:17-20.

37. Fetsch JF, Sesterhenn IA, Miettinen M, Davis CJ Jr. Epithelioid hemangioma of the penis: a clinicopathologic and immunohistochemical analysis of 19 cases, with special reference to exuberant examples often confused with epithelioid hemangioendothelioma and epithelioid angiosarcoma. Am J Surg Pathol 2004;28:523-533.

38. Srigley JR, Ayala AG, Ordóñez NG, van Nostrand AW. Epithelioid hemangioma of the penis. A rare and distinctive lesion. Arch Pathol Lab Med 1985;109:51-54.

39. Mehregan AH, Shapiro L. Angiolymphoid hyperplasia with eosinophilia. Arch Dermatol 1971;103:50-57.

40. Brenn T, Fletcher CD. Cutaneous epithelioid angiomatous nodule: a distinct lesion in the morphologic spectrum of epithelioid vascular tumors. Am J Dermatol 2004;26:14-21.

41. Deyrup AT, Tighiouart M, Montag AG, Weiss SW. Epithelioid hemangioendothelioma of soft tissue: a proposal for risk stratification based on 49 cases. Am J Surg Pathol 2008;32:924-927.

42. Mentzel T, Beham A, Calonje E, Katenkamp D, Fletcher CD. Epithelioid hemangioendothelioma of skin and soft tissues: clinicopathologic and immunohistochemical study of 30 cases. Am J Surg Pathol 1997;21:363-374.

43. Weiss SW, Enzinger FM. Epithelioid hemangioendothelioma: a vascular tumor often mistaken for a carcinoma. Cancer 1982;50:970-981.

44. Weiss SW, Ishak KG, Dail Dh, Sweet DE, Enzinger FM. Epithelioid hemangioendothelioma and related lesions. Semin Diagn Pathol 1986;3:259-287.

45. Eusebi V, Carcangiu ML, Dina R, Rosai J. Keratin-positive epithelioid angiosarcoma of the thyroid. A report of four cases. Am J Surg Pathol 1990;14:737-747.

46. Meis-Kindblom JM, Kindblom LG. Angiosarcoma of soft tissue: a study of 80 cases. Am J Surg Pathol 1998;22:683-697.

47. Wenig BM, Abbondanzo SL, Heffess CS. Epithelioid angiosarcoma of the adrenal glands. A clinicopathologic study of nine cases with a discussion of the implications of finding "epithelial-specific" markers. Am J Surg Pathol 1994;18:62-73.

Glomeruloid Hemangioma

48. Chan PT, Lee KC, Chong LY, Lo KK, Cheung YF. Glomeruloid haemangioma with cerebriform morphology in a patient with POEMS syndrome. Clin Exp Dermatol 2006;31:775-777.

49. Chung WK, Lee DW, Yang JH, Lee MW, Choi JH, Moon KC. Glomeruloid hemangioma as a very early presenting sign of POEMS syndrome. J Cutan Pathol 2009;36:1126-1128.

50. Ferran M, Gimenez-Arnau AM. Multiple eruptive angiomatous lesions in a patient with multiple myeloma. Glomeruloid hemangiomas associated with POEMS syndrome. Arch Dermatol 2006;142:1501-1506.

51. Lee H, Meier FA, Ma CK, Ormsby AH, Lee MW. Eosinophilic globules in 3 cases of glomeruloid hemangioma of the head and neck: a characteristic offering more evidence for thanatosomes with or without POEMS. Am J Dermatol 2008;30:539-544.

52. Perdaens C, De Raeve H, Goossens A, Sennesael J. POEMS syndrome characterized by glomeruloid angioma, osteosclerosis and multicentric Castleman disease. J Eur Acad Dermatol Venereol 2006;20:480-481.

53. Phillips JA, Dixon JE, Richardson JB, Fabre VC, Callen JP. Glomeruloid hemangioma leading to a diagnosis of POEMS syndrome. J Am Acad Dermatol 2006;55:149-152.

54. Obermoser G, Larcher C, Sheldon JA, Sepp N, Zelger B. Absence of human herpesvirus-8 in glomeruloid hemangiomas associated with POEMS syndrome and Castleman's disease. Br J Dermatol 2003;148:1276-1278.

55. Forman SB, Tyler WB, Ferringer TC, Elston DM. Glomeruloid hemangiomas without POEMS syndrome: series of three cases. J Cutan Pathol 2007;34:956-957.

56. González-Guerra E, Haro MR, Fariña MC, Martín L, Manzarbeitia L, Requena L. Glomeruloid haemangioma is not always associated with POEMS syndrome. Clin Exp Dermatol 2009;34:800-803.

57. Piña-Oviedo S, López-Patiño S, Ortiz-Hidalgo C. Glomeruloid hemangioma localized to the skin of the trunk with no clinical features of POEMS syndrome. Int J Dermatol 2006;45:1449-1450.

58. Vélez D, Delgado-Jiménez Y, Fraga J. Solitary glomeruloid haemangioma without POEMS syndrome. J Cutan Pathol 2005;32:449-452.

59. Dispenzieri A, Kyle RA, Lacy MQ, et al. POEMS syndrome: definitions and long-term outcome. Blood 2003;101:2496-2506.

60. Frizzera G. Castleman's disease and related disorders. Semin Diagn Pathol 1988;5:346-364.

61. Nakanishi T, Sobue I, Toyokura Y, et al. The Crow-Fukase syndrome: a study of 102 cases in Japan. Neurology 1984;34:712-720.

62. Takatsuki K, Sanada I. Plasma cell dyscrasia with polyneuropathy and endocrine disorder: clinical and laboratory features of 109 reported cases. Jpn J Clin Oncol 1983;13:543-556.

63. Scheers C, Kolivras A, Corbisier A, et al. POEMS syndrome revealed by multiple glomeruloid angiomas. Dermatology 2002;204:311-314.

64. Chan JK, Fletcher CD, Hicklin GA, Rosai J. Glomeruloid hemangioma. A distinctive cutaneous lesion of multicentric Castleman's disease associated with POEMS syndrome. Am J Surg Pathol 1990;14:1036-1046.

65. Zak FG, Solomon A, Fellner MJ. Vicero-cutaneous angiomatosis with dysproteinaemic phagocytosis: its relation to Kaposi's sarcoma and lymphoproliferative disorders. J Pathol 1966;92:594-599.

66. Ide F, Mishima K, Saito I. Papillary hemangioma on the face. J Cutan Pathol 2009;36:601-602.

67. Suurmeijer AJ, Fletcher CD. Papillary hemangioma. A distinctive cutaneous haemangioma of the head and neck area containing eosinophilic hyaline globules. Histopathology 2007;51:638-648.

Hobnail Hemangioma

68. Trindade F, Kutzner H, Tellechea O, Requena L, Colmenero I. Hobnail hemangioma reclassified as superficial lymphatic malformation: a study of 52 cases. J Am Acad Dermatol 2012;66:112-115.

69. Mentzel T, Partanen T, Kutzner H. Hobnail hemangioma ("targetoid hemosiderotic hemangioma"): clinicopathologic and immunohistochemical analysis of 62 cases. J Cutan Pathol 1999;26:279-286.

70. Franke FE, Steger K, Marks A, Kutzner H, Mentzel T. Hobnail hemangiomas (targetoid hemosiderotic hemangiomas) are true lymphangiomas. J Cutan Pathol 2004;31:362-367.

71. Santa-Cruz DJ, Aronberg J. Targetoid hemosiderotic hemangioma. J Am Acad Dermatol 1988;19:550-558.

72. Guillou L, Calonje E, Speight P, Rosai J, Fletcher CD. Hobnail hemangioma: a pseudomalignant vascular lesion with a reappraisal of targetoid hemosiderotic hemangioma. Am J Surg Pathol 1999;23:97-105.

Juvenile Capillary Hemangioma

73. Coffin CM, Dehner LP. Vascular tumors in children and adolescents: a clinicopathologic study of 228 tumors in 222 patients. Pathol Annu 1993;1:97-120.

74. Takahashi K, Mulliken JB, Kozakewich HP, Rogers RA, Folkman J, Ezekowitz RA. Cellular markers that distinguish the phases of hemangioma during infancy and childhood. J Clin Invest 1994;93:2357-2364.

75. Smolinski KN, Yan AC. Hemangiomas of infancy: clinical and biological characteristics. Clin Pediatr (Phila) 2005;44:747-766.

76. Enjolras O, Riche MC, Merland JJ, Escande JP. Management of alarming hemangiomas of infancy: a review of 25 cases. Pediatrics 1990;85:491-498.

77. North PE, Waner M, Mizeracki A, Mihm M Jr. GLUT1: a newly discovered immunohistochemical marker for juvenile hemangiomas. Hum Pathol 2000;31:11-22.

78. North PE, Waner M, Mizeracki A, et al. A unique microvascular phenotype shared by juvenile hemangiomas and human placenta. Arch Dermatol 2001;137:559-570.

79. Gonzalez-Crussi F, Reyes-Mugica M. Cellular hemangiomas of infancy ("hemangioendotheliomas"). Light microscopic, immunohistochemical, and ultrastructural observations. Am J Surg Pathol 1991;15.769-778.

80. Berenguer B, Mulliken JB, Enjolras O, et al. Rapidly involuting congenital hemangioma: clinical and histopathologic features. Pediatr Dev Pathol 2003;6:495-510.

81. North PE, Waner M, James CA, Mizeracki A, Frieden IJ, Mihm MC Jr. Congenital nonprogressive hemangioma. A distinct clinicopathologic entity unlike infantile hemangioma. Arch Pathol 2001;137:1607-1620.

Lobular Capillary Hemangioma

82. Patrice SJ, Wiss K, Mulliken J. Pyogenic granuloma (lobular capillary hemangioma) pathologic study of 178 cases. Pediatr Dermatol 1991;8:267-276.

83. Bhaskar SN, Jacoway JR. Pyogenic granuloma—clinical features, incidence, histology, and result of treatment: report of 242 cases. J Oral Surg 1966;24:391-398.

84. Puxeddu R, Berlucchi M, Ledda GP, Parodo G, Farina N, Nicolai P. Lobular capillary hemangioma of the nasal cavity: a retrospective study on 40 patients. Am J Rhinol 2006;20:480-484.

85. Mills SE, Cooper PH, Fechner RE. Lobular capillary hemangioma: the underlying lesion of pyogenic granuloma. A study of 73 cases from the oral and nasal mucous membranes. Am J Surg Pathol 1980;4:471-479.

86. Cooper PH, Mills SE. Subcutaneous granuloma pyogenicum. Lobular capillary hemangioma. Arch Dermatol 1982;118:30-33.

87. Warner J, Jones EW. Pyogenic granuloma with multiple satellites. A report of 11 cases. Br J Dermatol 1968;80:218-227.

88. Toida M, Hasegawa T, Watanabe F, et al. Lobular capillary hemangioma of the oral mucosa: clinicopathological study of 43 cases with a special reference to immunohistochemical characterization of the vascular elements. Pathol Int 2003;53:1-7.

89. Cooper PH, McAllister HA, Helwig EB. Intravenous pyogenic granuloma. A study of 18 cases. Am J Surg Pathol 1979;3:221-228.

90. Ulbright TM, Santa Cruz DJ. Intravenous pyogenic granuloma: case report with ultrastructural findings. Cancer 1980;45:1646-1652.

Spindle Cell Hemangioma

91. Weiss SW, Enzinger FM. Spindle cell hemangioendothelioma. A low-grade angiosarcoma resembling a cavernous hemangioma and Kaposi's sarcoma. Am J Surg Pathol 1986;10:521-530.

92. Perkins P, Weiss SW. Spindle cell hemangioendothelioma. An analysis of 78 cases with reassessment of its pathogenesis and biologic behavior. Am J Surg Pathol 1996;20:1196-1204.

93. Scott GA, Rosai J. Spindle cell hemangioendothelioma. Report of seven additional cases of a recently described vascular neoplasm. Am J Dermatopathol 1988;10:281-288.

94. Ding J, Hashimoto H, Imayama S, Tsuneyoshi M, Enjoji M. Spindle cell haemangioendothelioma: probably a benign vascular lesion not a low-grade angiosarcoma. A clinicopathological, ultrastructural and immunohistochemical study. Virchows Arch A Pathol Anat Histopathol 1992;420:77-85.

95. Fukunaga M, Ushigome S, Nikaido T, Ishikawa E, Nakamori K. Spindle cell hemangioendothelioma: an immunohistochemical and flow cytometric study of six cases. Pathol Int 1995;45:589-595.

96. Fanburg JC, Meis-Kindblom JM, Rosenberg AE. Multiple enchondromas associated with spindle cell hemangioendotheliomas. An overlooked variant of Maffucci's syndrome. Am J Surg Pathol 1995;19:1029-1038.

97. Lewis RJ, Ketcham AS. Mafucci's syndrome: functional and neoplastic sugnificance. Case report and review of the literature. J Bone Joint Surg Am 1973;55A:1465-1479.

97a. Pansuriya TC, van Eijk R, d'Adamo P, et al. Somatic mosaic IDH1 and IDH2 mutations are associated with enchondroma and spindle cell hemangioma in Ollier disease and Maffucci syndrome. Nat Genet 2011;43:1256-1261.

97b. Kurek KC, Pansuriya TC, van Ruler MA, et al. R132C IDH1 mutations are found in spindle cell hemangiomas and not in other vascular tumors or malformations. Am J Pathol 2013;182:1494-1500.

Tufted Angioma

98. Jones EW, Orkin M. Tufted angioma (angioblastoma). A benign progressive angioma not to be confused with Kaposi's sarcoma or low-grade angiosarcoma. J Am Acad Dermatol 1989;20(Pt 1):214-225.

99. Alessi E, Bertani E, Sala F. Acquired tufted angioma. Am J Dermatopathol 1986;8:426-429.

100. Padilla RS, Orkin M, Rosai J. Acquired "tufted" angioma (progressive capillary hemangioma). A distinctive clinicopathologic entity related to lobular capillary hemangioma. Am J Dermatopathol 1987;9:292-300.

101. Cho KH, Kim SH, Park KC, et al. Angioblastoma (Nakagawa)—is it the same as tufted angioma? Clin Exp Dermatol 1991;16:110-113.

102. Seo SK, Suh JC, Na GY, Kim IS, Sohn KR. Kasabach-Merritt syndrome: identification of platelet trapping in a tufted angioma by immunohistochemicstry technique using monoclonal antibody to CD61. Pediatr Dermatol 1999;16:392-394.

103. Osio A, Fraitag S, Hadj-Rabia S, Bodemer C, de Prost Y, Hamel-Teillac D. Clinical spectrum of tufted angiomas in childhood: a report of 13 cases and a review of the literature. Arch Dermatol 2010;146:758-763.

Verrucous Hemangioma

104. Imperial R, Helwig EB. Verrucous hemangioma. A clinicopathological study of 21 cases. Arch Dermatol 1967;96:247-253.

105. Cruces MJ, De la Torre C. Multiple eruptive verrucous hemangiomas: a variant of multiple hemangiomatosis. Dermatologica 1985;171:106-111.

106. Puig L, Llistosella E, Moreno A, de Moragas JM. Verrucous hemangioma. J Dermatol Surg Oncol 1987;13:1089-1092.
107. Yang CH, Ohara K. Successful surgical treatment of verrucous hemangioma: a combined approach. Dermatol Surg 2002;28:913-919.
108. Tennant LB, Mulliken JB, Perez-Atayde AR, Kozakewich HP. Verrucous hemangioma revisited. Pediatr Dermatol 2006;23:208-215.

Lymphangioma (Lymphatic Malformation)

109. Radhakrishnan K, Rockson SG. The clinical spectrum of lymphatic disease. Ann NY Acad Sci 2008;1131:155-184.
110. Flanagan BP, Helwig EB. Cutaneous lymphangioma. Arch Dermatol 1977;113:24-30.
111. Alquahtani A, Nguyen LT, Flageole H, Shaw K, Laberge JM. 25 years' experience with lymphangiomas in children. J Pediatr Surg 1999:34:1164-1168.
112. Allen JG, Riall TS, Cameron JL, Askin FB, Hruban RH, Campbell KA. Abdominal lymphangiomas in adults. J Gastrointest Surg 2006;10:746-751.
113. Byrne J, Blanc WA, Warburton D, Wigger J. The significance of cystic hygroma in fetuses. Hum Pathol 1984;15:61-67.
114. Hornick JL, Fletcher CD. Intraabdominal cystic lymphangiomas obscured by marked superimposed reactive changes: analysis of a series. Hum Pathol 2005;36:426-432.
115. Partanen TA, Alitalo K, Miettinen M. Lack of lymphatic vascular specificity of vascular endothelial growth factor receptor 3 in 185 vascular tumors. Cancer 1999;86:2406-2412.
116. Kahn HJ, Bailey D, Marks A. Monoclonal antibody D2-40, a new marker of lymphatic endothelium, reacts with Kaposi sarcoma and a subset of angiosarcomas. Mod Pathol 2002;15:434-440.
117. Perkins JA, Manning SC, Tempero RM, et al. Lymphatic malformations: review of current treatment. Otolaryngol Head Neck Surg 2010:142:795-803.

Lymphangiomatosis

118. Blei F. Lymphangiomatosis: clinical overview. Lymphat Res Biol 2011;9:185-190.
119. Ramani P, Shah A. Lymphangiomatosis. Histologic and immunohistochemical analysis of four cases. Am J Surg Pathol 1993;17:329-335.
120. Gomez CS, Calonje E, Ferrar DW, Browse NL, Fletcher CD. Lymphangiomatosis of the limbs. Clinicopathologic analysis of a series with a good prognosis. Am J Surg Pathol 1995;19:125-133.

Benign Lymphangioendothelioma (Acquired Progressive Lymphangioma)

121. Watanabe M, Kishiyama K Ohkawara A. Acquired progressive lymphangioma. J Am Acad Dermatol 1983;8:663-667.
122. Tadaki T, Aiba S, Masu S, Tagami H. Acquired progressive lymphangioma as a flat erythematous patch on the abdominal wall of a child. Arch Dermatol 1988;124:699-701.
123. Ramani P, Shah A. Lymphangiomatosis. Histologic and immunohistochemical analysis of four cases. Am J Surg Pathol 1993;17:329-335.
124. Jones EW, Winkelmann RK, Zachary CB, Reda AM. Benign lymphangioendothelioma. J Am Acad Dermatol 1990;23:229-235.
125. North PE, Kahn T, Kordisco MR, Dadras SS, Detmar M, Frieden IJ. Multifocal lymphangioendotheliomatosis with thrombocytopenia: a newly recognized clinicopathological entity. Arch Dermatol 2004;140:599-606.
126. Guillou L, Fletcher CD. Benign lymphangioendothelioma (acquired progressive lymphangioma): a lesion not to be confused with well-differentiated angiosarcoma and patch stage Kaposi's sarcoma: clinicopathologic analysis of a series. Am J Surg Pathol 2000;24:1047-1057.
127. Ramani P, Shah A. Lymphangiomatosis. Histologic and immunohistochemical analysis of four cases. Am J Surg Pathol 1993;17:329-335.
128. Gomez CS, Calonje E, Ferrar DW, Browse NL, Fletcher CD. Lymphangiomatosis of the limbs. Clinicopathologic analysis of a series with a good prognosis. Am J Surg Pathol 1995; 19:125-133.

Retiform Hemangioendothelioma

129. Calonje E, Fletcher CD, Wilson-Jones E, Rosai J. Retiform hemangioendothelioma. A distinctive form of low-grade angiosarcoma delineated in a series of 15 cases. Am J Surg Pathol 1994;18:115-125.
130. Duke D, Dvorak AM, Harris TJ, Cohen LM. Multiple retiform hemangioendotheliomas. A low-grade angiosarcoma. Am J Dermatopathol 1996;18:606-610.
131. Fukunaga M, Endo Y, Masui F, Yoshikawa T, Ishikawa T, Ushigome S. Retiform hemangioendothelioma. Virchows Arch 1996;482:301-304.
132. Miettinen M, Wang ZF. Prox1 transcription factor as a marker for vascular tumors—evaluation of 314 vascular and 1086 nonvascular tumors. Am J Surg Pathol 2012;36:351-359.
133. Sanz-Trelles A, Rodrigo-Fernandez I, Ayala-Carbonero A, Contreras-Rubio F. Retiform hemangioendothelioma. A new case in a child with diffuse endovascular papillary endothelial proliferation. J Cutan Pathol 1997;24:440-444.

Papillary Intralymphatic Angioendothelioma

134. Dabska M. Malignant endovascular papillary angioendothelioma of the skin in childhood. Clinicopathologic study of 6 cases. Cancer 1969;24:503-510.
135. Schwartz RA, Dabski C, Dabska M. The Dabska tumor: a thirty-year retrospect. Dermatology 2000;201:1-5.
136. Fanburg-Smith JC, Michal M, Partanen TA, Alitalo K, Miettinen M. Papillary intralymphatic angioendothelioma (PILA): a report of twelve cases of a distinctive vascular tumor with phenotypic features of lymphatic vessels. Am J Surg Pathol 1999;23:1004-1010.
137. Emanuel PO, Lin R, Silver L, Birge MB, Shim H, Phelps RG. Dabska tumor arising in lymphangioma circumscriptum. J Cutan Pathol 2008;35:65-69.

Kaposiform Hemangioendothelioma

138. Lyons LL, North PE, Mac Moune LF, Stoler MH, Folpe AL, Weiss SW. Kaposiform hemangioendothelioma: a study of 33 cases emphasizing the pathologic, immunophenotypic, and biologic uniqueness from juvenile hemangioma. Am J Surg Pathol 2004;28:559-568.
139. Mentzel T, Mazzoleni G, Dei Tos AP, Fletcher CD. Kaposiform hemangioendothelioma in adults. Clinicopathologic and immnohistochemical analysis of three cases. Am J Clin Pathol 1997;108:450-455.
140. Deraedt K, Vander Poorten V, Van Geet C, Renard M, De Wever I, Sciot R. Multifocal Kaposiform hemangioendothelioma. Virchows Arch 2006;448:843-846.
141. Sarkar M, Mulliken JB, Kozakewich HP, Robertson RL, Burrows PE. Thrombocytopenic coagulopathy (Kasabach-Merritt phenomenon) is associated with Kaposiform hemangioendothelioma and not with common infantile hemangioma. Plastic Reconstr Surg 1997;100:1377-1386.
142. Enroljas O, Wassef M, Mazoyer E, et al. Infants with Kasabach-Merritt syndrome do not have "true" hemangiomas. J Pediatr 1997;30:631-640.
143. Debelenko LV, Perez-Atayde AR, Mulliken JB, Liang MG, Archibald TH, Kozakewich HP. D2-40 immunohistochemical analysis of pediatric vascular tumors reveals positivity in Kaposiform hemangioendothelioma. Mod Pathol 2005;18:1454-1460.

Epithelioid Hemangioendothelioma

144. Weiss SW, Enzinger FM. Epithelioid hemangioendothelioma: a vascular tumor often mistaken for a carcinoma. Cancer 1982;50:970-981.
145. Weiss SW, Ishak KG, Dail DH, Sweet DE, Enzinger FM. Epithelioid hemangioendothelioma and related lesions. Semin Diagn Pathol 1986;3:259-287.
146. Mentzel T, Beham A, Calonje E, Katenkamp D, Fletcher CD. Epithelioid hemangioendothelioma of skin and soft tissues: clinicopathologic and immunohistochemical study of 30 cases. Am J Surg Pathol 1997;21:363-374.
147. Ishak KG, Sesterhenn IA, Goodman ZD, Rabin L, Stromeyer FW. Epithelioid hemangioendothelioma of the liver: a clinicopathologic and follow-up study of 32 cases. Hum Pathol 1984;15:839-852.
148. Verbeken E, Beyls J, Moerman P, Knoackaert D, Goddeeris P, Lauweryns JM. Lung metastasis of malignant epithelioid hemangioendothelioma mimicking a primary intravascular bronchioalveolar tumor. A histologic, ultrastructural, and immunohistochemical study. Cancer 1985;55:1741-1746.
149. Zhang PJ, Livolsi VA, Brooks JJ. Malignant epithelioid vascular tumors of the pleura: report of a series and literature review Hum Pathol 2000;31:29-34.
150. Miettinen M, Fetsch JF. Distribution of keratins in normal endothelial cells and in a spectrum of vascular tumors: implications in tumor diagnosis. Hum Pathol 2000;31:1062-1067.
151. Mendlick MR, Nelson M, Pickering D, et al. Translocation t(1;3)(p36.3;q25) is a nonrandom aberration in epithelioid hemangioendothelioma. Am J Surg Pathol 2001;25:684-687.
152. Errani C, Zhang L, Sung YS, et al. A novel WWTR1-CAMTA1 gene fusion is a consistent abnormality in epithelioid hemangioendothelioma of different anatomic sites. Genes Chromosomes Cancer 2011;50:644-653.
153. Tanas MR, Sboner A, Oliveira AM, et al. Identification of a disease-defining gene fusion in epithelioid hemangioendothelioma. Sci Transl Med 2011;3:98ra82.
154. Deyrup AT, Tighiouart M, Montag AG, Weiss SW. Epithelioid hemangioendothelioma of soft tissue: a proposal for risk stratification based on 49 cases. Am J Surg Pathol 2008;32:924-927.

Epithelioid Sarcoma-Like Hemangioendothelioma

155. Billings SD, Folpe AL, Weiss SW. Epithelioid sarcoma-like hemangioendothelioma. Am J Surg Pathol 2003;27:48-57.
156. Hornick JL, Fletcher CD. Pseudomyogenic hemangioendothelioma: a distinctive, often multicentric tumor with indolent behavior. Am J Surg Pathol 2011;35:190-201.

Angiosarcoma

157. Toro JR, Travis LB, Wu HJ, Zhu K, Fletcher CD, Devesa SS. Incidence patterns of soft tissue sarcomas, regardless of primary site, in the surveillance, epidemiology, and end results program, 1978-2001: an analysis of 26,758 cases. Int J Cancer 2006;119:2922-2930.

158. Fury MG, Antonescu CR, Van Zee KJ, Brennan MF, Maki RG. A 14-year retrospective review of angiosarcoma: clinical characteristics, prognostic factors, and treatment outcomes with surgery and chemotherapy. Cancer J 2005;11:241-247.

159. Abraham JA, Hornicek EJ, Kaufman AM, et al. Treatment and outcome of 82 patients with angiosarcoma. Ann Surg Oncol 2007;14:1953-1967.

160. Fayette J, Martin E, Piperno-Neumann S, et al. Angiosarcoma: a heterogeneous group of sarcomas with specific behavior depending on primary site: a retrospective study of 161 cases. Ann Oncol 2007;18:2030-2036.

161. Morgan MB, Swann M, Somach S, Eng W, Smoller B. Cutaneous angiosarcoma: a case series with prognostic correlation. J Am Acad Dermatol 2004;50:867-874.

162. Deyrup AT, McKenney JK, Tighiouart M, Folpe AL, Weiss SW. Sporadic cutaneous angiosarcomas: a proposal for risk stratification based on 69 cases. Am J Surg Pathol 2008;32:72-77.

163. Lezama-del Valle P, Gerald WL, Tsai J, Meyers P, La Quaglia MP. Malignant vascular tumors in young patients. Cancer 1998;83:1634-1639.

164. Deyrup AT, Miettinen M, North PE, et al. Pediatric cutaneous angiosarcomas: a clinicopathologic study of 10 cases. Am J Surg Pathol 2011;35:70-75.

165. Leake J, Sheehan MP, Rampling D, Ramani P, Atherton DJ. Angiosarcoma complicating zeroderma pigmentosum. Histopathology 1992;21:179-181.

166. Moskaluk CA, Merino MJ, Danforth DN, Medeiros LJ. Low-grade angiosarcoma of the skin of the breast: a complication of lumpectomy and radiation therapy for breast carcinoma. Hum Pathol 1992;23:710-714.

167. Strobbe LJ, Peterse HL, van Tinteren H, Wijnmaalen A, Rutgers EJ. Angiosarcoma of the breast after conservation therapy for invasive cancer, the incidence and outcome. An unforeseen sequela. Breast Cancer Res Treat 1998;47:101-109.

168. Monroe AT, Feigenberg SJ, Mendenhall NP. Angosarcoma after breast-conserving therapy. Cancer 2003;97:1832-1840.

169. Billings SD, McKenney JK, Folpe AL, Hardacre MC, Weiss SW. Cutaneous angiosarcoma following breast-conserving surgery and radiation: an analysis of 27 cases. Am J Surg Pathol 2004;28:781-788.

170. Fodor J, Orosz Z, Szabo E, et al. Angiosarcoma after conservation treatment for breast carcinoma: our experience and review of the literature. J Am Acad Dermatol 2006;54:499-504.

171. Fineberg S, Rosen PP. Cutaneous angiosarcoma and atypical vascular lesions of the skin and breast after radiation therapy for breast carcinoma. Am J Clin Pathol 1994;102:757-763.

172. Sener SF. Milos S, Feldman JL, et al. The spectrum of vascular lesions in the mammary skin, including angiosarcoma, after breast conservation treatment for breast cancer. J Am Coll Surg 2001;193:22-28.

173. Brenn T, Fletcher CD. Radiation-associated cutaneous atypical vascular lesions and angiosarcoma: clinicopathological analysis of 42 cases. Am J Surg Pathol 2005;29:983-996.

174. Patton KT, Deyrup AT, Weiss SW. Atypical vascular lesions after surgery and radiation of the breast: a clinicopathologic study of 32 cases analyzing histologic heterogeneity and association with angiosarcoma. Am J Surg Pathol 2008;32:943-950.

175. Stewart FW, Treves N. Lymphangiosarcoma in postmastectomy lymphedema: a report of six cases in elephantiasis chirurgica. Cancer 1948;1:64-81.

176. Woodward AH, Ivins JC, Soule EH. Lymphangiosarcoma arising in chronic lymphedematous extremities. Cancer 1972;30:562-572.

177. Sordillo P, Chapman R, Hajdu SI, Magill GB, Golbey RB. Lymphangiosarcoma. Cancer 1981;48:1674-1679.

178. Grobmyer SR, Daly JM, Glotzback RE, Grobmyer AJ 3rd. Role of surgery in the management of postmastectomy extremity angiosarcoma (Stewart-Treves syndrome). J Surg Oncol 2000;73:182-188.

179. Meis-Kindblom JM, Kindblom LG. Angiosarcoma of soft tissue: a study of 80 cases. Am J Surg Pathol 1998;22:683-697.

180. Fletcher CD, Beham A, Bekir S, Clarke AM, Marley NJ. Epithelioid angiosarcoma of deep soft tissue: a distinctive tumor readily mistaken for an epithelial neoplasm. Am J Surg Pathol 1991;15:915-924.

181. McCaughey WT, Dardick I, Barr JR. Angiosarcoma of serous membranes. Arch Pathol Lab Med 1983;107:304-307.

182. Wolov RB, Sato N, Azumi N, Lack EE. Intraabdominal "angiosarcomatosis": report of two cases after pelvic irradiation. Cancer 1991;67:2275-2279.

183. Suzuki F, Saito A, Ishi K, Koyatsu J, Maruyama T, Suda K. Intra-abdominal angiosarcomatosis after radiotherapy. J Gastroenterol Hepatol 1999;14:289-292.

184. Lin BT, Colby T, Gown AM, et al. Malignant vascular tumors of the serous membranes mimicking mesothelioma. A report of 14 cases Am J Surg Pathol 1996;20:1431-1439.

185. Zhang PJ, Livolsi VA, Brooks JJ. Malignant epithelioid vascular tumors of the pleura: report of a series and literature review. Hum Pathol 2000;31:29-34.

186. Del Frate C, Mortele K, Zanardi R, et al. Pseudo-mesotheliomatous angiosarcoma of the chest wall and pleura. J Thorac Imaging 2003;18:200-203.

187. Jennings TA, Peterson L, Axiotis CA, Friedlander GE, Cooke RA, Rosai J. Angiosarcoma associated with foreign body material. A report of three cases. Cancer 1988;62:2436-2444.

188. Ben-Izhak O, Kerner H, Brenner B, Lichtig C. Angiosarcoma of the colon developing in a capsule of a foreign body. Report of a case with associated hemorrhagic diathesis. Am J Clin Pathol 1992;97:416-420.

189. Mentzel T, Katenkamp D. Intraneural angiosarcoma and angiosarcoma arising in benign and malignant nerve sheath tumours: clinicopathological and immunohistochemical analysis of four cases. Histopathology 1999;35:114-120.

190. Morphopoulos GD, Banerjee SS, Ali HH, et al. Malignant peripheral nerve sheath tumour with vascular differentiation: a report of four cases. Histopathology 1996;28:401-410.

191. Malagon HD, Valdez AM, Moran CA, Suster S. Germ cell tumors with sarcomatous components: a clincopathologic and immunohistochemical study of 46 cases. Am J Surg Pathol 2007;31:1356-1362.

192. Kuzu I, Bicknell R, Harris AL, Jones M, Gatter KC, Mason DY. Heterogeneity of vascular endothelial cells with relevance to diagnosis of vascular tumours. J Clin Pathol 1992;45:143-148

193. Miettinen M, Lindenmayer AE, Chaubal A. Endothelial cell markers CD31, CD34, and BNH9 antibody to H- and Y-antigens—evaluation of their specificity and sensitivity in the diagnosis of vascular tumors and comparison with von Willebrand factor. Mod Pathol 1994; 7:82-90.

194. Miettinen M, Wang ZF, Paetau A, et al. ERG transcription factor as an immunohistochemical marker for vascular endothelial tumors and prostatic carcinoma. Am J Surg Pathol 2011;35:432-441.

195. Breiteneder-Geleff S, Soleiman A, Kowalski H, et al. Angiosarcomas express mixed endothelial phenotypes of blood and lymphatic capillaries: podoplanin as a specific marker for lymphatic endothelium. Am J Pathol 1999;154:385-394.

196. Kahn HJ, Bailey D, Marks A. Monoclonal antibody D2-40, a new marker of lymphatic endothelium, reacts with Kaposi sarcoma and a subset of angiosarcomas. Mod Pathol 2002;15:434-440.

197. Miettinen M, Fetsch JF. Distribution of keratins in normal endothelial cells and in a spectrum of vascular tumors: implications in tumor diagnosis. Hum Pathol 2000;31:1062-1067.

197a. Manner J, Radlwimmer B, Hohenberger P, et al. MYC high level gene amplification is a distinctive feature of angiosarcomas after irradiation or chronic lymphedema.Am J Pathol 2010;176:34-39.

197b. Guo T, Zhang L, Chang NE, Singer S, Maki RG, Antonescu CR. Consistent MYC and FLT4 gene amplification in radiation-induced angiosarcoma but not in other radiation-associated atypical vascular lesions. Genes Chromosomes Cancer 2011;50:25-33.

197c. Mentzel T, Schildhaus HU, Palmedo G, Büttner R, Kutzner H. Postradiation cutaneous angiosarcoma after treatment of breast carcinoma is characterized by MYC amplification in contrast to atypical vascular lesions after radiotherapy and control cases: clinicopathological, immunohistochemical and molecular analysis of 66 cases. Mod Pathol 2012;25:75-85.

197d. Fernandez AP, Sun Y, Tubbs RR, Goldblum JR, Billings SD. FISH for MYC amplification and anti-MYC immunohistochemistry: useful diagnostic tools in the assessment of secondary angiosarcoma and atypical vascular proliferations. J Cutan Pathol 2012;39:234-242.

Kaposi Sarcoma

198. Tappero JW, Conant MA, Wolfe SF, Berger TG. Kaposi's sarcoma. Epidemiology, pathogenesis, histology, clinical spectrum, staging criteria and therapy. J Am Acad Dermatol 1993;28:371-395.

199. Antman K, Chang Y. Kaposi's sarcoma. N Engl J Med 2000;342:1027-1038.

200. Schwartz RA, Micali G, Nasca MR, Scuderi L. Kaposi sarcoma: a continuing conundrum. J Am Acad Dermatol 2008;59:179-206.

201. Iscovich J, Boffetta P, Franceschi S, Azizi E, Sarid R. Classic Kaposi sarcoma: epidemiology and risk factors. Cancer 2000;88:500-517.

202. Hiatt KM, Nelson AM, Lichy J, Fanburg-Smith JC. Classic Kaposi sarcoma in the United States over the last two decades: a clinicopathologic and molecular study of 438 non-HIV-related Kaposi sarcoma patients with comparison to HIV-related Kaposi sarcoma. Mod Pathol 2008;21:572-582.

203. Slavin G, Cameron HM, Forbes C, Mitchell RM. Kaposi's sarcoma in East African children: A report of 51 cases. J Pathol 1970;100:198-199.

204. Penn I. Kaposi's sarcoma in transplant recipients. Transplantation 1997;64:669-673.

205. Lebbe C, Legendre C, Frances C. Kaposi sarcoma in transplantation. Transplant Rev (Orlando) 2008;22:252-61.

206. Ackerman AB. Subtle clues to diagnosis by conventional microscopy. The patch stage of Kaposi's sarcoma. Am J Dermatopathol 1979;1:165-172.

207. Chor PJ, Santa Cruz DJ. Kaposi's sarcoma. A clinicopathologic review and differential diagnosis. J Cutan Pathol 1992;19:6-20.

208. Kao G, Johnson FB, Sulica VI. The nature of hyaline (eosinophilic) globules and vascular slits in Kaposi's sarcoma. Am J Dermatopathol 1990;12:256-267.

209. Nickoloff BJ. The human progenitor cell antigen (CD34) is localized on endothelial cells, dermal dendritic cells, and perifollicular cells in formalin-fixed normal skin, and on proliferatin endothelial cells and stromal spindle-shaped cells in Kaposi's sarcoma. Arch Dermatol 1991;127:523-529.

210. Cheuk W, Wong KO, Wong CS, Dinkel JE, Ben-Dor D, Chan JK. Immunostaining for human herpesvirus 8 latent nuclear antigen-1 helps distinguish Kaposi sarcoma from its mimickers. Am J Clin Pathol 2004;121:335-342.

211. Patel RM, Goldblum JR, Hsi ED. Immuno-histochemical detection of human herpes virus-8 latent nuclear antigen-1 is useful in the diagnosis of Kaposi sarcoma. Mod Pathol 2004;17:456-460.

212. Weninger W, Partanen TA, Breiteneder-Geleff S, et al. Expression of vascular endothelial growath factor receptor-3 and podoplanin suggests a lymphatic endothelial cell origin of Kaposi's sarcoma tumor cells. Lab Invest 1999;79:243-251.

213. Cook PD, Czerniak B, Chan JK, et al. Nodular spindle-cell vascular transformation of lymph nodes. A benign process occurring predominantly in retroperitoneal lymph nodes draining carcinomas that can simulate Kaposi's sarcoma or metastatic tumor. Am J Surg Pathol 1995;19:1010-1020.

214. Chan JK, Frizzera G, Fletcher CD, Rosai J. Primary vascular tumors of lymph nodes other than Kaposi's sarcoma. Analysis of 39 cases and delineation of two new entities. Am J Surg Pathol 1992;16:335-358.

8 SOFT TISSUE TUMORS WITH CARTILAGINOUS OR OSSEOUS DIFFERENTIATION

This chapter discusses benign and malignant lesions that have cartilaginous or osseous differentiation, or in some cases, have names referring to the presence of cartilage (extraskeletal myxoid chondrosarcoma) or metaplastic bone (ossifying fibromyxoid tumor). Osteocartilaginous differentiation also occurs in other settings, such as benign lipomatous tumors, dedifferentiated liposarcoma, and metaplastic carcinomas, and these entities must be considered in the differential diagnosis.

SOFT TISSUE CHONDROMA

Definition. *Soft tissue chondromas* are benign, extraskeletal, extrasynovial tumors composed of mature chondrocytes in a hyaline cartilage matrix. Synonyms include *chondroma of soft parts* and *juxta-articular chondroma*.

Clinical Features. Soft tissue chondromas are rare tumors, although the precise incidence is difficult to estimate. Chondromas most often occur in middle-aged adults of either sex, in the fourth to seventh decades, but may occur in patients of any age (1–6). Chondromas most often involve the distal extremities, in particular, the fingers, but also occur adjacent to large joints (juxta-articular chondroma). Involvement of the head, neck, or trunk is uncommon (1–6). Chondromas typically present as small, superficial, painless, freely moveable masses, which may show radiographic evidence of calcification (7).

Gross Findings. Most soft tissue chondromas measure less than 2 cm. Grossly, they often closely resemble well-differentiated cartilaginous tumors in osseous locations, with a lobulated appearance and a glistening, gray to white cut surface. Grossly visible or palpable calcifications are sometimes present. Tumors that have undergone extensive calcification may appear less obviously cartilaginous.

Microscopic Findings. Most soft tissue chondromas are well-circumscribed, vaguely lobular lesions, closely resembling normal hyaline cartilage (fig. 8-1, left). The tumors are composed of small, amitotic chondrocytes variably showing mild nuclear enlargement with small nucleoli within well-formed lacunae, often with accentuated cell clustering (fig. 8-1, right) (1–6). The overall level of cellularity is typically greater than in normal articular cartilage and may be similar to that seen in grade 1 chondrosarcoma of bone. Myxoid change may be seen.

Stromal calcification is frequently present and may be extensive (fig. 8-2, left). Such calcification may incite an osteoclast and foreign body giant cell–rich reaction, occasionally almost completely obscuring the underlying tumor. So-called *chondroblastoma-like soft tissue chondromas* have higher cellularity, have less abundant extracellular matrix, and contain epithelioid chondrocytes, similar to those seen in chondroblastoma of bone (fig. 8-2, right) (8).

Special Studies. Soft tissue chondromas typically express S-100 protein. They are negative for markers of epithelial or myoepithelial differentiation, including cytokeratins, epithelial membrane antigen, smooth muscle actin, and calponin.

Differential Diagnosis. Distinguishing soft tissue chondroma from synovial chondromatosis or enchondroma of bone may be impossible on morphologic grounds alone, and requires clinical and radiographic correlation. Hyaline-type chondrosarcomas are rare in soft tissue and are typically much larger and more proximally located. Extraskeletal myxoid chondrosarcomas do not produce true hyaline-type cartilage. Calcifying aponeurotic fibroma usually occurs in young children, and is an infiltrative tumor composed of fibromatosis-like fascicles of spindled cells, in addition to foci of punctate calcification. Tumoral calcinosis most commonly involves larger, more proximal joints and lacks well-formed cartilage. Myoepitheliomas and mixed tumors may contain mature cartilage, but also often show epithelial differentiation and cytokeratin expression.

Treatment and Prognosis. Soft tissue chondromas are benign neoplasms requiring only simple excision.

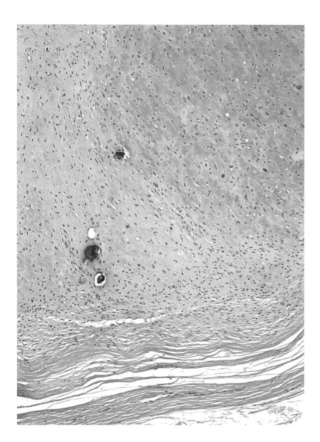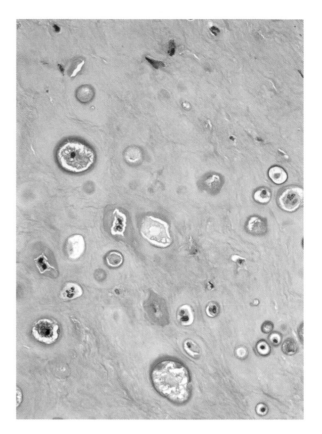

Figure 8-1

SOFT TISSUE CHONDROMA

Left: Most soft tissue chondromas are well-circumscribed, lobular proliferations of mature cartilage, resembling enchondroma of long bones.

Right: Mildly increased cellularity and nuclear enlargement may be present in soft tissue chondromas.

EXTRASKELETAL MYXOID CHONDROSARCOMA

Definition. *Extraskeletal myxoid chondrosarcoma* is a myxoid malignant mesenchymal neoplasm composed of spindled or epithelioid cells in a trabecular or net-like cellular arrangement and lacking markers of epithelial differentiation. In contrast with the name, the tumor does not contain differentiated cartilage; the name is based on historical assertions.

Clinical Features. Extraskeletal myxoid chondrosarcoma has a predilection to middle-aged adults of a median age of around 50 years and 2 to 1 male predominance. Isolated cases have been reported in children. The most common site is the thigh (more than 50 percent), with the rest evenly divided between the shoulder region, foot, and trunk wall; occasional cases are reported in body cavities and intracranial

spaces. Most extraskeletal myxoid chondrosarcomas are large intramuscular masses, but some are subcutaneous (9–15).

Gross Findings. The median tumor size in different series varies between 7 and 11 cm, and only rare cases are smaller than 5 cm. Grossly, the tumor is gelatinous and often hemorrhagic and may even simulate a hematoma.

Microscopic Findings. Histologically, the tumor is typically lobulated by fibrous septa and often contains intratumoral hemorrhage, hemosiderin, and stromal fibrosis. The tumor cells are arranged in interconnected cords or trabeculae or form a net-like pattern. Some cases contain clusters of round cells associated with the corded patterns (fig. 8-3). The tumor cells vary from round to stellate or spindled, with uniform nuclei and scant, variably eosinophilic cytoplasm. The cartilaginous component is only

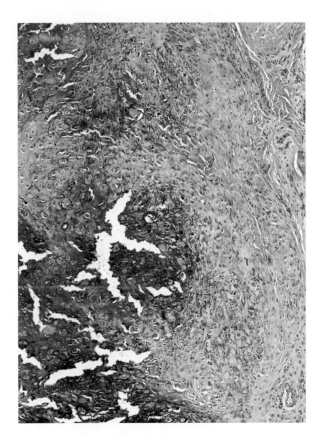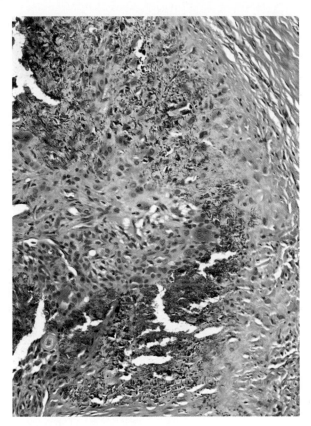

Figure 8-2

SOFT TISSUE CHONDROMA

Left: Soft tissue chondromas often undergo calcification, which is here extensive.
Right: Heavily calcified chondromas elicit an osteoclastic giant cell reaction and contain plump epithelioid chondrocytes, reminiscent of chondroblastoma of bone.

rarely detectable, but well-differentiated hyaline cartilage is not present.

Mitotic activity is usually low; however, highly cellular solid areas with substantial mitotic activity occur in tumors with high-grade transformation (16,17). Such tumors are generally only diagnosable if a conventional component or genetic documentation is available.

Special Studies. Extraskeletal myxoid chondrosarcoma contains abundant Alcian blue–positive acid mucopolysaccharides (best shown at pH 4.0). Immunohistochemically, the tumor cells are variably and inconsistently positive for S-100 protein (30 percent of cases) but are often positive for synaptophysin. They are generally negative for keratins and glial fibrillary acidic protein (GFAP), and occasional cases are focally positive for desmin or epithelial membrane antigen (11–13,18). Rare examples with rhabdoid cy-

tology are negative for the INI1/SMARCB1 gene product, similar to epithelioid sarcoma (19).

Ultrastructural studies have found intracisternal microtubules in the endoplasmic reticulum system, and some investigators have detected neuroendocrine-like dense core granules (13,18,20).

Genetics. Genetically typical is a gene fusion translocation *EWSR1-NR4A3*, which corresponds to the t(9;22)(q22;q12) chromosomal translocation seen in approximately 75 percent of cases. A rare variant fusion of *TAF2N-NR4A3*, corresponding to the t(9;7)(q22;q11) chromosomal translocation, occurs in a minority of cases (21–24). Classic cytogenetics or molecular genetic testing for these alterations by fluorescence in situ hybridization [FISH] or polymerase chain reaction [PCR]) may be diagnostically useful (25).

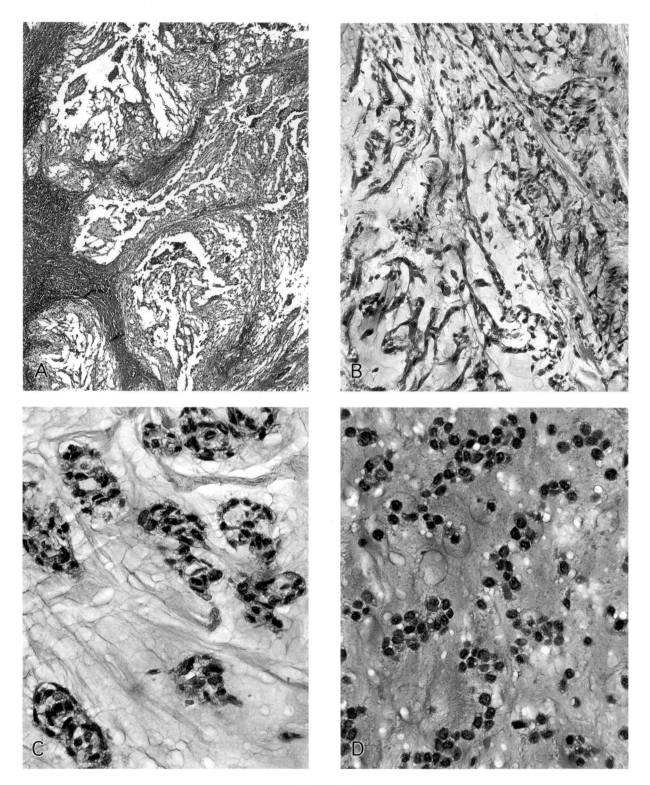

Figure 8-3

EXTRASKELETAL MYXOID CHONDROSARCOMA

A: At low magnification, the lobular organization is seen.
B–D: The tumor cells vary from spindled to round, and are organized in trabeculae or small clusters.

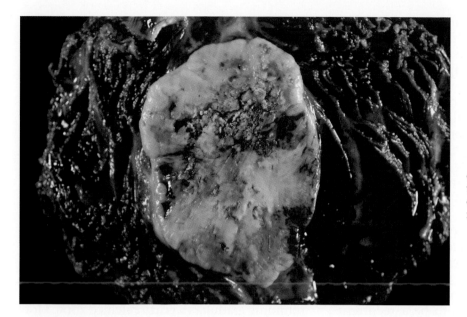

Figure 8-4

EXTRASKELETAL MESENCHYMAL CHONDROSARCOMA

A well-demarcated intramuscular mass is formed. It has a whitish cut surface and calcified cartilage is seen in the upper middle portion.

Differential Diagnosis. The most difficult problem is separating extraskeletal myxoid chondrosarcoma from malignant mixed tumor/myoepithelioma. Criteria that favor the latter include the presence of an epithelial ductal component, and immunohistochemical positivity for keratins, GFAP, and p63. Extraskeletal myxoid chondrosarcoma is usually more easily separated from cartilaginous neoplasms, such as variants of chondroma and typical chondrosarcoma, because it lacks a differentiated cartilaginous component. Metastatic chordoma may have a trabecular arrangement, but is keratin positive. In difficult cases, the demonstration of tumor-specific translocations is helpful.

Treatment and Prognosis. Extraskeletal myxoid chondrosarcoma often recurs and sometimes metastasizes to lung, often years after the primary tumor is diagnosed. Nevertheless, many patients live long even with lung metastases. Tumors with high-grade features have a higher metastatic rate and more aggressive course. High cellularity, pleomorphism, high mitotic activity, older patient age, larger tumor size, metastases, and proximal location have been cited as adverse prognostic factors.

Wide local excision, with consideration to adjuvant therapy, especially for tumors with high-grade features, is the preferred treatment. The largest series found 5- and 10-year overall survival rates of less than 80 percent and 65 percent (11,14).

EXTRASKELETAL MESENCHYMAL CHONDROSARCOMA

Definition. *Extraskeletal mesenchymal chondrosarcoma* is a high-grade sarcoma primarily arising in soft tissue and containing a primitive round cell component and foci of differentiated cartilage.

Clinical Features. Extraskeletal mesenchymal chondrosarcoma is less common than its osseous counterpart and comprises approximately 30 percent of all mesenchymal chondrosarcomas. There is a predilection to young adults, and two thirds occur in the second to fourth decades, with a 2 to 1 female predominance. The most commonly reported extraskeletal sites are head and neck region and thigh. Of head and neck sites, most tumors occur in the orbit and in intracranial soft tissues (meninges, skull basis) or in paraspinal neck tissues. Less often, the trunk wall, body cavities, and upper extremity are involved. Peripheral soft tissue examples usually form a 5 to 10-cm deep, intramuscular mass (26–32).

Gross Findings. Grossly, mesenchymal chondrosarcoma typically forms a well-demarcated mass. On sectioning, it contains a fleshy white component and variably prominent, often focally calcified, cartilaginous foci (fig. 8-4).

Microscopic Findings. Histologically, mesenchymal chondrosarcoma has a biphasic histology containing cartilaginous and primitive round cell components. The latter is dominant in most cases and is composed of sheets of medium-sized cells with round nuclei and scant cytoplasm, but some cases show some spindling. A hemangiopericytoma-like vascular pattern is often present and the collagenous matrix can be more prominent than generally observed in other small round cell tumors. The cartilaginous component may form small nests or larger islands that typically transition abruptly from the round cell component. The appearance varies from hyaline cartilage-like and basophilic to fibrocartilage-like, and variable calcification and metaplastic bone formation may be present (fig. 8-5).

Special Studies. Immunohistochemically, the small round cell component may show focal desmin positivity and is often CD99 positive. S-100 protein and SOX9 immunostains highlight the cartilaginous component (33–35). A *HEY1-NCOA2* gene fusion seems to be a recurrent molecular genetic change and may be a future genetic marker for this tumor type (36).

Treatment and Prognosis. This tumor is considered high grade by definition, and it has a high potential for both local recurrence and distant, especially pulmonary, metastases. In the largest series containing both osseous and extraskeletal cases, the 5-year survival rate was 55 percent and the 10-year rate was 27 percent.

MYOSITIS OSSIFICANS AND RELATED OSTEOCARTILAGINOUS PSEUDOTUMORS

Definition. *Myositis ossificans* is a non-neoplastic, self-limited pseudotumor characterized by myofibroblastic proliferation with associated bone and cartilage matrix production (37,38). It typically develops in skeletal muscle following trauma, and is presumed to be reactive in nature. Identical processes occur in the superficial soft tissue, adipose tissue, and mesentery (39–42). Related lesions include *panniculitis ossificans, fasciitis ossificans, fibro-osseous pseudotumor of the digits*, and *heterotopic mesenteric ossification*.

General Considerations. The clinical and pathologic features of myositis ossificans and related lesions vary depending on the length of time between the inciting injury and biopsy. Early lesions (within the first few weeks) are often dominated by myofibroblastic proliferation, mimicking various spindle cell sarcomas, whereas older lesions grow more bone and cartilage.

Clinical Features. Myositis ossificans typically occurs in young adults, equally in males and females. Patients usually present with a less than 3-month history of pain and swelling in the affected area. A history of trauma is sometimes, but not always, present. Greater than 75 percent of cases occur in the large skeletal muscles of the proximal extremities (37,38,42).

Fibro-osseous pseudotumors of the digits more often occur in young women, typically in the soft tissues of the fingers and less often the toes (41). Heterotopic mesenteric ossification generally occurs in elderly patients, often with a history of prior intra-abdominal surgery (39).

Gross Findings. Myositis ossificans typically measures less than 6 cm. Lesions examined early in their natural history show a gelatinous to hemorrhagic-appearing center, with a surrounding granular to gritty calcified zone. More mature examples consist largely of mature-appearing bone (37,38,42).

Fibro-osseous pseudotumors of the digits are usually much smaller and less well defined. Heterotopic mesenteric ossification may be larger than 10 cm at the time of diagnosis, and typically consists of areas of fat necrosis admixed with irregular zones of hemorrhage and metaplastic ossification (39–42).

Microscopic Findings. The microscopic features of myositis ossificans and related lesions are very similar. In the early phase, these pseudotumors demonstrate a close resemblance to nodular fasciitis, with a highly cellular proliferation of cytologically bland myofibroblasts in short, somewhat randomly arranged fascicles within a variably myxoid background. Mitotic activity may be high (fig. 8-6). Necrosis is usually absent.

By definition, the various fibro-osseous pseudotumors differ from nodular fasciitis by the presence of islands or trabeculae of immature-appearing cartilage and osteoid, often showing "maturation" transition into thicker trabeculae of woven bone at the periphery of the lesion. Older lesions may show lamellar bone (37,38,42). This evolution from fasciitis-like zones through immature cartilage and woven bone to mature lamellar bone is referred to as the "zoning phenomenon," and is one of the key histologic hallmarks of myositis ossificans (fig. 8-7). Occasionally, multiple overlapping areas of zonation

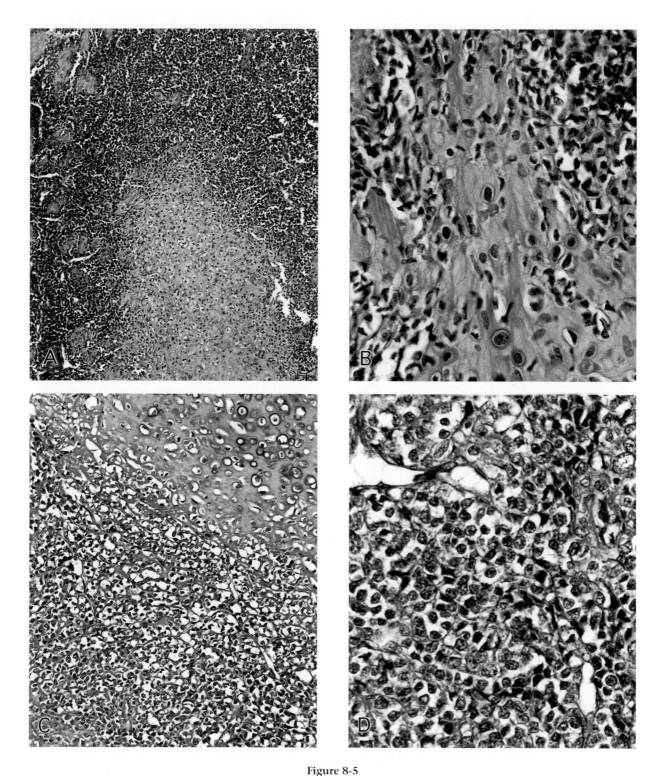

Figure 8-5

EXTRASKELETAL MESENCHYMAL CHONDROSARCOMA

A–C: This tumor contains a dominant primitive round cell component and a differentiated cartilaginous component that has hyaline cartilage or fibrocartilage-like features.

D: The primitive round cell component is composed of uniform medium-sized cells. A hemangiopericytoma-like vascular pattern may be present as seen here.

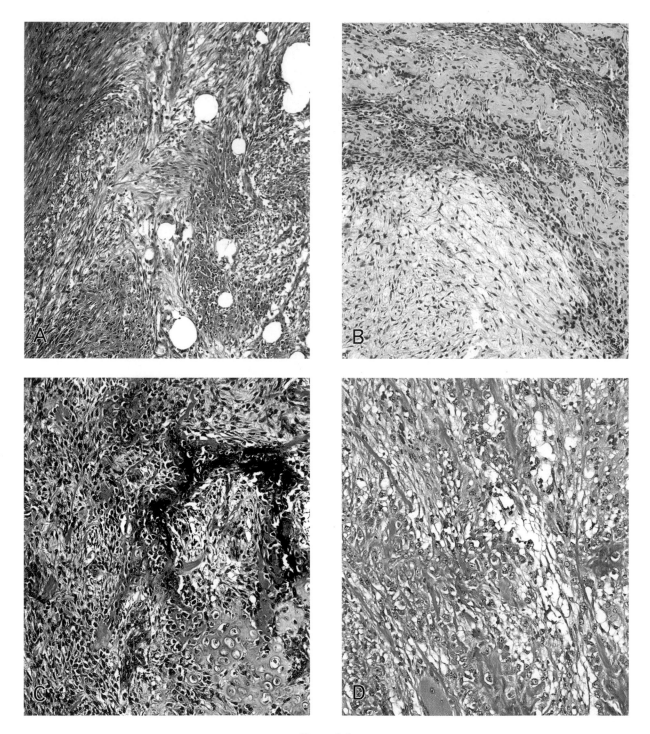

Figure 8-6

MYOSITIS OSSIFICANS

A: The most central zone in myositis ossificans typically consists of a highly cellular, loosely textured proliferation of mitotically active myofibroblasts, identical to nodular fasciitis.

B: These fasciitis-like zones typically merge with areas showing osteoid matrix production.

C: Osteocartilaginous matrix production in myositis ossificans.

D: Higher-power view of a bone-producing area. Although the lesion is highly cellular and mitotically active, and is producing "lace-like" osteoid, the proliferating osteoblasts are uniform and normochromatic.

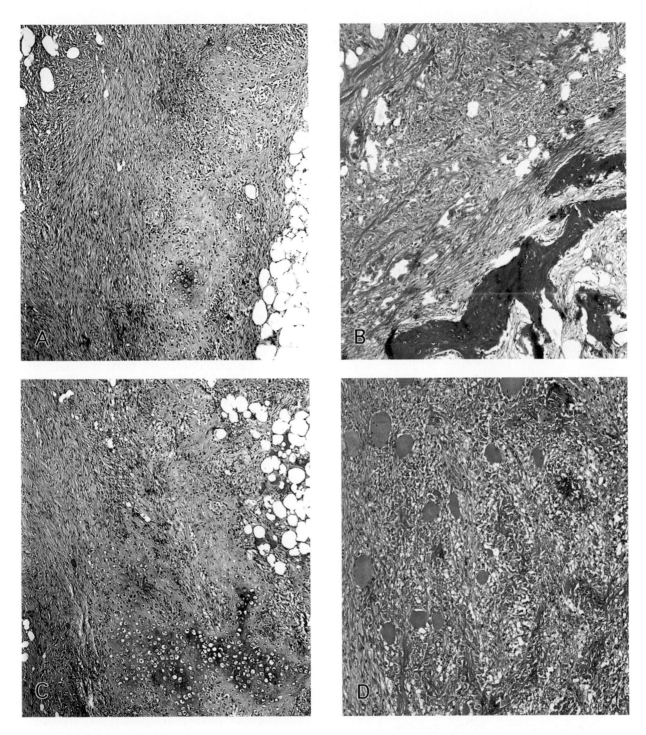

Figure 8-7

MYOSITIS OSSIFICANS

A: Myositis ossificans typically shows a "zonated" pattern of growth, with the most mature osteocartilaginous tissues at the periphery of the lesion.

B: In older examples, a shell of woven bone surrounds the tumor.

C: Some examples show overlapping zones of maturation, such that fasciitis-like spindled cells, cellular cartilage, and new bone production are seen together. It is important not to mistake such areas for soft tissue chondroblastic osteosarcoma.

D: Skeletal muscle is often entrapped at the periphery.

are present, somewhat complicating the recognition of this distinctive pattern.

Special Studies. Immunohistochemistry is generally of little value in the diagnosis of myositis ossificans and related lesions. In intra-abdominal cases, where the differential diagnosis includes carcinosarcoma, cytokeratin immunostains may be of some value, although care should be taken not to mistake the normal cytokeratin-positive submesothelial stromal cell population for tumor cells (43).

Genetics. *USP6* rearrangements, as seen in aneurysmal bone cyst and nodular fasciitis, have recently been shown in a small number of cases of myositis ossificans (44–46).

Differential Diagnosis. The distinction of myositis ossificans from nodular fasciitis and other reactive myofibroblastic proliferations rests solely on the identification of an osteocartilaginous matrix. Extraskeletal osteosarcoma differs from myositis ossificans by its occurrence in older patients, larger size, cytologic atypia and pleomorphism, atypical mitotic figures, and necrosis (47). Osteosarcomas often show a "reversed" pattern of zonation from myositis ossificans, with the least mature zones at the periphery. Similarly, carcinosarcomas, melanomas, and mesotheliomas with heterologous osteosarcomatous differentiation show a much greater degree of cytologic atypia than is seen in myositis ossificans. In selected cases, immunohistochemistry for epithelial, melanocytic, or mesothelial markers is of value.

Treatment and Prognosis. Myositis ossificans and the various fibro-osseous pseudotumors of the digits are benign, self-limited conditions requiring only simple excision. In some patients, it is necessary to let the lesions "mature" before attempting complete resection. The prognosis for patients with heterotopic mesenteric ossification is poor, usually because of multiple other medical problems and the local effects on gastrointestinal function.

EXTRASKELETAL OSTEOSARCOMA

Definition. *Extraskeletal osteosarcoma (soft tissue osteosarcoma)* is a malignant mesenchymal tumor showing osteoblastic differentiation and production of neoplastic osteoid matrix. As in skeletal osteosarcomas, there are fibroblastic, chondroblastic, and telangiectatic variants. By definition, extraskeletal osteosarcomas must arise primarily within the soft tissues, without attachment to underlying bone. Secondary bone involvement may, however, be seen in advanced tumors.

Clinical Features. Extraskeletal osteosarcoma occurs in older adults, with a peak incidence in the fifth and sixth decades (48–54). This is in contrast with the largely pediatric occurrence of skeletal osteosarcomas. These tumors are twice as common in men as women. Most arise in the deep soft tissues of the extremities, most often the thigh and buttock. Rare cases arise from the superficial soft tissues and the skin (55–59). Many cases of extraskeletal osteosarcoma have been reported as examples of postirradiation sarcoma (53,60–63).

Gross Findings. Extraskeletal osteosarcomas are typically large at the time of diagnosis (over 10 cm), and are grossly heterogeneous, fleshy tumors showing hemorrhage and/or necrosis (48–54). Grossly detectable bone is usually absent, although they may have a "gritty" quality on sectioning.

Microscopic Findings. Extraskeletal osteosarcomas show identical histologic features to their more common osseous counterparts. Most are obviously malignant, pleomorphic sarcomas composed of a highly cellular proliferation of spindled, epithelioid, and/or plasmacytoid cells, resembling, at least in part, non-neoplastic osteoblasts. Necrosis and atypical mitotic figures are typically present. The production of neoplastic osteoid matrix, outlining individual cells or in a lace-like to sheet-like pattern, is definitional of extraskeletal osteosarcoma in an otherwise undifferentiated pleomorphic sarcoma (fig. 8-8). Chondroblastic and fibroblastic differentiation is common. Rare tumors show morphologic features identical to small cell and telangiectatic osteosarcoma of bone (48–54). Unusual soft tissue tumors resembling low-grade fibroblastic osteosarcoma of bone (parosteal osteosarcoma or central low-grade osteosarcoma) have been reported (64); recent genetic data suggest that these may represent instead unusual variants of dedifferentiated liposarcoma with inapparent or easily overlooked areas of well-differentiated liposarcoma (65).

Special Studies. As in osteosarcoma of bone, immunohistochemistry plays a limited role in the diagnosis. Anomalous expression

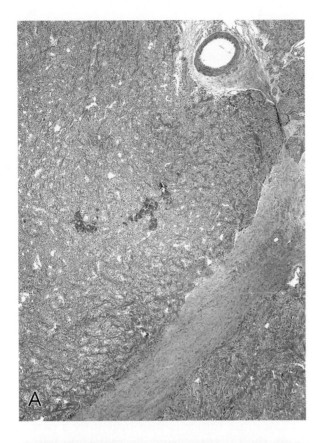

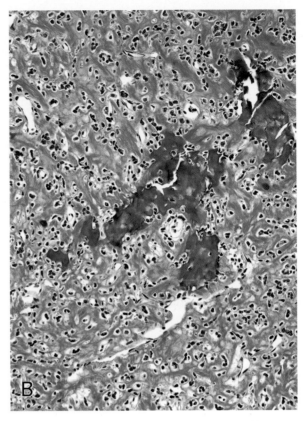

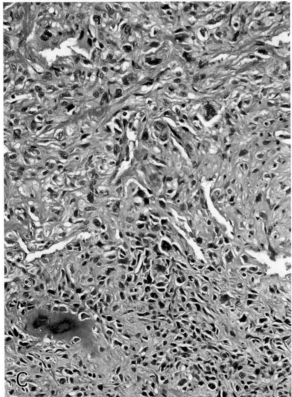

Figure 8-8

EXTRASKELETAL OSTEOSARCOMA

A: A large, heavily calcified mass in the thigh.

B: Production of "lace-like" osteoid by malignant-appearing epithelioid cells is characteristic of osteosarcoma in any location.

C: In many cases, osteoid production is limited in extent, with much of the tumor resembling undifferentiated pleomorphic sarcoma.

of cytokeratins, smooth muscle actin, desmin, and S-100 protein may be seen in a minority of tumors. Osteocalcin expression has been suggested to be of some value in the diagnosis of poorly differentiated osteosarcoma, but has not been widely adopted (66).

Differential Diagnosis. The differential diagnosis of extraskeletal osteosarcoma is principally with other pleomorphic sarcomas and with myositis ossificans. As noted above, the presence of neoplastic osteoid production is definitional of extraskeletal osteosarcoma. However, osteosarcomatous differentiation may be seen in other high-grade soft tissue sarcomas, including dedifferentiated liposarcoma and malignant peripheral nerve sheath tumors. The identification of areas of well-differentiated liposarcoma in the latter two is obviously essential for these particular diagnoses.

The distinction of extraskeletal osteosarcoma from metastatic carcinomas or melanomas showing osteoblastic differentiation rests on a combination of clinical history and identification of areas showing epithelial or melanocytic differentiation. The distinction of soft tissue osteosarcoma from primary osteosarcoma of bone showing secondary soft tissue involvement, or from metastatic osteosarcoma, requires clinical and radiographic correlation.

Myositis ossificans may be highly cellular and produce bone in a somewhat "lace-like" pattern, but lacks the obvious cytologic atypia seen in almost all extraskeletal osteosarcomas. Myositis ossificans also tends to show maturation toward the periphery, whereas the least differentiated zones in extraskeletal osteosarcoma are typically found at the leading edge of the tumor.

Treatment and Prognosis. Extraskeletal osteosarcomas are high-grade sarcomas conferring a poor prognosis. Many patients present with high-stage disease, and most die of metastatic disease in less than 5 years (48–54). Multiagent chemotherapeutic protocols, successful in primary osteosarcoma of bone, do not appear to be as valuable in extraskeletal osteosarcoma, possibly owing to the differences in patient age between these two groups of osteosarcomas.

OSSIFYING FIBROMYXOID TUMOR

Definition. *Ossifying fibromyxoid tumor* is a mesenchymal neoplasm of uncertain histogenesis. The tumor is typically composed of uniform oval to epithelioid cells and often surrounded by discontinuous bands of metaplastic bone. The tumor cells are almost always S-100 protein positive.

General Comments. The histogenesis remains uncertain, and neither nerve sheath nor cartilaginous differentiation of the main cellular component has been proven, despite some immunophenotypic similarity, especially the S-100 protein positivity.

Clinical Features. The tumor occurs in adults of all ages and is occasionally reported in children. The median age is around 50 years and there is a 1.5 to 1.0 male predominance. The tumor primarily involves the subcutis, although it may extend into skeletal muscle in the head and neck. The most commonly involved site is the lower extremity (especially thigh), but almost any external site can be involved. The commonly long history of the presence of tumor (over 10 years) indicates slow growth and much earlier onset than the date of surgery (67–74).

Gross Findings. Ossifying fibromyxoid tumor forms an oval to round, well-circumscribed mass varying in size from less than 1 cm to more than 10 cm (median, 3 cm). In 80 percent of cases, the tumor is surrounded by a partial bony shell that occasionally makes up half of the tumor volume (fig. 8-9).

Microscopic Findings. Histologically, the tumor typically contains peripheral bone spicules that sometimes extend into the center. There is variably developed lobulation (fig. 8-9). A fibrous pseudocapsule usually surrounds the tumor, but small satellite nodules may be present within or around the pseudocapsule.

The tumor cells often form diffuse arrangements within a moderately collagenous, focally myxoid matrix. Some tumors contain cords or trabecular arrangements of cells. Cytologically, the cells have epithelioid morphology and contain round, fairly uniform nuclei with small nucleoli, but focal atypia may be present. The cytoplasm is variably eosinophilic and is sometimes surrounded by a shrinkage space (fig. 8-10). Mitotic activity varies from 0 to over 10 mitoses per 10 high-power fields. Tumors with a mitotic rate of greater than 2 mitoses per 10 high-power fields have an increased risk for recurrence. There is no correlation, however, between prognosis and tumor size, presence of satellite nodules, or coagulation necrosis.

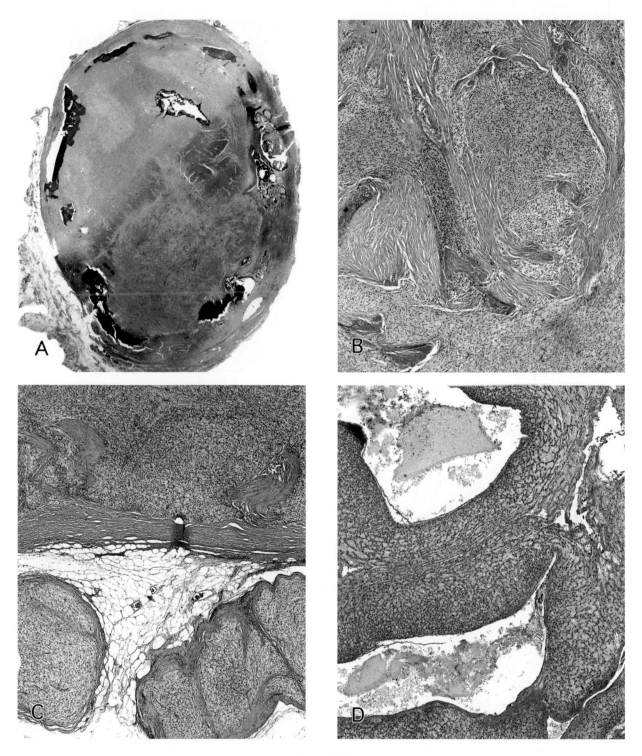

Figure 8-9

OSSIFYING FIBROMYXOID TUMOR

Low magnification images of ossifying fibromyxoid tumor.
A: An incomplete bony shell surrounds the tumor.
B,C: The tumor is multinodular and satellite nodules are present in the surrounding fat.
D: Focal cystic change is present.

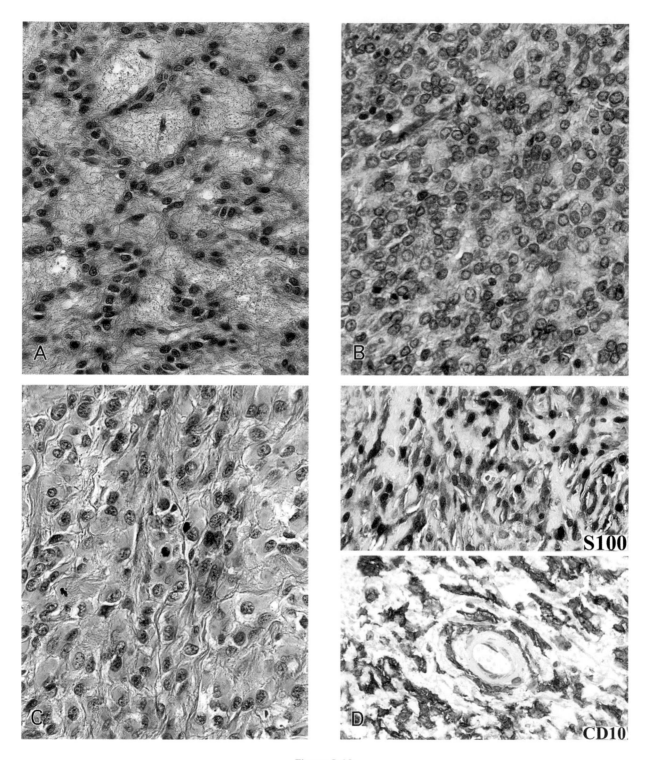

Figure 8-10

OSSIFYING FIBROMYXOID TUMOR

A: Corded pattern and uniform cytologic appearance in ossifying fibromyxoid tumor.

B: A more cellular example.

C: A tumor with significant mitotic activity (two mitotic figures seen to the right of center).

D: The tumor cells are immunohistochemically positive for S-100 protein and CD10.

Atypical variants with metastatic risk have been reported. Such tumors differ from classic ossifying fibromyxoid tumor by their often overt sarcomatous features, deep location, and low or no expression of S-100 protein (75,76). As some of these tumors do not contain conventional ossifying fibromyxoid tumor components, the relationship of these tumors with the latter is questionable.

Special Studies. Immunohistochemically typical is expression of vimentin and S-100 protein (in nearly 100 percent of cases), and CD10, at least focally. A minority of cases is focally positive for keratin cocktail, desmin, or GFAP (69). One tumor studied cytogenetically had a simple karyotype with a loss of chromosome 6 and an unbalanced t(6;14) translocation (77). *PHF1* gene rearrangements have been recently identified as a recurrent change (78,79).

Differential Diagnosis. Highly cellular and mitotically active and atypical overtly sarcomatous tumors, sometimes considered *malignant ossifying fibromyxoid tumor,* almost invariably represent other entities with focal metaplastic bone formation and a corded pattern. These entities include progression variants of low-grade fibromyxoid sarcomas and extraskeletal osteosarcoma variants. Tumors involving bones should not be classified as ossifying fibromyxoid tumors.

Tumors with neoplastic epithelial elements or significant keratin positivity are more consistent with mixed tumors (myoepithelioma variants). Some smooth muscle actin–positive myofibroblastic neoplasms resemble the nonossifying variants of ossifying fibromyxoid tumor. Their immunohistochemical profile, including negativity for S-100 protein, helps to separate them.

Treatment and Prognosis. There is a 20 to 30 percent risk of recurrence after local excision, and most recurrences occur 10 or more years after surgery. The development of metastases is exceptional; therefore, complete excision and follow-up are generally sufficient.

REFERENCES

Soft Tissue Chondroma

1. Chung EB, Enzinger FM. Chondroma of soft parts. Cancer. 1978;41:1414-1424.
2. Makino Y. A clinicopathological study on soft tissue tumors of the head and neck. Acta Pathol Jpn 1979;29:389-408.
3. Humphreys S, Pambakian H, McKee PH, Fletcher CD. Soft tissue chondroma—a study of 15 tumours. Histopathology 1986;10:147-159.
4. Fletcher CD, Krausz T. Cartilaginous tumours of soft tissue. Appl Pathol 1988;6:208-220.
5. Dahlin DC, Salvador AH. Cartilaginous tumors of the soft tissues of the hands and feet. Mayo Clin Proc 1974;49:721-726.
6. Reiman HM, Dahlin DC. Cartilage- and bone-forming tumors of the soft tissues. Semin Diagn Pathol 1986;3:288-305.
7. Floyd WE 3rd, Troum S. Benign cartilaginous lesions of the upper extremity. Hand Clin 1995;11:119-132.
8. Cates JM, Rosenberg AE, O'Connell JX, Nielsen GP. Chondroblastoma-like chondroma of soft tissue: an underrecognized variant and its differential diagnosis. Am J Surg Pathol 2001;25:661-666.

Extraskeletal Myxoid Chondrosarcoma

9. Enzinger FM, Shiraki M. Extraskeletal myxoid chondrosarcoma. An analysis of 34 cases. Hum Pathol 1972;3:421-435.
10. Saleh G, Evans HL, Ro JY, Ayala AG. Extraskeletal myxoid chondrosarcoma. A clinicopathologic study of ten patients with long-tern follow-up. Cancer 1992;70:2827-2830.
11. Meis-Kindblom JM, Bergh P, Gunterberg B, Kindblom LG. Extraskeletal myxoid chondrosarcoma. A reappraisal of its morphologic spectrum and prognostic factors based on 117 cases. Am J Surg Pathol 1999;23:636-650.
12. Oliveira AM, Sebo TJ, McGrory JE, Gaffey TA, Rock MG, Nascimento AG. Extraskeletal myxoid chondrosarcoma: A clinicopathological, immunohistochemical, and ploidy analysis of 23 cases. Mod Pathol 2000;13:900-908.
13. Okamoto S, Hisaoka M, Ishida T, et al. Extraskeletal myxoid chondrosarcoma: a clinicopathologic, immunohistochemical, and molecular analysis of 18 cases. Hum Pathol 2001;32:1116-1124.

14. Drilon AD, Popat S, Bhuchar G, et al. Extraskeletal myxoid chondrosarcoma: a retrospective review from 2 referral centers emphasizing long-term outcomes with surgery and chemotherapy. Cancer 2008;113:3364-3371.
15. Hachitanda Y, Tsuneyoshi M, Daimaru Y, et al. Extraskeletal myxoid chondrosarcoma in young children. Cancer 1988;61:2521-2526.
16. Lucas DR, Fletcher CD, Adsay NV, Zalupski MM. High-grade extraskeletal myxoid chondrosarcoma: a high-grade epithelioid malignancy. Histopathology 1999;35:201-208.
17. Ramesh K, Gahukamble L, Sarma NH, Al Fituri OM. Extraskeletal myxoid chondrosarcoma with dedifferentiation. Histopathology 1995;27:381-382.
18. Goh YW, Spagnolo DV, Platten M, et al. Extraskeletal myxoid chondrosarcoma: a light microscopic, immunohistochemical, ultrastructural, and immuno-ultrastructural study indicating neuroendocrine differentiation. Histopathology 2001;39:514-524.
19. Kohashi K, Oda Y, Yamamoto H, et al. SMARCB1/INI1 protein expression in round cell soft tissue sarcomas associated with chromosomal translocations involving EWS: a special reference to SMARCB1/INI1 negative variant extraskeletal myxoid chondrosarcoma. Am J Surg Pathol 2008;32:1168-1174.
20. Suzuki T, Kaneko H, Kojima K, Takatoh M, Hasebe K. Extraskeletal myxoid chondrosarcoma characterized by microtubular aggregates in the rough endoplasmic reticulum and tubulin immunoreactivity. J Pathol 1988;156:51-57.
21. Stenman G, Andersson H, Mandahl N, Meis-Kindblom JM, Kindblom LG. Translocation t(9;22)(q22;q12) is a primary cytogenetic abnormality in extraskeletal myxoid chondrosarcoma. Int J Cancer 1995;62:398-402.
22. Hirabayashi Y, Ishida T, Yoshida MA, et al. Translocation (9;22)(q22;q12). A recurrent chromosome abnormality in extraskeletal myxoid chondrosarcoma. Cancer Genet Cytogenet 1995;81:33-37.
23. Sciot R, Dal Cin P, Fletcher C, et al. t(9;22)(q22-31;q11-12) is a consistent marker of extraskeletal myxoid chondrosarcoma: evaluation of three cases. Mod Pathol 1995;8:765-768.
24. Sjogren H, Meis-Kindblom J, Kindblom L-G, Aman P, Stenman G. Fusion of the EWS-related gene TAF2N to TEC in extraskeletal myxoid chondrosarcoma. Cancer Res 1999;59:5064-5067.
25. Wang WL, Mayordomo E, Czerniak BA, et al. Fluorescence in situ hybridization is a useful ancillary diagnostic tool for extraskeletal myxoid chondrosarcoma. Mod Pathol 2008;21:1303-1310.

Extraskeletal Mesenchymal Chondrosarcoma

26. Guccion JG, Font RL, Enzinger FM, Zimmerman LW. Extraskeletal mesenchymal chondrosarcoma. Arch Pathol 1973;95:336-340.
27. Nakashima Y, Unni KK, Shives TC, Swee RG, Dahlin DC. Mesenchymal chondrosarcoma of bone and soft tissue. A review of 111 cases. Cancer 1986;57:2444-2453.
28. Rushing EJ, Armonda RA, Ansari Q, Mena H. Mesenchymal chondrosarcoma: a clinicopathologic and flow cytometry study of 13 cases presenting in the central nervous system. Cancer 1996;77:1884-1891.
29. Hashimoto N, Ueda T, Joyama S, Araki N, Beppu Y, Tatezaki S. Extraskeletal mesenchymal chondrosarcoma: an imaging review of ten new patients. Skeletal Radiol 2005;34:785-792.
30. Cesari M, Bertoni F, Bacchini P, Mercuri M, Palmerini E, Ferrari S. Mesenchymal chondrosarcoma. An analysis of patients treated at a single institution. Tumori 2007;93:423-427.
31. Dantonello TM, Int-Veen C, Leuschner I, et al. Mesenchymal chondrosarcoma of soft tissues and bone in children, adolescents, and young adults: experiences of the CWS and COSS study groups. Cancer 2008;112-2424-2431.
32. Shakked RJ, Geller DS, Gorlick R, Dorfman HD. Mesenchymal chondrosarcoma: clinicopathologic study of 20 cases. Arch Pathol Lab Med 2012;136:61-75.
33. Wehrli BM, Huang W, De Crombrugghe B, Ayala AG, Czerniak B. Sox9, a master regulator for chondrogenesis, distinguishes mesenchymal chondrosarcoma from other small blue round cell tumors. Hum Pathol 2003;34:263-269.
34. Fanburg-Smith JC, Auerbach A, Marwaha JS, Wang ZF, Rushing EJ. Reappraisal of mesenchymal chondrosarcoma: novel morphological observations of the hyaline cartilage and enchondral ossification and beta-catenin, Sox9, and osteocalcin immunostaining of 22 cases. Hum Pathol 2010;41:653-662.
35. Fanburg-Smith JC, Auerbach A, Marwaha JS, et al. Immunoprofile of mesenchymal chondrosarcoma: aberrant desmin and EMA expression, retention of INI-1, and negative estrogen reeptor in 22 female predominant central nervous system and musculoskeletal cases. Ann Diagn Pathol 2010;14:8-14.
36. Wang L, Motoi T, Khanin R, et al. Identification of a novel, recurrent HEY1-NCOA2 fusion in mesenchymal chondrosarcoma based on genome-wide screen of exon-level expression data. Genes Chromosomes Cancer 2012;51:127-139.

Myositis Ossificans and Related Osteocartilaginous Pseudotumors

37. Angervall L, Stener B, Stener I, Ahren C. Pseudo-malignant osseous tumour of soft tissue. A clinical, radiological and pathological study of five cases. J Bone Joint Surg Br 1969;51:654-663.
38. Ackerman LV. Extra-osseous localized non-neoplastic bone and cartilage formation (so-called myositis ossificans): clinical and pathological confusion with malignant neoplasms. J Bone Joint Surg Am. 1958 Apr;40-A:279-298.
39. Patel RM, Weiss SW, Folpe AL. Heterotopic mesenteric ossification: a distinctive pseudosarcoma commonly associated with intestinal obstruction. Am J Surg Pathol 2006;30:119-122.
40. Bovo G, Romano F, Perego E, Franciosi C, Buffa R, Uggeri F. Heterotopic mesenteric ossification ("intraabdominal myositis ossificans"): a case report. Int J Surg Pathol 2004;12:407-409.
41. Meneses MF, Unni KK, Swee RG. Bizarre parosteal osteochondromatous proliferation of bone (Nora's lesion). Am J Surg Pathol 1993;17:691-697.
42. Unni KK, McLeod RA, Dahlin DC. Conditions that simulate primary neoplasms of bone. Pathology Annual 1980;15(Pt 1):91-131.
43. Van Muijen GN, Ruiter DJ, Warnaar SO. Coexpression of intermediate filament polypeptides in human fetal and adult tissues. Lab Invest 1987;57:359-369.
44. Sukov WR, Franco MF, Erickson-Johnson M, et al. Frequency of USP6 rearrangements in myositis ossificans, brown tumor, and cherubism: molecular cytogenetic evidence that a subset of "myositis ossificans-like lesions" are the early phases in the formation of soft-tissue aneurysmal bone cyst. Skeletal Radiol 2008;37:321-327.
45. Oliveira AM, Hsi BL, Weremowicz S, et al. USP6 (Tre2) fusion oncogenes in aneurysmal bone cyst. Cancer Res 2004;64:1920-3.
46. Erickson-Johnson MR, Chou MM, Evers BR, et al. Nodular fasciitis: a novel model of transient neoplasia induced by MYH9-USP6 gene fusion. Lab Invest 2011;91:1427-1433.
47. Lidang Jensen M, Schumacher B, Myhre Jensen O, Steen Nielsen O, Keller J. Extraskeletal osteosarcomas: a clinicopathologic study of 25 cases. Am J Surg Pathol 1998;22:588-594.

Extraskeletal Osteosarcoma

48. Fine G, Stout AP. Osteogenic sarcoma of the extraskeletal soft tissues. Cancer 1956;9:1027-1043.
49. Allan CJ, Soule EH. Osteogenic sarcoma of the somatic soft tissues. Clinicopathologic study of 26 cases and review of literature. Cancer 1971;27:1121-1133.
50. Sordillo PP, Hajdu SI, Magill GB, Golbey RB. Extraosseous osteogenic sarcoma. A review of 48 patients. Cancer 1983;51:727-734.
51. Chung EB, Enzinger FM. Extraskeletal osteosarcoma. Cancer 1987;60:1132-1142.
52. Fang Z, Yokoyama R, Mukai K, Beppu Y, Fukuma H. Extraskeletal osteosarcoma: a clinicopathologic study of four cases. Jpn J Clin Oncol 1995;25:55-60.
53. Lidang Jensen M, Schumacher B, Myhre Jensen O, Steen Nielsen O, Keller J. Extraskeletal osteosarcomas: a clinicopathologic study of 25 cases. Am J Surg Pathol 1998;22:588-594.
54. Lee JS, Fetsch JF, Wasdhal DA, Lee BP, Pritchard DJ, Nascimento AG. A review of 40 patients with extraskeletal osteosarcoma. Cancer 1995;76:2253-2259.
55. Park SG, Song JY, Song IG, Kim MS, Shin BS. Cutaneous extraskeletal osteosarcoma on the scar of a previous bone graft. Ann Dermatol 2011;23(Suppl 2):S160-164.
56. Larsen S, Davis DM, Comfere NI, Folpe AL, Sciallis GF. Osteosarcoma of the skin. Int J Dermatol 2010;49:532-540.
57. Riddle ND, Bowers JW, Bui MM, Morgan MB. Primary cutaneous osteoblastic osteosarcoma: a case report and review of the current literature. Clin Exp Dermatol 2009;34:e879-880.
58. Kobos JW, Yu GH, Varadarajan S, Brooks JS. Primary cutaneous osteosarcoma. [see comments]. Am J Dermatopathol 1995;17:53-57.
59. Kuo TT. Primary osteosarcoma of the skin. J Cutan Pathol 1992;19:151-155.
60. Wiklund TA, Blomqvist CP, Raty J, Elomaa I, Rissanen P, Miettinen M. Postirradiation sarcoma. Analysis of a nationwide cancer registry material. Cancer 1991;68:524-531.
61. Laskin WB, Silverman TA, Enzinger FM. Postradiation soft tissue sarcomas. An analysis of 53 cases. Cancer 1988;62:2330-2340.
62. Alpert LI, Abaci IF, Werthamer S. Radiation-induced extraskeletal osteosarcoma. Cancer 1973;31:1359-1363.
63. Boyer CW, Jr., Navin JJ. Extraskeletal osteogenic sarcoma; a late complication of radiation therapy Cancer 1965;18:628-633.
64. Abramovici LC, Hytiroglou P, Klein RM, et al. Well-differentiated extraskeletal osteosarcoma: report of 2 cases, 1 with dedifferentiation. Hum Pathol 2005;36:439-443.
65. Yoshida A, Ushiku T, Motoi T, Shibata T, Fukayama M, Tsuda H. Well-differentiated liposarcoma with low-grade osteosarcomatous component: an underrecognized variant. Am J Surg Pathol 2010;34:1361-1366.

66. Fanburg-Smith JC, Bratthauer GL, Miettinen M. Osteocalcin and osteonectin immunoreactivity in extraskeletal osteosarcoma: A study of 28 cases. Hum Pathol 1999;30:32-8.

Ossifying Fibromyxoid Tumor

67. Enzinger FM, Weiss SW, Liang CY. Ossifying fibromyxoid tumor of soft parts. A clinicopathologic analysis of 59 cases. Am J Surg Pathol 1989;13:817-827.

68. Miettinen M, Finnell V, Fetsch JF. Ossifying fibromyxoid tumor of soft parts. Clinicopathological analysis of 104 cases and a critical review of literature. Am J Surg Pathol 2008;32:995-1005.

69. Schofield JB, Krausz T, Stamp GW, Fletcher CD, Fisher C; Azzopardi JG. Ossifying fibromyxoid tumour of soft parts: immunohistochemical and ultrastructural analysis. Histopathology 1993; 22:101-112.

70. Miettinen M. Ossifying fibromyxoid tumor of soft parts. Additional observations of a distinctive soft tissue tumor. Am J Clin Pathol 1991;95:142-149.

71. Zamecnik M, Michal M, Simpson RH, et al. Ossifying firbromyxoid tumor of soft parts: a report of 17 cases with emphasis on unusual histologic features. Ann Diagn Pathol 1997;1:73-81.

72. Williams SB, Ellis GL, Meis JM, et al. Ossifying fibromyxoid tumour (of soft parts) of the head and neck: a clinicopathological and immunohistochemical study of nine cases. J Laryngol Otol 1993;107:75-80.

73. Hanski V, Lewicki Z. New observations on three cases of ossifying fibromyxoid tumor of soft parts. Pat Pol 1994;45:231-238.

74. Holck S, Pederson JG, Ackermann T, et al. Ossifying fibromyxoid tumour of soft parts, with focus on unusual clinicopathological features. Histopathology 2003;42:599-604.

75. Kilpatrick SE, Ward WG, Mozes M, Miettinen M, Fukunaga M, Fletcher CD. Atypical and malignant variants of ossifying fibromyxoid tumor. Clinicopathologic analysis of six cases. Am J Surg Pathol 1995;19:1039-1046.

76. Folpe AL, Weiss SW. Ossifying fibromyxoid tumor of soft parts. A clinicopathologic study of 70 cases with emphasis on atypical and malignant variants. Am J Surg Pathol 2003;27:421-431.

77. Sovani V, Velagaleti GVN, Filipowicz E, Gatalica Z, Knisely AS. Ossifying fibromyxoid tumor of soft parts: report of a case with novel cytogenetic findings. Cancer Genet Cytogenet 2001;127:1-6.

78. Gebre-Medhin S, Nord KH, Möller E, et al. Recurrent rearrangement of the PHF1 gene in ossifying fibromyxoid tumors. Am J Pathol 2012;181:1069-1077.

79. Graham RP, Weiss SW, Sukov WR, et al. PHF1 rearrangements in ossifying fibromyxoid tumors of soft parts: a fluorescence in situ hybridization study of 41 cases with emphasis on the malignant variant. Am J Surg Pathol 2013;37:1751-1755.

9

SOFT TISSUE TUMORS WITH EPITHELIAL DIFFERENTIATION

This chapter discusses four different, mostly unrelated, entities that are characterized by variable epithelial differentiation, either morphologically or immunohistochemically: synovial sarcoma, epithelioid sarcoma, extrarenal rhabdoid tumor, and mixed tumor/myoepithelioma. Of these, epithelioid sarcoma and extrarenal rhabdoid tumor have overlapping features and, in fact, may be difficult to distinguish under certain circumstances. Metastatic carcinomas and mesothelioma may show similar immunohistochemical features and sometimes also overlapping morphology. Thorough morphologic evaluation and extended panels of immunohistochemical stains are necessary for the differential diagnosis.

SYNOVIAL SARCOMA

Definition. *Synovial sarcoma* is a clinically, histopathologically, and genetically distinct sarcoma showing epithelial differentiation at either the light microscopic level (*biphasic synovial sarcoma*) or by immunohistochemistry or ultrastructural analysis (*monophasic synovial sarcoma*). It has no re-

lationship to non-neoplastic synovial tissue, and may occur at essentially any location. Archaic synonyms include *tendosynovial sarcoma, synovial cell sarcoma, carcinosarcoma of soft tissues, malignant synovioma*, and *synovioblastic sarcoma*.

Clinical Features. Synovial sarcomas are common tumors, accounting for up to 10 percent of soft tissue sarcomas (1–5). They usually occur in young adults (median age, 34 years), although they are seen at any age. The tumors are more common in males (fig. 9-1). The usual location for synovial sarcoma is adjacent to the knee, although this tumor may occur in any somatic soft tissue location, as well as, rarely, within the viscera (fig. 9-2). For unknown reasons, synovial sarcomas are very rare in the retroperitoneum (6). Approximately 10 percent involve the head and neck (7–11).

Synovial sarcoma typically presents as a nonspecific soft tissue mass or swelling, sometimes with associated pain. The tumors often grow slowly and are not felt to represent malignancies clinically. Calcifications may be radiographically apparent in some tumors.

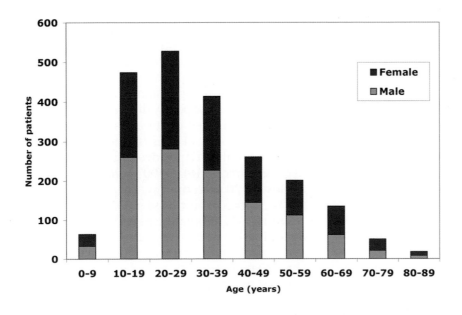

Figure 9-1

SYNOVIAL SARCOMA

Age and sex distribution of 2,130 patients with synovial sarcoma.

Gross Findings. Most synovial sarcomas appear as nonspecific soft tissue masses. Calcified examples may have a gritty texture. Many tumors are well circumscribed, although infiltration of adjacent structures, in particular tendons and joint capsules, is invariably present. Cystic change may be prominent. Most synovial sarcomas are small at the time of diagnosis (3 to 6 cm).

Microscopic Findings. Monophasic fibrous synovial sarcoma accounts for approximately 70 percent of synovial sarcomas. It is characterized by moderately long fascicles of uniform, hyperchromatic spindled cells, with variable myxoid change, creating an appearance of alternating zones of hypercellularity and hypocellularity ("marbled pattern") (fig. 9-3). The tumor cells lack pleomorphism and have "carrot-shaped" nuclei with small or indistinct nucleoli. The presence of pleomorphic cells within a biphasic soft tissue tumor should suggest the possibility of metastatic carcinosarcoma, rather than synovial sarcoma. Mitotic activity is often deceptively low. Branching, "hemangiopericytoma-like" vessels, wiry collagen, stromal calcifications, and numerous mast cells are frequently present (12–16).

Biphasic synovial sarcomas have scattered foci of glandular differentiation, usually in the form of small glands lined by low cuboidal to columnar epithelium, often with intraluminal necrotic eosinophilic debris (fig. 9-4). Rarely, squamous differentiation is present. Glandular differentiation may be difficult to appreciate by light microscopy, requiring cytokeratin immunostains for confirmation (occult glandular differentiation) or may, rarely, be extensive, obscuring the underlying spindle cell component (monophasic epithelial synovial sarcoma). It is unlikely that purely epithelial synovial sarcomas truly exist.

Poorly differentiated synovial sarcoma is best considered a form of tumor progression in monophasic fibrous or biphasic synovial sarcoma, rather than a distinct variant. Poorly differentiated synovial sarcomas are characterized by round cell differentiation, rhabdoid features, geographic necrosis, and elevated mitotic activity (fig. 9-5A,B) (12,13,16,17). The hemangiopericytoma-like vascular pattern is often accentuated in poorly differentiated synovial sarcomas, and it is likely that many tumors previously reported as malignant hemangiopericytomas represent instead synovial sarcomas

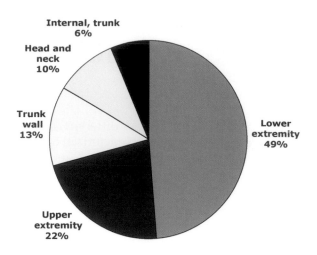

Figure 9-2

SYNOVIAL SARCOMA

Anatomic distribution of 2,130 synovial sarcomas.

(18). Some synovial sarcomas are extensively myxoid (fig. 9-5C,D).

Special Studies. Biphasic synovial sarcomas do not require immunohistochemistry for diagnosis, although occasionally distinguishing biphasic synovial sarcomas with only focal glandular differentiation from monophasic tumors requires cytokeratin immunostains. Monophasic synovial sarcomas express cytokeratins of both simple and complex epithelial types (low and high molecular weight cytokeratins), and antibodies to high molecular weight cytokeratins may be helpful in the diagnosis of poorly differentiated tumors (12,16,17,19,20). Expression of CK7 and CK19 help distinguish monophasic synovial sarcoma from malignant peripheral nerve sheath tumors (21). Cytokeratin expression is typically limited in monophasic and poorly differentiated synovial sarcomas, and often confined to individual cells and small groups of cells (fig. 9-3C). Epithelial membrane antigen is positive in some cytokeratin-negative tumors (16). S-100 protein is expressed in close to 20 percent of synovial sarcomas, but CD34 expression is not seen (17,21).

Expression of putative nerve sheath markers, including nerve growth factor receptor, CD57, and neurofilament protein may be seen (16,23). Over 70 percent of synovial sarcomas are CD99 positive, particularly poorly differentiated tumors

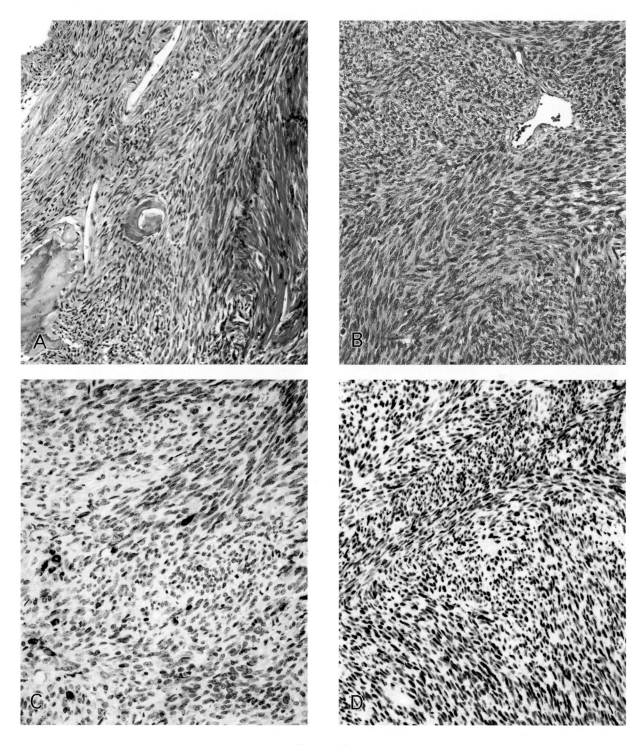

Figure 9-3

MONOPHASIC FIBROUS SYNOVIAL SARCOMA

A: The characteristic "marbled" pattern, with alternating zones of hypercellularity and hypocellularity, is seen.

B: The cellular areas consist of a monomorphic proliferation of uniform, hyperchromatic spindled cells with "carrot-shaped" nuclei.

C: By immunohistochemistry, monophasic fibrous synovial sarcomas typically show only scattered cytokeratin-positive cells.

D: Diffuse expression of transducin-like enhancer (TLE)-1 protein is characteristic.

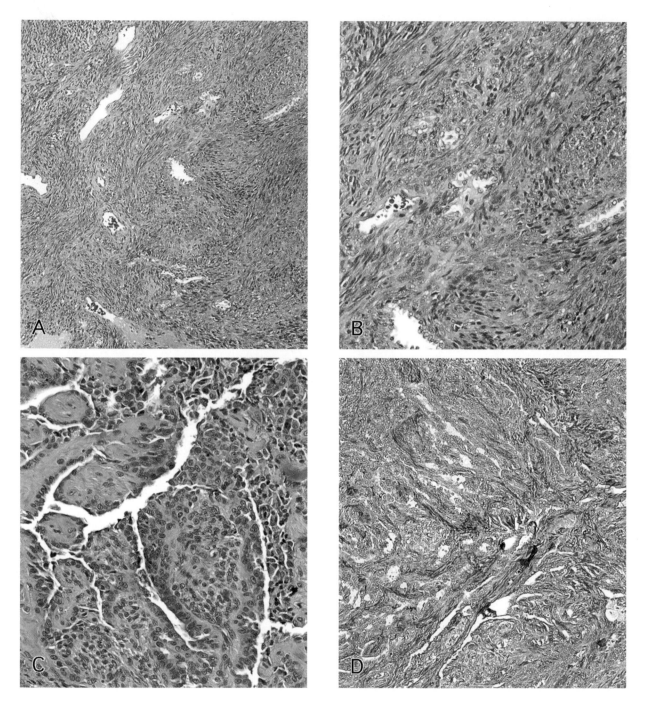

Figure 9-4

BIPHASIC SYNOVIAL SARCOMA

A: Most biphasic synovial sarcomas consist predominantly of spindled cells, identical to monophasic fibrous synovial sarcoma, with scattered small glands.

B: The glands are typically lined by small, uniform, cuboidal epithelial cells, and may contain intraluminal eosinophilic, necrotic debris.

C: In some cases, glandular differentiation takes the form of elongated, branching glandular structures, creating a pseudopapillary appearance.

D: In rare instances, the epithelial component of biphasic synovial sarcoma may predominate, with only a minor component of spindled cells. Such cases likely account for those rare tumors reported as examples of monophasic epithelioid synovial sarcoma.

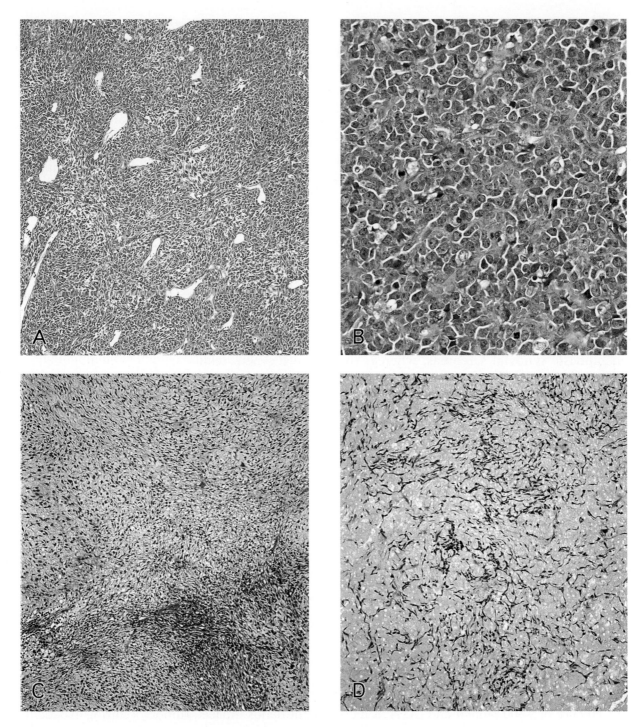

Figure 9-5

POORLY DIFFERENTIATED SYNOVIAL SARCOMA

A: Poorly differentiated synovial sarcomas often show an accentuated "hemangiopericytoma-like" vascular pattern, and may be mistaken for malignant hemangiopericytoma. The poorly differentiated histology represents a form of tumor progression in both monophasic and biphasic synovial sarcomas, rather than a distinct subtype.

B: There is a highly cellular proliferation of mitotically active primitive round cells.

C: In some cases, the hypocellular myxoid zones predominate.

D: Purely myxoid synovial sarcomas may appear deceptively bland, mimicking a variety of other myxoid soft tissue tumors.

(16,17,24,25). Many synovial sarcomas are positive for bcl-2, a nonspecific maker of questionable use (26). Diffuse nuclear expression of tranducin-like element-1 (TLE-1) protein is a highly sensitive marker of all types of synovial sarcoma, although more limited expression may be seen in a variety of other soft tissue tumors, in particular, nerve sheath tumors (fig. 9-3D) (27–29).

Genetics. Synovial sarcomas are characterized genetically by the presence of balanced, reciprocal translocations, including t(X;18)(p11.23;q11)(SS18-SSX1) in approximately 65 percent of cases, t(X;18)(p11.21;q11)(SS18-SSX2) in approximately 35 percent of cases, and t(X;18)(p11;q11)(SS18-SSX4), t(X;20)(p11;q13.3)(SS18L1-SSX1) in less than 1 percent of cases (30–34). These translocations are detected by traditional cytogenetics, reverse transcriptase polymerase chain reaction (RT-PCR) or fluorescence in situ hybridization (FISH) and are specific for synovial sarcoma (35,36). *SS18-SSX1* fusions are more common in biphasic synovial sarcomas, whereas the monophasic variant more often contains the *SS18-SSX2* fusion (37–41). It has been suggested (38–42) that patients with the *SS18-SSX2* fusion may have a better prognosis than those with the *SS18-SSX1* variant, although this has not been confirmed in other studies.

Differential Diagnosis. Monophasic synovial sarcomas should be distinguished from other monomorphic spindle cell sarcomas, including malignant peripheral nerve sheath tumor, adult-type fibrosarcoma, and solitary fibrous tumors. The histologic features of monophasic synovial sarcoma and malignant peripheral nerve sheath tumor overlap significantly, and there are no histopathologic features, with the exceptions of pleomorphism, occurrence in a patient with known neurofibromatosis type 1, or clear-cut origin from a neurofibroma, that definitively allow this distinction. Both synovial sarcoma and malignant peripheral nerve sheath tumor may arise from nerves. Expression of cytokeratins, in the absence of S-100 protein and CD34, is most characteristic of synovial sarcoma, although up to 20 percent express S-100 protein. Cytogenetic or molecular genetic evidence of a synovial sarcoma–associated translocation is thus considered the "gold standard" for this distinction.

Adult-type fibrosarcoma is by definition a diagnosis of exclusion and many tumors previously so classified represent instead monophasic synovial sarcomas. Immunohistochemistry for TLE-1 may be valuable in the distinction of cytokeratin-negative monophasic synovial sarcoma from adult-type fibrosarcoma. Although both synovial sarcomas and solitary fibrous tumors contain wiry collagen and hemangiopericytoma-like vasculature, solitary fibrous tumors lack the fascicular arrangement, alternating hypocellularity and hypercellularity, and hyperchromatism exhibited by monophasic synovial sarcomas, and are CD34 positive. Small synovial sarcomas of the hands and feet may be deceptively bland appearing, thus mimicking benign fibrous histiocytomas. The presence of stromal calcifications and the demonstration of epithelial marker expression are of value in this distinction.

Poorly differentiated synovial sarcomas are distinguished from other round cell sarcomas by the identification of areas of conventional monophasic or biphasic synovial sarcoma and with genetic tests.

Biphasic synovial sarcomas must be distinguished from carcinosarcomas and mesotheliomas, particularly in intra-abdominal and mediastinal locations. Carcinosarcomas typically arise in much older patients than do synovial sarcomas and show much greater pleomorphism. Biphasic mesotheliomas typically show diffuse cytokeratin expression and expression of mesothelial markers, such as calretinin and WT-1. Specific translocations are not seen in carcinosarcomas or mesotheliomas.

Treatment and Prognosis. Synovial sarcomas are considered to be at least grade II sarcomas under the National Cancer Institute and French Federation of Cancer Centers (FNCLCC) sarcoma grading systems (43), with cases showing poorly differentiated histology having the worst prognosis (12,13,15). Thus all synovial sarcomas are considered high grade for purposes of clinical management, with the possible exception of very hypocellular, heavily calcified tumors of the hands and feet. Tumors occurring in patients under 15 years of age, less than 5 cm in size, and containing massive calcification with few tumor cells appear to confer the best prognosis (13,15). The 5-year survival rate for patients with synovial sarcoma is approximately 55 percent (12,13,15,44). Synovial sarcomas are treated with aggressive multimodality therapy.

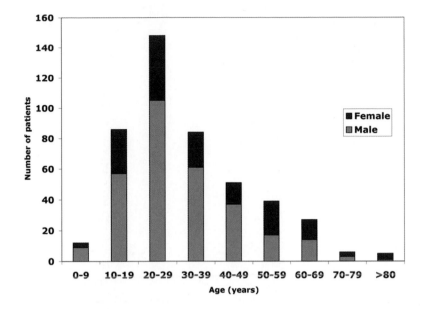

Figure 9-6

EPITHELIOID SARCOMA

Age and sex distribution of 458 patients with epithelioid sarcoma.

EPITHELIOID SARCOMA

Definition. *Epithelioid sarcoma* is a distinctive sarcoma with epithelial differentiation that most often involves the distal extremities of young patients.

General Considerations. Epithelioid sarcoma was first formally described by Enzinger in 1970 (45). It had previously been considered part of the spectrum of "tendosynovial sarcoma," a term previously used to describe what we now consider to represent epithelioid sarcoma, clear cell sarcoma, and synovial sarcoma.

Clinical Features. Classic epithelioid sarcomas most commonly occur in adolescents and young adults, with a median age of 26 years. The tumor is approximately twice as common in males as females (fig. 9-6). Epithelioid sarcomas usually involve the hands and fingers, followed by the wrist and lower arm, and lower leg and knee, but may occur in any location (45–47). Involvement of tendons and aponeuroses is common (fig. 9-7). Most are small (less than 5 cm) at the time of diagnosis. Proximal-type epithelioid sarcomas tend to occur in older adults; most often involve the deep soft tissues of the perineum, genital region, and pelvic soft tissues; and present as much larger masses than do classic epithelioid sarcomas (48).

Classic epithelioid sarcoma often presents as a small, indurated, sometimes ulcerated nodule or nodules, frequently present for several weeks

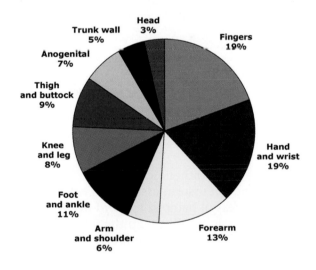

Figure 9-7

EPITHELIOID SARCOMA

Anatomic distribution of 458 epithelioid sarcomas.

or longer before coming to clinical attention. The clinical index of suspicion for a malignant lesion is often low, and many classic epithelioid sarcomas are initially thought to represent abscesses, warts, and other non-neoplastic processes (46). Proximal-type epithelioid sarcoma presents as a nonspecific soft tissue mass (47,48).

Gross Findings. Epithelioid sarcomas are typically small, ulcerated, firm, single or multiple nodules, sometimes with overlying ulceration.

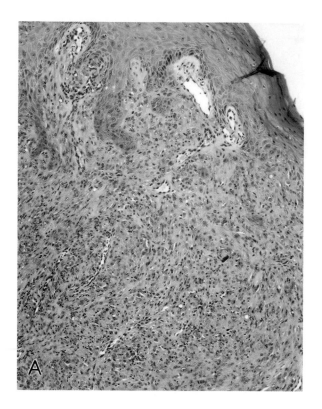 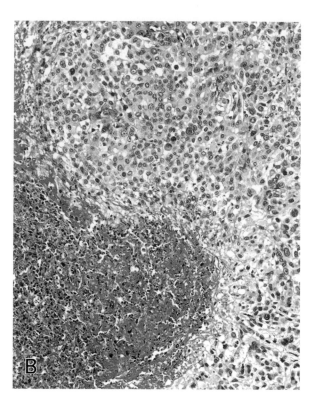

Figure 9-8

EPITHELIOID SARCOMA INVOLVING THE SKIN

A: Such tumors appear to arise from the epidermis, potentially resulting in a misdiagnosis as squamous cell carcinoma.
B: Necrosis within epithelioid sarcoma tumor cell nests may mimic a rheumatoid nodule or other necrobiotic processes. The cells are usually small and fairly bland, although nuclear irregularity and hyperchromasia are apparent on close inspection.

Proximal-type epithelioid sarcomas are larger, nonspecific soft tissue masses, often with grossly apparent areas of hemorrhage and necrosis.

Microscopic Findings. Epithelioid sarcomas may appear fairly circumscribed at low-power magnification, but are invariably highly infiltrative tumors, frequently extending into the surrounding connective tissue in the form of small nests and single files of individual tumor cells (45–47). Tumor nodules often show central necrosis, mimicking necrobiotic granulomas. When individual tumor nodules grow along tendons and fuse, they produce a "garland-like" appearance. The neoplastic cells may appear small and epithelioid, or show greater pleomorphism and a rhabdoid appearance, particularly in larger, more proximally located tumors (47,48).

Although an epithelioid morphology is always at least focally present, many epithelioid sarcomas also show cellular spindling, and this "modulation" from epithelioid to spindled cells is a charac-teristic finding (fig. 9-8). Rare epithelioid sarcomas consist chiefly of spindled cells (fibroma-like variant), potentially mimicking fibrous histiocytoma and other low-grade spindle cell lesions (49).

The nuclei of epithelioid sarcoma cells are uniform appearing, but invariably show hyperchromatism, chromatin abnormalities, and irregular nuclear contours. The nucleoli are usually small or inapparent.

Unusual morphologic changes include pseudovascular change, pseudogland formation, myxoid change, calcification, and bone formation (50,51). A mixed chronic inflammatory cell infiltrate is typically present, and may occasionally be so pronounced as to obscure the underlying tumor, or to suggest a hemato-lymphoid neoplasm instead (fig. 9-9).

Special Studies. Epithelioid sarcomas express cytokeratins, including those of low and high molecular weights (47,48). They are generally negative, however, for CK5/6, a finding that

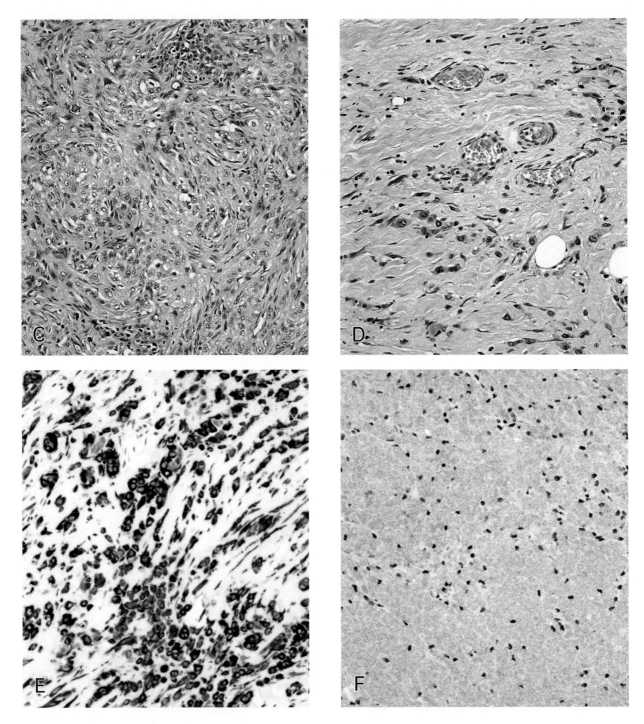

Figure 9-8, continued

C: The neoplastic cells tend to "modulate" from epithelioid to spindled, a characteristic finding.

D: Although epithelioid sarcomas appear circumscribed at scanning magnification, higher-power magnification invariably reveals infiltrative growth of small tumor nests and single cells into the surrounding soft tissues, particularly at the periphery of the lesion. This growth pattern likely accounts for the high local recurrence rate of epithelioid sarcoma.

E: By immunohistochemistry, epithelioid sarcomas express cytokeratins (seen here), vimentin, and in approximately 50 percent of cases, CD34.

F: Loss of SMARCB1/INI1 protein expression is seen in approximately 90 percent of cases, and helps to distinguish epithelioid sarcomas from carcinomas and other cytokeratin-positive sarcomas.

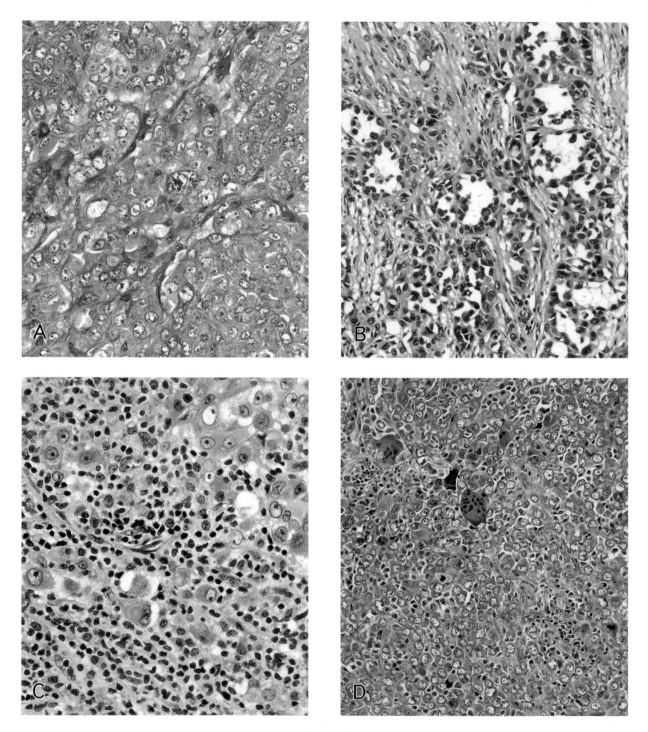

Figure 9-9

EPITHELIOID SARCOMA: MORPHOLOGIC VARIATION

A: Proximal-type epithelioid sarcoma shows greater nuclear pleomorphism and rhabdoid cytomorphology.

B: Loss of cellular cohesion in nests of epithelioid sarcoma tumor cells creates a pseudoglandular or pseudovascular appearance.

C: Many epithelioid sarcomas elicit a chronic inflammatory cell infiltrate, and in some cases, this infiltrate is dense enough to largely obscure the underlying neoplasm.

D: Osteoclast-rich epithelioid sarcoma.

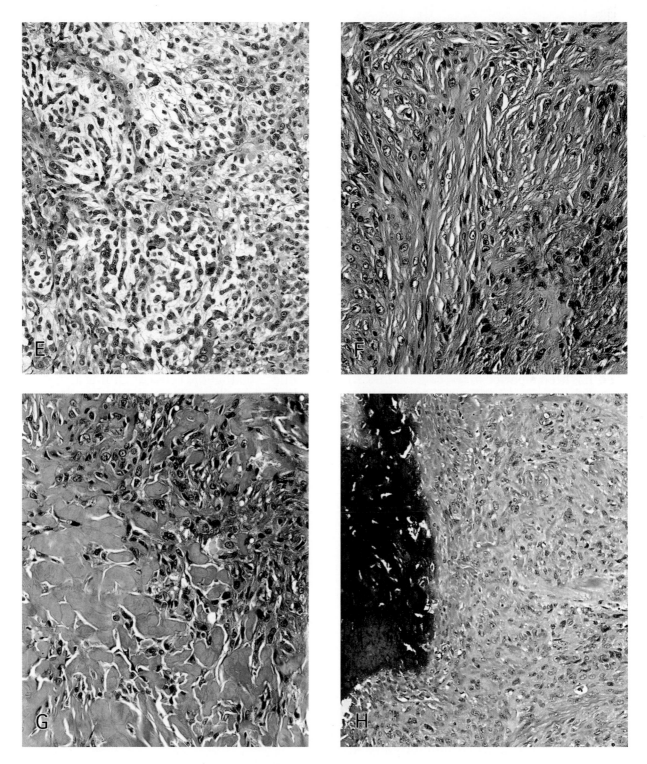

Figure 9-9, continued

E: Rare myxoid change mimics other myxoid soft tissue tumors.

F: Epithelioid sarcomas with a principally spindled pattern of growth ("fibroma-like") mimic benign fibrous histiocytomas and other low-grade spindle cell tumors.

G: Extensive collagen deposition may mimic the stromal changes that accompany fibrous histiocytomas.

H: Bone production is an uncommon finding.

may be of value in their distinction from cutaneous squamous cell carcinoma (52). Rarely, epithelioid sarcomas show limited expression of cytokeratins, or are even cytokeratin negative. Epithelioid sarcomas are also frequently positive for epithelial membrane antigen and GLUT-1, findings that have suggested the possibility of perineurial differentiation in these tumors (53,54). CD34 is expressed by approximately 50 percent of cases, in contrast with less than 2 percent of carcinomas (48,55,56). Epithelioid sarcomas do not express other markers of endothelial differentiation, such as CD31, FLI-1, or vWF. Over 90 percent of epithelioid sarcomas of both classic and proximal type show loss of expression of SMARCB1/INI1/BAF47, a finding that is useful in their distinction from carcinomas and other cytokeratin-positive sarcomas (53,57).

Genetics. The few cytogenetic studies of epithelioid sarcomas show nonspecific chromosomal gains and losses (58–64). However, loss of 22q11, the location of the *SMARCB1/INI1/BAF47* gene, has been reported in few cases. *SMARCB1/INI1/BAF47* homozygous gene deletions have also been reported in epithelioid sarcomas of both classic and proximal type (51,65–67).

Differential Diagnosis. Epithelioid sarcomas differ from granulomatous processes by the infiltrative growth pattern, the presence of true tumor cell necrosis as opposed to necrobiosis, the presence of hyperchromatic cells expressing cytokeratins, and the loss of SMARCB1/INI1 expression. Loss of SMARCB1/INI1 expression is also helpful in the distinction of epithelioid sarcomas from primary and metastatic carcinomas. Pseudovascular epithelioid sarcomas often express high molecular weight cytokeratins, unlike endothelial cell neoplasms, and lack expression of CD31, FLI-1 protein, vWF, and SMARCB1/INI-1.

Fibroma-like epithelioid sarcomas may be bland in appearance, closely mimicking cellular fibrous histiocytoma and other low-grade spindle cell tumors of the distal extremities. Cytokeratin immunostains help differentiate these tumors. Factor XIIIa immunostains are not helpful in this setting.

Calcified epithelioid sarcomas may mimic calcifying aponeurotic fibroma, but lack the distinctive chondroid nodules seen in that entity, and show cytokeratin expression. Synovial sarcomas bear little, if any, resemblance to epithelioid sarcomas, beyond sharing cytokeratin expression.

Treatment and Prognosis. Epithelioid sarcomas recur in over 70 percent of cases, often as multiple subcutaneous nodules in the more proximal extremity. Nearly 50 percent of epithelioid sarcomas eventually metastasize distantly, most often to lymph nodes and lungs, but also to skin and soft tissue sites (45–47). Metastatic epithelioid sarcomas are almost uniformly fatal.

Epithelioid sarcomas are not graded. The adverse prognostic features are chiefly clinical and include male sex, proximal location, size over 5 cm, and deep location. Pathologic parameters such as high mitotic rate, necrosis, and vascular invasion are also been associated with worse outcome in some studies, but their prognostic value is outweighed by clinical variables.

EXTRARENAL RHABDOID TUMOR

Extrarenal rhabdoid tumor is analogous to a similar tumor in the kidney that is composed of round to epithelioid cells containing abundant intermediate filament material as inclusions (fig. 9-10A–C). The tumor is positive for keratins and other epithelial markers and characteristically immunohistochemically lacks INI1/SMARCB1 gene product expression (fig. 9-10D).

Extrarenal rhabdoid tumor is rare and has features that overlap with those of epithelioid sarcoma. It usually occurs in young children and is clinically very aggressive. Many other sarcomas and even nonsarcomatous tumors (some carcinomas, mesothelioma, and malignant melanoma) contain similar intermediate filament inclusions, so that the rhabdoid appearance is not sufficient for diagnosis. An extensive immunohistochemical work-up to rule out other possibilities should be performed. This diagnosis should be considered for tumors primarily occurring in young children and showing a prominent rhabdoid cytomorphology, keratin and epithelial membrane antigen expression, and lack of INI1/SMARCB1 gene product.

MIXED TUMOR/MYOEPITHELIOMA

Definition. *Mixed tumor/myoepithelioma* is a soft tissue tumor that is analogous to similar tumors in skin and salivary glands. Mixed tumor refers to examples with recognizable tubular epithelial components, whereas myoepithelioma

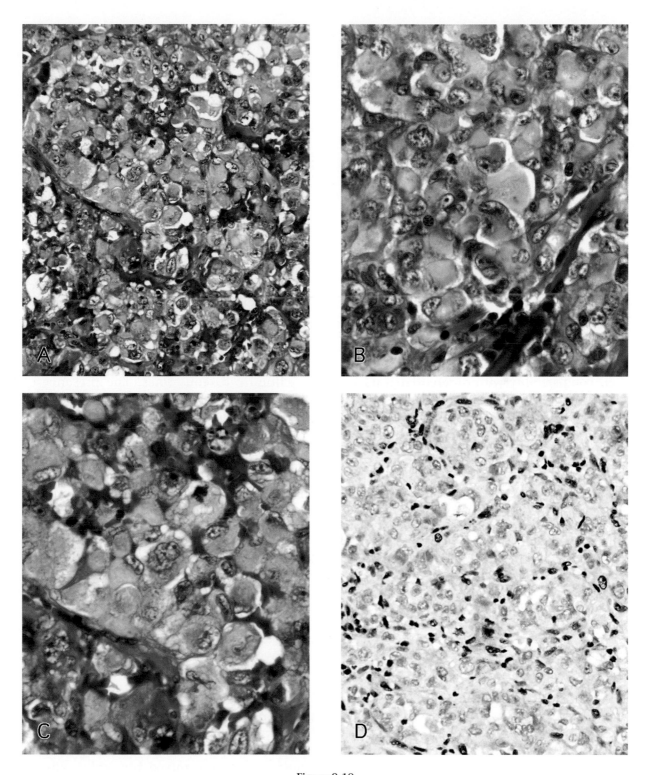

Figure 9-10

EXTRARENAL RHABDOID TUMOR

A-C: Extrarenal rhabdoid tumor shows epithelioid cytology. Higher magnification reveals eosinophilic, inclusion-like cytoplasm in many cells.

D: Tumor cells lack Integrase Interactor 1 (INI1/SMARCB1) protein seen in the stromal cells.

is a spindle cell neoplasm with a myoepithelial phenotype as determined by immunohistochemistry or other means. *Chondroid syringoma* is synonymous, and *parachordoma* is a histologic variant.

General Comments. Most mixed tumors of soft tissue are probably of skin adnexal origin and are centered in the subcutis. Some, however, arise from deeper soft tissues or even bone. Initially reported as mixed tumors of the skin of salivary gland type (68) and chondroid syringomas (69), the literature is now using myoepithelioma a catch-all term to also include mixed tumors (70–74). Here we use the designation mixed tumor/myoepithelioma.

Mixed tumors/myoepitheliomas have a spectrum from benign to malignant, and the latter have also been called *myoepithelial carcinomas*. Some tumors diagnosed as myoepithelial carcinomas in children are primitive round cell tumors (75), and we consider their classification as myoepithelial carcinomas controversial and their comparability with differentiated mixed tumor/myoepitheliomas as questionable.

Clinical Features. Mixed tumors/myoepitheliomas of soft tissue occur at all ages but have a predilection for adults of 30 to 50 years. Malignant myoepitheliomas (myoepithelial carcinomas) have been reported in children from infancy on (73–77). Tumors containing tubular epithelial elements and therefore qualifying as mixed tumors have a predilection for the head and neck area, whereas myoepitheliomas preferentially occur in the extremities and trunk wall. Distal sites, especially fingers and toes, are also frequently involved.

The tumor varies from a small nodule of 1 cm or less to a mass over 10 cm, but most examples are smaller than 4 cm. The larger tumors have generally occurred in deep soft tissues.

Gross Findings. Grossly, mixed tumor/myoepithelioma forms a circumscribed mass that is white to gray-white on sectioning and may have a cartilaginous or myxoid texture.

Microscopic Findings. Histologically, these tumors vary. At one end of the spectrum is a tumor containing tubular epithelial elements, along with solid sheets of epithelioid cells (fig. 9-11). Mixed tumors are divided into eccrine and apocrine types (the latter is more common), but this does not seem to have great clinical signifi-

cance (78). Some examples contain only solid sheets of epithelioid cells, or are composed of epithelioid cells arranged in cords or clusters in a fibrosclerosing or focally myxoid matrix. Some variants contain cells with a plasmacytoid morphology or "rhabdoid" cytoplasmic inclusions in intermediate filaments (fig. 9-11C) (79).

Parachordoma is a benign morphologic variant containing cords or vacuolated epithelioid cells resembling the epithelioid cells of chordoma. In general, both nuclear atypia and mitotic activity are limited (80–82). The World Health Organization (WHO) classification has concluded that it is reasonably similar to the mixed tumor/myoepithelioma group to be included as a variant (83).

The most convincing malignant examples contain elements recognizable as a benign mixed tumor or spindle cell myoepithelioma (84). The malignant elements vary from carcinomatous epithelial components to those containing mesenchymoid components, such as chondro-osseous ones. The presence of significant nuclear atypia and mitotic activity signal malignant potential, although there is no definite cut-off level for distinguishing benign from malignant (fig. 9-12).

Special Studies. Mixed tumors/myoepitheliomas are almost always immunohistochemically positive for S-100 protein. Most have also at least focally keratin-positive components, and many are extensively keratin positive with the AE1/AE3 cocktail antibody and epithelial membrane antigen. Patchy positivity for glial fibrillary acidic protein (GFAP) is a typical, although not ubiquitous, feature. Expression of myoepithelial markers, such as smooth muscle actin and calponin, is variable, and only a minority of cases contains cells positive for p63 and myoepithelial/basal cell keratins (CK5 and CK14), usually only focally.

Genetics. A subset of mixed tumor myoepitheliomas contains the Ewing sarcoma gene (*EWSR1*) involving fusion translocations, such as *EWSR1-POU5F1*, *EWSR1-PBX1*, and *EWSR1-ZNF444*. These translocations are different from those seen in the mixed tumors of salivary glands and the *EWSR1* fusion partners are different from those of Ewing sarcoma (85,86). Recently, *PLAG1* gene rearrangements have also been shown to be common in both cutaneous

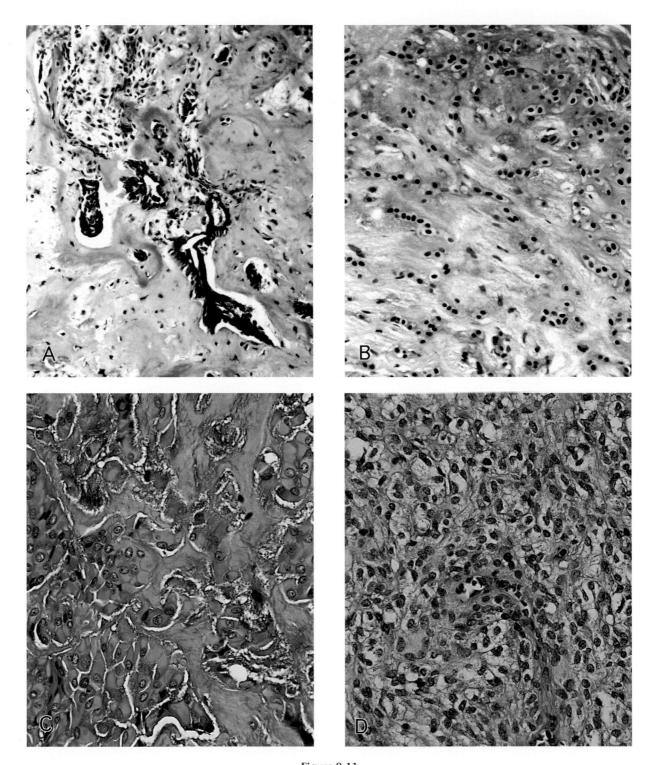

Figure 9-11

MIXED TUMOR/MYOEPITHELIOMA

A: This tumor with ductal elements and chondromyxoid matrix resembles mixed tumor of salivary glands.

B: Trabecular pattern with myxoid matrix.

C: Epithelioid cells with rhabdoid cytoplasmic inclusions.

D: Solid ovoid to spindle cell pattern of myoepithelioma.

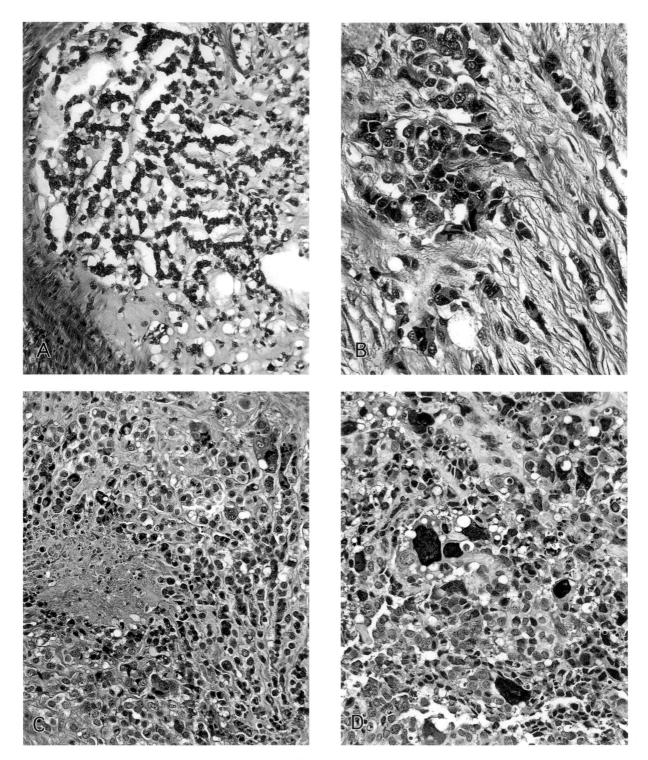

Figure 9-12

MALIGNANT MYOEPITHELIOMA

A: A tumor lobule contains cords of cells in a myxoid matrix.
B: Highly atypical cells form invasive cords in desmoplastic stroma.
C: Necrosis and mitotic activity are present.
D: Marked nuclear pleomorphism in the epithelioid component.

and soft tissue myoepitheliomas/mixed tumors with ductal differentiation similar to corresponding salivary gland tumors. PLAG1 immunohistochemistry may be useful for the identification of such tumors (87,88).

Differential Diagnosis. While the diagnosis of benign mixed tumors is usually straightforward, the examples with lesser or no obvious epithelial differentiation have to be separated from other S-100 protein- and GFAP-positive tumors. Epithelioid peripheral nerve sheath tumors lack both epithelial- and myoepithelial-specific markers. In the facial region, salivary gland mixed tumor has been ruled out before diagnosing a primary soft tissue tumor. Variants with corded patterns and myxoid matrix are difficult to separate from extraskeletal myxoid chondrosarcoma because of additional antigenic overlap. In such cases, detection of the *NR4A3* gene rearrangement supports the latter diagnosis (89).

Malignant examples pose greater diagnostic problems. They should be separated from biphasic synovial sarcoma, which has a distinctive combination of epithelial and spindle cell elements. Metaplastic carcinosarcomas from various origins (gynecologic, lung) and chordoma should be ruled out with clinicopathologic correlation before making the diagnosis of malignant soft tissue myoepithelioma. Malignant examples in body cavities should be separated from other aggressive epithelial tumors, such as germ cell tumors and NUT midline carcinoma.

Treatment and Prognosis. Complete excision is generally sufficient. More attention should be paid to documenting complete excision in atypical and malignant cases, including a strong consideration for re-excision after incomplete excision.

REFERENCES

Synovial Sarcoma

1. Toro JR, Travis LB, Wu HJ, Zhu K, Fletcher CD, Devesa SS. Incidence patterns of soft tissue sarcomas, regardless of primary site, in the surveillance, epidemiology and end results program, 1978-2001: an analysis of 26,758 cases. Int J Cancer 2006;119:2922-2930.

2. Yuceturk G, Sabah D, Kececi B, Kara AD, Yalcinkaya S. Prevalence of bone and soft tissue tumors. Acta Orthop Traumatol Turc 2011;45:135-143.

3. Fang ZW, Chen J, Teng S, Chen Y, Xue RF. Analysis of soft tissue sarcomas in 1118 cases. Chin Med J (Engl) 2009;122:51-53.

4. Hayes-Jordan AA, Spunt SL, Poquette CA, et al. Nonrhabdomyosarcoma soft tissue sarcomas in children: is age at diagnosis an important variable? J Pediatr Surg 2000;35:948-53; discussion 53-54.

5. Gustafson P. Soft tissue sarcoma. Epidemiology and prognosis in 508 patients. Acta Orthop Scand Suppl 1994;259:1-31.

6. Fisher C, Folpe AL, Hashimoto H, Weiss SW. Intra-abdominal synovial sarcoma: a clinicopathological study. Histopathology 2004;45:245-253.

7. Simunjak B, Petric V, Bedekovic V, Cupic H, Hat J. Dimensions and outcome of synovial sarcoma of the head and neck: case presentation and review of the literature. J Otolaryngol 2005;34:420-423.

8. Bentz BG, Singh B, Woodruff J, Brennan M, Shah JP, Kraus D. Head and neck soft tissue sarcomas: a multivariate analysis of outcomes. Ann Surg Oncol 2004;11:619-628.

9. Sturgis EM, Potter BO. Sarcomas of the head and neck region. Curr Opin Oncol 2003;15:239-252.

10. Potter BO, Sturgis EM. Sarcomas of the head and neck. Surg Oncol Clin N Am 2003;12:379-417.

11. Pandey M, Chandramohan K, Thomas G, et al. Soft tissue sarcoma of the head and neck region in adults. Int J Oral Maxillofac Surg 2003;32:43-48.

12. van de Rijn M, Barr FG, Xiong QB, Hedges M, Shipley J, Fisher C. Poorly differentiated synovial sarcoma: an analysis of clinical, pathologic, and molecular genetic features. Am J Surg Pathol 1999;23:106-112.

13. Skytting B, Meis-Kindblom JM, Larsson O, et al. Synovial sarcoma—identification of favorable and unfavorable histologic types: a Scandinavian sarcoma group study of 104 cases. Acta Orthop Scand 1999;70:543-554.

14. Krane JF, Bertoni F, Fletcher CD. Myxoid synovial sarcoma: an underappreciated morphologic subset. Mod Pathol 1999;12:456-462.

15. Bergh P, Meis-Kindblom JM, Gherlinzoni F, et al. Synovial sarcoma: identification of low and high risk groups. Cancer 1999;85:2596-2607.

16. Folpe AL, Schmidt RA, Chapman D, Gown AM. Poorly differentiated synovial sarcoma: immunohistochemical distinction from primitive neuroectodermal tumors and high-grade malignant peripheral nerve sheath tumors. Am J Surg Pathol 1998;22:673-682.

17. Pelmus M, Guillou L, Hostein I, Sierankowski G, Lussan C, Coindre JM. Monophasic fibrous and poorly differentiated synovial sarcoma: immunohistochemical reassessment of 60 t(X;18) (SYT-SSX)-positive cases. Am J Surg Pathol 2002;26:1434-440.

18. Enzinger FM, Smith BH. Hemangiopericytoma. An analysis of 106 cases. Hum Pathol 1976;7:61-82.

19. Miettinen M, Nobel MP, Tuma BT, Kovatich AJ. Keratin 17: Immunohistochemical mapping of its distribution in human epithelial tumors and its potential applications. Applied Immunohistochem 1997;5:152-159.

20. Fisher C. Synovial sarcoma. Ann Diagn Pathol 1998;2:401-421.

21. Guillou L, Wadden C, Kraus MD, Dei Tos AP, Fletcher CD. S-100 protein reactivity in synovial sarcomas—A potentially frequent diagnostic pitfall. Immunohistochemical analysis of 100 cases. Applied Immunohistochemistry. 1996;4(3):167-175.

22. Smith TA, Machen SK, Fisher C, Goldblum JR. Usefulness of cytokeratin subsets for distinguishing monophasic synovial sarcoma from malignant peripheral nerve sheath tumor. Am J Clin Pathol 1999;112:641-648.

23. Fanburg-Smith JC, Miettinen M. Low-affinity nerve growth factor receptor (p75) in dermatofibrosarcoma protuberans and other nonneural tumors: a study of 1,150 tumors and fetal and adult normal tissues. Hum Pathol 2001;32:976-983.

24. Sun B, Sun Y, Wang J, et al. The diagnostic value of SYT-SSX detected by reverse transcriptase-polymerase chain reaction (RT-PCR) and fluorescence in situ hybridization (FISH) for synovial sarcoma: a review and prospective study of 255 cases. Cancer Sci 2008;99:1355-1361.

25. Renshaw AA. O13 (CD99) in spindle cell tumors. Reactivity with hemangiopericytoma, solitary fibrous tumor, synovial sarcoma, and meningioma but rarely with sarcomatoid mesothelioma. Appl Immunohistochem 1995;3:250-256.

26. Antonescu CR, Kawai A, Leung DH, et al. Strong association of SYT-SSX fusion type and morphologic epithelial differentiation in synovial sarcoma. Diagn Mol Pathol 2000;9:1-8.

27. Kosemehmetoglu K, Vrana JA, Folpe AL. TLE1 expression is not specific for synovial sarcoma: a whole section study of 163 soft tissue and bone neoplasms. Mod Pathol 2009;22:872-878.

28. Jagdis A, Rubin BP, Tubbs RR, Pacheco M, Nielsen TO. Prospective evaluation of TLE1 as a diagnostic immunohistochemical marker in synovial sarcoma. Am J Surg Pathol 2009;33:1743-1751.

29. Terry J, Saito T, Subramanian S, et al. TLE1 as a diagnostic immunohistochemical marker for synovial sarcoma emerging from gene expression profiling studies. Am J Surg Pathol 2007;31:240-246.

30. Amary MF, Berisha F, Bernardi Fdel C, et al. Detection of SS18-SSX fusion transcripts in formalin-fixed paraffin-embedded neoplasms: analysis of conventional RT-PCR, qRT-PCR and dual color FISH as diagnostic tools for synovial sarcoma. Mod Pathol 2007;20:482-496.

31. Panagopoulos I, Mertens F, Isaksson M, et al. Clinical impact of molecular and cytogenetic findings in synovial sarcoma. Genes Chromosomes Cancer 2001;31:362-372.

32. Ladanyi M. Fusions of the SYT and SSX genes in synovial sarcoma. Oncogene 2001;20:5755-5762.

33. Argani P, Zakowski MF, Klimstra DS, Rosai J, Ladanyi M. Detection of the SYT-SSX chimeric RNA of synovial sarcoma in paraffin-embedded tissue and its application in problematic cases. Mod Pathol 1998;11:65-71.

34. Fligman I, Lonardo F, Jhanwar SC, Gerald WL, Woodruff J, Ladanyi M. Molecular diagnosis of synovial sarcoma and characterization of a variant SYT-SSX2 fusion transcript. Am J Pathol 1995;147:1592-1599.

35. Ladanyi M, Woodruff JM, Scheithauer BW, et al. Re: O'Sullivan MJ, Kyriakos M, Zhu X, Wick MR, Swanson PE, Dehner LP, Humphrey PA, Pfeifer JD: malignant peripheral nerve sheath tumors with t(X;18). A pathologic and molecular genetic study. Mod pathol 2000;13:1336-46. Mod Pathol 2001;14:733-737.

36. Coindre JM, Hostein I, Benhattar J, Lussan C, Rivel J, Guillou L. Malignant peripheral nerve sheath tumors are t(X;18)-negative sarcomas. Molecular analysis of 25 cases occurring in neurofibromatosis type 1 patients, using two different RT-PCR-based methods of detection. Mod Pathol 2002;15:589-592.

37. ten Heuvel SE, Hoekstra HJ, Bastiaannet E, Suurmeijer AJ. The classic prognostic factors tumor stage, tumor size, and tumor grade are the strongest predictors of outcome in synovial sarcoma: no role for SSX fusion type or ezrin expression. Appl Immunohistochem Mol Morphol 2009;17:189-195.

38. Takenaka S, Ueda T, Naka N, et al. Prognostic implication of SYT-SSX fusion type in synovial sarcoma: a multi-institutional retrospective analysis in Japan. Oncol Rep 2008;19:467-476.

39. Ladanyi M, Antonescu CR, Leung DH, et al. Impact of SYT-SSX fusion type on the clinical behavior of synovial sarcoma: a multi-institutional retrospective study of 243 patients. Cancer Res 2002;62:135-140.

40. Ladanyi M. Correlates of SYT-SSX fusion type in synovial sarcoma: getting more complex but also more interesting? J Clin Oncol 2005;23:3638-9; author reply 9-40.

41. Guillou L, Benhattar J, Bonichon F, et al. Histologic grade, but not SYT-SSX fusion type, is an important prognostic factor in patients with synovial sarcoma: a multicenter, retrospective analysis. J Clin Oncol 2004;22:4040-4050.

42. Antonescu CR, Kawai A, Leung DH, et al. Strong association of SYT-SSX fusion type and morphologic epithelial differentiation in synovial sarcoma. Diagn Mol Pathol 2000;9:1-8.

43. Deyrup AT, Weiss SW. Grading of soft tissue sarcomas: the challenge of providing precise information in an imprecise world. Histopathology 2006;48:42-50.

44. Carrillo R, Rodriguez-Peralto JL, Batsakis JG. Synovial sarcomas of the head and neck. Ann Otol Rhinol Laryngol 1992;101:367-370.

Epithelioid Sarcoma

45. Enzinger FM. Epithelioid sarcoma: a sarcoma simulating a granuloma or a carcinoma. Cancer 1970;26:1029-1041.

46. Chase DR, Enzinger FM. Epithelioid sarcoma. Diagnosis, prognostic indicators, and treatment. Am J Surg Pathol 1985;9:241-263.

47. Chbani L, Guillou L, Terrier P, et al. Epithelioid sarcoma: a clinicopathologic and immunohistochemical analysis of 106 cases from the French sarcoma group. Am J Clin Pathol 2009;131:222-227.

48. Guillou L, Wadden C, Coindre JM, Krausz T, Fletcher CD. "Proximal-type" epithelioid sarcoma, a distinctive aggressive neoplasm showing rhabdoid features. Clinicopathologic, immunohistochemical, and ultrastructural study of a series. Am J Surg Pathol 1997;21:130-146.

49. Mirra JM, Kessler S, Bhuta S, Eckardt J. The fibroma-like variant of epithelioid sarcoma. A fibrohistiocytic/myoid cell lesion often confused with benign and malignant spindle cell tumors. Cancer 1992;69:1382-1395.

50. Koplin SA, Nielsen GP, Hornicek FJ, Rosenberg AE. Epithelioid sarcoma with heterotopic bone: a morphologic review of 4 cases. Int J Surg Pathol 2010;18:207-212.

51. Raoux D, Peoc'h M, Pedeutour F, Vaunois B, Decouvelaere AV, Folpe AL. Primary epithelioid sarcoma of bone: report of a unique case, with immunohistochemical and fluorescent in situ hybridization confirmation of INI1 deletion. Am J Surg Pathol 2009;33:954-958.

52. Lin L, Skacel M, Sigel JE, et al. Epithelioid sarcoma: an immunohistochemical analysis evaluating the utility of cytokeratin 5/6 in distinguishing superficial epithelioid sarcoma from spindled squamous cell carcinoma. J Cutan Pathol 2003;30:114-117.

53. Orrock JM, Abbott JJ, Gibson LE, Folpe AL. INI1 and GLUT-1 expression in epithelioid sarcoma and its cutaneous neoplastic and nonneoplastic mimics. Am J Dermatopathol 2009;31:152-156.

54. Smith ME, Brown JI, Fisher C. Epithelioid sarcoma: presence of vascular-endothelial cadherin and lack of epithelial cadherin. Histopathology 1998;33:425-431.

55. Laskin WB, Miettinen M. Epithelioid sarcoma: new insights based on an extended immunohistochemical analysis. Arch Pathol Lab Med 2003;127:1161-1168.

56. Miettinen M, Fanburg-Smith JC, Virolainen M, Shmookler BM, Fetsch JF. Epithelioid sarcoma: an immunohistochemical analysis of 112 classical and variant cases and a discussion of the differential diagnosis. Hum Pathol 1999;30:934-942.

57 Hornick JL, Dal Cin P, Fletcher CD. Loss of INI1 expression is characteristic of both conventional and proximal-type epithelioid sarcoma. Am J Surg Pathol 2009;33:542-550.

58. Stenman G, Kindblom LG, Willems J, Angervall L. A cell culture, chromosomal and quantitative DNA analysis of a metastatic epithelioid sarcoma. Deletion 1p, a possible primary chromosomal abnormality in epithelioid sarcoma. Cancer 1990;65:2006-2013.

59. Reeves BR, Fisher C, Smith S, Courtenay VD, Robertson D. Ultrastructural, immunocytochemical, and cytogenetic characterization of a human epithelioid sarcoma cell line (RM-HS1). J Nation Cancer Instit 1987;78:7-18.

60. Modena P, Lualdi E, Facchinetti F, et al. SMARCB1/INI1 tumor suppressor gene is frequently inactivated in epithelioid sarcomas. Cancer Res 2005;65:4012-4019.

61. Iwasaki H, Ohjimi Y, Ishiguro M, et al. Epithelioid sarcoma with an 18q aberration. Cancer Genet Cytogenet 1996;91:46-52.

62. Feely MG, Fidler ME, Nelson M, Neff JR, Bridge JA. Cytogenetic findings in a case of epithelioid sarcoma and a review of the literature. Cancer Genet Cytogenet 2000;119:155-157.

63. Cordoba JC, Parham DM, Meyer WH, Douglass EC. A new cytogenetic finding in an epithelioid sarcoma, t(8;22)(q22;q11). Cancer Genet Cytogenet 1994;72:151-154.

64. Brassesco MS, Valera ET, Castro-Gamero AM, et al. Cytogenetic findings in an epithelioid sarcoma with angiomatoid features. A case report. Genet Mol Res 2009;8:1211-1217.

65. Modena P, Lualdi E, Facchinetti F, et al. SMARCB1/ INI1 tumor suppressor gene is frequently inactivated in epithelioid sarcomas. Cancer Res 2005; 65:4012-4019.

66. Kosemehmetoglu K, Kaygusuz G, Bahrami A, et al. Intra-articular epithelioid sarcoma showing mixed classic and proximal-type features: report of 2 cases, with immunohistochemical and molecular cytogenetic INI-1 study. Am J Surg Pathol 2011;35:891-897.

67. Sullivan LM, Folpe AL, Pawel BR, Judkins AR, Biegel JA. Epithelioid sarcoma is associated with a high percentage of SMARCB1 deletions. Mod Pathol 2013;26:385-392.

Mixed Tumor/Myoepithelioma

68. Stout AP, Gorman G. Mixed tumors of the skin of the salivary gland type. Cancer 1959;12:537-543.

69. Hirsch P, Helwig EB. Chondroid syringoma. Mixed tumor of skin, salivary gland type. Arch Dermatol 1961;84:835-847.

70. Kilpatrick SE, Hitchcock MG, Kraus MD, Calonje E, Fletcher CD. Mixed tumors and myoepitheliomas of soft tissue: a clinicopathologic styudy of 19 cases with a unifying concept. Am J Surg Pathol 1997;21:13-22.

71. Michal M, Miettinen M. Myoepitheliomas of skin and soft tissues. Virchows Arch 1999;434:393-400.

72. Hornick JL, Fletcher CD. Myoepithelial tumors of soft tissue: a clinicopathologic and immunohistochemical study of 101 cases with evaluation of prognostic parameters. Am J Surg Pathol 2003;27:1183-1196.

73. Mentzel T, Requena L, Kaddu S, Soares de Aleida LM, Sangueza OP, Kutzner H. Cutaneous myoepithelial neoplasms: clinicopathologic and immunohistochemical study of 20 cases suggesting a continuous spectrum ranging from benign mixed tumor of the skin to cutaneous myoepithelioma and myoepithelial carcinoma. J Cutan Pathol 2003;30:294-302.

74. Hornick JL, Fletcher CD. Cutaneous myoepithelioma: a clinicopathologic and immunohistochemical study of 14 cases. Hum Pathol 2004;35:14-24.

75. Gleason BC, Fletcher CD. Myoepithelial carcinoma of soft tissue in children: an aggressive neoplasm analyzed in a series of 29 cases. Am J Surg Pathol 2007;31:1813-1824.

76. Kunikane H, Ishikura H, Yamaguchi J, Yoshiki T, Itoh T, Aizawa M. Chondroid syringoma (mixed tumor of the skin). A clinicopathologic study of 13 cases. Acta Pathol Jpn 1987;37:615-625.

77. Hassab-El-Naby HM, Tam S, White WL, Ackerman AB. Mixed tumors of the skin. A histological and immunohistochemical study. Am J Dermatopathol 1989;11:413-428.

78. Headington JT. Mixed tumor of the skin: eccrine and apocrine type. Arch Dermatol 1961;84:989-996.

79. Ferreiro JA, Nascimento AG. Hyaline-cell rich chondroid syringoma. A tumor mimicking malignancy. Am J Surg Pathol 1995;19:912-917.

80. Dabska M. Parachordoma—a new clinical entity. Cancer 1977;40:1586-1592

81. Fisher C, Miettinen M. Parachordoma: clinicopathologic and immunohistochemical study of four cases of an unusual soft tissue neoplasm. Ann Diagn Pathol 1997;1:3-10

82. Folpe AL, Agoff SN, Willis J, Weiss SW. Parachordoma is immunohistochemically and cytogenetically distinct from axial chordoma and extraskeletal myxoid chondrosarcoma. Am J Surg Pathol 1999;23:1059-1067.

83. Fletcher CD, Antonescu CR, Hornick JL, Heim S. Mixed tumor/myoepithelioma/parachordoma. In: WHO classification of tumours of soft tissue and bone. IARC Press, Lyon, France. (In press)

84. Ishimura E, Iwamoto H, Kobashi Y, Yamabe H, Ichijima K. Malignant chondroid syringoma. Report of a case with widespread metastasis and review of pertinent literature. Cancer 1983;52:1966-1973.

85. Brandal P, Panagopoulos I, Bjerkehagen B, et al. Detection of a t(1;22)(q23;q12) translocation leading to an EWSR1-PBX1 fusion gene in myoepithelioma. Genes Chromosomes Cancer 2008;47:558-654.

86. Antonescu CR, Zhang L, Chang NE, et al. EWSR1-POU5FI fusion in soft tissue myoepithelial tumots. A molecular analysis of sixty-six cases, including soft tissue, bone, and visceral lesions, showing common involvement of the EWSR1 gene. Genes Chromosomes Cancer 2010;49:1114-1124.

87. Bahrami A, Dalton JD, Krane JF, Fletcher CD. A subset of cutaneous and soft tissue mixed tumors are genetically linked to their salivary gland counterpart. Genes Chromosomes Cancer 2012;51:140-148.

88. Antonescu CR, Zhang L, Shao SY, et al. Frequent PLAG1 gene rearrangements in skin and soft tissue myoepithelioma with ductal differentiation. Genes Chromosomes Cancer 2013;52:675-682.

89. Flucke U, Tops BB, Verdijk MA, et al. NR4A3 rearrangement reliably distinguished between the clinicopathologically overlapping entities myoepithelial carcinoma of soft tissue and cellular extraskeletal myxoid chondrosarcoma. Virchows Arch 2012;460:621-628.

10 MISCELLANEOUS TRANSLOCATION SARCOMAS

This chapter contains five sarcoma types, common to which is the lack of defined histogenesis, usual occurrence in children and young adults, and content of characteristic tumor-associated translocations, many of which involve the Ewing sarcoma gene (*EWSR1*). These are all rare tumors and include aggressive malignancies, such as Ewing sarcoma family tumors, desmoplastic small round cell tumor, and clear cell sarcoma. Angiomatoid fibrous histiocytoma is a very low-grade, nearly clinically benign tumor, whereas alveolar soft part sarcoma often metastases but has a protracted clinical course.

EWING SARCOMA/PERIPHERAL NEUROECTODERMAL TUMOR

Definition. *Ewing sarcoma* is an undifferentiated small blue round cell tumor involving bone and soft tissue and primarily affecting children and young adults. Genetically, Ewing sarcoma is defined by gene fusion translocations involving the Ewing sarcoma gene *EWSR1*, and the *ETS* transcription factor gene family, most commonly *FLI1*. Variants belonging to Ewing sarcoma family include *peripheral neuroectodermal tumor (PNET)*, *Askin tumor*, and *non-EWSR1 rearranged small blue round cell tumors*.

Clinical Features. In children, Ewing sarcoma is predominantly a bone tumor, while in adults it occurs more commonly in soft tissue. Ewing sarcoma is the second most common primary bone sarcoma, after osteosarcoma (1). Extraskeletal Ewing sarcoma usually affects the deep soft tissues of the trunk and extremity, but unusual sites such as head and neck or retroperitoneum have also been described (fig. 10-1).

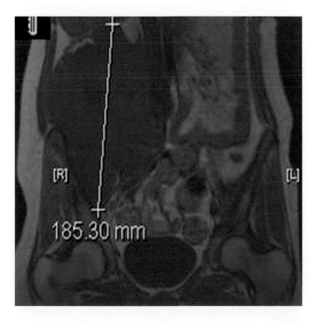 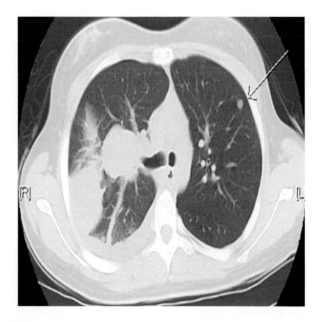

Figure 10-1

EWING SARCOMA

Left: Radiographic appearance of a large right-sided pelvic soft tissue mass in a 15-year-old female. T1-weighted magnetic resonance imaging (MRI) shows a large, fairly homogeneous right pelvic lesion measuring over 18 cm.

Right: The chest computerized tomography (CT) shows the presence of lung nodules, consistent with disease metastatic to the lung at presentation.

The term Askin tumor was initially applied to lesions limited to thoracopulmonary and chest wall locations and thought to represent a distinct entity with neuroepithelial differentiation and preferential occurrence in females (2). Similar to PNET (see below), Askin tumors are now classified as Ewing sarcomas, based on their similar immunoprofile and genetic signature. There is no gender predominance of this form of the disease, and the median age at presentation is higher than for those patients with bone primaries.

Ewing sarcoma affects children, adolescents, and young adults, with most cases occurring in the second and third decades of life. The median age at diagnosis ranges from 13 to 19 years in studies not restricted to pediatric recruitment (3). The few patients older than 30 years have a similar spectrum of *EWSR1-ETS* fusions (4).

Adolescents and young adults fare more poorly than children diagnosed with this disease. Ewing sarcoma is more common in Caucasians and occurs only rarely in patients of African and, to a lesser extent, Asian descent. Ewing sarcoma displays a high propensity for metastasis, most commonly to lung and bone.

Gross Findings. On gross examination, Ewing sarcomas present as well-circumscribed nodular masses, with a nonencapsulated pushing border, within skeletal muscle. On cross sectioning, the tumors have a soft, tan-yellow cut surface, with areas of hemorrhage and necrosis.

Microscopic Findings. Microscopically, most tumors are composed of a strikingly uniform cytomorphology, with round nuclei showing smooth nuclear contour and vesicular fine chromatin (fig. 10-2). Lesional cells are arranged in solid sheets and show ill-defined cell borders with scant, often clear cytoplasm (fig. 10-2). The presence of spindled, pleomorphic, or multinucleated tumor cells is typically not in keeping with a diagnosis of Ewing sarcoma. Mitotic figures are readily noted, as are areas of necrosis and hemorrhagic loose stroma (fig. 10-2). The presence of a more sclerotic stroma or prominent myxoid change is uncommon.

Ewing sarcomas occasionally show subtle cytologic variability, such as a more irregular nuclear contour, slight variation in the size and shape of the nuclei without obvious pleomorphism, more conspicuous nucleoli, and

moderate amount of cytoplasm (fig. 10-3). These histologic features have been used in the past to define the term *atypical Ewing sarcoma*, which typically requires molecular confirmation for a definitive diagnosis.

PNET is a histologic variant of Ewing sarcoma showing distinctive rosette formation (fig.10-4, left). The lesional cells share an almost identical morphology with the cells of classic Ewing sarcoma, except that they are separated by an eosinophilic fibrillary stroma that forms the center of the rosette. Immunohistochemically, PNET has a similar membranous pattern of CD99 reactivity (fig. 10-4, right), and at the molecular level, similar genetic abnormalities.

Special Studies. The cells of Ewing sarcoma are strongly and diffusely positive (with a distinctive membranous pattern) for CD99, which recognizes the p30/32MIC2 glycoprotein on the membrane of the tumor cells (5). Although CD99 is far from being a specific marker, being positive in other small blue round cell tumors, it is highly sensitive for Ewing sarcoma (fig. 10-5, left) (6). The diagnosis of Ewing sarcoma in a tumor that shows negative or only focal, patchy, weak, or cytoplasmic staining for CD99 should be seriously questioned. Conversely, other small blue round cell tumors can express this marker, including alveolar rhabdomyosarcoma, desmoplastic small round cell tumor, angiomatoid fibrous histiocytoma, and lymphoblastic lymphoma, typically with a more nonspecific cytoplasmic pattern. Nuclear FLI1 reactivity (fig. 10-5, right) and ERG reactivity are seen in FLI1- and ERG-rearranged Ewing sarcomas, respectively, however, this result should be distinguished from angiosarcomas as well as from ERG-fusion positive leukemias. In a subset of cases, Ewing sarcoma expresses either low or high molecular weight cytokeratins (7). Rare cases express desmin and S-100 protein. Neuron-specific enolase and CD56 are often positive, while synaptophysin and chromogranin are consistently negative.

Genetics. At the molecular genetic level, Ewing sarcoma is characterized by a balanced reciprocal translocation, t(11;22)(q24;q12), in 85 percent of cases (8), which encodes an oncogenic fusion protein and transcription factor EWSR1-FLI1. This tumor-specific chimeric fusion retains the amino terminus of EWSR1, a member of the TET (TLS/EWS/TAF15) family

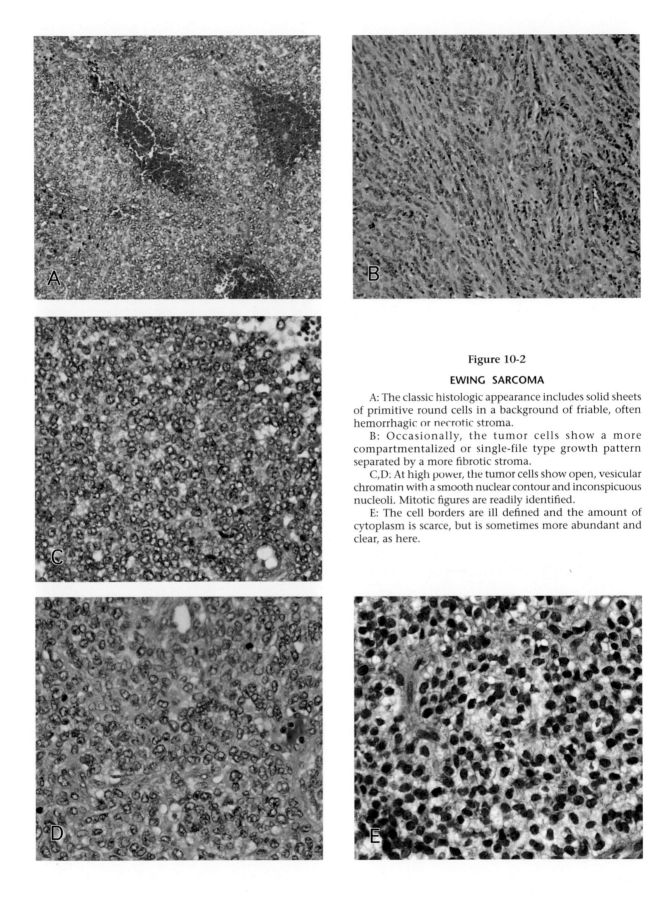

Figure 10-2

EWING SARCOMA

A: The classic histologic appearance includes solid sheets of primitive round cells in a background of friable, often hemorrhagic or necrotic stroma.

B: Occasionally, the tumor cells show a more compartmentalized or single-file type growth pattern separated by a more fibrotic stroma.

C,D: At high power, the tumor cells show open, vesicular chromatin with a smooth nuclear contour and inconspicuous nucleoli. Mitotic figures are readily identified.

E: The cell borders are ill defined and the amount of cytoplasm is scarce, but is sometimes more abundant and clear, as here.

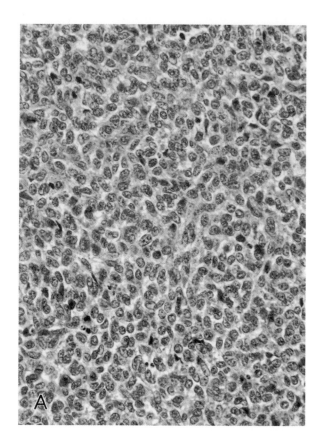

Figure 10-3

ATYPICAL EWING SARCOMA

A: A variation of the classic morphology, referred to as atypical Ewing sarcoma, is this abdominal wall tumor in a 78-year-old female. A mixture of round to oval undifferentiated cells with small nucleoli and fine, salt and pepper chromatin is seen.

B: Due to the clinical presentation and focal cytokeratin positivity the diagnosis was a Merkel cell carcinoma.

C: Subsequent resection showed diffuse reactivity for CD99. Reverse transcriptase-polymerase chain reaction (RT-PCR) detected the presence of an *EWSR1-FLI1* fusion transcript.

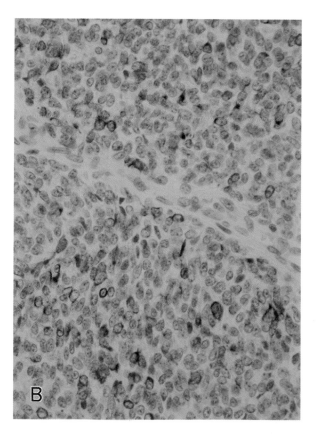

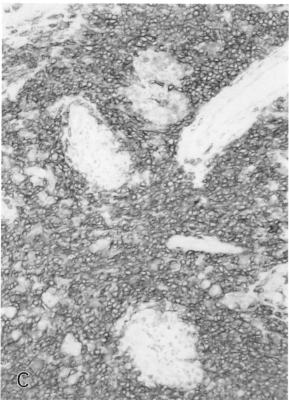

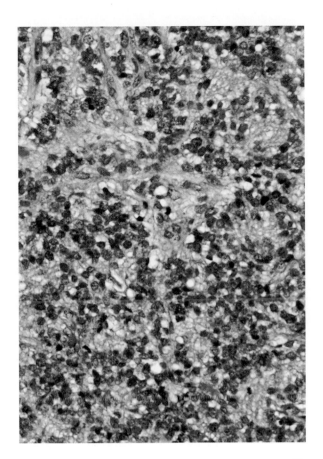 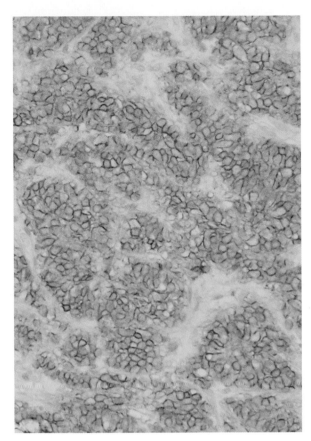

Figure 10-4

EWING SARCOMA/PERIPHERAL NEUROECTODERMAL TUMOR

Left: This histologic variant of Ewing sarcoma shows distinctive rosette formation, reminiscent of Flexner rosettes. Nevertheless, the cytology of the lesional cells closely resembles that of classic Ewing sarcoma tumor cells, with monotonous round cells and fine, vesicular chromatin.

Right: This histologic variant also shares the strong and membranous pattern of CD99 staining.

of RNA-binding proteins, and the carboxy terminus of FLI1, a member of the ETS family of transcription factors (9). The EWSR1 promoter is strongly and broadly activated, leading to relatively unrestricted high level expression of the resulting fusion genes (10,11). In contrast, expression of native FLI1 is tightly regulated and lineage restricted (12).

The second most common translocation variant includes *EWSR1* fused to *ERG* on chromosome 21q22 (10 percent). Rare cases with fusions of *EWSR1* to other *ETS* family genes, such as *ETV1*, *E1AF*, and *FEV*, have been identified, but their clinicopathologic similarity to classic Ewing sarcomas remains unclear (13,14). Since *FUS* may substitute for the *EWSR1* gene in certain translocation-associated sarcomas, it is not surprising

that a subset of Ewing sarcomas show recurrent *FUS-ERG* gene fusions (three of the four cases reported involved the chest wall) (15).

Rare Ewing sarcomas harbor noncanonical *EWSR1* fusions to either *ZSG* (16) or *SP3* (14) zinc-finger DNA-binding domains, NFATc2 transcription factor (17), or the chromatin remodeling gene *SMARCA5* (18). Since most of these variants are case reports or small case series, it is difficult to compare their similarities and differences to classic Ewing sarcoma tumors.

In addition to the *EWSR1*- or *FUS*-rearranged Ewing sarcoma, two other genetic subgroups have recently emerged, characterized by non-*TET/ETS* fusions. Although their morphologic appearance is characterized by monotonous small blue round cells, resembling at least in

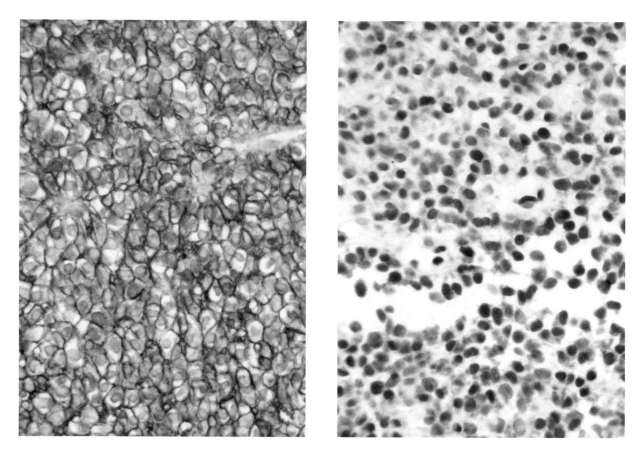

Figure 10-5

EWING SARCOMA

Left: The tumor cells show strong and diffuse reactivity for O13 with a distinctive membranous pattern of staining.
Right: Nuclear reactivity for FLI1 is typically present and further supports the diagnosis.

part the prototypical *EWSR1-ETS*-positive Ewing sarcoma, they also exhibit certain distinctive phenotypic and immunohistochemical features that set them apart. Further studies incorporating larger number of cases, with longer follow-up, will hopefully determine whether these tumors should be classified as Ewing sarcoma-like tumors or categorized as a separate nosologic entity. The first group in this class is characterized by a *CIC-DUX4* fusion, the result of either t(4;19)(q35;q13) or t(10;19)(q26,q13). The *DUX4* retrogene is evolutionary duplicated and is present at 4q35 and 10q26 subtelomeric regions. In a recent series, approximately two thirds of *EWSR1* rearrangement-negative small blue round cell tumors were positive for the *CIC-DUX4* fusion (20). Tumors positive for the *CIC-DUX4* fusion occur mainly in male young adult patients (median age, 29 years), with

the soft tissues of the extremities being the most frequent location. Microscopically, *CIC-DUX4*-positive sarcomas demonstrate small to medium-sized round to oval cells, packed in solid sheets with minimal or absent intervening collagen (20). Distinct areas of spindle-shaped cells are only occasionally noted. Most tumor cells have an ill-defined cell border, with a scant amount of amphophilic or lightly eosinophilic cytoplasm, vesicular nuclei, and distinct, often enlarged, nucleoli (fig. 10-6A,B). Geographic areas of necrosis are commonly seen, as well as individual cell necrosis with a starry-sky appearance (fig. 10-6C). Overall, these tumors show a higher degree of heterogeneity in nuclear shape and size than the rather monotonous cytomorphology seen in classic Ewing sarcoma. CD99 expression appears much more variable, being either diffuse or patchy, and the tumors

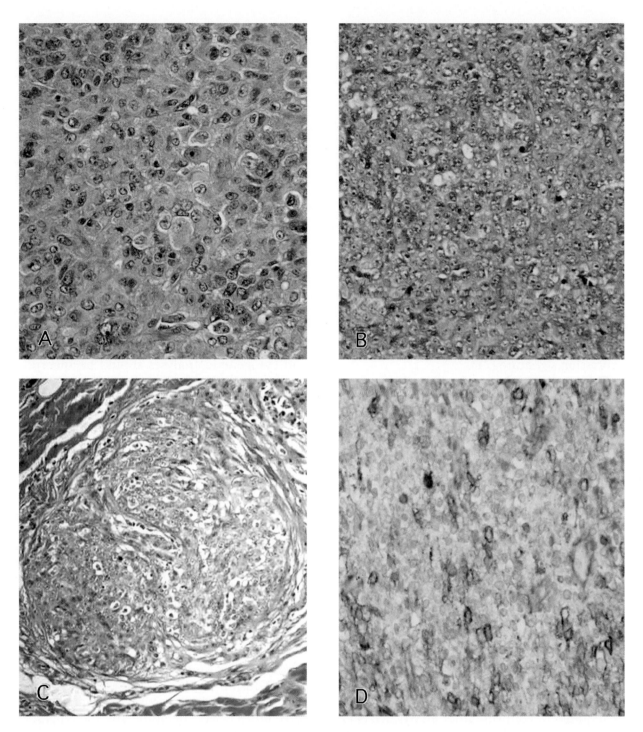

Figure 10-6

CIC-DUX4-POSITIVE EWING SARCOMA-LIKE TUMOR

A,B: These small blue round cell tumors show more variability in cytomorphology, with variations in nuclear size and shape (A), more prominent nucleoli (B), and sometimes more abundant eosinophilic cytoplasm, reminiscent of a plasmacytoid neoplasm (A) than classic Ewing sarcoma.

C: Individual tumor necrosis, resembling the starry-sky appearance seen in Burkitt lymphomas, is occasionally seen, as well a vague whorling growth pattern.

D: Only focal or patchy O13 reactivity has been reported in these tumors.

mostly lack other markers of differentiation (fig. 10-6D) (20).

A novel intrachromosomal X-chromosome paracentric inversion, resulting in a *BCOR-CCNB3* fusion, was recently described in mainly Ewing sarcoma-like tumors of the bone; it was identified from a screen of 594 sarcomas lacking *EWSR1* rearrangement or other known sarcoma fusion products (21). These tumors are also identified by CCNB3 immunohistochemistry. *BCOR* is a gene encoding a ubiquitously expressed transcriptional co-repressor that binds bcl-6 and proteins involved in chromatin dynamics, while *CCNB3* encodes an otherwise testis-specific meiotic cyclin. Despite remarkable clinical and pathologic similarities to the Ewing sarcoma group of tumors, gene profiling and single nucleotide polymorphism (SNP) array analyses indicate that this new group of tumors is biologically distinct from Ewing sarcoma and, in particular, does not share the *EWSR1-ETS* expression signature (21).

Differential Diagnosis. The differential diagnosis includes mainly tumors with a small blue round cell phenotype. Alveolar rhabdomyosarcoma with a predominantly solid growth pattern may closely resemble Ewing sarcoma morphologically, however, it typically shows more irregular nuclear contours, scant eosinophilic cytoplasm, diffuse staining for desmin and myogenin, as well as a *FOXO1* gene rearrangement by fluorescence in situ hybridization (FISH), allowing a correct diagnosis. Desmoplastic small round cell tumor, especially when arising in unusual anatomic locations or expressing an incomplete multiphenotypic immunoprofile, can be confused with Ewing sarcoma. Further uncertainty occurs when Ewing sarcoma tumors express cytokeratins or desmin. The presence of an *EWSR1* gene rearrangement by FISH does not allow distinction between the two entities, and reverse transcriptase-polymerase chain reaction (RT-PCR) analysis may be required to confirm either an *EWSR1-WT1* fusion transcript, characteristic of desmoplastic small round cell tumor, or *EWSR1-FLI1* or *EWSR1-ERG*, typical for Ewing sarcoma, for a correct interpretation.

Since cytokeratin expression is present either focally or diffusely in up to 20 percent of genetically confirmed Ewing sarcoma cases (7), the differentiation from a small cell neuroendocrine carcinoma (i.e., Merkel cell carcinoma or small cell neuroendocrine undifferentiated carcinoma) may be difficult, especially in unusual clinical presentations, such as older patients, cutaneous/superficial soft tissue, or sinonasal sites. Positivity for CK20 and/or reactivity for chromogranin/synaptophysin is typically seen in neuroendocrine carcinomas, but is negative in Ewing sarcoma.

One additional pitfall is the morphologic and immunohistochemical overlap of Ewing sarcoma with lymphoblastic lymphoma. Although both tumors may express CD99 and FLI1, CD45 and terminal deoxynucleotidyltransferase (TdT) are positive only in lymphoblastic lymphoma and should be routinely included in all immunopanels for small blue round cell tumors. As immunohistochemical studies are not always definitive, with significant overlap between different small blue round cell tumors, molecular and cytogenetic analyses should be incorporated into the routine work-up of cases with either atypical morphology or immunoprofile, or unusual clinical presentation.

On a cautionary note, the presence of an *EWSR1* gene rearrangement does not qualify a tumor as an Ewing sarcoma or round cell sarcoma. *EWSR1* rearrangements are present in a variety of other sarcoma types, such as extraskeletal myxoid chondrosarcoma, clear cell sarcoma of soft parts and gastrointestinal locations (22–24), and even in benign tumors, some exhibiting a more undifferentiated/small round cell morphology, such as angiomatoid fibrous histiocytoma (25) and myoepithelial tumors (26). As FISH studies have been made widely available and are now increasingly used by practicing pathologists even in the absence of a soft tissue expert consultation, we have encountered misinterpretations of the positive *EWSR1* fusion result as being Ewing sarcoma. In some instances, these diagnostic errors triggered unnecessary chemotherapy and radiation therapy to the patient. Any molecular and cytogenetic results should be always correlated with the clinicopathologic findings as well as with the immunohistochemical results before rendering a definitive diagnosis. If unexpected FISH results are encountered, they should then be validated with a different molecular technique,

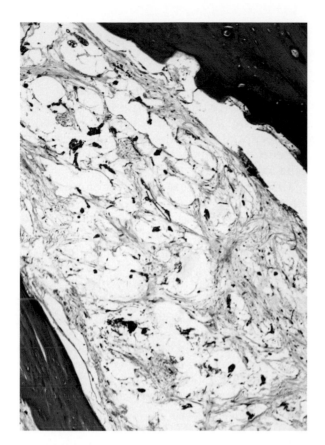 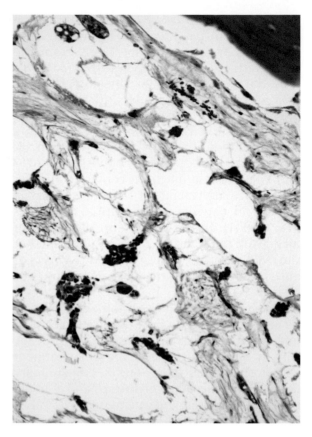

Figure 10-7

EWING SARCOMA

Postchemotherapy changes include dense stromal fibrosis and less tumor necrosis. Good responders, defined as greater than 90 percent necrosis/fibrosis, show only scattered small nests of microscopic residual Ewing sarcoma cells (left). Frequently, the viable nests are artifactual empty spaces, suggestive of lymphovascular invasion (right). When in doubt, CD99 immunohistochemistry confirms these scattered microscopic foci of residual tumor.

such as RT-PCR, or a second opinion obtained from a sarcoma expert.

Treatment and Prognosis. The primary management of patients with the Ewing sarcoma family of tumors entails a multidisciplinary team approach, including neoadjuvant chemotherapy and surgery, followed by adjuvant chemotherapy and, occasionally, radiation therapy. Historical data demonstrate that the survival rate for patients with primary Ewing sarcoma treated with local therapy alone is poor, on the range of 15 percent. This is most likely due to the fact that most patients harbor micrometastatic disease, as the relapse rate for surgically resected Ewing sarcoma in the absence of systemic chemotherapy is about 90 percent (27–29). The addition of systemic chemotherapy has increased the cure rate to about 75 percent in children with primary disease, but only to about 50 percent in adults. With current treatment options, the 5-year overall survival rate for patients with nonmetastatic disease is 60 to 70 percent. The survival rate for the 25 percent of patients who present with metastatic disease, however, is approximately 20 percent (30,31), and for those who develop relapsed and/or refractory disease, no more than 10 percent.

Independent reports suggest that tumor size over 8 cm and the presence of metastasis are strong predictors of negative outcome. Good histologic response (necrosis over 90 percent) after neoadjuvant chemotherapy appears to be a significant predictor of a positive outcome (fig. 10-7). Other established prognostic factors are high tumor volume, presence of serum lactate dehydrogenase, axial location, and age greater than 15 years (32).

The effect of *EWSR1-ETS* fusion on disease progression in patients with Ewing sarcoma/PNET was evaluated prospectively from the co-operative Euro-E.W.I.N.G. 99 trial (33). This prospective study found no correlation between fusion type and prognosis, and refuted two previous smaller retrospective studies that suggested a positive correlation (34). This finding was also substantiated by a Children's Oncology Group prospective study published in 2010 (35). Metastasis at diagnosis conferred a 5-year relapse-free survival rate of 22 percent versus 55 percent for patients without initial metastasis (p < 0.0001). In the group with metastasis at diagnosis, multivariate analysis showed that site (axial or other) and age cohort (15 years or older) had a significant effect on relapse-free survival (36).

The current standard chemotherapy options include doxorubicin, vincristine, cyclophosphamide, and dactinomycin or experimental therapy with these four drugs alternating with treatment with ifosfamide and etoposide (37). Preliminary data regarding neoadjuvant therapy and response in metastatic disease indicate the *CIC-DUX4* Ewing sarcoma subtype is less sensitive than classic Ewing sarcoma to standard chemotherapy agents (20), while data are yet to be published on the clinical behavior of *BCOR-CCNB3* Ewing-like sarcomas. Thus, it is presently not clear from these data whether this new tumor category should be considered enough like an Ewing sarcoma to mandate systemic chemotherapy.

Other exploratory therapies include targeting the IGF1R-signaling pathway, either by IGF1R antibodies (IgG1: R1507 and AMG479; IgG2: figitumumab) or small molecule tyrosine kinase inhibitors. Striking clinical responses for most IGF1R inhibitors in Ewing sarcoma patients have been documented. In a multicentered phase II trial using R1507 (38), however, there was a 10 percent overall complete/partial response rate of the 113 patients with recurrent or refractory Ewing sarcoma/PNET, with a median duration of response of 29 weeks and median survival period of 7.6 months. Of 11 responses observed, 10 were in patients who had presented with primary osseous tumors. Mechanisms of drug resistance and predictors of medication sensitivity need to be refined for IGF1R-directed therapeutics in this disease.

DESMOPLASTIC SMALL ROUND CELL TUMOR

Definition. *Desmoplastic small round cell tumor* (DSRCT) is a multiphenotypic primitive tumor characterized by extensive reactive fibrosis surrounding nests of tumor cells. It occurs with predilection in the abdominal cavity of young males and it is characterized by a *EWRS1-WT1* gene fusion.

Clinical Features. This tumor primarily affects adolescents and young adults, usually presenting with widespread intra-abdominal serosal involvement not related to a particular organ system. Presenting symptoms are typically related to the primary site, such as pain, abdominal distention, palpable mass, acute abdomen, ascites, and organ obstruction. The computerized tomography (CT) or magnetic resonance imaging (MRI) scans reveal multiple, large, dense masses in the abdomen, sometimes with central necrosis. There is a strong male predominance (about 5 to 1), and the tumor nearly always affects the peritoneum as multifocal/metastatic disease.

Gross Findings. Patients often present with diffuse abdominal metastatic disease, similar in gross appearance to carcinomatosis. A dominant tumor mass is often noted, surrounded by smaller lesions studding the peritoneum (fig. 10-8A). On sectioning, the nodular masses have a white-tan, firm cut surface, with variable areas of necrosis and hemorrhage (fig. 10-8B,C).

Microscopic Findings. Microscopically, DSRCT is characterized by nests and trabeculae of undifferentiated small neoplastic cells within an abundant desmoplastic stroma. The ratio between the tumor and stroma is variable, but most tumors are composed of small to medium-sized nests separated by dense fibrous stroma (fig. 10-9A). Comedo-type necrosis is often noted within the center of the tumor nests (fig. 10-9B). Only occasionally are lesions composed either of predominantly sclerotic stroma with only minute clusters or scattered individual tumor cells (fig. 10-9C) or conversely, by mainly solid tumor growth with minimal intervening stroma (fig. 10-9D,E). Rare examples show tubular or rosette-type structure formation (fig. 10-10).

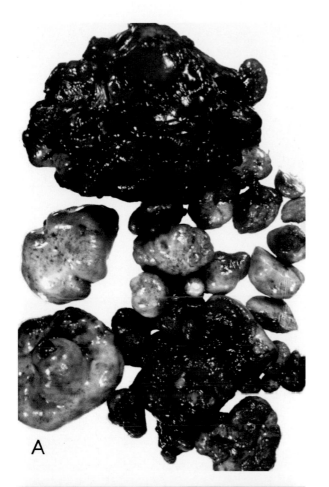

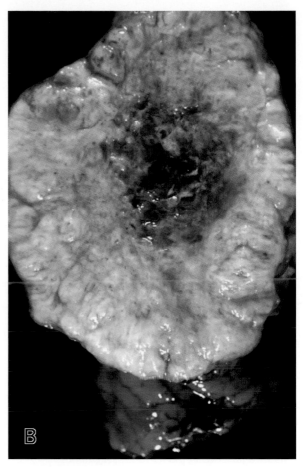

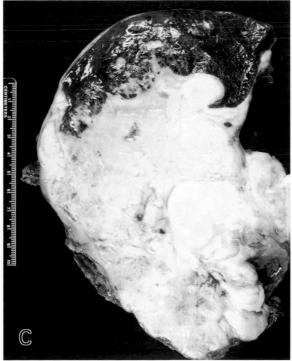

Figure 10-8

DESMOPLASTIC SMALL ROUND CELL TUMOR

A: A bulky intra-abdominal tumor is composed of multiple nodules that stud the peritoneal surface.

B: A dominant nodule has white-tan firm, uniform cut surface and focal areas of hemorrhage.

C: The tumor directly extends into the intra-abdominal organs, such as spleen parenchyma.

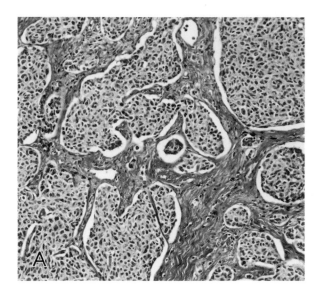

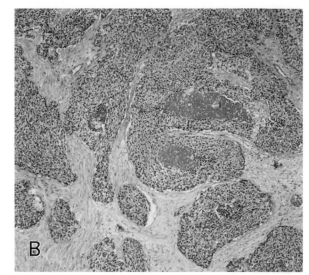

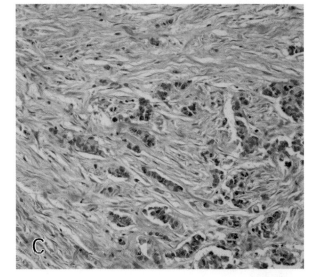

Figure 10-9

DESMOPLASTIC SMALL ROUND CELL TUMOR

A: Variably sized and shaped tumor nests are separated by a desmoplastic stroma.

B: Comedo-type necrosis is seen in the centers of the nests.

C: Less often, the stromal component shows overgrowth with only minute small clusters. Single-file or individual cells are embedded in the sclerotic background.

D,E: The tumor has more solid and confluent nests (D) or, in rare cases, lacks the desmoplastic stroma (E) and suggests alternative diagnoses (such as lymphoma, carcinoma).

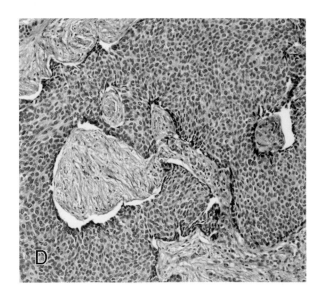

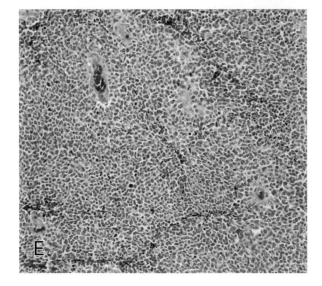

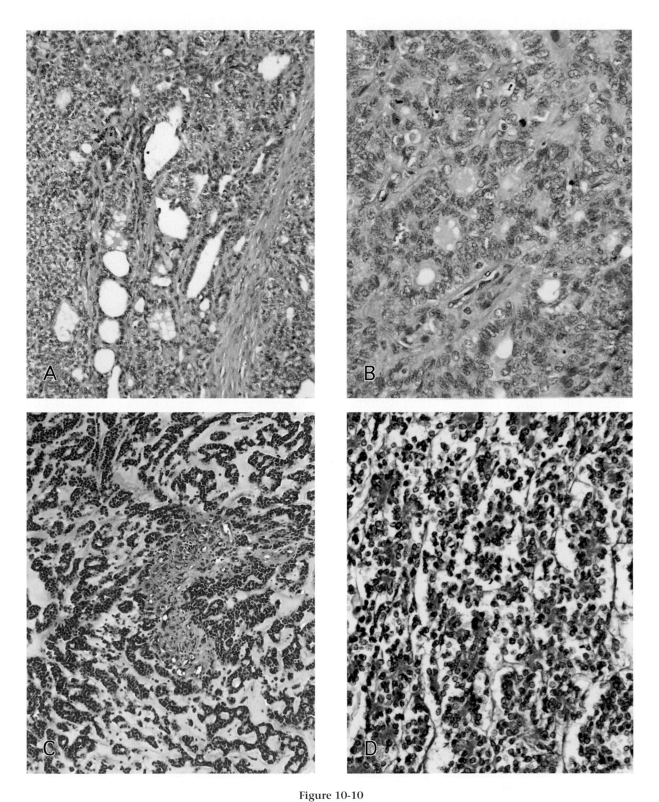

Figure 10-10

DESMOPLASTIC SMALL ROUND CELL TUMOR

Unusual histologic features include the presence of tubular structures (A–C) or rosette formation (D). Occasionally, glomeruloid-like vascular hyperplasia is noted within the stroma adjacent to the tumor nests (C).

These unusual microscopic appearances are under-recognized by the practicing pathologist and may suggest alternative diagnoses, such as Ewing sarcoma/PNET, adenocarcinoma, or mesothelioma (see Differential Diagnosis). Lesional cells have a primitive appearance with scant cytoplasm and round to oval nuclei, with coarse chromatin and mild pleomorphism. Mitotic figures are readily appreciated. The stroma is primarily fibroblastic with variable collagen deposition (fig. 10-9C). Occasionally, there is vascular hyperplasia (fig. 10-10C).

Special Studies. The tumor cells have complex multi-immunophenotype–expressing proteins associated with epithelial, muscular, and neural differentiation. Both cytokeratin and desmin reactivities are commonly seen (fig. 10-11A,B), sometimes with distinctive dot-like cytoplasmic localization, which translates to the paranuclear arrays of intermediate filaments seen ultrastructurally. Immunohistochemical analysis using an antibody directed to the carboxy terminus of *WT1* (Wilms tumor gene) is reactive within the nucleus of the tumor cells, consistent with the proposed transcription factor activity of the fusion molecule (fig. 10-11C) (39,40). Other markers often expressed include epithelial membrane antigen, vimentin, and neuron-specific enolase. O13 or CD99 may also be positive, with nonspecific cytoplasmic staining rather than a crisp membranous pattern. Myogenin and MyoD1 are consistently negative, as are synaptophysin and chromogranin.

Genetics. DSRCT is characterized by a recurrent chromosomal translocation, t(11;22) (p13;q12), which occurs in most cases (41–43). The translocation is unique to DSRCT, but the breakpoints involve two chromosomal regions previously implicated in other malignant developmental tumors: Ewing sarcoma gene (*EWSR1*) on 22q12 and Wilms tumor gene, *WT1*, on 11p13. The chimeric protein containing the potential transactivation domain of *EWSR1* is fused to zinc fingers 2-4 of the Wilms tumor suppressor and transcriptional repressor *WT1* (44–46). The *EWSR1-WT1* gene fusion is a sensitive and specific molecular marker for DSRCT that is especially useful in cases with unusual clinical or histologic features (47).

The oncogenic fusion of *EWSR1* to *WT1* in DSRCT results in the induction of platelet-de-rived growth factor alpha (PDGFα), a potent fibroblast growth factor that contributes to the characteristic reactive fibrosis associated with this unique tumour (48). Interestingly, the serosal lining of body cavities, the most common site of DSRCT, has high transient fetal expression of *WT1* gene. WT1 protein is expressed in tissues derived from the intermediate mesoderm, primarily those undergoing transition from mesenchyme to epithelium (49,50). This pattern recapitulates the epithelial differentiation noted in DSRCT.

Differential Diagnosis. The main entities in the differential diagnosis are other small blue round cell sarcomas, such as Ewing sarcoma and rhabdomyosarcoma. Since DSRCT sometimes lacks reactivity for WT1 or desmin, as well as expresses O13, the distinction from an intra-abdominal Ewing sarcoma can be challenging. Furthermore, demonstration of *EWSR1* gene rearrangement by FISH cannot distinguish between the two entities and requires further molecular confirmation of the fusion transcript: either *EWSR1-WT1* for DSRCT or *EWSR1-Fli1* or *EWSR1-ERG* for Ewing sarcoma by RT-PCR. An alveolar rhabdomyosarcoma is distinguished by the diffuse and strong reactivity for myogenin, which is typically negative in DSRCT.

Occasionally, malignant mesothelioma or small cell carcinoma of ovary are considered in the differential diagnosis, due to some immunohistochemical overlap and an undifferentiated appearance. In these instances, FISH analysis for the presence of a *EWSR1* gene rearrangement helps in the distinction.

Treatment and Prognosis. Patients with DSRCT have a dismal prognosis, with a 15 percent overall survival rate at 5 years (51). Patients presenting with abdominal disease almost always have tumors at an advanced stage with regional dissemination, with large masses or extensive seeding of the peritoneum and metastasis to locoregional lymph nodes. Combined modality therapy with chemotherapy and surgery is the standard of care, but is clearly inadequate based on the poor overall survival rate (52). Patients with the best outcome are those who have both a good response to chemotherapy (using agents typically employed for Ewing sarcoma) and successful surgical debulking.

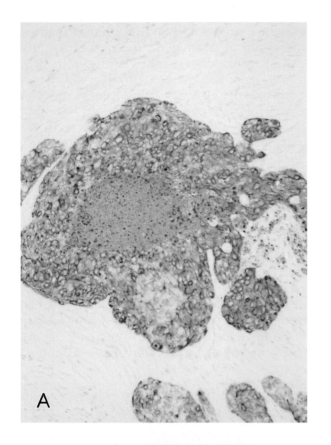

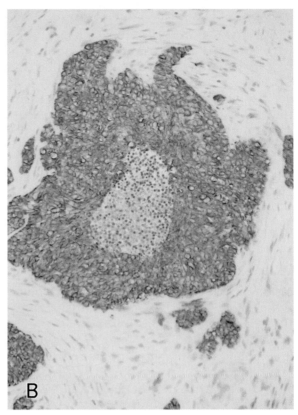

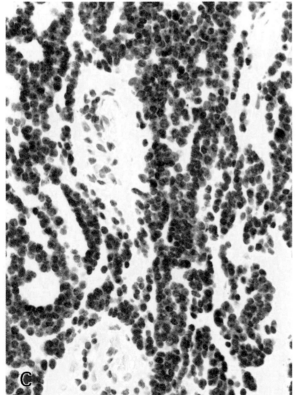

Figure 10-11

DESMOPLASTIC SMALL ROUND CELL TUMOR

The immunoprofile includes strong reactivity for cytokeratin such as AE1:AE3 (A) and desmin (B), and nuclear expression of the C-terminus WT1 antibody (C).

CLEAR CELL SARCOMA

Definition. *Clear cell sarcoma* is a rare tumor with an epithelioid to spindled morphology showing melanocytic differentiation and *EWSR1* gene fusions, usually with the *ATF1* gene. It involves the soft tissues of the extremities, especially tendons and aponeuroses. A gastrointestinal variant with lesser melanocytic differentiation exists.

General Considerations. Clear cell sarcoma has been designated in the past as *malignant melanoma of soft parts* due to its considerable morphologic overlap with metastatic melanoma and consistent expression of melanocytic markers (53). However, the two pathologic entities have distinct genetic abnormalities, with clear cell sarcoma showing recurrent *EWSR1-ATF1* fusion, and melanoma harboring *BRAF* mutations. More recently, similar translocations have been found in gastrointestinal tumors, which show partial morphologic overlap and incomplete melanocytic differentiation (54). The relationship between the gastrointestinal clear cell sarcoma and the more common soft tissue tumor remains controversial and requires further investigation.

Clinical Features. Clear cell sarcoma is a rare tumor that affects young adults. The peak incidence is in the third and fourth decades of life, with no sex predilection. Most cases occur in the extremity, with the foot/ankle region accounting for 40 percent. It is often intimately associated with tendons or aponeuroses. The tumor may extend to the subcutis, but the skin is typically uninvolved. The head and neck and trunk wall are rarely affected (53,55–58). Isolated examples have been reported in the retroperitoneum, viscera, and bone. In the gastrointestinal tract, the tumor most often involves the small bowel and, less commonly, stomach and colon. The tumor usually presents as a slowly growing mass that is present for several weeks to several years.

Gross Findings. Most are fairly small (less than 5 cm), however, lesions larger than 10 cm have been described. The cut surface is lobulated and gray-white with a well-circumscribed, pushing border. Pigmentation, necrosis, and cystic changes are rarely encountered.

Microscopic Findings. Microscopically, clear cell sarcoma shows a characteristic nested growth pattern, with fibrous septa dividing the tumor in distinct compartments (fig. 10-12A,B). Most have a predominantly epithelioid morphology, but areas of spindling may be intermixed (fig. 10-12D). Some tumors show an alveolar growth pattern or rhabdoid features.

Despite its name, clear cell sarcoma cells commonly display a pale eosinophilic or amphophilic cytoplasm, with true clearing present only in a minority of the neoplastic cells. Although the tumor cells show vesicular nuclei with macronucleoli, there is significantly less nuclear pleomorphism and lower mitotic activity compared to metastatic melanoma (fig. 10-12C). The presence of scattered multinucleated giant cells with nuclei arranged in a horseshoe pattern is a useful diagnostic clue. Melanin is often not detected histologically, but can be highlighted by a Fontana stain in two thirds of the cases.

Compared to the classic soft tissue lesions, gastrointestinal clear cell sarcoma is composed of monotonous round to epithelioid cells arranged in solid, nested, or pseudopapillary growth patterns (fig. 10-13A–C). The cells have scant clear to light eosinophilic cytoplasm, fine chromatin, with much smaller, often inconspicuous nucleoli. Osteoclast-like giant cells are present in half of the cases (fig. 10-13D).

Special Studies. There is strong and diffuse staining for S-100 protein, HMB-45, microphthalmia-associated transcription factor (MITF) and other melanoma antigens (fig. 10-14A–C) (59). Gastrointestinal clear cell sarcoma shows similar strong S-100 protein reactivity, but rare expression for other melanocytic markers (fig. 10-15, left) (54,60). Melanosomes in varying stages of development are detected ultrastructurally (61,62).

Genetics. The typical finding is the presence of a reciprocal translocation, t(12;22)(q13;q12), resulting in the fusion of genes *EWSR1* with *ATF1* in over 90 percent of cases (fig. 10-14D) (63,64). The most common fusion transcript is type 1, having exon 8 of *EWSR1* fused in frame with *ATF1* codon 65. A related variant translocation, t(2;22)(q32.3;q12), resulting in *EWSR-CREB1* fusion, was recently reported in a small subset (6 percent) of clear cell sarcoma (59,65). No significant association between the transcript type and immunohistochemical profile or patient's outcome was found (59,66). Similar to

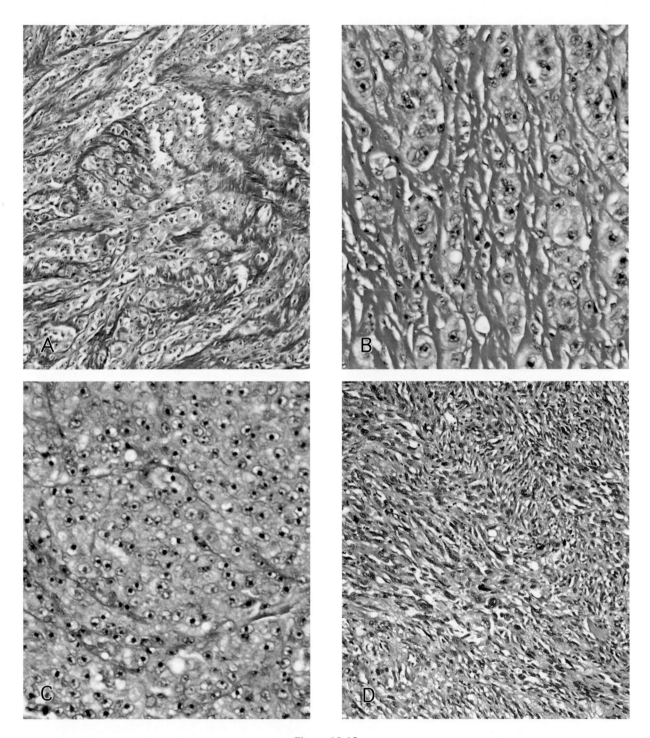

Figure 10-12

CLEAR CELL SARCOMA

A: There is an intimate relationship of the tumor with the aponeurotic structures, from which thick fibrous bands extend to divide into solid compartments.

B: High power shows single cells and small nests separated by hyalinized stroma.

C: The epithelioid cells show ill-defined cell borders, gray amphophilic cytoplasm, and nuclei with distinct macronucleoli but minimal nuclear pleomorphism.

D: Areas of spindling are also noted.

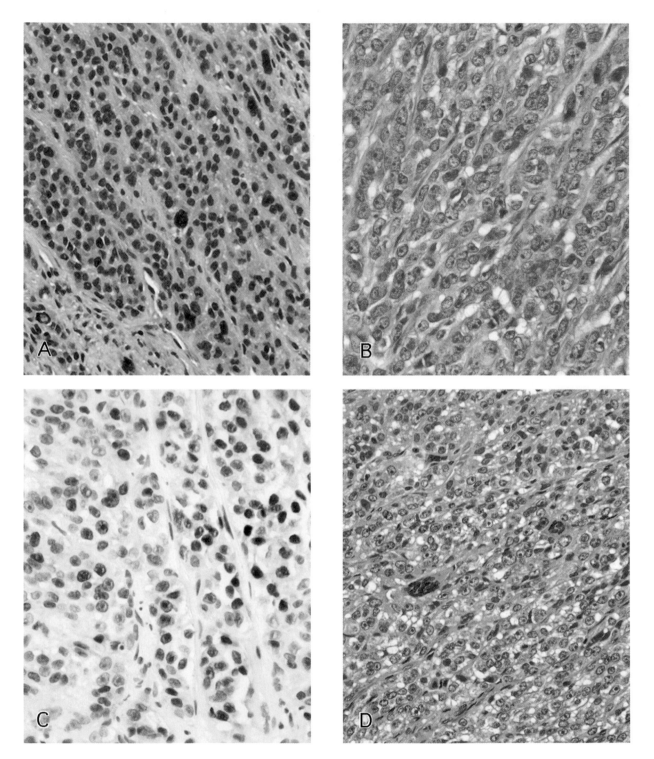

Figure 10-13

GASTROINTESTINAL CLEAR CELL SARCOMA

A,B: There is a distinctive nested growth pattern (A), composed of monotonous round to epithelioid cells with fine chromatin and inconspicuous nucleoli (B).

C: A peculiar pseudopapillary growth pattern may be mistaken for a papillary carcinoma.

D: Scattered osteoclast-type giant cells are present in some but not all cases.

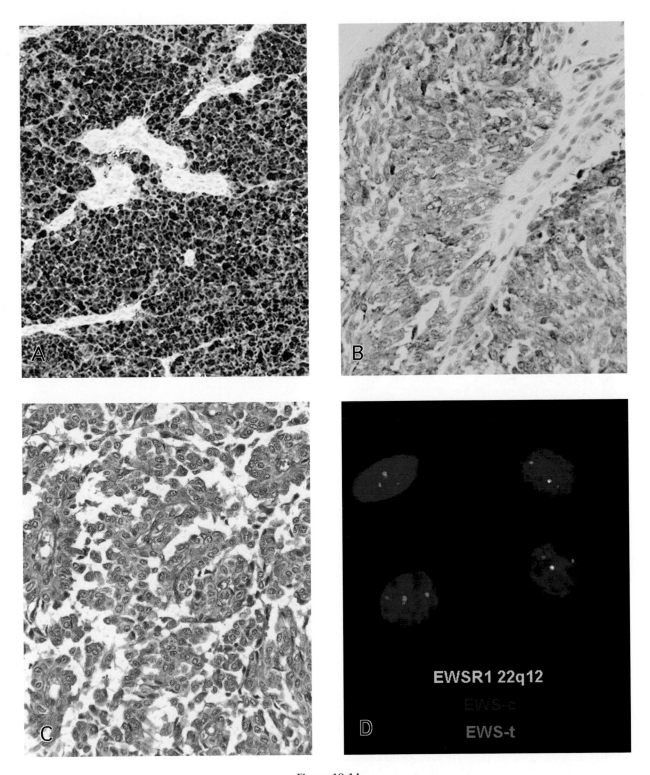

Figure 10-14

CLEAR CELL SARCOMA

Ancillary techniques are helpful in confirming the diagnosis. Strong and diffuse reactivity for S-100 protein (A), HMB-45 (B), and MITF (C), is seen. Fluoresence in situ hybridization (FISH) analysis confirms the presence of *EWSR1* gene rearrangement in challenging cases, particularly to distinguish the tumor from metastatic melanoma (D).

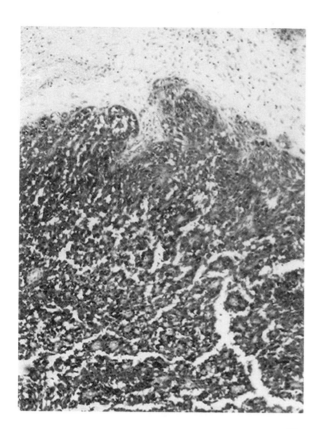 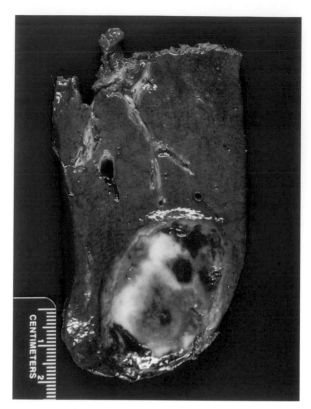

Figure 10-15

GASTROINTESTINAL CLEAR CELL SARCOMA

Left: Special studies show strong reactivity for S-100 protein, not for other more specific melanocytic markers.

Right: These tumors are very aggressive, with a high propensity to locoregional lymph node spread as well as liver metastases.

the soft tissue counterpart, the gastrointestinal variant displays *EWSR1* rearrangements involving either *ATF1* or *CREB1* (54,67–69).

Differential Diagnosis. The differential diagnosis of clear cell sarcoma includes other deep soft tissue sarcomas with an epithelioid nested morphology and either clear or eosinophilic cytoplasm and S-100 protein expression. Epithelioid malignant peripheral nerve sheath tumor may have a similar appearance, although the cells exhibit distinctive, densely eosinophilic cytoplasm in a variably myxoid stroma, and typically do not express melanocytic markers. Soft tissue myoepithelial tumors may exhibit a similar nested growth pattern and cytoplasmic clearing, however, they typically have inconspicuous nucleoli and usually coexpress epithelial membrane antigen or cytokeratins in addition to S-100 protein. Melanocytic schwannomas share the clear cell sarcoma cytomorphology with nested

growth and macronucleoli, but in addition exhibit a high degree of melanin pigmentation and often psammomatous calcifications. An epithelioid PEComa may also have a nested growth pattern, clear to eosinophilic cytoplasm, and melanocytic differentiation; however, most PEComas do not express S-100 protein and commonly express myoid markers.

Particularly due to its clinical presentation as well as its nested and monomorphic cytomorphology, gastrointestinal clear cell sarcoma may be misdiagnosed as either a gastrointestinal carcinoid or a gastrointestinal stromal tumor. Immunohistochemical studies help in this distinction: gastrointestinal clear cell sarcoma is strongly positive for S-100 protein but is negative for CD117, Ano1/DOG1, chromogranin, and epithelial markers (70); in contrast, melanoma frequently coexpresses melanocytic markers (HMB-45, melan A). Clinical correlation and a more organized architecture (packeting in clear cell sarcoma) also help to separate this tumor from melanoma. In challenging cases, FISH analysis for the presence of *EWSR1* gene rearrangement helps to separate clear cell sarcoma from melanoma.

Treatment and Prognosis. Despite an often prolonged clinical course, clear cell sarcoma is associated with a poor prognosis, with survival rates at 5, 10, and 20 years of 67 percent, 33 percent, and 10 percent, respectively (58,59). Nodal metastasis develops in half of the patients. The lung and bone are the other frequent sites of dissemination. The 5-year survival rates overestimate the long-term survival, since many patients develop recurrences and metastases, sometimes more than 10 years after diagnosis. Tumor size (greater than 5 cm), necrosis, and local recurrence are unfavorable prognostic markers (71). The gastrointestinal variant is a highly aggressive tumor with early spread to locoregional lymph nodes, liver, and peritoneum (fig. 10-15, right).

ANGIOMATOID FIBROUS HISTIOCYTOMA

Definition. *Angiomatoid fibrous histiocytoma* is an unusual and mostly benign mesenchymal neoplasm with distinctive morphologic features. These are varying proportions of spindle histiocytoid cells, pseudovascular spaces, and prominent lymphocytic rimming, simulating a lymph node. It typically involves the *EWSR1* gene in fusion translocations.

Clinical Features. Angiomatoid fibrous histiocytoma typically occurs in children and adolescents, with an equal sex distribution. There is a peak incidence in the second decade of life, although rare cases have been described from birth (72) to 79 years old (73). The limbs are the most common sites, followed closely by the trunk and head and neck. About two thirds of cases occur in areas where normal lymph nodes are found (antecubital fossa, popliteal fossa, axilla, inguinal areas, and neck).

Patients typically present with a painless soft tissue lump, which could be mistaken clinically for enlarged lymph nodes. Occasionally, systemic symptoms, such as severe anemia and weight loss, have been described and may precede the detection of the soft tissue mass (74,75).

Gross Findings. On gross examination, angiomatoid fibrous histiocytomas are well-circum-scribed, firm subcutaneous nodules, simulating a lymph node. On cut surface, the lesions show a multilocular hemorrhagic appearance, simulating a hematoma or intranodal hemorrhage. The tumors are usually small, with a median of 2 cm, but a wide range in size distribution has been reported (0.7 to 12.0 cm) (74,75).

Microscopic Findings. Microscopically, four key morphologic features are typically found in varying proportions: 1) pseudoangiomatoid spaces filled with blood and surrounded by tumor cells (fig. 10-16A–C); 2) nodular or cannon-ball proliferations of either spindle or more epithelioid/small cells, with a distinctive syncytial growth pattern (fig. 10-16D); 3) thick fibrous pseudocapsule; and 4) pericapsular cuffing of lymphoplasmacytic cells with occasional germinal centers, mimicking a lymph node metastasis (fig. 10-16D,E). There are two histologic subtypes described, having either a predominantly spindle cell or round cell growth pattern (76). The predominantly spindle cell subtype typically shows uniform cytomorphology with eosinophilic or clear cytoplasm, vesicular nuclei, and low proliferation activity (fig. 10-17A). More pleomorphic examples with brisk mitotic activity have been described without prognostic implications, but may masquerade as a more aggressive pleomorphic sarcoma and may require confirmation at the molecular level (fig. 10-17B). The small cell component is typically composed of dark, hyperchromatic nuclei, with scant eosinophilic cytoplasm (fig. 10-17C).

The common location of angiomatoid fibrous histiocytoma in areas of normal lymphoid tissue, as well as the scattered desmin-positive cells within the adjacent lymphoid tissue, similar to cells seen within the tumor, raise the possibility that some of these lesions may be related to a subset of fibroblastic reticulum cells of normal lymphoid tissue, which are positive for vimentin and desmin (76).

Special Studies. Angiomatoid fibrous histiocytoma is often positive for desmin, CD68, epithelial membrane antigen, and CD99 (fig. 10-18) (76,77). The tumors are negative for myogenin, S-100 protein, HMB-45, CD21, CD35, CD34, and CD31. The ultrastructural findings are nonspecific.

Genetics. The most common genetic abnormality is the t(2;22) translocation, resulting in *EWSR1-CREB1* fusion in more than 90 percent of cases (fig. 10-19) (73,78). Rare cases may

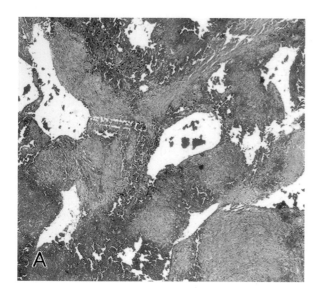

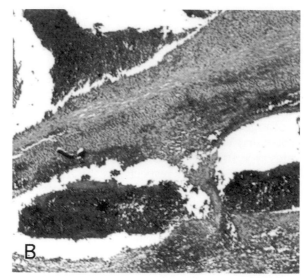

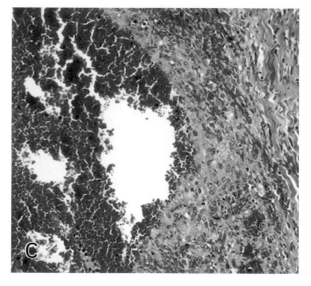

Figure 10-16

ANGIOMATOID FIBROUS HISTIOCYTOMA

A,B: Distinctive histopathologic features include large, ectatic pseudovascular spaces filled with blood, which may be mistaken for a hematoma.

C: Some of these cystic structures are lined by strips of tumor cells.

D,E: An additional characteristic finding is the prominent inflammatory component, typically present as a lymphoid aggregate with reactive germinal centers, reminiscent of a lymph node.

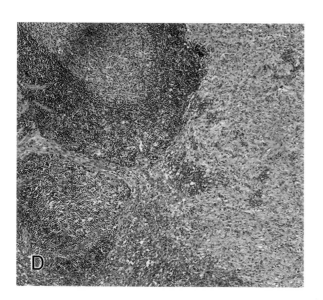

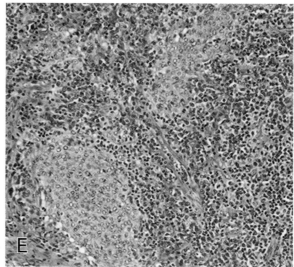

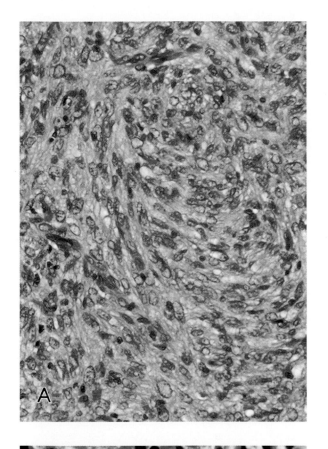

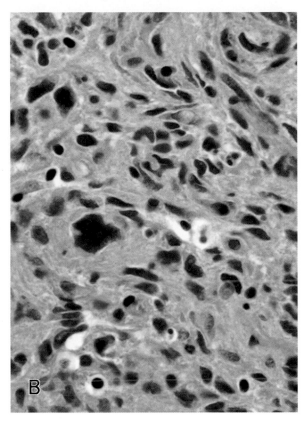

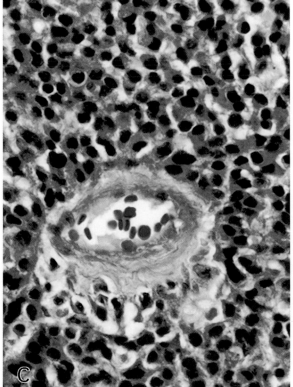

Figure 10-17

ANGIOMATOID FIBROUS HISTIOCYTOMA

A: Two distinct morphologic variants are noted: the most common is the spindle cell type, in which monotonous and bland fusiform cells are tightly arranged in a syncytial or vague whorling pattern.

B: Occasionally, this variant shows more pronounced nuclear pleomorphism, which may suggest a high-grade pleomorphic sarcoma.

C: The least common and under-recognized variant is the small cell variant, which is composed of round, primitive cells with scant eosinophilic cytoplasm and hyperchromatic, pyknotic nuclei.

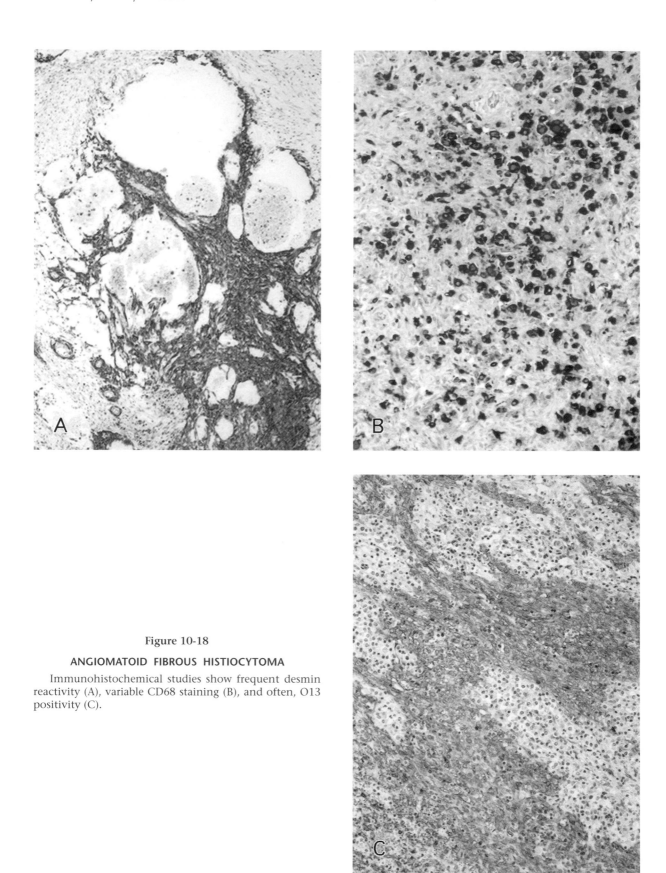

Figure 10-18

ANGIOMATOID FIBROUS HISTIOCYTOMA

Immunohistochemical studies show frequent desmin reactivity (A), variable CD68 staining (B), and often, O13 positivity (C).

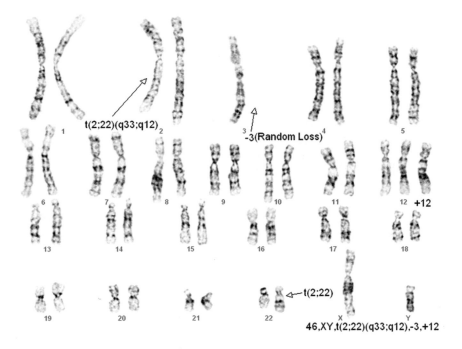

t(2;22)(q33;q12)

-3(Random Loss)

+12

<—t(2;22)

46,XY,t(2;22)(q33;q12),-3,+12

Figure 10-19

ANGIOMATOID FIBROUS HISTIOCYTOMA

Karyotype showing the characteristic t(2;22) (q33;q12) translocation.

show instead a *FUS-ATF1* (79,80) or *EWSR1-ATF1* fusion (81–83). The transcript structure is composed of exon 7 of *EWSR1* fused to exon 7 of *CREB1*. The predicted protein structure of EWSR1-CREB1 parallels closely that of EWSR1-ATF1 (84). No obvious correlations between fusion transcript type and patient demographics, tumor location, or immunoprofile are noted. Identical fusions involving *ATF1* and *CREB1* are found in clear cell sarcoma as well (84–86).

Differential Diagnosis. Particularly underrecognized is the angiomatoid fibrous histiocytoma composed mainly of a small blue cell phenotype, which may be confused with a high-grade undifferentiated sarcoma. The distinction from Ewing sarcoma is especially challenging, based on a constellation of overlapping findings, such as the undifferentiated/small cell morphology, CD99 immunoreactivity, and presence of an *EWSR1* gene rearrangement. The frequent small size and superficial location in the subcutis are important clues against a diagnosis of Ewing sarcoma. RT-PCR for confirming the fusion partner of the *EWSR1* gene is indicated in challenging cases.

In the rare cases where the spindle cell variant of angiomatoid fibrous histiocytoma shows more pronounced nuclear pleomorphism and hyperchromasia and is sometimes associated with increased mitotic activity, it becomes more problematic to distinguish from a malignant fibrous histiocytoma. Important clues are the clinical presentation, including the much younger age of patients with angiomatoid fibrous histiocytoma, as well as the lack of lymphoid aggregates with conspicuous germinal centers in malignant fibrous histiocytoma.

Aneurysmal fibrous histiocytoma is a rare variant of benign fibrous histiocytoma that has rapid growth due to its spontaneous intralesional hemorrhage. Similar to angiomatoid fibrous histiocytoma, the aneurysmal variant is characterized by blood-filled spaces lined by discohesive tumor cells at low power. In contrast, they lack the brisk lymphoid cuffing and are typically centered in the dermis.

Treatment and Prognosis. Angiomatoid fibrous histiocytoma is an indolent tumor, with 2 to 10 percent local recurrences and less than 1 percent metastases, usually to the loco-regional lymph nodes (76). Rare deaths due to late distant metastases have been reported (74,75,87,88). In some of those cases, the aggressive tumors may be other entities. There are no known clinical or morphologic factors that correlate with outcome or predict metastasis. Wide local excision is the treatment of choice for primary tumors (75,76). These tumors are prone to local recurrence if incompletely excised (typically within 1 year from the initial resection).

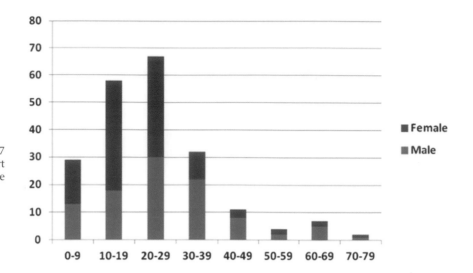

Figure 10-20

ALVEOLAR SOFT PART SARCOMA

Age and sex distribution of 207 patients with alveolar soft part sarcoma (Armed Forces Institute of Pathology [AFIP] data).

ALVEOLAR SOFT PART SARCOMA

Definition. *Alveolar soft part sarcoma* is a malignant mesenchymal neoplasm characterized by epithelioid, variably eosinophilic cells often arranged in pseudoalveolar compartments, surrounded by fibrovascular septa. The tumor typically carries the *ASPL-TFE3* gene fusion and expresses TFE3 transcription factor.

Clinical Features. Alveolar soft part sarcoma is rare, comprising less than 1 percent of all soft tissue sarcomas. Based on Armed Forces Institute of Pathology (AFIP) data, it has a strong predilection to children and young adults of a median age of 21 years. There is a mild (1.1 to 1.0) female predominance, but patients under 21 years have a 1.6 to 1.0 female predominance and patients 21 years and older have a 1.3 to 1.0 male predominance (fig. 10-20).

The most commonly involved locations are the lower extremity, especially thigh (38 percent), followed by head and neck (31 percent), trunk wall/body cavities (18 percent), and upper extremity (13 percent). Orbit and tongue are the most commonly involved sites in the head and neck (fig. 10-21). Cases considered primary tumors have also been reported in a variety of internal organs and in bones (89–94).

Gross and Microscopic Findings. Grossly, alveolar soft part sarcoma typically shows a homogeneous yellowish surface on sectioning. Histologically typical is compartmental, nested, or microlobular organization spaced by vascular septa. The compartments contain epithelioid tumor cells with a moderate amount of pale eosinophilic to partially clear cytoplasm. In many cases, the center is free of cells, imparting an alveolar appearance (fig. 10-22). The compartment size varies. Especially in young patients, the compartments are small and often lack central alveolar spaces.

Cytologically typical are moderate size nuclei with small nucleoli and limited overall nuclear atypia, but rare atypical variants have been reported (95). Marked nuclear pleomorphism and marked mitotic activity are rare and if present should lead to a serious consideration of an alternative diagnosis. Calcification is present in some cases. Lymphovascular invasion is particularly common in this entity.

Special Studies. Periodic acid–Schiff (PAS)-positive and diastase-resistant cytoplasmic crystals or amorphous globules are present in most cases (fig. 10-23, left). By electron microscopy, the crystals have a distinctive lattice-like internal structure with 100-angstrom periodicity (96,97). The most important immunohistochemical study is for TFE3 transcription factor, which is detectable in tumor cell nuclei in virtually all cases (fig. 10-23, right) (98). Approximately half of cases show variable, usually focal, desmin positivity, and focal smooth muscle actin and S-100 protein positivity may be detected. The tumor cells are negative for keratins and do not show nuclear staining for myogenic determination

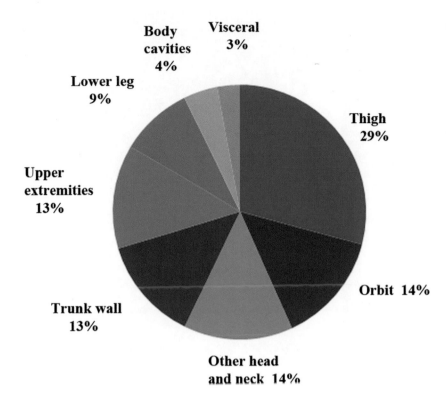

Figure 10-21

ALVEOLAR SOFT PART SARCOMA

Anatomic distribution of 205 alveolar soft part sarcomas (AFIP data).

markers (MyoD1, myogenin) (99–102). The cytoplasmic crystals contain monocarboxylate transporter 1 and CD147 (103).

ASPL-TFE3 gene fusion translocation is typical of this tumor and can be detected by PCR-based fusion transcript tests, or FISH via TFE3 break-apart probe (104–109). The corresponding nonbalanced t(17q25.3 Xp11.2) translocation is observed cytogenetically.

Differential Diagnosis. Alveolar soft part sarcoma should be separated from other epithelioid neoplasms with compartmental patterns, especially malignant melanoma and related tumors, renal cell carcinoma, granular cell tumor, PEComa, and paraganglioma. Prominent nuclear atypia and mitotic activity direct the search to such alternative diagnoses; helpful auxiliary tests to rule out the above-mentioned tumors include melanoma markers, keratins, epithelial membrane antigen, and the neuroendocrine markers chromogranin A and synaptophysin. PEComas are variably positive for HMB-45. Regarding genetic testing, the same *ASPL-TFE3* gene fusion (but with a balanced translocation) also occurs in the so-called Xp11.2 translocation renal carcinomas (especially in young age groups), and these tumors are also immunohistochemically positive for TFE3 (110,111).

Treatment and Prognosis. In general, the course of disease is slow, but metastases develop over time in a majority of patients. Up to 10 percent of patients present with lung or other metastases. Nevertheless, surgical excision of pulmonary and brain metastases has been found beneficial. Targeted therapies, such as various tyrosine kinase inhibitors, are being explored (111). In the largest series, the 5-, 10-, and 15-year survival rates for patients presenting with localized tumors were 60 percent, 38 percent, and 15 percent (112).

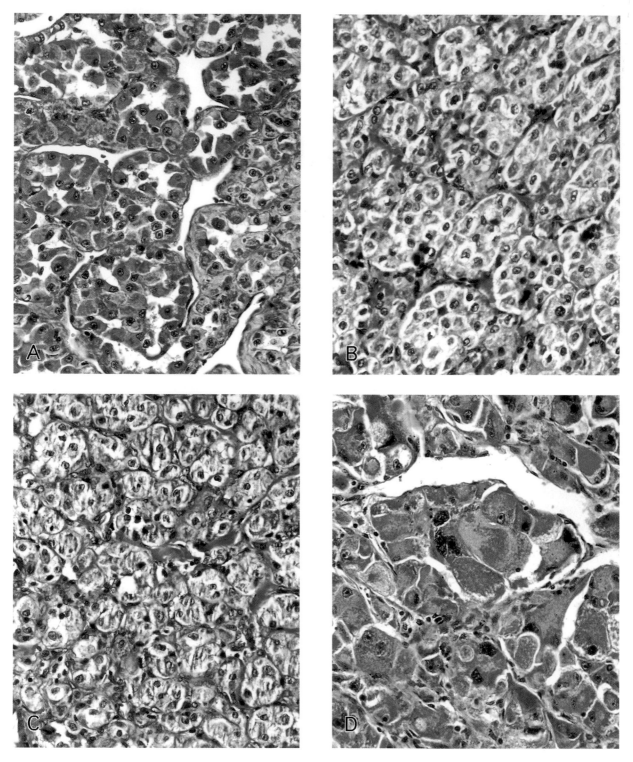

Figure 10-22

ALVEOLAR SOFT PART SARCOMA

A: Alveolar soft part sarcoma shows a variably developed compartmental pattern, often with central alveolar spaces.
B,C: Some tumors are composed of smaller compartments, which lack central alveolar spaces.
D: Focal pleomorphism is a rare finding.

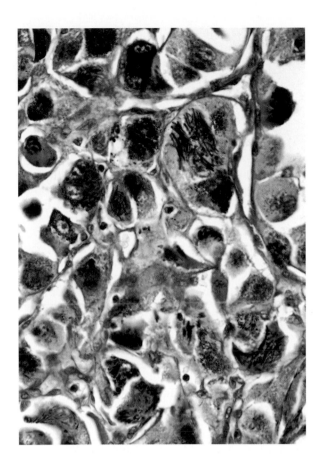 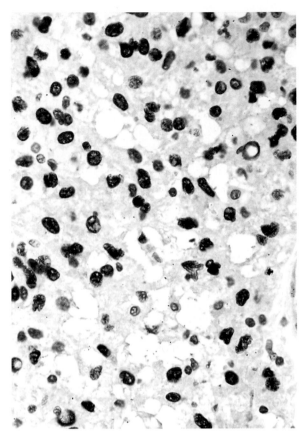

Figure 10-23

ALVEOLAR SOFT PART SARCOMA

Left: The tumor cells typically contain periodic acid–Schiff (PAS)-positive cytoplasmic crystals.
Right: Tumor cell nuclei are immunohistochemically positive for transcription factor E3 (TFE3).

REFERENCES

Ewing Sarcoma/Peripheral Neuroectodermal Tumor

1. Gurney JG, Davis S, Severson RK, Fang JY, Ross JA, Robison LL. Trends in cancer incidence among children in the U.S. Cancer 1996;78:532-541.
2. Askin FB, Rosai J, Sibley RK, Dehner LP, McAlister WH. Malignant small cell tumor of the thoracopulmonary region in childhood: a distinctive clinicopathologic entity of uncertain histogenesis. Cancer 1979;43:2438-2451.
3. Paulussen M, Frohlich B, Jurgens H. Ewing tumour: incidence, prognosis and treatment options. Paediatr Drugs 2001;3:899-913.
4. Lawlor ER, Mathers JA, Bainbridge T, et al. Peripheral primitive neuroectodermal tumors in adults: documentation by molecular analysis. J Clin Oncol 1998;16:1150-1157.
5. Kovar H, Dworzak M, Strehl S, et al. Overexpression of the pseudoautosomal gene MIC2 in Ewing's sarcoma and peripheral primitive neuroectodermal tumor. Oncogene 1990;5:1067-1070.
6. Scotlandi K, Serra M, Manara MC, et al. Immunostaining of the p30/32MIC2 antigen and molecular detection of EWS rearrangements for the diagnosis of Ewing's sarcoma and peripheral neuroectodermal tumor. Hum Pathol 1996;27:408-416.
7. Gu M, Antonescu CR, Guiter G, Huvos AG, Ladanyi M, Zakowski MF. Cytokeratin immunoreactivity in Ewing's sarcoma: prevalence in 50 cases confirmed by molecular diagnostic studies. Am J Surg Pathol 2000;24:410-416.

8. Turc-Carel C, Aurias A, Mugneret F, et al. Chromosomes in Ewing's sarcoma. I. An evaluation of 85 cases of remarkable consistency of t(11;22)(q24;q12). Cancer Genet Cytogenet 1988;32:229-238.

9. Delattre O, Zucman J, Plougastel B, et al. Gene fusion with an ETS DNA-binding domain caused by chromosome translocation in human tumours. Nature 1992;359:162-165.

10. Plougastel B, Zucman J, Peter M, Thomas G, Delattre O. Genomic structure of the EWS gene and its relationship to EWSR1, a site of tumor-associated chromosome translocation. Genomics 1993;18:609-615.

11. Aman P, Panagopoulos I, Lassen C, et al. Expression patterns of the human sarcoma-associated genes FUS and EWS and the genomic structure of FUS. Genomics 1996;37:1-8.

12. Truong AH, Ben-David Y. The role of Fli-1 in normal cell function and malignant transformation. Oncogene 2000;19:6482-6489.

13. Ng TL, O'Sullivan MJ, Pallen CJ, et al. Ewing sarcoma with novel translocation t(2;16) producing an in-frame fusion of FUS and FEV. J Mol Diagn 2007;9:459-463.

14. Wang L, Bhargava R, Zheng T, et al. Undifferentiated small round cell sarcomas with rare EWS gene fusions: identification of a novel EWS-SP3 fusion and of additional cases with the EWS-ETV1 and EWS-FEV fusions. J Mol Diagn 2007;9:498-509.

15. Shing DC, McMullan DJ, Roberts P, et al. FUS/ERG gene fusions in Ewing's tumors. Cancer Res 2003;63:4568-4576.

16. Mastrangelo T, Modena P, Tornielli S, et al. A novel zinc finger gene is fused to EWS in small round cell tumor. Oncogene 2000;19:3799-3804.

17. Szuhai K, Ijszenga M, de Jong D, Karseladze A, Tanke HJ, Hogendoorn PC. The NFATc2 gene is involved in a novel cloned translocation in a Ewing sarcoma variant that couples its function in immunology to oncology. Clin Cancer Res 2009;15:2259-2268.

18. Sumegi J, Nishio J, Nelson M, Frayer RW, Perry D, Bridge JA. A novel t(4;22)(q31;q12) produces an EWSR1-SMARCA5 fusion in extraskeletal Ewing sarcoma/primitive neuroectodermal tumor. Mod Pathol 2011;24:333-342.

19. Lemmers RJ, van der Vliet PJ, Klooster R, et al. A unifying genetic model for facioscapulohumeral muscular dystrophy. Science 2010;329:1650-1653.

20. Italiano A, Sung YS, Zhang L, et al. High prevalence of CIC fusion with double-homeobox (DUX4) transcription factors in EWSR1-negative undifferentiated small blue round cell sarcomas. Genes Chromosomes Cancer 2012;51:207-218.

21. Pierron G, Tirode F, Lucchesi C, et al. A new subtype of bone sarcoma defined by BCOR-CCNB3 gene fusion. Nat Genet 2012;44:461-466.

22. Antonescu CR, Gerald WL, Magid MS, Ladanyi M. Molecular variants of the EWS-WT1 gene fusion in desmoplastic small round cell tumor. Diagn Mol Pathol 1998;7:24-28.

23. Antonescu CR, Tschernyavsky SJ, Woodruff JM, Jungbluth AA, Brennan MF, Ladanyi M. Molecular diagnosis of clear cell sarcoma: detection of EWS-ATF1 and MITF-M transcripts and histopathological and ultrastructural analysis of 12 cases. J Molec Diagn 2002;4:44-52.

24. Antonescu CR, Nafa K, Segal NH, Dal Cin P, Ladanyi M. EWS-CREB1: a recurrent variant fusion in clear cell sarcoma—association with gastrointestinal location and absence of melanocytic differentiation. Clin Cancer Res 2006;12:5356-5362.

25. Antonescu CR, Dal Cin P, Nafa K, et al. EWSR1-CREB1 is the predominant gene fusion in angiomatoid fibrous histiocytoma. Genes Chromosomes Cancer 2007;46:1051-1060.

26. Antonescu CR, Zhang L, Chang NE, et al. EWSR1-POU5F1 fusion in soft tissue myoepithelial tumors. A molecular analysis of sixty-six cases, including soft tissue, bone, and visceral lesions, showing common involvement of the EWSR1 gene. Genes Chromosomes Cancer 2010;49:1114-1124.

27. Wang CC, Schulz MD. Ewing's sarcoma; a study of fifty cases treated at the Massachusetts General Hospital, 1930-1952 inclusive. N Engl J Med 1953;248:571-576.

28. Dahlin DC, Coventry MB, Scanlon PW. Ewing's sarcoma. A critical analysis of 165 cases. J Bone Joint Surg Am 1961;43-A:185-192.

29. Lahl M, Fisher VL, Laschinger K. Ewing's sarcoma family of tumors: an overview from diagnosis to survivorship. Clin J Oncol Nursing 2008;12:89-97.

30. Terrier P, Llombart-Bosch A, Contesso G. Small round blue cell tumors in bone: prognostic factors correlated to Ewing's sarcoma and neuroectodermal tumors. Semin Diagn Pathol 1996;13:250-257.

31. Rodriguez-Galindo C, Navid F, Liu T, Billups CA, Rao BN, Krasin MJ. Prognostic factors for local and distant control in Ewing sarcoma family of tumors. Ann Oncology 2008;19:814-820.

32. Paulussen M, Bielack S, Jurgens H, Casali PG. ESMO clinical recommendations. On behalf of the ESMO Guidelines Working Group., 2009.

33. Le Deley MC, Delattre O, Schaefer KL, et al. Impact of EWS-ETS fusion type on disease progression in Ewing's sarcoma/peripheral primitive neuroectodermal tumor: prospective results from the cooperative Euro-E.W.I.N.G. 99 trial. J Clin Oncol 2010;28:1982-1988.

34. Zoubek A, Dockhorn-Dworniczak B, Delattre O, et al. H. Does expression of different EWS chimeric transcripts define clinically distinct risk groups of Ewing tumor patients? J Clin Oncol 1996;14:1245-1251.

35. van Doorninck JA, Ji L, Schaub B, et al. Current treatment protocols have eliminated the prognostic advantage of type 1 fusions in Ewing sarcoma: a report from the Children's Oncology Group. J Clin Oncol 2010;28:1989-1994.

36. Cotterill SJ, Ahrens S, Paulussen M, et al. Prognostic factors in Ewing's tumor of bone: analysis of 975 patients from the European Intergroup Cooperative Ewing's Sarcoma Study Group. J Clin Oncol 2000;18:3108-3114.

37. Grier HE, Krailo MD, Tarbell NJ, et al. Addition of ifosfamide and etoposide to standard chemotherapy for Ewing's sarcoma and primitive neuroectodermal tumor of bone. N Engl J Med 2003;348:694-701.

38. Pappo AS, Patel SR, Crowley J, et al. R1507, a monoclonal antibody to the insulin-like growth factor 1 receptor, in patients with recurrent or refractory Ewing sarcoma family of tumors: results of a phase II Sarcoma Alliance for Research through Collaboration study. J Clin Oncol 2011; 29:4541-4547.

Desmoplastic Small Round Cell Tumor

39. Barnoud R, Sabourin JC, Pasquier D, et al. Immunohistochemical expression of WT1 by desmoplastic small round cell tumor: a comparative study with other small round cell tumors. Am J Surg Pathol 2000;24:830-836.

40. Hill DA, Pfeifer JD, Marley EF, et al. WT1 staining reliably differentiates desmoplastic small round cell tumor from Ewing sarcoma/primitive neuroectodermal tumor. An immunohistochemical and molecular diagnostic study. Am J Clin Pathol 2000;114:345-353.

41. Sawyer JR, Tryka AF, Lewis JM. A novel reciprocal chromosome translocation t(11;22)(p13;q12) in an intraabdominal desmoplastic small round-cell tumor. Am J Surg Pathol 1992;16:411-416.

42. Biegel JA, Conard K, Brooks JJ. Translocation (11;22)(p13;q12): primary change in intra-abdominal desmoplastic small round cell tumor. Genes Chromosomes Cancer 1993;7:119-121.

43. Rodriguez E, Sreekantaiah C, Gerald W, Reuter VE, Motzer RJ, Chaganti RS. A recurring translocation, t(11;22)(p13;q11.2), characterizes intra-abdominal desmoplastic small round-cell tumors. Cancer Genet Cytogenet 1993;69:17-21.

44. Ladanyi M, Gerald W. Fusion of the EWS and WT1 genes in the desmoplastic small round cell tumor. Cancer Res 1994;54:2837-2840.

45. de Alava E, Ladanyi M, Rosai J, Gerald WL. Detection of chimeric transcripts in desmoplastic small round cell tumor and related developmental tumors by reverse transcriptase polymerase chain reaction. A specific diagnostic assay. Am J Pathol 1995;147:1584-1591.

46. Gerald WL, Rosai J, Ladanyi M. Characterization of the genomic breakpoint and chimeric transcripts in the EWS-WT1 gene fusion of desmoplastic small round cell tumor. Proc Natl Acad Sci U S A 1995;92:1028-1032.

47. Gerald WL, Ladanyi M, de Alava E, et al. Clinical, pathologic, and molecular spectrum of tumors associated with t(11;22)(p13;q12): desmoplastic small round-cell tumor and its variants. J Clin Oncol 1998;16:3028-3036.

48. Lee SB, Kolquist KA, Nichols K, et al. The EWS-WT1 translocation product induces PDGFA in desmoplastic small round-cell tumour. Nat Genet 1997;17:309-313.

49. Pritchard-Jones K, Fleming S. Cell types expressing the Wilms' tumour gene (WT1) in Wilms' tumours: implications for tumour histogenesis. Oncogene 1991;6:2211-2220.

50. Ramani P, Cowell JK. The expression pattern of Wilms' tumour gene (WT1) product in normal tissues and paediatric renal tumours. J Pathol 1996;179:162-168.

51. Lal DR, Su WT, Wolden SL, Loh KC, Modak S, La Quaglia MP. Results of multimodal treatment for desmoplastic small round cell tumors. J Pediatr Surg 2005;40:251-255.

52. Philippe-Chomette P, Kabbara N, Andre N, et al. Desmoplastic small round cell tumors with EWS-WT1 fusion transcript in children and young adults. Pediatr Blood Cancer 2012;58:891-897.

Clear Cell Sarcoma

53. Chung EB, Enzinger FM. Malignant melanoma of soft parts. A reassessment of clear cell sarcoma. Am J Surg Pathol 1983;7:405-413.

54. Antonescu CR, Nafa K, Segal NH, Dal Cin P, Ladanyi M. EWS-CREB1: a recurrent variant fusion in clear cell sarcoma—association with gastrointestinal location and absence of melanocytic differentiation. Clin Cancer Res 2006;12:5356-5362.

55. Enzinger FM. Clear-cell sarcoma of tendons and aponeuroses. An analysis of 21 cases. Cancer 1965;18:1163-1174.

56. Deenik W, Mooi WJ, Rutgers EJ, Peterse JL, Hart AA, Kroon BB. Clear cell sarcoma (malignant melanoma) of soft parts: A clinicopathologic study of 30 cases. Cancer 1999;86:969-975.

57. Eckardt JJ, Pritchard DJ, Soule EH. Clear cell sarcoma. A clinicopathologic study of 27 cases. Cancer 1983;52:1482-1488.

58. Lucas DR, Nascimento AG, Sim FH. Clear cell sarcoma of soft tissues. Mayo Clinic experience with 35 cases. Am J Surg Pathol 1992;16:1197-1204.

59. Hisaoka M, Ishida T, Kuo TT, et al. Clear cell sarcoma of soft tissue: a clinicopathologic, immunohistochemical, and molecular analysis of 33 cases. Am J Surg Pathol 2008;32:452-460.

60. Comin CE, Novelli L, Tornaboni D, Messerini L. Clear cell sarcoma of the ileum: report of a case and review of literature. Virchows Arch 2007;451:839-845.

61. Kindblom LG, Lodding P, Angervall L. Clear-cell sarcoma of tendons and aponeuroses. An immunohistochemical and electron microscopic analysis indicating neural crest origin. Virchows Arch A Pathol Anat Histopathol 1983;401:109-128.

62. Mukai M, Torikata C, Iri H, et al. Histogenesis of clear cell sarcoma of tendons and aponeuroses. An electron-microscopic, biochemical, enzyme histochemical, and immunohistochemical study. Am J Pathol 1984;114:264-272.

63. Antonescu CR, Tschernyavsky SJ, Woodruff JM, Jungbluth AA, Brennan MF, Ladanyi M. Molecular diagnosis of clear cell sarcoma: detection of EWS-ATF1 and MITF-M transcripts and histopathological and ultrastructural analysis of 12 cases. J Mol Diagn 2002;4:44-52.

64. Zucman J, Delattre O, Desmaze C, et al. EWS and ATF-1 gene fusion induced by t(12;22) translocation in malignant melanoma of soft parts. Nat Genet 1993;4:341-345.

65. Wang WL, Mayordomo E, Zhang W, et al. Detection and characterization of EWSR1/ATF1 and EWSR1/CREB1 chimeric transcripts in clear cell sarcoma (melanoma of soft parts). Mod Pathol 2009;22:1201-1209.

66. Coindre JM, Hostein I, Terrier P, et al. Diagnosis of clear cell sarcoma by real-time reverse transcriptase-polymerase chain reaction analysis of paraffin embedded tissues: clinicopathologic and molecular analysis of 44 patients from the French sarcoma group. Cancer 2006;107:1055-1064.

67. Covinsky M, Gong S, Rajaram V, Perry A, Pfeifer J. EWS-ATF1 fusion transcripts in gastrointestinal tumors previously diagnosed as malignant melanoma. Hum Pathol 2005;36:74-81.

68. Lyle PL, Amato CM, Fitzpatrick JE, Robinson WA. Gastrointestinal melanoma or clear cell sarcoma? Molecular evaluation of 7 cases previously diagnosed as malignant melanoma. Am J Surg Pathol 2008;32:858-866.

69. Davis IJ, Kim JJ, Ozsolak F, et al. Oncogenic MITF dysregulation in clear cell sarcoma: defining the MiT family of human cancers. Cancer Cell 2006;9:473-484.

70. Stockman DL, Miettinen M, Suster S, et al. Malignant gastrointestinal neuroectodermal tumor: clinicopathological, immunohistochemical, ultrastructural, and molecular analysis of 16 cases with a reappraisal of clear cell sarcoma-like tumors of the gastrointestinal tract. Am J Surg Pathol 2012;36:857-868.

71. Sara AS, Evans HL, Benjamin RS. Malignant melanoma of soft parts (clear cell sarcoma). A study of 17 cases, with emphasis on prognostic factors. Cancer 1990;65:367-374.

Angiomatoid Fibrous Histiocytoma

72. Argenyi ZB, Van Rybroek JJ, Kemp JD, Soper RT. Congenital angiomatoid malignant fibrous histiocytoma. A light-microscopic, immunopathologic, and electron-microscopic study. Am J Dermatopathol 1988;10:59-67.

73. Antonescu CR, Dal Cin P, Nafa K, et al. EWSR1-CREB1 is the predominant gene fusion in angiomatoid fibrous histiocytoma. Genes Chromosomes Cancer 2007;46:1051-1060.

74. Enzinger FM. Angiomatoid malignant fibrous histiocytoma: a distinct fibrohistiocytic tumor of children and young adults simulating a vascular neoplasm. Cancer 1979;44:2147-2157.

75. Costa MJ, Weiss SW. Angiomatoid malignant fibrous histiocytoma. A follow-up study of 108 cases with evaluation of possible histologic predictors of outcome. Am J Surg Pathol 1990;14:1126-1132.

76. Fanburg-Smith JC, Miettinen M. Angiomatoid "malignant" fibrous histiocytoma: a clinicopathologic study of 158 cases and further exploration of the myoid phenotype. Hum Pathol 1999;30:1336-1343.

77. Hasegawa T, Seki K, Ono K, Hirohashi S. Angiomatoid (malignant) fibrous histiocytoma: a peculiar low-grade tumor showing immunophenotypic heterogeneity and ultrastructural variations. Pathol Int 2000;50:731-738.

78. Rossi S, Szuhai K, Ijszenga M, et al. EWSR1-CREB1 and EWSR1-ATF1 fusion genes in angiomatoid fibrous histiocytoma. Clin Cancer Res 2007;13:7322-7328.

79. Waters BL, Panagopoulos I, Allen EF. Genetic characterization of angiomatoid fibrous histiocytoma identifies fusion of the FUS and ATF-1 genes induced by a chromosomal translocation involving bands 12q13 and 16p11. Cancer Genet Cytogenet 2000;121:109-116.

80. Raddaoui E, Donner LR, Panagopoulos I. Fusion of the FUS and ATF1 genes in a large, deep-seated angiomatoid fibrous histiocytoma. Diagn Mol Pathol 2002;11:157-162.

81. Hallor KH, Mertens F, Jin Y, et al. Fusion of the EWSR1 and ATF1 genes without expression of the MITF-M transcript in angiomatoid fibrous histiocytoma. Genes Chromosomes Cancer 2005;44:97-102.

82. Hallor KH, Micci F, Meis-Kindblom JM, et al. Fusion genes in angiomatoid fibrous histiocytoma. Cancer Lett 2007;251:158-163.

83. Somers GR, Viero S, Nathan PC, Teshima I, Pereira C, Zielenska M. Association of the t(12;22)(q13;q12) EWS/ATF1 rearrangement with polyphenotypic round cell sarcoma of bone: a case report. Am J Surg Pathol 2005;29:1673-1679.

84. Antonescu CR, Nafa K, Segal NH, Dal Cin P, Ladanyi M. EWS-CREB1: a recurrent variant fusion in clear cell sarcoma—association with gastrointestinal location and absence of melanocytic differentiation. Clin Cancer Res 2006;12:5356-5362.

85. Antonescu CR, Tschernyavsky SJ, Woodruff JM, Jungbluth AA, Brennan MF, Ladanyi M. Molecular diagnosis of clear cell sarcoma: detection of EWS-ATF1 and MITF M transcripts and histopathological and ultrastructural analysis of 12 cases. J Mol Diagn 2002;4:44-52.

86. Panagopoulos I, Mertens F, Debiec-Rychter M, et al. Molecular genetic characterization of the EWS/ATF1 fusion gene in clear cell sarcoma of tendons and aponeuroses. Int J Cancer 2002;99:560-567.

87. Pettinato G, Manivel JC, De Rosa G, Petrella G, Jaszcz W. Angiomatoid malignant fibrous histiocytoma: cytologic, immunohistochemical, ultrastructural, and flow cytometric study of 20 cases. Mod Pathol 1990;3:479-487.

88. Matsumura T, Yamaguchi T, Tochigi N, Wada T, Yamashita T, Hasegawa T. Angiomatoid fibrous histiocytoma including cases with pleomorphic features analysed by fluorescence in situ hybridisation. J Clin Pathol 2010;63:124-128.

Alveolar Soft Part Sarcoma

89. Anderson ME. Hornicek FJ, Gebhardt MC, Raskin KA, Mankin HJ. Alveolar soft part sarcoma. A rare and enigmatic entity. Clin Orthop Rel Res 2005;438:144-148.

90. Portera CA Jr, Ho V, Patel SR, et al. Alveolar soft part sarcoma. Clinical course and patterns of metastasis in 70 patients treated at a single institution. Cancer 2001;91:585-591.

91. Ogose A, Yazawa Y, Ueda T, et al. Alveolar soft part sarcoma in Japan: multi-institutional study of 57 patients from the Japanese Musculoskeletal Oncology Group. Oncology 2003;65:7-13.

92. Kayton ML, Meyers P, Wexler LH, Gerald WL, LaQuaglia MP. Clinical presentation, treatment, and outcome of alveolar soft part sarcoma in children, adolescents, and young adults. J Pediatr Surg 2006;41:187-193.

93. Fanburg-Smith JF, Miettinen M, Folpe AL, Weiss SW, Childers EL. Lingual alveolar soft part sarcoma, 14 cases:novel clinical and morphologica observations. Histopathology 2004;45:526-537.

94. Aisner SC, Beebe K, Blacksin M, Mirani N, Hameed M. Primary alveolar soft part sarcoma of fibula demonstrating ASPL-TFE3 fusion: a case report and review of the literature. Skeletal Radiol 2008;37:1047-1051.

95. Evans HL. Alveolar soft-part sarcoma. A study of 13 typical examples and one with a histologically atypical component. Cancer 1985;55:912-917.

96. Ordonez NG, Ro JY, Mackay B. Alveolar soft part sarcoma. An ultrastructural and immunocytochemical investigation of its histogenesis. Cancer 1989;63:1721-1736

97. Mukai M, Torikata C, Iri H, et al. Alveolar soft part sarcoma. An elaboration of a three-dimensional configuration of the crystalloids by digital image processing. Am J Pathol 1984;116:398-406.

98. Argani P, Lai P, Hutchinson B, Lui MY, Reuter VE, Ladanyi M. Aberrant nuclear immunoreactivity for TFE3 in neoplasms with TFE3 gene fusions: a sensitive and specific immunohistochemical assay. Am J Surg Pathol 2003;27:750-761.

99. Persson S, Willems JS, Kindblom LG, Angervall L. Alveolar soft part sarcoma. An immunohistochemical, cytologic and electron-microscopic study and a quantitative DNA analysis. Virchows Arch A Pathol Anat Histopathol 1988;412:499-513.

100. Mukai M, Torikata C, Shimoda T, Iri H. Alveolar soft-part sarcoma. Assessment of immunohistochemical demonstration of desmin using paraffin sections and frozen sections. Virchows Arch A Pathol Anat Histopathol 1989;414:503-509.

101. Matsuno Y, Mukai K, Itabashi M, et al. Alveolar soft-part sarcoma. A clinicopathologic and immunohistochemical study of 12 cases. Acta Pathol Jpn 1990;40:199-205.

102. Miettinen M, Ekfors T. Alveolar soft part sarcoma. Immunohistochemical evidence for muscle cell differentiation. Am J Clin Pathol 1990;93:32-38.

103. Ladanyi M, Antonescu CR, Drobnjak M, et al. The precrystalline cytoplasmic granules of alveolar soft part sarcoma contain monocarboxylate transporter 1 and CD147. Am J Pathol 2002;160:1215-1221.

104. Sciot R, Dal Cin P, De Vos R, et al. Alveolar soft-part sarcoma: evidence for its myogenic origin and for the involvement of 17q25. Histopathology 1993;23:439-444.

105. van Echten J, van den Berg E, van Baarlen J, et al. An important role for chromosome 17, band q25, in the histogenesis of alveolar soft part sarcoma. Cancer Genet Cytogenet 1995;82:57-61.

106. Heimann P, Devalck C, Debusscher C, Sariban E, Vamos E. Alveolar soft-part sarcoma: further evidence by FISH for the involvement of chromosome band 17q25. Genes Chromosomes Cancer 1998;23:194-197.

107. Joyama S, Ueda T, Shimizu K, et al. Chromosome rearrangement at 17q25 and Xp11.2 in alveolar soft-part sarcoma. A case report and review of the literature. Cancer 1999;86:1246-1250.

108. Ladanyi M, Lui MY, Antonescu CR, et al. The der(17)t(X;17)(p11;q25) of human alveolar soft part sarcoma fuses the TFE3 transcription factor gene to ASPL, a novel gene at 17q25. Oncogene 2001,20:48-57.

109. Aulmann S, Longerich T, Schirmacher P, Mechtersheimer G, Penzel R. Detection of the ASPSCR1-TFE3 gene fusion in paraffin-embedded alveolar soft part sarcomas. Histopathology 2007;50:881-886.

110. Argani P, Antonescu CR, Illei PB, et al. Primary renal neoplasms with the ASPL-TFE3 gene fusion of alveolar soft part sarcoma: a distinctive tumor entity previously included among renal cell carcinomas of children and adolescents. Am J Pathol 2001;159:179-192.

111. Mitton B, Federman N. Alveolar soft part sarcomas: Molecular pathogenesis and implications for novel targeted therapies. Sarcoma 2012;2012:428789.

112. Lieberman PH, Brennan MF, Kimmel M, Erlandson RA, Garin-Chesa P, Flehinger BY. Alveolar soft-part sarcoma. A clinico-pathologic study of half a century. Cancer 1989;63:1-13.

11 MISCELLANEOUS TUMORS

This chapter contains three unrelated clinicopathologic entities that cannot be conveniently included in any other chapters. Two of these are rare tumors: perivascular epithelioid cell tumor (PEComa) and phosphaturic mesenchymal tumor. Tenosynovial giant cell tumor is a relatively common tumor with multiple clinicopathologic variants.

PERIVASCULAR EPITHELIOID CELL TUMOR

Definition. *Perivascular epithelioid cell tumors (PEComas)* are mesenchymal tumors composed of histologically distinctive perivascular epithelioid cells showing a characteristic myomelanocytic immunophenotype (1). PEComas occur in viscera (e.g., angiomyolipoma), soft tissue, bone, and cutaneous locations. Only soft tissue and cutaneous PEComas are disscussed here. Synonyms include *abdominal pelvic sarcoma of perivascular epithelioid cells* and *clear cell myomelanocytic tumor*.

General Considerations. The concept of a family of neoplasms derived from perivascular epithelioid cells was first proposed by Bonetti et al. in 1992 (2). PEComas are defined both by their characteristic morphologic features and by their unusual immunophenotype, with expression of both smooth muscle markers and markers of melanocytic differentiation.

Members of the PEComa family of tumors include *renal* and *extrarenal angiomyolipomas, clear cell "sugar" tumors of the lung, lymphangioleiomyomatosis,* and a variety of unusual soft tissue, cutaneous, and bone tumors described under several names (3). PEComas span a spectrum from histologically and clinically benign tumors, to "pseudomalignant" tumors and histologically and clinically malignant tumors.

Clinical Features. Soft tissue and cutaneous PEComas occur most often in middle-aged patients, show a striking female predominance even in nongynecologic locations, and are only rarely associated with the tuberous sclerosis complex, unlike angiomyolipoma and lymphangioleiomyomatosis (4). Soft tissue PEComas occur in many sites, but are particularly common in the omentum and mesentery (3). Cutaneous PEComas do not seem to have a predilection for any one location (5).

Gross and Microscopic Findings. Grossly, PEComas present as nonspecific, sometimes highly vascular soft tissue or skin masses. Histologically, the perivascular epithelioid cells are characterized by a perivascular location and a radial arrangement around the vascular lumen. Typically, the cells in an immediate perivascular location are the most epithelioid, while spindled cells resembling smooth muscle are seen at some distance from the vessels. Lipid-distended cells, mimicking adipocytes or lipoblasts, are also usually found distant from blood vessels.

Great variation is seen in the proportion of epithelioid, spindled, and lipid-distended cells, and PEComas may mimic carcinomas (6), smooth muscle tumors (7), and adipocytic tumors (8). The perivascular epithelioid cells have clear to lightly eosinophilic cytoplasm and may show a perinuclear eosinophilic zone, with surrounding clear cell change. Nuclei are typically small, centrally placed, round to oval, and normochromatic, with small nucleoli (fig. 11-1). On occasion, however, striking nuclear hyperchromasia and irregularity are seen, reminiscent of the degenerative changes seen in symplastic uterine leiomyomas and ancient schwannomas (4).

Soft tissue and cutaneous PEComas generally fall into one of two morphologic subtypes: a spindle cell subtype similar to clear cell myomelanocytic tumor as originally described (9), and an epithelioid form essentially identical to epithelioid angiomyolipoma of the kidney. The *spindle cell type of PEComa* is composed of uniform, moderate-sized spindled perivascular epithelioid cells arranged in fascicles and nests, surrounded by an elaborate capillary-sized vasculature (9). Spindled PEComas show stromal calcifications, hemosiderin-laden macrophages, and rarely, intracytoplasmic melanin pigment (fig. 11-2A,B). A subset of spindled PEComas,

435

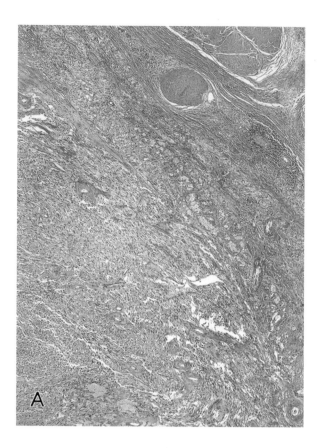

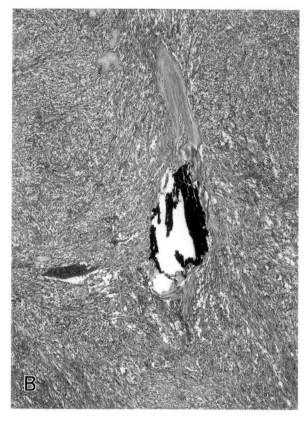

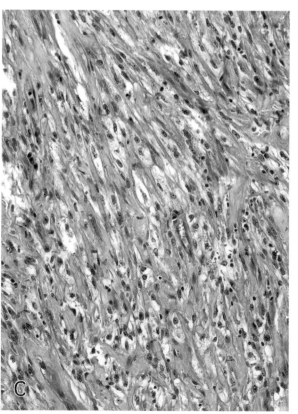

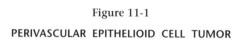

Figure 11-1

PERIVASCULAR EPITHELIOID CELL TUMOR

A: A circumscribed but microscopically infiltrative growth pattern is seen.

B: The neoplastic cells grow in a nested and fascicular pattern, with a well-developed, arborizing capillary network. Stromal calcifications are present.

C: Most soft tissue PEComas are of spindle cell type, and are composed of uniform spindled cells with clear to lightly eosinophilic cytoplasm, ovoid nuclei with small nucleoli, and little if any pleomorphism or mitotic activity.

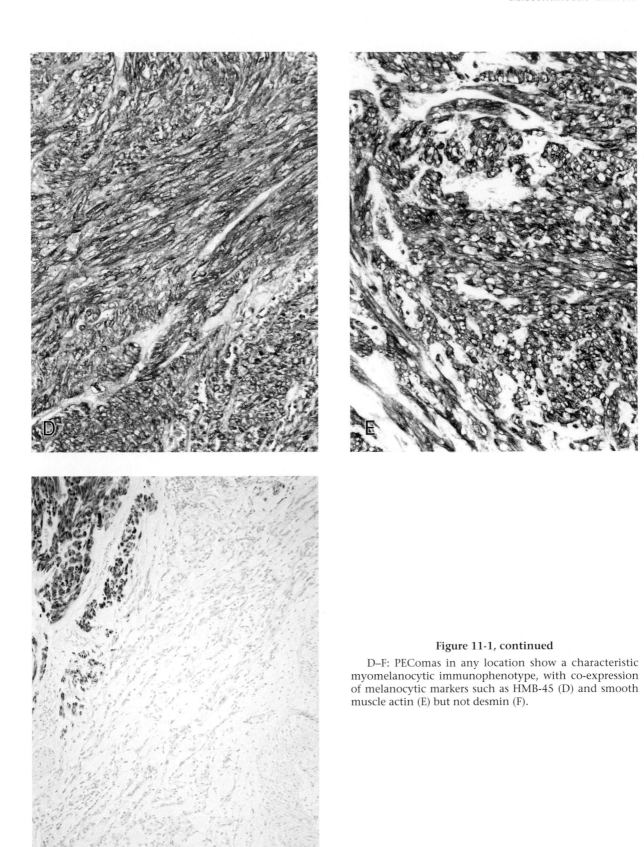

Figure 11-1, continued

D–F: PEComas in any location show a characteristic myomelanocytic immunophenotype, with co-expression of melanocytic markers such as HMB-45 (D) and smooth muscle actin (E) but not desmin (F).

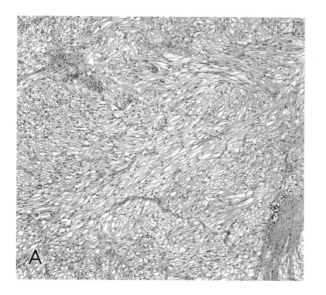

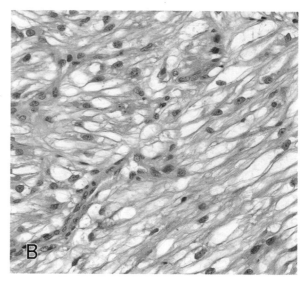

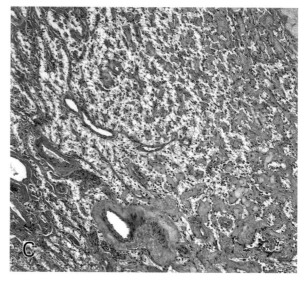

Figure 11-2

INTRA-ABDOMINAL PERIVASCULAR EPITHELIOID CELL TUMOR

A,B: As in deep soft tissue, most intra-abdominal PEComas are of spindle cell type, displaying similar low- (A) and high-power (B) appearances.

C,D: A distinctive morphologic variant of intra-abdominal PEComa, referred to as sclerosing PEComa, is characterized by thick-walled, hyalinized blood vessels (C) and generally more epithelioid cytomorphology (D). Such tumors are more likely to express desmin.

E: Epithelioid PEComas may show a variety of potentially worrisome pseudomalignant cytomorphologic features, including multinucleated tumor giant cells, "spider cell-like" cells, and nuclear pleomorphism in the absence of mitotic activity ("symplastic change").

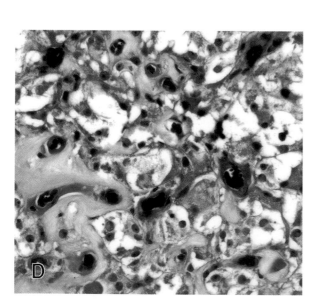

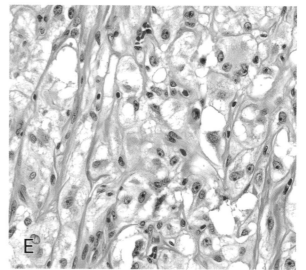

particularly those in the retroperitoneum and elsewhere in the abdomen, has striking stromal sclerosis, with broad zones of perivascular sclerosis separating the neoplastic cells into discrete nests; such tumors are referred to as *sclerosing PEComas* and often feature epithelioid cytology (fig. 11-2C,D) (10).

Epithelioid PEComas are essentially identical to epithelioid angiomyolipomas of the kidney, being composed of sheets and nests of typical perivascular epithelioid cells. Unusual features, seen in a few tumors, include multinucleated giant cells, "spider cell-like" cells, and scattered markedly atypical cells (fig. 11-2E). Malignancy in PEComas is discussed below (Treatment and Prognosis)

Special Studies. PEComas are characterized in most instances by a myomelanocytic immunophenotype, with co-expression of melanocytic markers, such as gp100 protein (HMB-45), melan-A, tyrosinase, and microphthalmia transcription factor (MITF), and muscle markers, such as smooth muscle actin, pan-muscle actin, muscle myosin, and calponin (2,4,11). Desmin expression is seen in approximately 30 percent of PEComas, particularly those of the sclerosing type (4,10). Patchy S-100 protein expression of variable intensity is present in about 30 percent as well. Expression of muscle markers is often limited in cutaneous PEComas and some sclerosing PEComas are actin negative (10). In general, the predominantly epithelioid tumors tend to express melanocytic markers more strongly than myoid markers, with the opposite found in the predominantly spindled PEComas.

Estrogen and progesterone receptors are frequently positive in classic renal angiomyolipoma but are only rarely positive in extrarenal PEComas (4,12). Rare PEComas are CD117 (c-kit) positive (4). TFE3 may expressed, usually in MITF-negative PEComas (4,13–16). Expression of CD1a in PEComas, reported to be of value for differentiating them from true smooth muscle tumors, has recently been shown to represent a technical artifact (17).

Genetics. Tuberous sclerosis complex is due to mutations in either the *TSC1* or *TSC2* genes (18). Complete loss of either TSC1 or TSC2 protein results in deregulated growth signaling due to unregulated mTORC1 activation. Inactivation of TSC2 has been shown in cases of lymphangioleiomyomatosis, and in variable percentages of renal angiomyolipomas (19–22). Loss of TSC2 protein expression has also been documented in a small number of soft tissue PEComas (9). By immunohistochemistry, PEComas have shown evidence of mTOR pathway activation, with expression of phospho-S6 kinase and phospho-S6 proteins (23,24).

Only a small number of PEComas have been studied for other types of genetic events. Losses of chromosomes 1p, 17p, 18p, and 19, and gains of chromosomes 2q, 3q, 5q, 12q, and X have recently been reported in a small number of studied renal angiomyolipomas and nonrenal PEComas (25,26). Some PEComas contain *TFE3* gene rearrangements (13).

Differential Diagnosis. The differential diagnosis of PEComas is fairly broad and is dictated by the morphology (spindled versus epithelioid) and the location of a given tumor. Both the morphologic and the immunophenotypic features of PEComa overlap to a degree with those of melanoma and clear cell sarcoma. In most cases, melanoma and clear cell sarcoma are distinguished from PEComa by their strong expression of S-100 protein and nonimmunoreactivity for smooth muscle actin. Clear cell sarcomas also have, in most cases, a specific t(12; 22)(q13; q13)(*EWS-ATF1*) gene fusion (27), not seen in PEComa or conventional melanoma.

Gastrointestinal stromal tumors (GIST) may show both epithelioid and spindled morphology, however, the cells of GIST tend to have fibrillar-appearing cytoplasm, and usually lack prominent clear cell change. By immunohistochemistry, over 90 percent of GISTs express CD117 (c-kit) and DOG1, markers seldom positive in PEComa, and lack expression of melanocytic markers.

Clear cell carcinomas typically have a higher nuclear grade than do PEComas, display diffuse expression of cytokeratins, and lack expression of melanocytic markers. Alveolar soft part sarcoma may mimic PEComa, although it usually shows a much higher nuclear grade with macronucleoli. Alveolar soft part sarcoma does not express smooth muscle actin or melanocytic markers (28). Immunohistochemistry or fluorescence in situ hybridization (FISH) for TFE3 (positive in alveolar soft part sarcoma) is of value in selected cases, although some PEComas show limited TFE3 expression (4).

Table 11-1

PROPOSED CLASSIFICATION CRITERIA FOR PECOMAS[a]

	Criteria	Percentage Fulfilling Criteria with Aggressive Behavior	Comment
Benign	No worrisome features (< 5 cm, non-infiltrative, non-high nuclear grade and cellularity, mitotic rate ≤1/50HPF,[b] no necrosis, no vascular invasion)	0 of 22 (0%)	
Uncertain malignant potential	1) Nuclear pleomorphism/multinucleated giant cells only; or	1) 0 of 6 (0%)	1) "Symplastic" PEComa—probably benign, but few reported cases
	2) Size >5cm only	2) 2 of 17 (12%)	2) Large tumors should be extensively sampled to exclude areas with other worrisome features
Malignant	Two or more worrisome features (>5 cm, infiltrative, high nuclear grade and cellularity, mitotic rate >1/50HPF, necrosis, vascular invasion)	12 of 17 (71%)	

[a]Adapted from reference #7.
[b]HPF = high-power field.

PEComas lack the diffuse cytoplasmic eosinophilia, perinuclear vacuoles, and cigar-shaped nuclei seen in true smooth muscle tumors. Epithelioid smooth muscle tumors may resemble epithelioid PEComas; careful inspection almost invariably reveals small spindled areas with the morphologic features of true smooth muscle (29). Some conventional smooth muscle tumors contain HMB-45-positive cells, and PEComas may express desmin (30), and thus immunohistochemistry cannot be used alone for this distinction.

Treatment and Prognosis. Criteria for malignancy in nonangiomyolipoma PEComas have recently been proposed (Table 11-1) (31). There is a significant association between a tumor size of over 5 cm, infiltrative growth pattern, high nuclear grade, necrosis, and mitotic activity of more than 1 mitosis per 50 high-power fields and subsequent aggressive clinical behavior (figs. 11-3, 11-4). Most previously reported PEComas with aggressive clinical behavior have shown some combination of these features, typically two or more. Owing to their rarity, there has been some debate as to whether any PEComas should be labeled as benign, or whether all PEComas should be considered to have uncertain malignant potential. As noted in Table 11-1, PEComas lacking any worrisome features have an extremely low risk for clinically aggressive behavior, and thus can be provisionally labeled as either "benign," or having a "very low risk for aggressive behavior." The term "PEComa

of uncertain malignant potential" should be reserved for tumors showing only one atypical feature, most often either large size or nuclear atypia. Although the latter group seems to be clinically benign ("symplastic PEComa"), our experience with such cases is limited.

Data as to the proper role for surgery, radiotherapy, and conventional chemotherapy in the treatment of PEComas are scarce. In general, most morphologically benign PEComas are cured with simple excision, whereas many morphologically malignant PEComas recur locally and spread distantly, despite aggressive surgical intervention and adjuvant radiotherapy and chemotherapy. Recently, promising results have been shown in the treatment of lymphangioleiomyomatosis with rapamycin, an inhibitor of the mTOR pathway, and such agents may prove valuable in the treatment of PEComas (32,33).

PHOSPHATURIC MESENCHYMAL TUMOR

Definition. *Phosphaturic mesenchymal tumors* (PMT) are morphologically distinctive neoplasms of both soft tissue and bone origin, which produce tumor-induced osteomalacia in most affected patients, usually through production of fibroblast growth factor-23 (FGF-23). *Phosphaturic mesenchymal tumor, mixed connective tissue type* is synonymous.

General Considerations. The term phosphaturic mesenchymal tumor, mixed connective

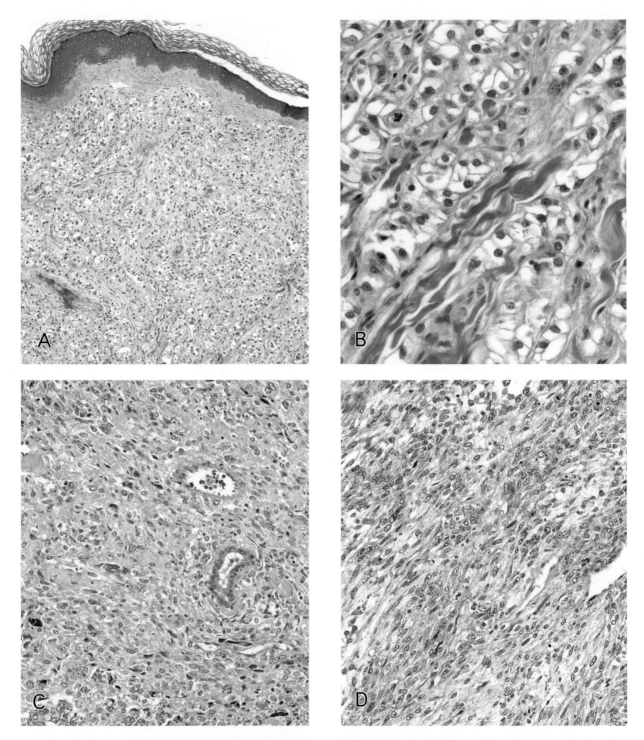

Figure 11-3

MALIGNANT PERIVASCULAR EPITHELIOID CELL TUMOR

A: Histologically malignant dermal PEComa grows as a nested proliferation of epithelioid cells with clear to lightly eosinophilic cytoplasm.

B: Although the most superficial parts of this tumor displayed little nuclear atypia, mitotic activity is appreciable.

C,D: Deeper portions of this tumor showed much higher cellularity, high nuclear grade, and frequent mitotic figures, fulfilling the criteria for malignancy.

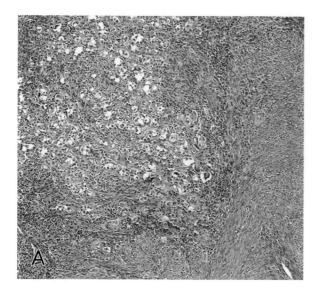

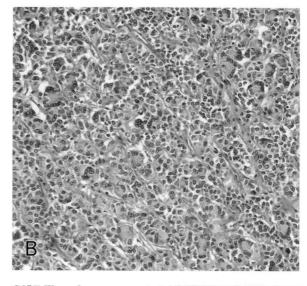

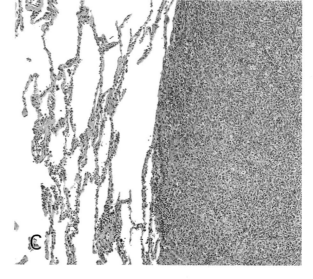

Figure 11-4

**UTERINE PERIVASCULAR
EPITHELIOID CELL TUMOR**

A: Uterine PEComa consists of an infiltrative proliferation of nests of epithelioid cells with clear to lightly eosinophilic cytoplasm.

B: Areas within this tumor show a more solid growth pattern and great cytologic atypia.

C: In the patient, lung metastases developed with a short period of time.

D,E: These metastases were identical to the more cellular portions of the uterine primary tumor (D) and continued to show strong expression of HMB-45.

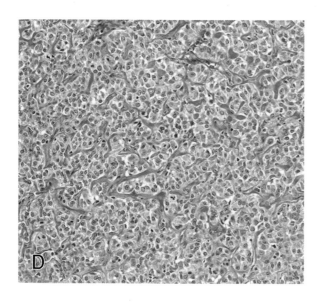

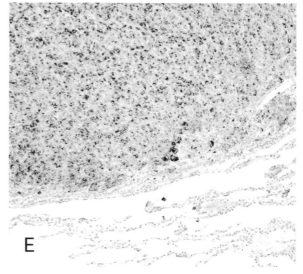

tissue variant, was first introduced by Weidner and Santa Cruz (34) as a unifying concept for what had previously been considered a heterogeneous group of tumor-induced osteomalacia-associated bone and soft tissue tumors. Further support for the existence of PMT as a discrete histopathologic entity was provided by Folpe et al. (35) and Bahrami et al. (36), who found that over 90 percent of tumor-induced osteomalacia-associated mesenchymal tumors correspond morphologically to PMT. Although Weidner and Santa Cruz originally described "osteoblastoma-like," "ossifying fibroma-like," and "nonossifying fibroma-like" variants of PMT in bone, these appear to represent minor morphologic variants, rather than discrete entities. Expression of FGF-23, a phosphaturic hormone known to inhibit phosphate re-uptake in the renal proximal tubule, is the pathogenetic mechanism underlying tumor-induced osteomalacia in most patients with this disorder (37).

Clinical Features. PMTs are rare tumors, most often occurring in middle-aged adults in soft tissue, bone, and sinonasal locations (35,36). Occasional tumors have been reported in infants (38). Most PMTs present as small, inapparent lesions that require careful clinical examination and radionuclide scans (octreotide scans, fluorodeoxyglucose [FDG]-positron emission tomography [PET]) for localization in some cases. A long history of osteomalacia is usually, but not always, present. *Nonphosphaturic PMTs* are in most instances superficial soft tissue tumors identified prior to becoming symptomatic, although for some patients, the osteomalacia is discovered following the identification of the tumor (36). Most PMTs are histologically and clinically benign, with complete excision resulting in dramatic improvement of phosphate wasting and osteomalacia.

Gross Findings. PMTs present as nonspecific soft tissue or bone masses, often with a component of fat. Some tumors are highly calcified.

Microscopic Findings. PMTs are characterized by a highly vascular proliferation of bland, spindled to stellate cells, which produce an unusual "smudgy" matrix. The tumor vasculature may be hemangiopericytoma-like, consist of arborizing capillaries, or rarely, resemble cavernous hemangioma. The matrix of PMT calcifies in a distinctive "grungy" or flocculent fashion,

and may resemble primitive cartilage or osteoid (34–36). This calcification serves as a stimulus for the recruitment of osteoclasts and bland fibrohistiocytic spindled cells, may undergo aneurysmal bone cyst-like changes, and occasionally ossifies. A variable component of mature adipose tissue is also frequently present (fig. 11-5). Lesions occurring in the craniofacial sinuses are less likely to contain calcified matrix (35), although typical PMT occurs in these locations (39).

Malignant PMTs show frankly sarcomatous features, such as high nuclear grade, high cellularity, necrosis, and elevated mitotic activity, resembling undifferentiated pleomorphic sarcoma in most instances (35). A preexisting component of benign-appearing PMT may be identified (fig. 11-6).

Special Studies. PMT expresses FGF-23, in the absence of other soft tissue cell-type markers (35). At the present time, however, commercially available antibodies specific to FGF-23 and applicable to formalin-fixed, paraffin-embedded tissues are not widely available. FGF-23 expression can be demonstrated by reverse transcriptase-polymerase chain reaction (RT-PCR) in routinely processed tissues, both in PMTs presenting with tumor-induced osteomalacia and those without such a history (36). Owing to the sensitivity of molecular assays, however, low level expression of FGF-23 is also occasionally identified in other tumors, including occasional cases of fibrous dysplasia (40), aneurysmal bone cyst, and chondromyxoid fibroma of bone (41).

Genetics. To date, a specific genetic event has not been identified in PMT.

Differential Diagnosis. In most cases, PMT resected expressly for treatment of known tumor-induced osteomalacia is easy to diagnose. Unsuspected PMT may be confused with hemangiopericytomas/solitary fibrous tumors, hemangiomas, giant cell tumors, spindle cell lipomas, and various cartilaginous tumors, among others. Recognition of the unique constellation of histologic features shown by PMT, in particular, the distinctive calcified matrix, is the key to distinguishing it from other tumors. Typical soft tissue hemangiopericytomas/solitary fibrous tumors show a uniformly distributed, thick-walled branching vasculature; contain bland round to ovoid cells; frequently

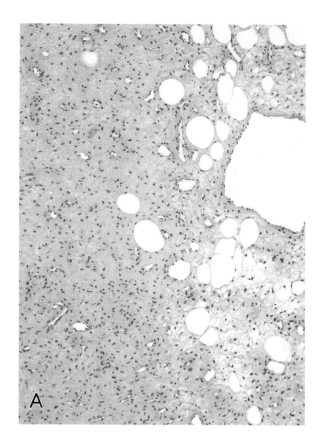

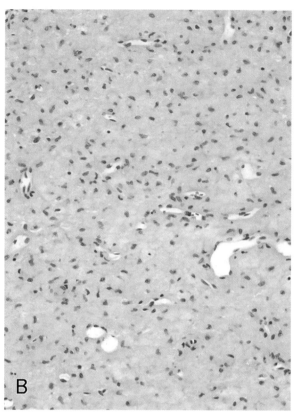

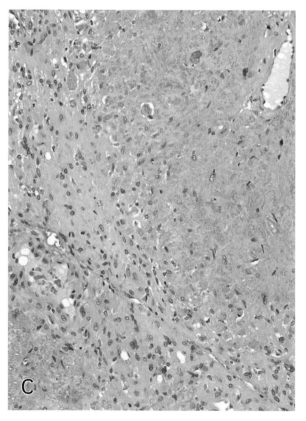

Figure 11-5

PHOSPHATURIC MESENCHYMAL TUMOR

A: These tumors are typically composed of a hypocellular, highly vascular proliferation of small, bland, featureless, spindled to slightly stellate cells, with a variable amount of mature fat.

B: Higher-power magnification shows bland, small cells and abundant "smudgy"-appearing matrix.

C: The matrix typically calcifies in an unusual flocculent or "grungy" pattern.

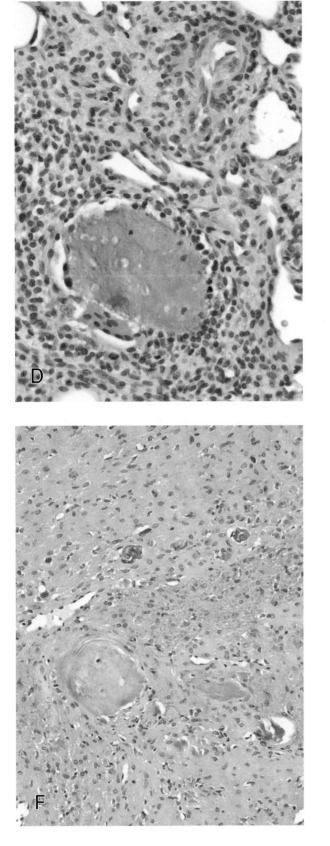

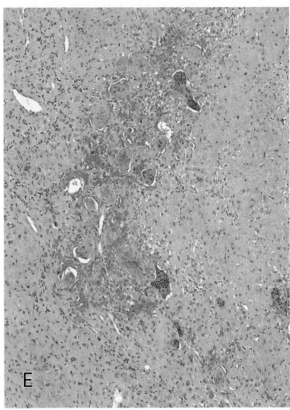

Figure 11-5, continued

D: Although most phosphaturic mesenchymal tumors (PMTs) contain abundant calcified matrix, occasional examples show only small collections of similar material.

E: This calcified matrix appears to act as a stimulus for the recruitment of osteoclast-like giant cells.

F: The production of bone and cartilage is seen.

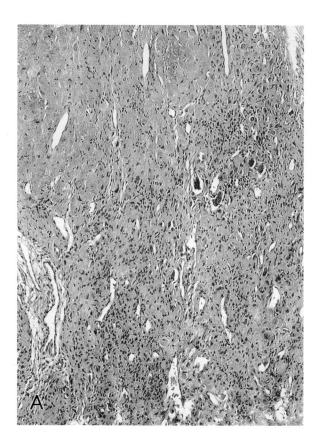

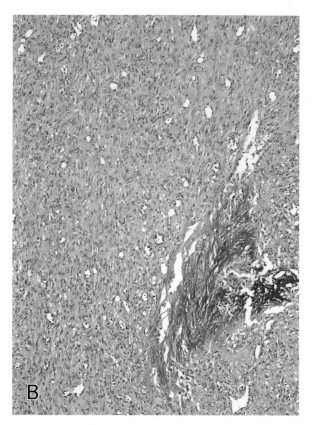

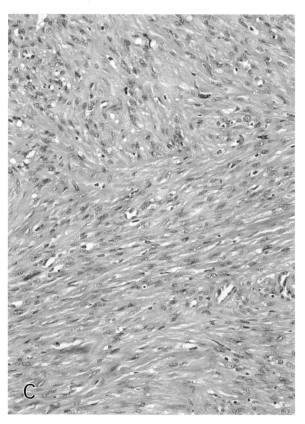

Figure 11-6

PHOSPHATURIC MESENCHYMAL TUMOR

A: Rarely, PMTs show histologic features of malignancy and behave in a clinically malignant fashion, with metastases and death from disease. This example consisted for the most part of typical hypocellular PMT.

B: An abrupt transition is seen from typical PMT areas into zones showing much greater cellularity and a fascicular growth pattern.

C: At higher power, the cells in these more cellular areas are pleomorphic and hyperchromatic, resembling an undifferentiated spindle cell sarcoma. This tumor metastasized to the lungs.

express CD34; and lack calcified matrix. Chondromas of soft parts may show a pattern of calcification that mimics PMT and they often contain osteoclast-like giant cells, but lack the bland spindle cells, myxoid change, and fat seen in many PMTs. Giant cell tumors of bone and soft tissue lack the distinctive spindle cells and matrix of PMT. Mesenchymal chondrosarcoma is an obviously malignant-appearing sarcoma that shows an admixture of round cells, hemangiopericytoma-like spindled areas, and relatively mature cartilage.

In histologically malignant cases, recognition of the unique histologic elements of PMT and awareness that they may contain chondroid or osteoid-like matrix allow their distinction from osteosarcoma, chondrosarcoma, and undifferentiated pleomorphic sarcoma.

Treatment and Prognosis. Histologically benign PMTs behave in a clinically benign fashion, although they frequently recur locally if incompletely excised. Histologically malignant PMTs have significant potential for aggressive local recurrence, distant metastasis, and adverse patient outcome (35).

TENOSYNOVIAL GIANT CELL TUMOR

Definition. *Tenosynovial giant cell tumor* includes localized (nodular) and diffuse variants typically associated with synovial and tenosynovial tissues. The tumor contains large numbers of mononuclear histiocytes and often multinucleated osteoclast-like giant cells, xanthoma cells, and a neoplastic epithelioid cell population often focally positive for desmin. Malignant variants are rare.

Clinical Features. Localized tenosynovial giant cell tumor occurs mostly in young adults, with a mild female predominance, although occasionally it is seen in children. Periarticular sites in fingers and other distal extremity sites, such as feet and ankles, are most common. Localized variants form circumscribed localized synovial or tenosynovial-associated nodules usually measuring 1 to 2 cm (42–47). In some cases, tenosynovial giant cell tumors erode adjacent bones (48).

Intra-articular localized examples usually present in the knee and, less commonly, in the hip joint. Rare examples occur in the elbow, arm, thigh, and around the spine. These are typically pedunculated 1- to 3-cm synovial masses, which may strangulate and undergo infarction.

Diffuse intra-articular variants are much less common than the localized variants and involve intra-articular synovia as innumerable separate or confluent nodules. They are also termed *diffuse pigmented villonodular synovitis* (49–53).

Diffuse extra-articular examples are rare and typically present in more proximal locations than the localized type (for example, forearm). They form larger masses, up to 10 cm or more (54,55).

Gross Findings. Tenosynovial giant cell tumors involving fingers are usually nodules of less than 2 cm, but those involving the foot are often larger. The nodules are yellowish brown, based on their content of hemosiderin and xanthoma cells. The diffuse extra-articular variants are often pale yellow.

Microscopic Findings. The localized variant forms a circumscribed ovoid mass that is often divided into lobules by prominent collagenous matrix. The dominant components are mononuclear histiocytes and xanthoma cells. There are variable numbers of multinucleated giant osteoclast-like cells, usually containing 10 to 50 nuclei. However, in some cases, these giant cells are scant or even absent. Hemosiderin is often present in some of the histiocytes (fig. 11-7). The actual neoplastic cell is an inconspicuous and often scant epithelioid cell, which blends into the histiocytic infiltration and is histologically difficult to detect.

Mitotic activity is common and can exceed 10 mitoses per 10 high-power fields. Higher mitotic counts are not associated with an increased risk of recurrence. Vascular invasion may be observed and has no adverse significance in this tumor. The diffuse intra-articular form (pigmented villonodular synovitis) is histologically similar but often richer in hemosiderin pigment (fig. 11-8A,B).

The diffuse extra-articular form can be difficult to recognize because of its lack of lobulation and few if any osteoclast-like giant cells. It typically contains extensive xanthoma cell infiltration, hemosiderin-laden histiocytes, and pseudoglandular or alveolar spaces with histiocytes and lymphocytes inside (fig. 11-8C,D).

Rare histologic findings include massive infarction (especially seen in intra-articular forms) and focal cartilaginous metaplasia (fig. 11-9).

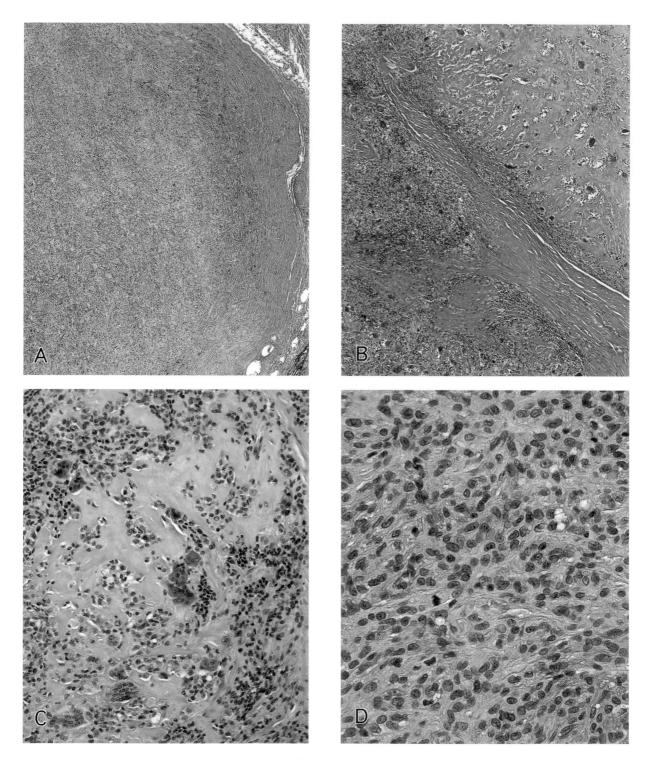

Figure 11-7

LOCALIZED TENOSYNOVIAL GIANT CELL TUMOR

A: Localized tenosynovial giant cell tumor typically forms a well-demarcated nodule.

B,C: The nodule contains mononuclear cells and multinucleated osteoclast-like cells, often in a sclerosing stroma, and sometimes with focal hemosiderin deposition.

D: The mononuclear cells are uniform and have moderate mitotic activity.

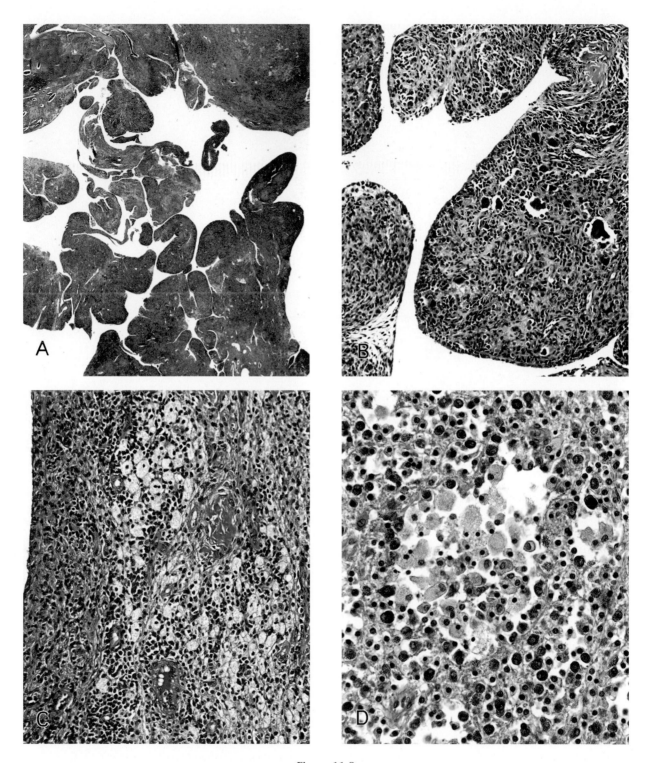

Figure 11-8

DIFFUSE TENOSYNOVIAL GIANT CELL TUMOR

A,B: Diffuse intra-articular tenosynovial giant cell tumor forms multiple polypoid protrusions in the synovium, which contain cellular components similar to localized tumors.

C,D: The diffuse extra-articular variant contains only a few giant cells, but xanthoma cells and hemosiderin-laden mononuclear cells are numerous. Pseudoglandular spaces are often prominent.

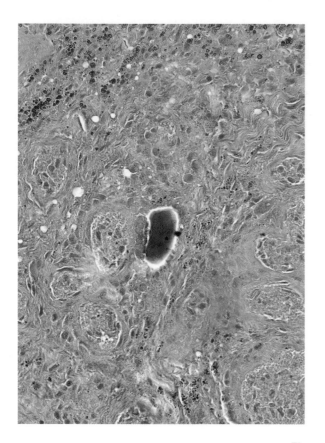 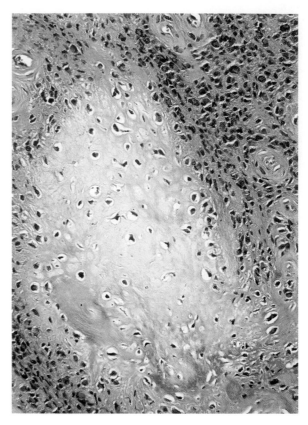

Figure 11-9

INFARCTED INTRA-ARTICULAR TENOSYNOVIAL GIANT CELL TUMOR

Left: Shadows of multinucleated osteoclast-like giant cells are seen.
Right: Focal cartilaginous metaplasia is present.

Malignant Tenosynovial Giant Cell Tumor. Extremely rare, histologically malignant tumors with severe nuclear atypia and atypical mitoses are recognized as *malignant tenosynovial giant cell tumors* only in the presence of a benign component or based on tumor developing at the site of a previously diagnosed tenosynovial giant cell tumor (56–60).

Two series of malignant tenosynovial giant cell tumors reported lymph node, lung, and bone metastases in 7 of 17 patients, and at least 5 patients died of disease (61,62). The patients were older than those with benign tumors (mean age, 61 years), the tumors were larger (mean, over 9 cm), had higher mitotic activity (18 versus 2 mitoses per 10 high-power fields), and often had atypical mitoses, tumor necrosis, and a higher Ki67 index (40 versus 13 percent) (62).

The histologic appearance of these tumors is often similar to malignant fibrous histiocytoma/pleomorphic undifferentiated sarcoma, so that the specific diagnosis is difficult histologically without synchronous or metachronous evidence of tenosynovial giant cell tumor at the same site.

Special Studies. The neoplastic epithelioid cells are often highlighted as desmin-positive cells with delicate dendritic processes (63). The histiocytic markers CD68 and CD163 highlight large numbers of histiocytes (64–66). The multinucleated forms are generally negative for CD163 (fig. 11-10).

Genetics. Fusion translocations *COL6A3-CSF1* (cytogenetically, t(1;2)(p11;q36-37)) cause overexpression of colony stimulating factor 1 (CSF1) under the control of collagen type 6 promoter. The end result is massive histiocytic recruitment causing the typical histiocytic dominance (67,68).

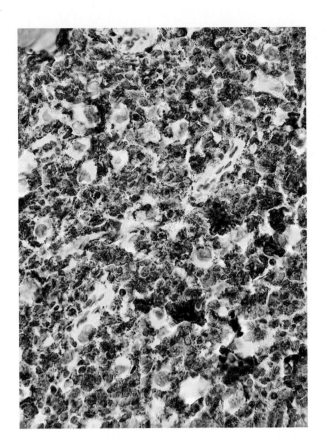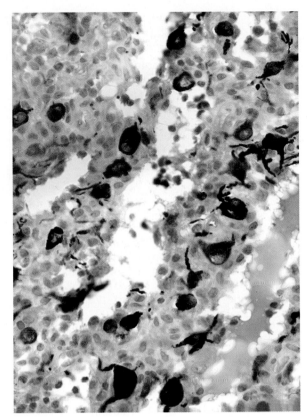

Figure 11-10

TENOSYNOVIAL GIANT CELL TUMOR

Left: Immunostaining for CD163 reveals an abundant histiocytic component.
Right: Scattered desmin-positive cells probably represent the true neoplastic cell population.

Differential Diagnosis. Giant cell tumor of soft tissues is typically more homogeneous and cellular and contains a less prominent histiocytic element without xanthoma cells than tenosynovial giant cell tumor. Metaplastic bone is often present. Soft tissue extension of giant cell tumor of bone may be seen near the large joints, especially the knee. As giant cell tumors of soft tissue are often histologically similar to giant cell tumors of bone, radiologic studies are often necessary for the differential diagnosis. Identifying the diffuse variant of tenosynovial giant cell tumor sometimes requires radiologic correlation, and the longitudinal diffuse tenosynovial involvement is not easily detectable histologically.

Epithelioid sarcoma may simulate localized tenosynovial giant cell tumors when containing numerous osteoclastic giant cells, but it also contains an atypical, eosinophilic epithelioid cell population that is keratin and epithelial membrane antigen positive. This differential diagnosis is especially relevant in the digital lesions.

Hemosiderotic synovitis is a consequence of intra-articular bleeding. Grossly and even histologically, it simulates diffuse villonodular synovitis as a brown, villous process. Although extensive hemosiderin deposition can be present, the villous projections are usually narrow and only contain paucicellular stroma with no multinucleated histiocytes.

The desmin-positive cells in tenosynovial giant cell tumor should not be mistaken of cells of myoid sarcomas, especially rhabdomyosarcoma.

Treatment and Prognosis. Local excision is sufficient in most cases, but recurrence is common. The diffuse intra-articular variant often justifies synovectomy for complete removal. Diffuse extra-articular examples are typically managed by wider resection involving tenosynovial tissues. Rare lung metastases occur unpredictably.

Malignant examples have been reported, but in some cases it is uncertain whether the malignancy is fully comparable with tenosynovial giant cell tumor. The reported examples often develop extensive locoregional recurrences and pulmonary metastases, and one series showed 50 percent tumor-related mortality (69).

REFERENCES

Perivascular Epithelioid Cell Tumor

1. Hornick JL, Pan CC. PEComa. In Fletcher CD, Bridge JA, Hogendoorn PC, Mertens F, eds. WHO classification of tumors of soft tissue and bone. Lyon, France: IARC Press; 2013:230-231.

2. Bonetti F, Pea M, Martignoni G, Zamboni G. PEC and sugar. Am J Surg Pathol 1992;16:307-308.

3. Folpe AL, Kwiatkowski DJ. Perivascular epithelioid cell neoplasms: pathology and pathogenesis. Hum Pathol 2010;41:1-15.

4. Folpe AL, Mentzel T, Lehr HA, Fisher C, Balzer BL, Weiss SW. Perivascular epithelioid cell neoplasms of soft tissue and gynecologic origin: a clinico-pathologic study of 26 cases and review of the literature. Am J Surg Pathol 2005;29:1558-1575.

5. Mentzel T, Reibhauer S, Rutten A, Hantschke M, Soares de Almeida LM, Kutzner H. Cutaneous clear cell myomelanocytic tumor: a new member of the growing family of perivascular epithelioid cell tumors (PEComas). Clinicopathological and immunohistochemical analysis of seven cases. Histopathology 2005;46:498-504.

6. Martignoni G, Pea M, Bonetti F, et al. Carcinoma-like monotypic epithelioid angiomyolipoma in patients without evidence of tuberous sclerosis: a clinicopathologic and genetic study. Am J Surg Pathol 1998;22:663-672.

7. Kulkarni B, Desai SB, Dave B, Tongaonkar HB, Kulkarni JN, Chinoy RF. Renal angiomyolipo-mas—a study of 18 cases. Indian J Pathol Microbiol 2005;48:459-463.

8. Hruban RH, Bhagavan BS, Epstein JI. Massive retroperitoneal angiomyolipoma. A lesion that may be confused with well-differentiated lipo-sarcoma. Am J Clin Pathol 1989;92:805-808.

9. Folpe AL, Goodman ZD, Ishak KG, et al. Clear cell myomelanocytic tumor of the falciform liga-ment/ligamentum teres: a novel member of the perivascular epithelioid clear cell family of tumors with a predilection for children and young adults. Am J Surg Pathol 2000;24:1239-1246.

10. Hornick JL, Fletcher CD. Sclerosing PEComa: clinicopathologic analysis of a distinctive variant with a predilection for the retroperitoneum. Am J Surg Pathol 2008;32:493-501.

11. Pea M, Bonetti F, Zamboni G, et al. Melano-cyte-marker HMB-45 is regularly expressed in angiomyolipoma of the kidney. Pathology 1991; 23:185-188.

12. Logginidou H, Ao X, Russo I, Henske EP. Frequent estrogen and progesterone receptor immunore-activity in renal angiomyolipomas from women with pulmonary lymphangioleiomyomatosis. Chest 2000;117:25-30.

13. Argani P, Aulmann S, Illei PB, et al. A distinctive subset of PEComas harbors TFE3 gene fusions. Am J Surg Pathol 2010;34:1395-1406.

14. Kuroda N, Goda M, Kazakov DV, Hes O, Michal M, Lee GH. Perivascular epithelioid cell tumor of the nasal cavity with TFE3 expression. Pathol Int 2009;59:769-770.

15. Tanaka M, Kato K, Gomi K, et al. Perivascular epithelioid cell tumor with SFPQ/PSF-TFE3 gene fusion in a patient with advanced neuroblas-toma. Am J Surg Pathol 2009;33:1416-1420.

16. Wen MC, Jan YJ, Li MC, Wang J, Lin A. Monotypic epithelioid angiomyolipoma of the liver with TFE3 expression. Pathology 2010;42:300-302.

17. Ahrens WA, Folpe AL. CD1a immunopositivity in perivascular epithelioid cell neoplasms: true expression or technical artifact? A streptavidin-biotin and polymer-based detection system immunohistochemical study of perivascular epi-thelioid cell neoplasms and their morphologic mimics. Hum Pathol 2011;42:369-374.

18. Dabora SL, Jozwiak S, Franz DN, et al. Mutational analysis in a cohort of 224 tuberous sclerosis patients indicates increased severity of TSC2, compared with TSC1, disease in multiple organs. Am J Hum Genet 2001;68:64-80.

19. Astrinidis A, Khare L, Carsillo T, et al. Mutational analysis of the tuberous sclerosis gene TSC2 in patients with pulmonary lymphangioleiomyo-matosis. J Med Genet 2000;37:55-57.

20. Carsillo T, Astrinidis A, Henske EP. Mutations in the tuberous sclerosis complex gene TSC2 are a cause of sporadic pulmonary lymphangioleiomyomatosis. Proc Natl Acad Sci U S A. 2000;97:6085-6090.

21. Strizheva GD, Carsillo T, Kruger WD, Sullivan EJ, Ryu JH, Henske EP. The spectrum of mutations in TSC1 and TSC2 in women with tuberous sclerosis and lymphangiomyomatosis. Am J Respir Crit Care Med 2001;163:253-258.

22. Henske EP, Neumann HP, Scheithauer BW, Herbst EW, Short MP, Kwiatkowski DJ. Loss of heterozygosity in the tuberous sclerosis (TSC2) region of chromosome band 16p13 occurs in sporadic as well as TSC-associated renal angiomyolipomas. Genes Chromosomes Cancer 1995;13:295-298.

23. Kenerson H, Folpe AL, Takayama TK, Yeung RS. Activation of the mTOR pathway in sporadic angiomyolipomas and other perivascular epithelioid cell neoplasms. Hum Pathol 2007;38:1361-1371.

24. Martignoni G, Pea M, Reghellin D, et al. Molecular pathology of lymphangioleiomyomatosis and other perivascular epithelioid cell tumors. Arch Pathol Lab Med 2010;134:33-40.

25. Pan CC, Chung MY, Ng KF, et al. Constant allelic alteration on chromosome 16p (TSC2 gene) in perivascular epithelioid cell tumour (PEComa): genetic evidence for the relationship of PEComa with angiomyolipoma. J Pathol 2008;214:387-393.

26. Pan CC, Jong YJ, Chai CY, Huang SH, Chen YJ. Comparative genomic hybridization study of perivascular epithelioid cell tumor: molecular genetic evidence of perivascular epithelioid cell tumor as a distinctive neoplasm. Hum Pathol 2006;37:606-612.

27. Reeves BR, Fletcher CD, Gusterson BA. Translocation t(12;22)(q13;q13) is a nonrandom rearrangement in clear cell sarcoma. Cancer Genet Cytogenet 1992;64:101-103.

28. Folpe AL, Deyrup AT. Alveolar soft-part sarcoma: a review and update. J Clin Pathol 2006;59:1127-1232.

29. Prayson RA, Goldblum JR, Hart WR. Epithelioid smooth-muscle tumors of the uterus: a clinicopathologic study of 18 patients. Am J Surg Pathol 1997;21:383-391.

30. Silva EG, Deavers MT, Bodurka DC, Malpica A. Uterine epithelioid leiomyosarcomas with clear cells: reactivity with HMB-45 and the concept of PEComa. Am J Surg Pathol 2004;28:244-249.

31. Folpe AL, Goldblum JR, Rubin BP, et al. Morphologic and immunophenotypic diversity in Ewing family tumors: a study of 66 genetically confirmed cases. Am J Surg Pathol 2005;29:1025-1033.

32. Krishnan A, Sandrini A, Yates D. Regression of pulmonary lymphangioleiomyomatosis (PLAM)-associated retroperitoneal angiomyolipoma post-lung transplantation with rapamycin treatment. J Heart Lung Transplant 2008;27:1268.

33. Morton JM, McLean C, Booth SS, Snell GI, Whitford HM. Regression of pulmonary lymphangioleiomyomatosis (PLAM)-associated retroperitoneal angiomyolipoma post-lung transplantation with rapamycin treatment. J Heart Lung Transplant 2008;27:462-5.

Phosphaturic Mesenchymal Tumor

34. Weidner N, Santa Cruz D. Phosphaturic mesenchymal tumors. A polymorphous group causing osteomalacia or rickets. Cancer 1987;59:1442-454.

35. Folpe AL, Fanburg-Smith JC, Billings SD, et al. Most osteomalacia-associated mesenchymal tumors are a single histopathologic entity: an analysis of 32 cases and a comprehensive review of the literature. Am J Surg Pathol 2004;28:1-30.

36. Bahrami A, Weiss SW, Montgomery E, et al. RT-PCR analysis for FGF23 using paraffin sections in the diagnosis of phosphaturic mesenchymal tumors with and without known tumor induced osteomalacia. Am J Surg Pathol 2009;33:1348-1354.

37. Kumar R. New insights into phosphate homeostasis: fibroblast growth factor 23 and frizzled-related protein-4 are phosphaturic factors derived from tumors associated with osteomalacia. Curr Opin Nephrol Hypertens 2002;11:547-553.

38. Jung GH, Kim JD, Cho Y, Chung SH, Lee JH, Sohn KR. A 9-month-old phosphaturic mesenchymal tumor mimicking the intractable rickets. J Pediatr Orthop B 2010;19:127-132.

39. Shelekhova KV, Kazakov DV, Michal M. Sinonasal phosphaturic mesenchymal tumor (mixed connective tissue variant): report of 2 cases. Am J Surg Pathol 2010;34:596-597.

40. Riminucci M, Collins MT, Fedarko NS, et al. FGF-23 in fibrous dysplasia of bone and its relationship to renal phosphate wasting. J Clin Invest 2003;112:683-692.

41. Krishnamurthy S, Inwards CY, Oliveira AM, Folpe AL. Frequent expression of fibroblast growth factor-23 (FGF-23) mRNA in aneurysmal bone cyst (ABC). Mod Pathol 2011;24(Suppl 1):17A.

Tenosynovial Giant Cell Tumor

42. Jaffe HL, Lichtenstein J, Sutro C. Pigmented villonodular synovitis, bursitis and tenosynovitis. Arch Pathol 1941;31:731-765.

43. Myers BW, Masi AT, Feigenbaum SL. Pigmented villonodular synovitis and tenosynovitis. a clinical and epidemiologic study of 166 cases and literature review. Medicine (Baltimore) 1980;59:223-238.

44. Monaghan H, Salter DM, Al-Nafussi A. Giant cell tumour of tendon sheath (localised nodular tenosynovitis): clinicopathological features of 71 cases. J Clin Pathol 2001;54:404-407.

45. Jones FE, Soule EH, Coventry MB. Fibrous xanthoma of synovium (giant cell tumor of tendon sheath, pigmented nodular synovitis). A study of one hundred and eighteen cases. J Bone Joint Surg Am 1969;51:76-86.

46. Ushijima M, Hashimoto H, Tsuneyoshi M, Enjoji M. Giant cell tumor of tendon sheath (nodular tenosynovitis). A study of 207 cases to compare the large joint group with the common digit group. Cancer 1986;57:875-884.

47. Rao AS, Vigorita VJ. Pigmented villonodular synovitis (giant cell tumor of the tendon sheath and synovial membrane). A review of eighty-one cases. J Bone Joint Surg Am 1984;66:76-94.

48. Karasick D, Karasick S. Giant cell tumor of tendon sheath: spectrum of radiologic changes. Skeletal Radiol 1992;21:219-224.

49. Granowitz SP, D'Antonio J, Mankin HL. The pathogenesis and long-term end results of pigmented villonodular synovitis. Clin Orthop Relat Res 1976;114:335-351.

50. Ushijima M, Hashimoto H, Tsuneyoshi M, Enjoji M. Pigmented villonodular synovitis. A clinicopathologic study of 52 cases. Acta Pathol Jpn 1986;36:317-326.

51. Schwartz HS, Unni KK, Pritchard DJ. Pigmented villonodular synovitis. A retrospective review of affected large joints. Clin Orthop Relat Res 1989;247:243-255.

52. Dorwart RH, Genant HK, Johnston WH, Morris JM. Pigmented villonodular synovitis of synovial joints: clinical, pathologic, and radiologic features. AJR Am J Roentgenol 1984;143:877-885.

53. Gonzalez Della Valle A, Piccaluga F, Potter HG, Salvati EA, Pusso R. Pigmented villonodular synovitis of the hip: 2- to 23-year follow-up study. Clin Orthop Relat Res 2001;388:187-199.

54. Rowlands CG, Roland B, Hwang WS, Sevick RJ. Diffuse variant tenosynovial giant cell tumor: a rare and aggressive lesion. Hum Pathol 1994;25:423-425.

55. Somerhausen NS, Fletcher CD. Diffuse-type giant cell tumor: clinicopathologic and immunohistochemical analysis of 50 cases with extraarticular disease. Am J Surg Pathol 2000;24:479-492.

56. Kahn LB. Malignant giant cell tumor of the tendon sheath. Ultrastructural study and review of the literature. Arch Pathol 1973;95:203-208.

57. Castens HP, Howell RS. Malignant giant cell tumor of tendon sheath. Virchows Arch A Pathol Anat Histol 1979;382:237-243.

58. Nielsen AL, Kiaer T. Malignant giant cell tumor of synovium and locally destructive pigmented villonodular synovitis: ultrastructural and immunohistochemical study and review of the literature. Hum Pathol 1989;20:765-771.

59. Choong PF, Willen H, Nilbert M, et al. Pigmented villonodular synovitis. Monoclonality and metastasis—a case for neoplastic origin? Acta Orthop Scand 1995;66:64-68.

60. Layfield LJ, Meloni-Ehrig A, Liu K, Shepard R, Harrelson JM. Malignant giant cell tumor of synovium (malignant pigmented villonodular synovitis). Arch Pathol Lab Med 2000;124:1636-1641.

61. Cupp JS, Miller MA, Montgomery KD, et al. Translocation and expression of CSF1 in pigmented villonodular synovitis, tenosynovial giant cell tumor, rheumatoid arthritis and other reactive synovitides. Am J Surg Pathol 2007;31:970-976.

62. Bertoni F, Unni KK, Beabout JW, Sim FH. Malignant giant cell tumor of tendon sheaths and joints (malignant pigmented villonodular synovitis). Am J Surg Pathol 1997;21:153-163.

63. Folpe AL, Weiss SW, Fletcher CD, Gown AM. Tenosynovial giant cell tumors: evidence for a esmin-positive dendritic cell subpopulation. Mod Pathol 1998;11:939-944.

64. Wood GS, Beckstead JH, Medeiros LJ, Kempson RL, Warnke RA. The cells of giant cell tumor of tendon sheath resemble osteoclasts. Am J Surg Pathol 1988;12:444-452.

65. O'Connell JX, Fanburg JC, Rosenberg AE. Giant cell tumor of tendon sheath and pigmented villonodular synovitis: immunophenotype suggests a synovial cell origin. Hum Pathol 1995;26:771-775.

66. Darling JM, Goldring SR, Harada Y, Handel ML, Glowacki J, Gravallese EM. Multinucleated cells in pigmented villonodular synovitis and giant cell tumor of tendon sheath express features of osteoclasts. Am J Pathol 1997;150:1383-1393.

67. West RB, Rubin BP, Miller MA, et al. A landscape effect in tenosynovial giant cell tumor from activation of CSF1 expression by a translocation in a minority of tumor cells. Proc Natl Acad Sci U S A 2006;103:690-695.

68. Möller E, Mandahl N, Mertens F, Panagopoulos I. Molecular identification of COL6A3-CSF1 fusion transcripts in tenosynovial giant cell tumors. Genes Chromosomes Cancer 2008;47:21-25.

69. Li CF, Wang JW, Huang WW, et al. Malignant diffuse-type tenosynovial giant cell tumors. A series of 7 cases comparing with 24 benign lesions with review of the literature. Am J Surg Pathol 2008;32:587-599.

12 CYTOPATHOLOGY OF SOFT TISSUE TUMORS AND TUMOR-LIKE LESIONS

The technique of fine needle aspiration (FNA) biopsy to diagnose soft tissue tumors is extremely demanding, difficult, and controversial; thus, its use on a regular basis is confined to a small number of medical centers because of the limitations imposed by the nature of the technique, and the infrequency, unfamiliarity, heterogeneity, and overlapping features of soft tissue neoplasms. Compounding these difficulties is an absence of spatial relationships in FNA in contrast to those appreciated in tissue sections, an inability to produce "mitotic counts" or extent of necrosis, and the chronic battle to procure a sufficient number of cells for evaluation (Table 12-1). Open biopsy remains the "gold standard" for the initial diagnosis of soft tissue neoplasms, yet most surgeons opt for core needle biopsies initially for a variety of reasons. Although we and others have demonstrated that FNA of soft tissue masses is sufficient in many instances to establish a correct and specific diagnosis, in some centers it does not approach the sensitivity and specificity of open biopsy (1). Even though there are many benefits to soft tissue FNA (Table 12-2), this is far from an infallible procedure. Its accuracy is dependent on several factors (Table 12-3), and, it cannot be overemphasized that correlation of cytologic morphology with clinical and imaging data is mandatory for successful results. A major benefit of first attempting FNA in our particular institution is the rapid, cheap, and harmless nature of the test that in many instances produces a result that allows the surgeon/clinician to proceed to more informed or even definitive management (2).

Many view FNA as only useful for locally recurrent and metastatic disease. Some have stated that it is a useful screening tool for soft tissue masses (3). It has been shown, however, that with experience and the judicious use of ancillary testing, FNA can separate benign from malignant soft tissue lesions. For many neoplasms, the correct subclassification into clinically relevant groups that permit practical patient management is possible with a high degree of accuracy in experienced centers (4–10). Our purpose in this chapter is to concentrate on the FNA cytomorphology of a variety of soft tissue neoplasms and discuss its limitations, pitfalls, and use in the differential diagnosis.

Table 12-1

REASONS FOR DIAGNOSTIC DIFFICULTY WITH SOFT TISSUE FNA CYTOLOGY

Infrequency of soft tissue tumors (except lipoma)
    Pathologists less familiar and thus less "comfortable" with such lesions
    Most clinicians do not perform or will not consider FNA for a patient with a soft tissue mass

Operator dependent

Overlapping morphologic features of many tumors (particularly spindle cell neoplasms)

Heterogeneity of architectural patterns and/or individual cell morphology within many soft tissue tumors
    Sampling error: proper sampling becomes a major issue in some lesions with different features in different areas
    Spatial relationships of vessels to tumor, and vascular pattern(s), typically lost
    Inability to accurately evaluate mitotic activity, presence/absence of a fibrous capsule, interface of lesion with surrounding nonlesional tissue, amount of necrosis (if any)
    Limited cellularity in fibrous lesions precludes sampling of adequate/diagnostic cells

---

Table 12-2

BENEFITS OF SOFT TISSUE FNA CYTOLOGY

Rapid turnaround time; facilitates triage of patient and specimen

Cost-effective; complications rare

Relatively painless; anesthetic unnecessary; office procedure

A single FNA allows for greater volumetric sampling than a single core needle biopsy

Does not contaminate a subsequent surgical site

Confirms a metastatic/recurrent lesion in a known cancer patient with a high degree of accuracy

---

Table 12-3

FACTORS DETERMINING ACCURACY OF SOFT TISSUE FNA CYTOLOGY

Clinical setting in which FNA is practiced: pathologist-performed FNA versus clinician-performed FNA; slides submitted with minimal to no clinical or radiographic history versus pathologist having full access to medical and radiologic records and discussion with surgeon or oncologist

Experience of pathologist, surgeon, radiologist

Evaluation of a primary tumor versus recurrent or metastatic neoplasm

Number of passes into the lesion

Type of neoplasm/lesion: certain neoplasm are much more recognizable than others

Whether material is also procured for cell block, immunophenotyping, FISH[a], or PCR

Whether one is evaluating the ability to separate a benign mass from a malignant one, or one is evaluating the ability of FNA to diagnose specific tumor type

[a]FISH = fluorescence in situ hybridization; PCR = polymerase chain reaction.

FIBROBLASTIC, MYOFIBROBLASTIC, AND FIBROHISTIOCYTIC TUMORS

Desmoid-Type Fibromatosis

The *fibromatoses* consist of several clinico-pathologic subtypes (*palmar, plantar, abdominal desmoid, fibromatosis colli, extra-abdominal desmoid*), yet the cytopathology is similar for each subtype and generally not distinguishable without clinical information. Smears, surprisingly, show a broad range of cellularity, from markedly hypocellular (11,12) to those with moderate-high cellularity (13,14). The smear background is clean, without necrosis. Spindle and stellate cells are in loose clusters, occasionally with a collagenous stroma or dispersed as single forms (fig. 12-1). Uniformly sized fibroblasts have oval to elongated, smoothly contoured nuclei possessing small nucleoli, finely dispersed chromatin, and thin delicate, wispy unipolar and bipolar cytoplasmic tendrils (12). Bare nuclei are common. The amount of metachromatic-staining collagenous stroma is variable, but usually scant. Entrapped atrophic myofibers with clustered nuclei, mimicking multinucleated giant cells, may be seen (fig. 12-2).

A large study of 69 patients with histologically proven desmoid tumors showed an accuracy of 94 percent using FNA in differentiating a benign from malignant process, and 51 percent in specifically recognizing desmoid fibromatosis (14). Hypertrophic scar is cytologically indistinguishable from fibromatosis. Other entities to consider for superficial masses include nodular fasciitis, and schwannoma. For deep-seated masses, gastrointestinal stromal tumor, leio-myoma, solitary fibrous tumor, and low-grade fibromyxoid sarcoma are potential mimickers.

Infantile Digital Fibroma/Fibromatosis

Infantile digital fibroma, also termed *inclusion body fibromatosis*, has characteristic clinical features and is rarely the subject of FNA cytology. Smears are markedly cellular with cells distributed primarily singly but with some loose clusters. At first glance, the smear is worrisome for a spindle cell sarcoma (fig. 12-3). Smoothly contoured fusiform nuclei have fine chromatin, indistinct nucleoli, and delicately tapered bipolar cytoplasmic processes. The most striking feature is a spherical, cytoplasmic glassy inclusion that has a sky blue color in R-stained smears (fig. 12-4). FNA confirms the diagnosis in the correct clinical context.

Nodular Fasciitis

Aspirates of *nodular fasciitis* show variable cellularity; most are hypercellular, but myxoid variants may be markedly hypocellular (15). Dispersed cells exist as single forms, but with much overlapping and in hypercellular aggregates (fig. 12-5). The jagged or feathery edges of these aggregates are not distinctive for any tumor type. Slender fibroblast-like cells have a small to moderate amount of pale-staining, short unipolar or bipolar cytoplasmic processes that are tapered or blunt ended (15,16). The nuclei are of similar size, are oval to markedly fusiform with finely granular chromatin, and have smooth or curved outer contours. Larger polygonal cells with macronuclei and single, enlarged nucleoli are a minor element in smears;

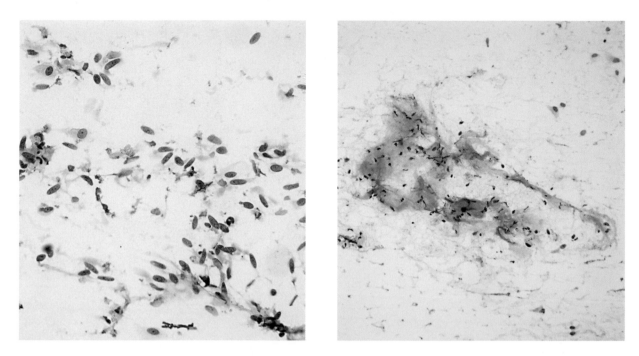

Figure 12-1

FIBROMATOSIS

Left: A modestly cellular smear with bland spindle, oval nuclei in a clean background.
Right: A hypocellular aspirate with wispy collagen matrix (left, right: Papanicolaou stain).

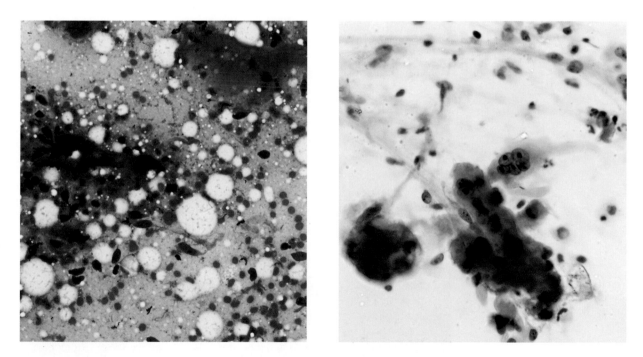

Figure 12-2

FIBROMATOSIS

Left: Stripped bare nuclei mix with those having imperceptible cytoplasmic tails (Romanowsky stain).
Right: Degenerating skeletal muscle mimics multinucleated giant cells (Papanicolaou stain).

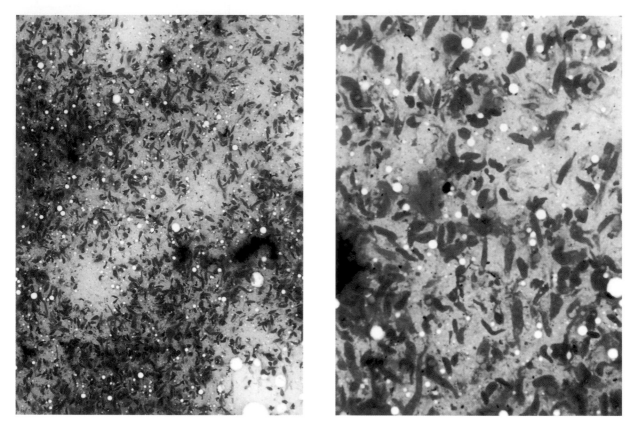

Figure 12-3

INFANTILE DIGITAL FIBROMA

Left: A markedly hypercellular smear suggests sarcoma.

Right: Spindle and serpiginous nuclei have minimal cytoplasm except for glassy light blue inclusions (left, right: Romanowsky stain).

Figure 12-4

INFANTILE DIGITAL FIBROMA

Multiple spherical inclusions are obvious; some indent cell nuclei (Romanowsky stain).

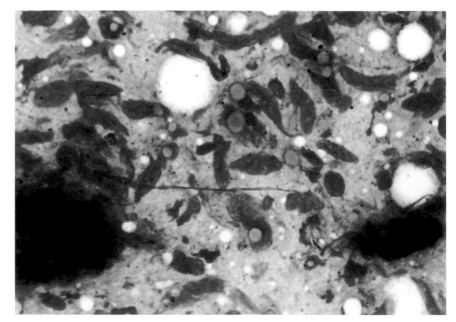

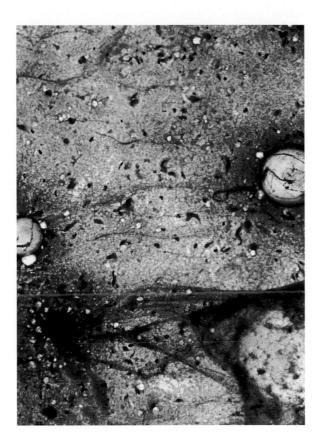 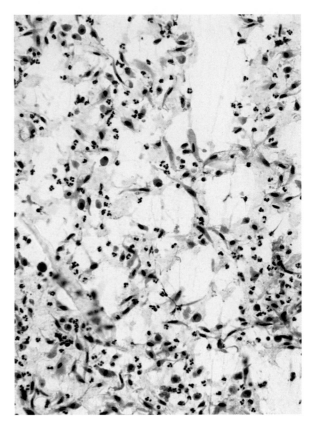

Figure 12-5

NODULAR FASCIITIS

Left: Myxoid foci are hypocellular, with abundant background stroma (Romanowsky stain).
Right: This smear with inflammatory cells mimics a "tissue-culture" appearance (Papanicolaou stain).

these often imitate the appearance of ganglion cells (15,17,18). The nucleoli are generally inconspicuous in most cells, and are small when present. A minor population has polygonal, stellate shapes with 2 to 3 nuclei or more per cell, and even foreign body–type giant cells. Myxoid stroma is obvious in some cases, and fibrous stroma varies from a few collagen strands to large dense fragments containing a variable number of embedded cells (19). Although some believe that a mixed inflammatory infiltrate is characteristic of nodular fasciitis, this is not universally present. Mitotic figures may be seen, but necrotic debris is absent.

The ease with which the well-circumscribed nodular architecture is appreciated in tissue sections is lost in smears. Because high cellularity produces a superficial resemblance to spindle cell sarcoma, misinterpretation of nodular fasciitis aspirates as malignant is common (fig. 12-6) (18). The differential diagnosis includes granulation tissue, proliferative fasciitis, dermatofibrosarcoma protuberans, low-grade myxofibrosarcoma, and synovial sarcoma. The presence of enlarged ganglion-type cells is more characteristic of proliferative fasciitis and proliferative myositis (16). Granulation tissue typically contains a much greater neutrophilic infiltrate, small visible capillaries, and foamy histiocytes (fig. 12-7).

Elastofibroma

Aspirates of *elastofibroma* are typically hypocellular or only moderately cellular, and contain a mixture of mature fat, collagen, and isomorphic bland spindle cells. The latter are pale with smooth slender or ovoid nuclei, even distributed nuclear chromatin, small nucleoli when visible, and pale thin cytoplasmic processes. Degenerated elastic fibers may be difficult

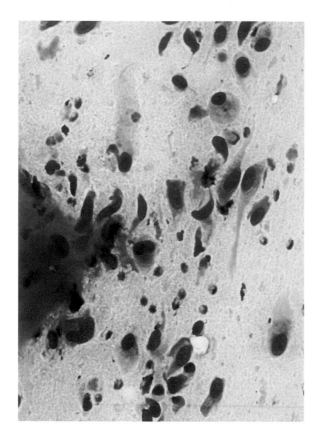
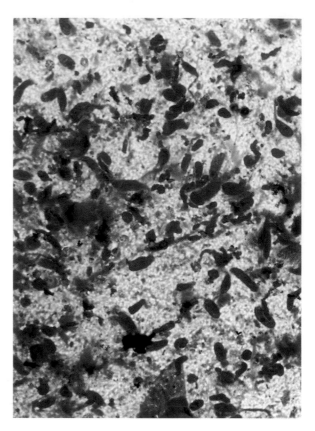

Figure 12-6

NODULAR FASCIITIS

Left: The cells have minimally contorted oval nuclei with a modest amount of cytoplasm.

Right: Many crooked nuclei can lead to a mistaken impression of sarcoma or neural neoplasm (left, right: Romanowsky stain).

Figure 12-7

GRANULATION TISSUE

A curved capillary winds through a collection of histiocytes, fibroblasts, and inflammatory cells (Romanowsky stain).

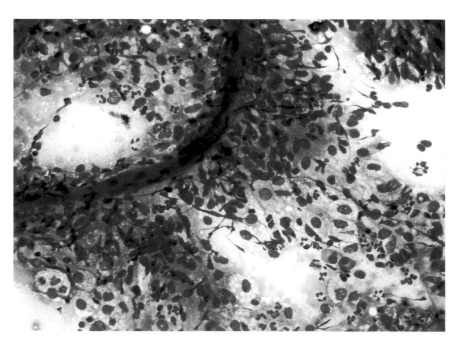

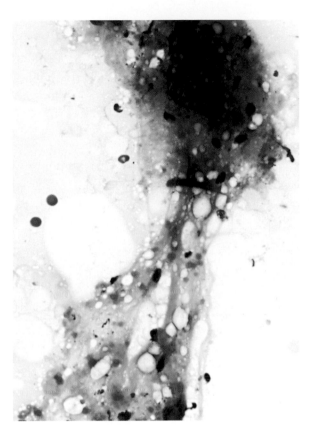
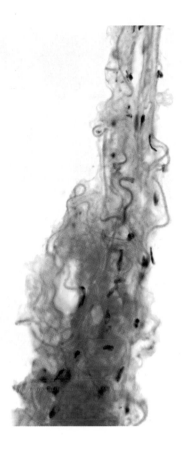

Figure 12-8

ELASTOFIBROMA

Left: The glassy bluish beads and a single vertical rod (center) of degenerated elastic fibers are easily overlooked (Romanowsky stain).

Right: Wiry filamentous elastic fibers are nearly transparent in this Papanicolaou stain.

to find or overlooked. They are glassy light blue (in R-stained smears), rod shaped, wiry, curved or globular with beaded, fern-like serrated outlines (fig. 12-8) (20–22). Staining of these extra-cellular fibers directly on the smear with an elastic stain is diagnostic (fig. 12-9) (21). Failure to find these fibers makes the distinction of elastofibroma from spindle cell lipoma nearly impossible.

Solitary Fibrous Tumor

Like many low-grade spindle cell proliferations, the cytopathology of *solitary fibrous tumor* is not sufficiently distinctive to allow a specific diagnosis without the use of a cell block preparation (especially, for CD34 immunochemistry). Smear cellularity varies from low to highly cellular, with a clean or bloody background. Banal-appearing cells in a dissociated pattern have isomorphic spindle- and oval-shaped nuclei, with thin cytoplasmic processes interspersed with stripped nuclei (fig. 12-10) (23). Anisonucleosis is usually minimal, and nuclear chromatin is evenly dispersed, finely granular, and hypochromic, while lacking enlarged nucleoli. Irregular ropy collagen fibers may contain embedded spindle cells (24).

Unlike large tissue specimens, cytopathology is unable to recognize hypercellular and hypocellular zones or a hemangiopericytomatous vascular pattern. Malignancy is difficult to recognize in these aspirates. Some reports show no difference in cellularity between benign and malignant examples (24). Others, however describe increased cellularity, individual cell necrosis, and round or epithelioid forms; yet the individual cytomorphology remains similar with minimal nuclear pleomorphism (25,26).

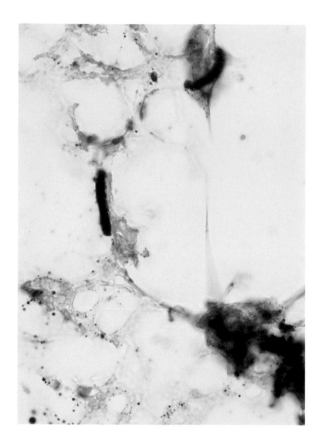 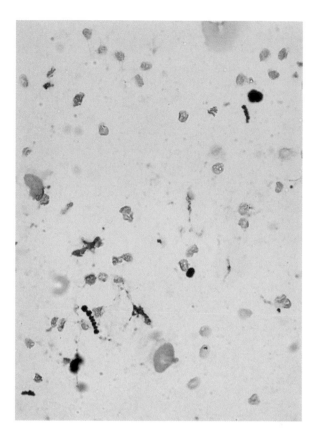

Figure 12-9

ELASTOFIBROMA

Left, Right: Curved, straight, and beaded elastic fibers are seen (Weigert elastic stain).

Dermatofibrosarcoma Protuberans

The localization of *dermatofibrosarcoma protuberans* primarily to the dermis and subcutis of the trunk and proximal extremities is a major factor in its recognition when a highly cellular aspirate dominated by spindle cells is found. Nonetheless, a specific diagnosis is difficult without immunohistochemical staining, or knowledge of a previous history of the tumor. Some claim to appreciate a storiform pattern in smears (27), but the authors' opinion, this is highly subjective, and does not seem to be useful in recognizing this neoplasm.

Hypercellular 3-dimensional aggregates are populated by fusiform cells showing minimal anisonucleosis, with short cytoplasmic processes or bare nuclei. Chromatin is evenly dispersed in oval to elliptical nuclei, with vague nucleoli (fig. 12-11) (28,29). Often, cells are embedded within a small to moderate amount of collagen.

Fibrosarcoma arising in dermatofibrosarcoma protuberans is probably impossible to distinguish from dermatofibrosarcoma protuberans alone or other spindle cell sarcomas using FNA-based cytologic preparations. In addition to spindle cell sarcoma, the differential diagnosis includes solitary fibrous tumor, nodular fasciitis, spindle cell melanoma, perineurioma, and cellular benign fibrous histiocytoma.

Spindle cell melanoma is extremely difficult to separate from spindle cell sarcoma when it lacks melanin deposition. Knowledge of a prior history of melanoma is probably the most helpful information for avoiding diagnostic error. In one large series, cytoplasmic pigment was present in only 15 percent of cases (30).

Tenosynovial Giant Cell Tumor

The cytopathology of *localized tenosynovial giant cell tumor,* also termed *giant cell tumor of tendon sheath,* consists of moderate to highly

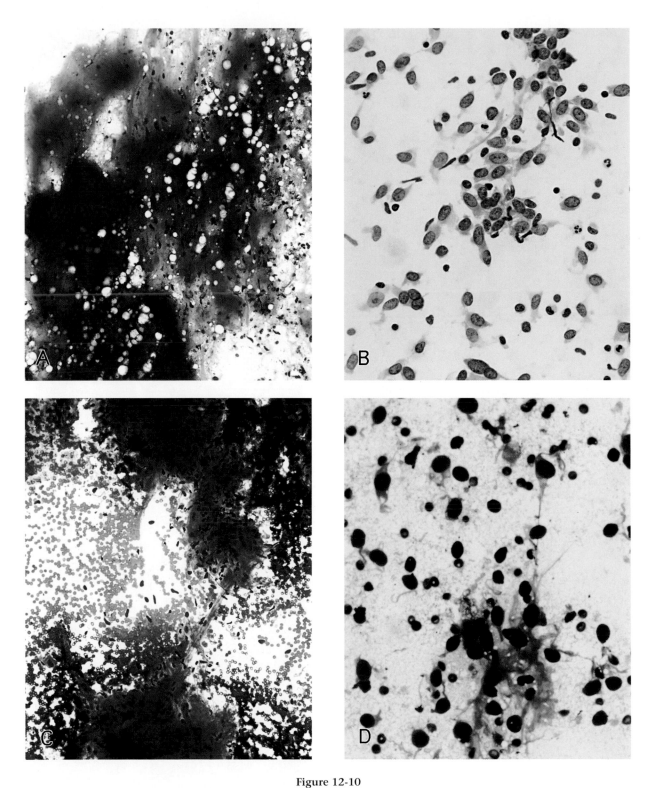

Figure 12-10

SOLITARY FIBROUS TUMOR

A: Seen are spindle cells and abundant stroma (Romanowsky stain).
B: The nuclei are rounded, oval, and hypochromic (Papanicolaou stain).
C,D: Thick cell clusters (C) alternate with smears having dissociated nuclei (D) (C,D: Romanowsky stain).

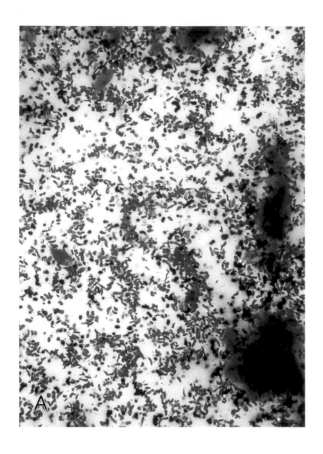

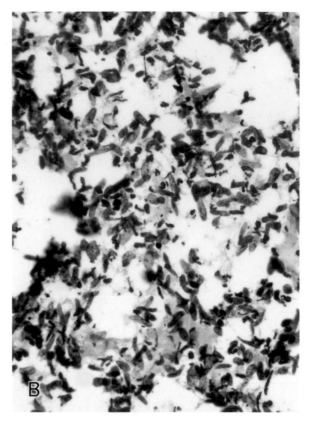

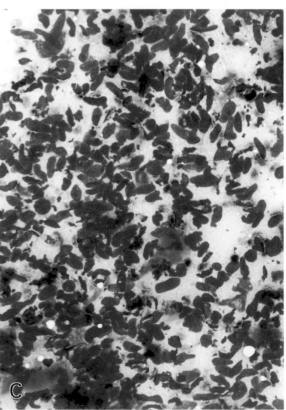

Figure 12-11

DERMATOFIBROSARCOMA PROTUBERANS

A: Three-dimensional clusters and an abundance of spindle cells are typical (Romanowsky stain).

B,C: There is marked overlapping of spindle-shaped nuclei with minimal cytoplasm (Papanicolaou and Romanowsky stains).

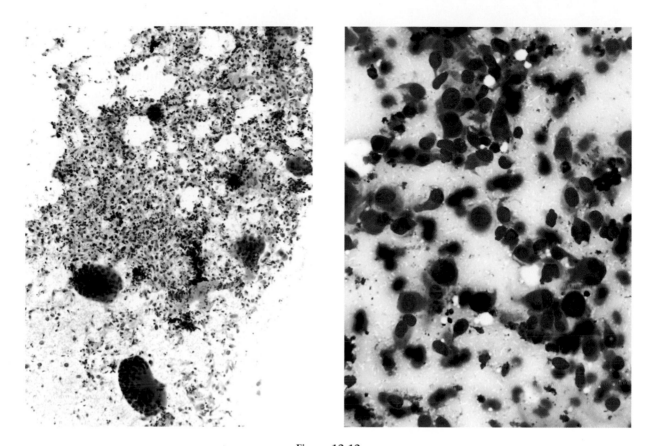

Figure 12-12

TENOSYNOVIAL GIANT CELL TUMOR

Left: Several multinucleated giant cells are scattered among single cells (Papanicolaou stain).
Right: The polygonal cells may be in clusters, or loosely dispersed as seen here (Romanowsky stain).

cellular smears with numerous single polygonal and spindle cells mixed with osteoclast-type multinucleated giant cells (31,32). Cell clusters are uncommon, and the smear background is clean (fig. 12-12). Polygonal cells are singly dispersed and many are binucleated with "mirror-image" nuclei, but lacking pseudoinclusions. They have a moderate amount of finely granular cytoplasm with sharp cell borders and occasional tapering. Single nuclei are uniform in size and shape, eccentrically placed in the cell, and round to oval, with fine pale chromatin and indistinct nucleoli. Nuclear grooves are seen in some P-stained slides, but are not appreciated in R-stained smears. Giant cell nuclei vary from as few as 3 to up to 50 per cell, and, importantly, faithfully duplicate the nuclear morphology of single cells. Hemosiderin-laden and foamy macrophages are variable in amount, but are usually a minor component of the aspirate (fig. 12-13).

Giant cell tumor of tendon sheath is reliably identifiable in a high percentage of cases in the correct clinical context (33). Binucleation and eccentric nuclear placement raise the possibility of clear cell sarcoma and metastatic melanoma. The latter typically has a known history, and lacks a predominance of osteoclastic giant cells. Clear cell sarcoma, however, may confusingly display multinucleated cells, but these are atypical tumor cells as opposed to the osteoclast-like giant cells in giant cell tumor. In some examples, cell block immunochemistry is necessary for diagnosis.

Giant Cell Tumor of Soft Parts

Giant cell tumor of soft parts cytologically imitates its osseous counterpart. Hypercellular smears contain an overabundance of multinucleated osteoclast-type giant cells found singly or in loose aggregates. The nuclei number from 6 to 50 per cell, averaging about 20 per

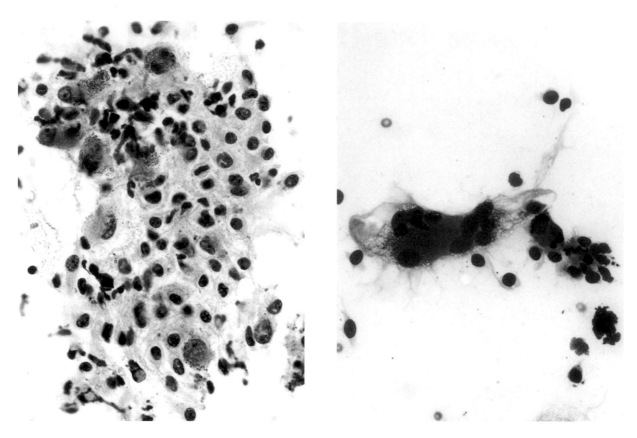

Figure 12-13

TENOSYNOVIAL GIANT CELL TUMOR

Hemosiderin deposition is variably present (left, Papanicolaou stain; right, Romanowsky stain).

cell with nuclear overlapping common (34). Nuclei within the giant cells are often similar in all respects to each other and to singly scattered cells (fig. 12-14). Some mononuclear cells, however, exhibit marked nuclear enlargement. The nuclei have a round to oval shape, smooth contour, evenly distributed granular chromatin, and small nucleoli or coarse chromatin (35). Microfragments of collagen stroma are present in some smears. Necrosis is unusual.

Isolated marked atypia may preclude a definitive diagnosis using cytology, but the cytology features imitate the histologic ones, which also show atypical nonosteoclastic binucleated or mononuclear cells. Unlike giant cell tumor of tendon sheath, which is a major consideration in the differential diagnosis, osteoclastic giant cells are so numerous they are found in virtually every mid-power field of the smear. The pleomorphism characteristic of the giant cell variant of undifferentiated pleomorphic sarcoma is absent.

Low-Grade Fibromyxoid Sarcoma

Low-grade fibromyxoid sarcoma must be considered in a hypocellular aspirate consisting of bland spindle cells and a myxoid background. The capillary network seen histologically is rarely demonstrable in aspiration smears (36). Most authors describe bland spindle cells in clusters and loose fascicles in a collagenous, myxoid matrix, but conclude that the cytologic findings are too nonspecific to allow a definitive diagnosis (fig. 12-15A,B) (36,37). Cytogenetic or molecular analysis for t(7;16)(q34;p11) is diagnostic.

The variant containing giant collagen rosettes has not been fully described in the cytology literature. Our unpublished experience shows hypocellular smears containing large, rounded fragments of metachromatic-staining fibrous tissue mimicking collagen rosettes containing cytologically banal spindle cells (fig. 12-15C). The cells embedded within the collagenous

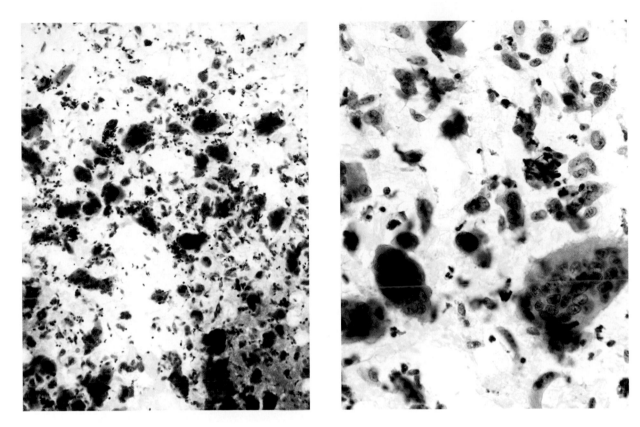

Figure 12-14

TENOSYNOVIAL GIANT CELL TUMOR

Left: Large numbers of osteoclast-type giant cells and single cells are seen.

Right: This image is identical to what is seen in giant cell tumor of tendon sheath, thus necessitating knowledge of the location and the clinical picture to avoid diagnostic error (left, right: Papanicolaou stain).

matrix are difficult to visualize, but surrounding this matrix are oval, rounded, and fusiform nuclei within scant cytoplasm and many stripped nuclei in a clean background.

Undifferentiated Pleomorphic Sarcoma

The abundantly cellular smears of *undifferentiated pleomorphic sarcoma* include cells distributed in aggregates and as single cells. The cell aggregates are loosely clustered or are organized into thick 3-dimensional fragments. These aspirates rarely demonstrate a well-developed storiform arrangement. The cells display a wide polymorphous spectrum of anaplasia with extreme variation in cell and nuclear size and shape, including spindle, stellate, rounded, and bizarre configurations. The cytologic features of malignancy are obvious and include enlarged dense nuclei, misshapen nucleoli, intranuclear pseudoinclusions, coarse chromatin, "tadpole"

cells with tapered cytoplasm, and cells with a high nuclear to cytoplasmic ratio (38,39). Cytoplasmic volume is variable: generally modest in spindle cells and more voluminous in pleomorphic cells (fig. 12-16). Multinucleated tumor giant cells are common. Inflammatory cells are variable in amount and include lymphocytes, neutrophils, and plasma cells.

In the correct clinical context, FNA cytology is highly successful in recognizing these high-grade sarcomas, with over 90 percent accuracy in some series (40). The differential diagnosis includes metastatic poorly differentiated carcinoma, anaplastic lymphoma, and melanoma. In most cases, a prior history of malignancy coupled with proper imaging suffices to recognize this malignancy. Kilpatrick et al. (41) assert that establishing a specific histologic subtype is not necessary for initiating adequate therapy for many high-grade adult sarcomas.

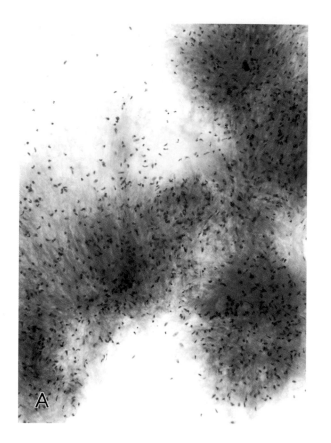

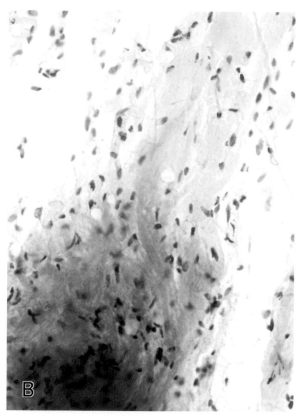

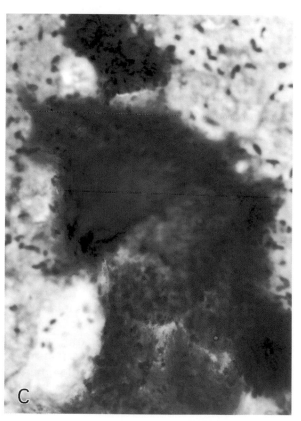

Figure 12-15

LOW-GRADE FIBROMYXOID SARCOMA

A: Moderately cellular myxocollagenous clusters lack architectural uniqueness.

B: Uniformly sized spindle cells are in a syncytial arrangement without discrete cell borders (A,B: Papanicolaou stain).

C: Giant collagen rosette variant. This 3-dimensional microfragment shows peripheral nuclear palisading surrounding an acellular collagenous center.

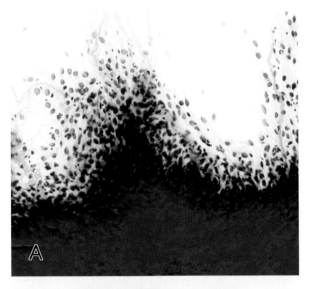

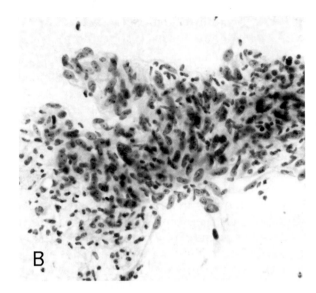

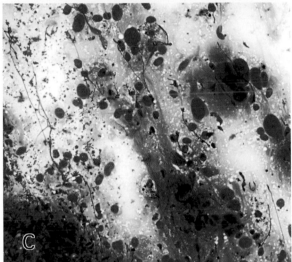

Figure 12-16

UNDIFFERENTIATED PLEOMORPHIC SARCOMA

A: The edge of a thick hypercellular microfragment with seemingly uniform cells.

B: A smaller fragment allows appreciation of nucleomegaly and discrete nucleoli.

C–E: Marked cytomegaly, nuclear pleomorphism, and multinucleation (Papanicolaou stain except C).

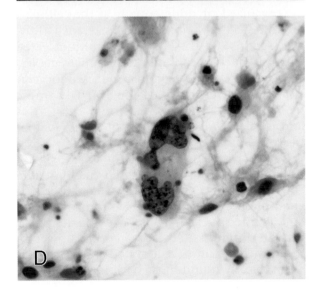

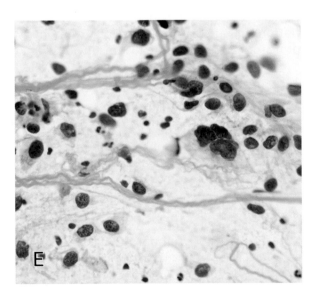

Myxofibrosarcoma (Myxoid Malignant Fibrous Histiocytoma)

The myxoid variant of undifferentiated pleomorphic sarcoma, *myxofibrosarcoma,* is divided into low- and high-grade variants, with an inverse relationship between smear cellularity, amount of myxoid stroma, and sarcoma grade. Low-grade myxofibrosarcoma consists of low to moderately cellular smears with a variable, but usually abundant, nonopaque myxoid stroma best seen in R-stained smears (42). Although short capillary branches are present, they generally do not approach the number or complex pattern observed in smears of myxoid liposarcoma. Many cells of low-grade myxofibrosarcoma are spindle or stellate, with modest nucleomegaly, dense nuclear chromatin, and no visible nucleoli. The key is definite evidence of nuclear atypia (nucleomegaly, pleomorphism, multinucleation), which is sometimes subtle and difficult to appreciate in smears. The major tumor to be confused with low-grade myxofibrosarcoma when it occurs in a deep location is intramuscular myxoma. The key features distinguishing them are increased cellularity and any degree of nuclear enlargement or atypia in the former (43).

Pronounced hypercellularity, myxoid stroma, and a myriad of pleomorphic, spindle, and tadpole-shaped cells underscore the cytomorphology of high-grade myxofibrosarcoma, which mimics undifferentiated pleomorphic sarcoma but with the addition of a myxoid background stroma (fig. 12-17) (44). Necrosis is a regular component of these aspirates. The distinctive multinodularity, elongated curved capillaries, and pattern of infiltration that are readily analyzable components of histologic sections are lost in smears.

LIPOMATOUS TUMORS

Lipoma/Hibernoma

Mature adipose tissue, when smeared, produces small discrete clear bubbles on the glass visible to the naked eye. Tight 3-dimensional lobules of lipocytes are readily recognizable as fat due to the large, single, optically clear cytoplasmic vacuole resulting in a thin sliver of cytoplasm sharply delineated from surrounding cells by a thin, easily visible cell border (fig. 12-18). The cell nuclei are small, indistinct, and placed at the cell edge without atypia. When viewed on end, the nucleus appears flattened and crescentic. Occasional short capillary segments are visible, but there is no vascular branching and the smear background is clean. The diagnosis of lipoma is inferred by the presence of a mass, since FNA cannot demonstrate a fibrous capsule. Intramuscular lipoma smears contain short segments of normal skeletal myofibers, but are otherwise similar to superficial lipoma. Many of the histologic variants of lipoma (angiolipoma, myolipoma, chondrolipoma) are not readily recognizable using FNA.

Hibernoma smears are easily mistaken for mature fat; once must recognize that the cytoplasm of many cells are filled with small uniform vacuoles rather than a single vacuole or just a few vacuoles, and that the nuclei are centrally rather than eccentrically placed in the cell (fig. 12-19) (45). Mature adipocytes are often mixed with brown fat cells.

Fat necrosis, with or without an associated lipoma, may produce a soft tissue mass. Aspirates are moderately cellular, with lipocytes having single and multivacuolated cytoplasm. Multinucleated giant cells, granular background cellular debris, macrophages, and inflammatory cells are usually present (fig. 12-20).

Pleomorphic Lipoma

Pleomorphic lipoma smears contain primarily individually scattered polygonal and spindle cells mixed with mature lipocytes. Multinucleated cells show some anisonucleosis, high nuclear to cytoplasmic ratios, and 2 to 5 hyperchromatic, partially overlapping nuclei per cell (46). These are organized circumferentially at the cell margin, mimicking their "floret" appearance in tissue sections (fig. 12-21). These multinucleated cells infrequently contain cytoplasmic vacuoles, however, intranuclear cytoplasmic pseudoinclusions have been reported (46,47). The smear background contains occasional capillaries and metachromatic stroma, but an absence of necrosis and mitotic figures.

The focus needs to be on the whole smear, not merely the multinucleated pleomorphic cells, because they have been confused for examples of pleomorphic sarcoma (48,49). Similar multinucleated floret cells are described in well-differentiated liposarcoma; however, mononuclear multivacuolated lipoblasts are also typically found in such aspirates (50).

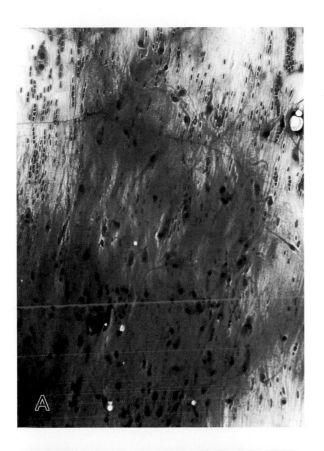

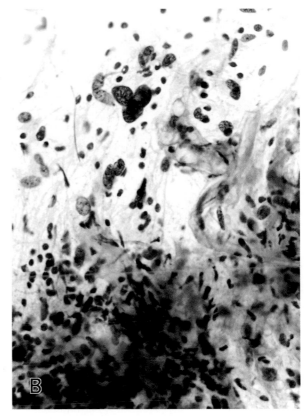

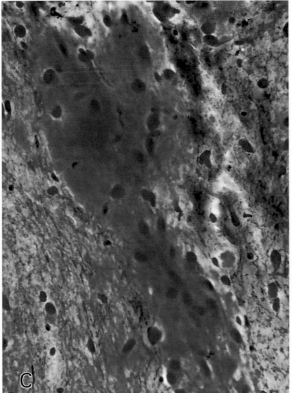

Figure 12-17

MYXOFIBROSARCOMA

A: High-grade myxofibrosarcoma shows obvious cellular pleomorphism and myxoid stroma (Romanowsky stain).

B: The myxoid background is less noticeable in P-stained smears.

C: A low-grade tumor has slightly enlarged polygonal cells in a dense myxoid stroma (Romanowsky stain).

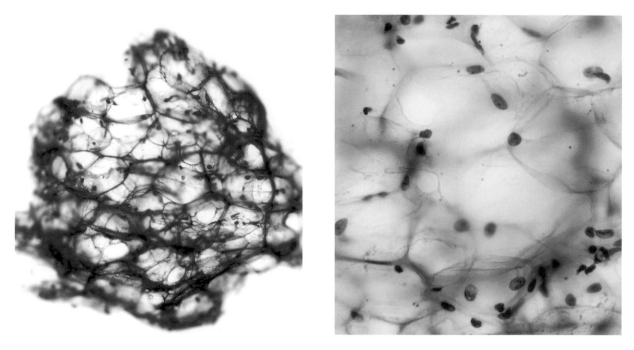

Figure 12-18

LIPOMA

Left: A lobule of mature fat has discrete cell borders and larger cytovacuoles (Romanowsky stain).
Right: The cell nuclei are larger than typically seen in tissue sections (Papanicolaou stain).

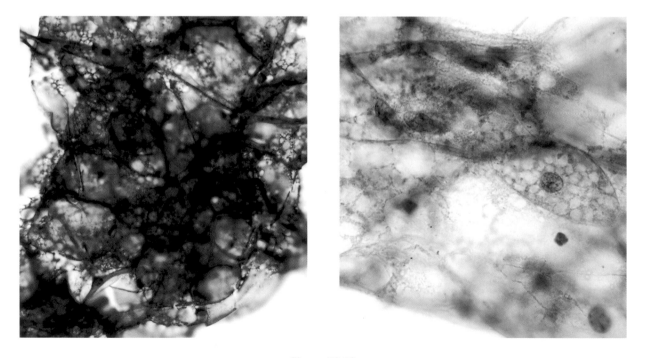

Figure 12-19

HIBERNOMA

The cell cytoplasm is distended by multiple lipid-filled vacuoles (left, Romanowsky stain; right, Papanicolaou stain).

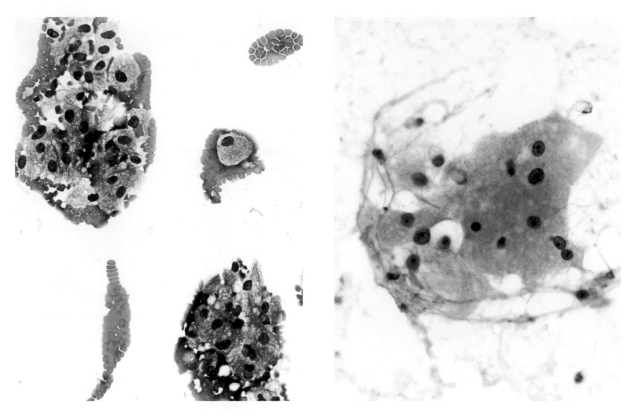

Figure 12-20

FAT NECROSIS

Left: There are small clusters of foamy macrophages (Romanowsky stain).
Right: Several macrophages are beginning to merge to form a multinucleated giant cell (Papanicolaou stain).

Spindle Cell Lipoma

Spindle cell lipoma may resemble unremarkable fibroadipose tissue due to the combination of collagenous fibers, lipocytes, and spindle cells. It is the presence of excessive numbers of bland spindle cells with oval or fusiform nuclei that should prompt a consideration of this neoplasm, particularly if it arises in the posterior neck/upper back location. Spindle cells are spread as single forms and in collective clusters, often embedded in collagen, with occasional nuclear grooves, indistinct nucleoli, smooth or undulating contours, and minimal cytoplasm (fig. 12-22) (51). The multinucleated floret-type giant cell may be seen as part of the overlap with pleomorphic lipoma. The background may show myxoid stroma, but rarely is it abundant, and there is an absence of necrotic debris.

The differential diagnosis includes other benign spindle cell proliferations including fibromatosis, nerve sheath tumors (52), solitary fibrous tumor, and low-grade myxofibrosarcoma in aspirates containing an abundant myxoid background.

Myxoid/Round Cell Liposarcoma

The three major features of *myxoid liposarcoma* seen in tissue—a plexiform vascular pattern, myxoid stroma, and bland mononuclear cells—are reproduced with stunning accuracy in most well-performed aspirates. Plexiform arborizing capillaries seen at low power closely mimic the "chicken-wire" or "crow's feet" pattern. The cells are dispersed as discrete aggregates surrounded by abundant metachromatic-staining stroma. In P-stained smears, the capillaries and myxoid stroma are more transparent and less readily appreciated (fig. 12-23). The stroma has a similar finely granular quality as that described for myxoma, but in areas may acquire a fibrillary opacity, and even appear as discrete fragments (53).

473

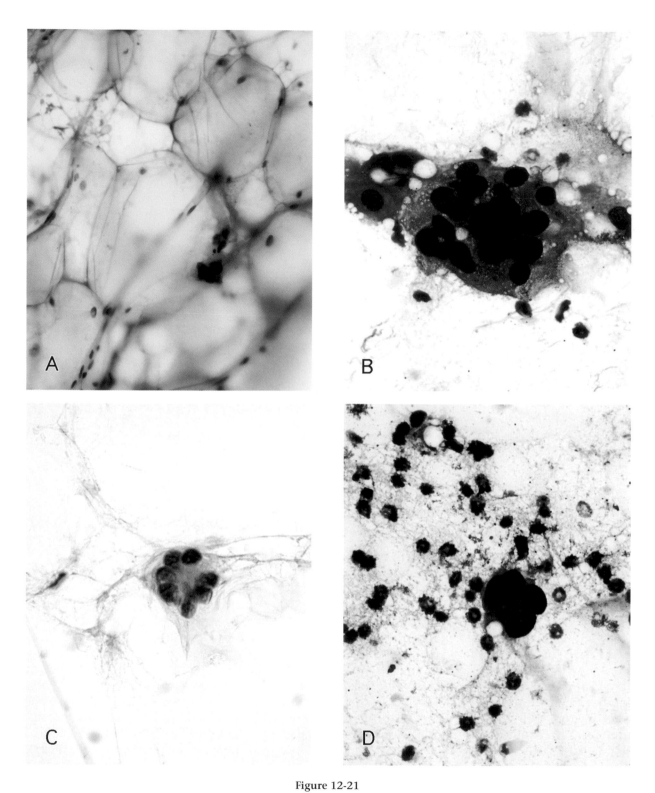

Figure 12-21

PLEOMORPHIC LIPOMA

A: Two multinucleated cells are embedded within mature adipose tissue.

B–D: Variations of multinucleated cells, some having the classic "floret" appearance (A,C: Papanicolaou stain); B,D: Romanowsky stain).

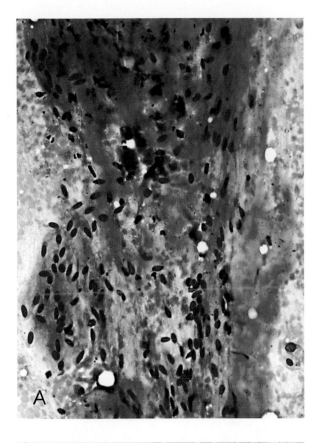

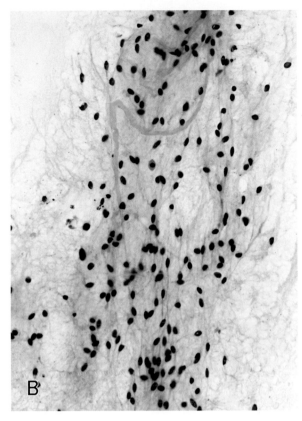

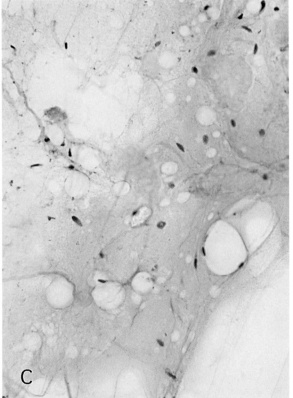

Figure 12-22

SPINDLE CELL LIPOMA

A: Monotonous spindle cells are embedded in a fibro-collagenous stroma with no visible adipose tissue (Romanowsky stain).

B: Spindle cells in a myxoid stroma (Papanicolaou stain).

C: Spindle cells in a lipomatous background (Papanicolaou stain).

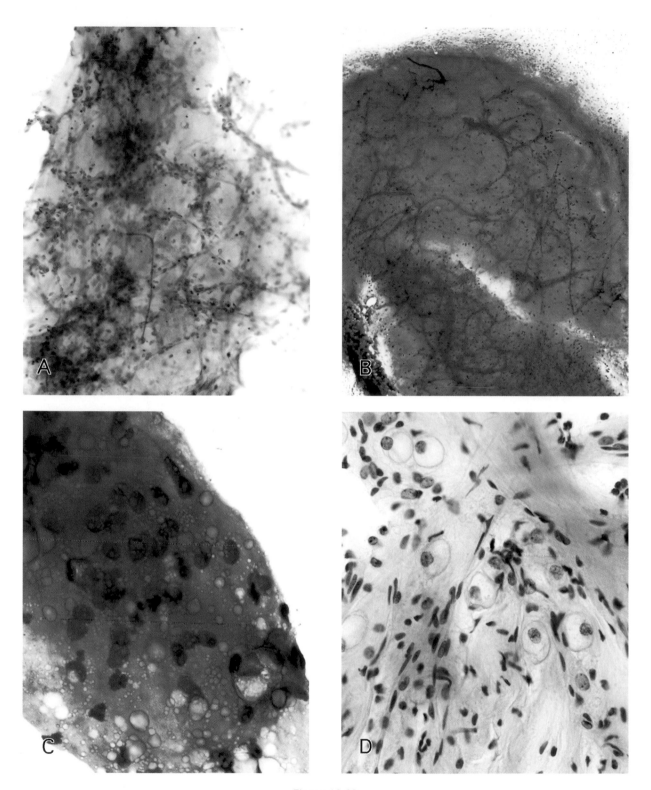

Figure 12-23

MYXOID LIPOSARCOMA

A,B: Numerous delicate branching capillaries are set in a myxoid background with inconspicuous cells.
C,D: Univacuolated lipoblasts (A,D: Papanicolaou stain; B,C: Romanowsky stain).

Most cells are nonlipoblastic, having isomorphic small, ovoid and fusiform nuclei lacking distinct nucleoli and meager amounts of cytoplasm (54). These cells merge into the vascular and stromal components on the smear. The lipoblasts have a slightly enlarged nucleus; a single cytoplasmic vacuole surrounds or pushes the nucleus to one edge. Nucleoli, when present, are more obvious in P-stained smears. The lipoblasts may be few in number and are more likely to be located in the vascular/myxoid stromal meshwork (55). Mitotic figures are nearly impossible to find.

A specific diagnosis of myxoid liposarcoma can be made from FNA cytopathology alone in most cases if adequate material is obtained. Because some cases may have a small number of recognizable lipoblasts, one study suggests that if other features of myxoid liposarcoma are present (myxoid stroma, proliferative branching capillary network, small undifferentiated mononuclear cells) then the lack of vacuolated lipoblasts does not exclude a diagnosis of liposarcoma (55). Conversely, a study using logistic regression analysis found that only the presence of lipoblasts on the smear was significant for the diagnosis of myxoid liposarcoma (43). Although lipoblasts and branching capillary segments were seen in the same percentage of cases (67 percent) in that study, a plexiform vascular pattern was also seen in 15 percent of low-grade myxofibrosarcomas and 6 percent of chondrosarcomas. Others found lipoblasts in less than 50 percent of cases (56).

The *round cell variant* (*highly cellular myxoid liposarcoma*) may coexist as part of the same mass. Whereas myxoid liposarcoma is characterized by its modestly cellular vascular and myxoid components, the round variant has increased cellularity and lacks both a myxoid stroma and fine capillary branching. The nuclei are larger and rounded, and may display a discrete nucleolus (fig. 12-24). Cell clusters may have numerous vacuoles, and nuclei, although small, display hyperchromasia, anisokaryosis, and discrete visible nucleoli (47). If areas of necrosis exist on a smear that is otherwise typical for myxoid liposarcoma, it should suggest possible round cell liposarcoma. Due to its hypercellular population of monotonous rounded cells, the differential diagnosis includes malignant small round cell tumors. A specific FNA-based diagnosis of myxoid/round cell liposarcoma using fluorescence in situ hybridization (FISH) analysis has been reported (57).

Atypical Lipomatous Tumor/ Well-Differentiated Liposarcoma

Aspirate smears of *atypical lipomatous tumor/ well-differentiated liposarcoma* are dominated by bubbly globules of mature lipocytes, reflecting the more common lipoma-like variant of this neoplasm (58). The lipoblasts are characterized by enlarged, densely chromatic, irregularly contoured and sometimes multilobated nuclei (59). The cytoplasm varies from large single vacuoles to multiple coarse vacuoles indenting the nucleus (fig. 12-25). Not all lipoblasts possess concave nuclear indentations; some appear as hyperchromatic misshapen nuclei with granular cytoplasm. Nondescript smaller round cells and spindle cells are seen also, but are usually difficult to confidently recognize as lipoblasts.

The lipoblasts may exhibit a spindle shape in the sclerosing variant of this neoplasm, creating a mistaken impression of a spindle cell sarcoma (56). Cells with multiple nuclei in a wreath or ring-like placement, as seen in pleomorphic lipoma, may be found (50). Well-differentiated liposarcoma is often mistaken for a benign lipoma, either because of sampling error or failure to locate abnormal nuclei in an abundance of mature fat (60,61).

Dedifferentiated Liposarcoma

Aspirates of *dedifferentiated liposarcoma* have foci of both well-differentiated liposarcoma and nonlipogenic pleomorphic sarcoma. Most arise in the retroperitoneum as large, bulky masses. The cytologic morphology imitates that of an undifferentiated pleomorphic sarcoma (fig. 12-26). If the well-differentiated component is also sampled, cells with large lipid-filled cytoplasmic vacuoles are seen in addition to large pleomorphic cells with bizarre nuclei (62).

Pleomorphic Liposarcoma

Smears of *pleomorphic liposarcoma* closely mimic, and in most instances, are indistinguishable from those of undifferentiated pleomorphic sarcoma since lipid differentiation is often difficult to appreciate. Cellular pleomorphism and

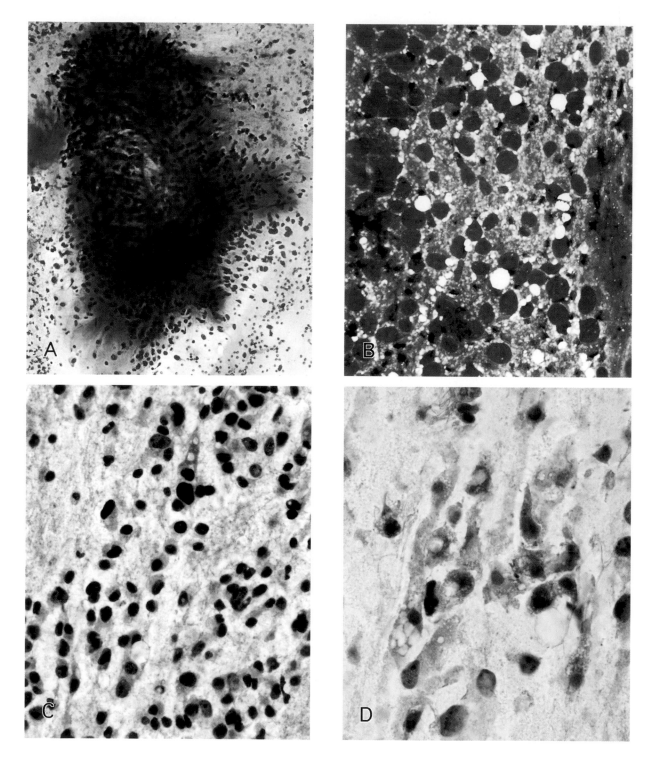

Figure 12-24

ROUND CELL LIPOSARCOMA

A: A hypercellular 3-dimensional cluster lacks a vascular pattern.

B,C: Monotonous lipoblasts are dissociated from each other and loosely clustered. Cytoplasmic lipid vacuoles are variably present.

D: Some cells show multivacuolation (A,B: Romanowsky stain; C,D: Papanicolaou stain).

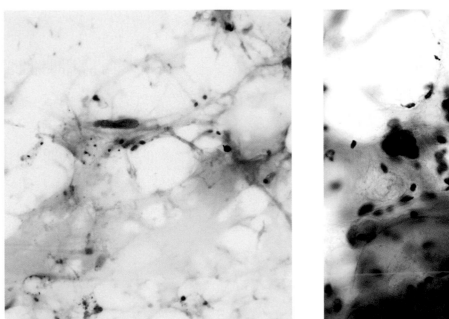
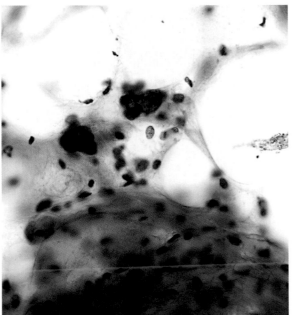

Figure 12-25

WELL-DIFFERENTIATED LIPOSARCOMA

Single (left) or multiple (right) hyperchromic, enlarged cells lacking cytoplasmic vacuoles are surrounded by mature fat (left, right: Papanicolaou stain).

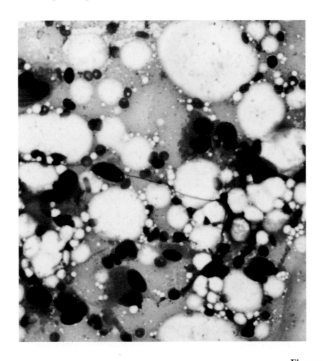
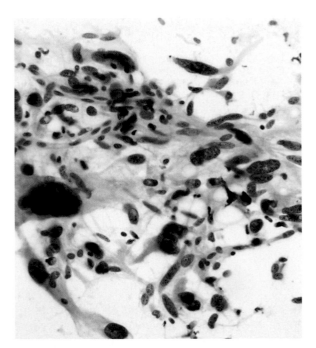

Figure 12-26

DEDIFFERENTIATED LIPOSARCOMA

Left: A focus of well-differentiated liposarcoma contains many lipoblasts (Romanowsky stain).

Right: A more typical example illustrates the malignant features of a nonlipogenic high-grade undifferentiated sarcoma (Papanicolaou stain).

479

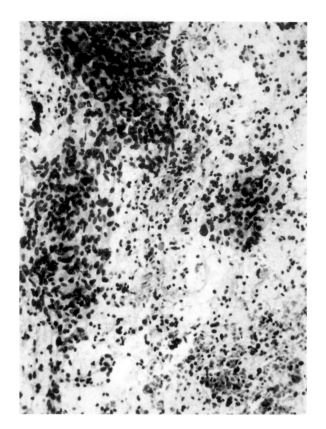
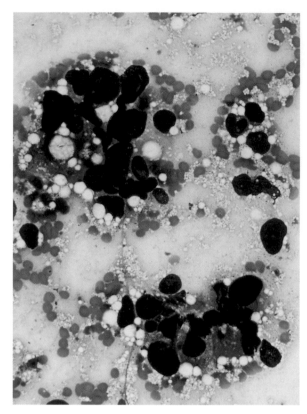

Figure 12-27

PLEOMORPHIC LIPOSARCOMA

Left: A highly cellular pleomorphic sarcoma with necrosis (upper left) (Papanicolaou stain).

Right: In this epithelioid variant, extremely large cells with multiple cytoplasmic lipid vacuoles. Cytologically, this variant cannot be differentiated from conventional pleomorphic liposarcoma (Romanowsky stain).

multinucleation are evident and large, coarse cytoplasmic vacuoles are the rule (47). Single cells are more common than cell clusters (fig. 12-27). The smears typically contain necrotic cellular debris. Unlike pleomorphic lipoma, nuclei with irregular contours are not arranged in a wreath-like fashion at the cell perimeter; rather, they are randomly situated within the cytoplasm.

MYOGENIC TUMORS

Leiomyoma

Leiomyoma of somatic soft tissue is uncommon. Most reports are from visceral organs, and some of these earlier reports may represent examples of gastrointestinal stromal tumor (63). Smears typically contain only a small number of tightly clustered microfragments. These contain banal spindle cell nuclei insinuated in an abundant fibrillar cytoplasmic syncytium, with few dissociated single cells (fig. 12-28). The syncytial clusters show nuclei in regular parallel alignment with little nuclear overlap (64). These aggregates do not display the high cellularity associated with other spindle cell sarcomas. The nuclei are oval to markedly elongated with minimal waviness, fine chromatin, and faint nucleoli. There is an absence of multinucleated cells, vascularity, and necrosis.

Leiomyosarcoma

Aspirates of *leiomyosarcoma* contain thick 3-dimensional hypercellular microfragments, loosely clustered cell monolayers, and isolated single cells (64). Spindle-shaped cells with minimal anisocytosis, long cytoplasmic processes, and increased cellularity exist in low-grade leiomyosarcoma smears. High-grade tumors mimic undifferentiated pleomorphic sarcoma: the dissociated cells are larger and have moderate to marked nuclear pleomorphism (rounded,

480

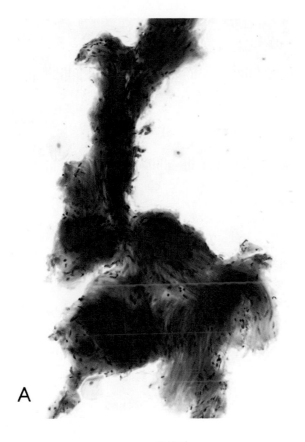

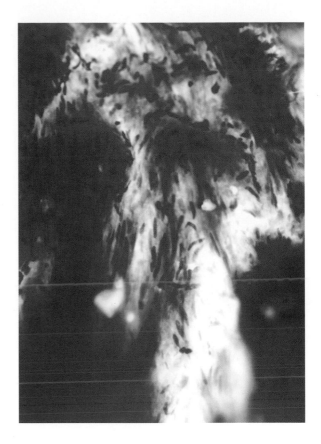

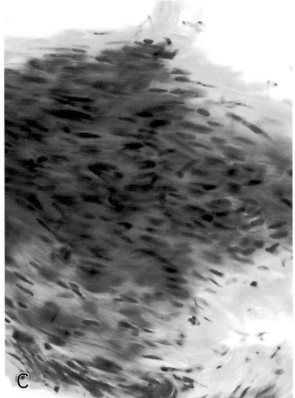

Figure 12-28

LEIOMYOMA

A: A tightly aggregated fragment of smooth muscle shows no single cells and a clean background.

B,C: Uniformly sized, thin rod-shaped nuclei are embedded in a syncytium, and often in parallel arrangement (A,C: Papanicolaou stain; B: Romanowsky stain).

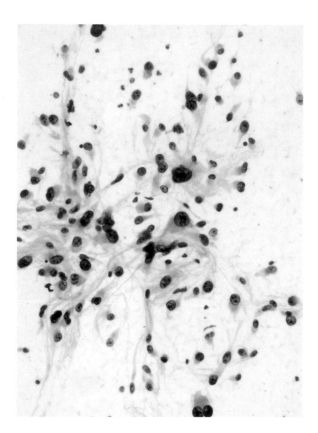
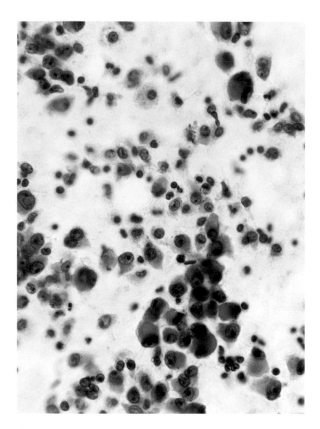

Figure 12-29

LEIOMYOSARCOMA

Left: This high-grade leiomyosarcoma has the characteristics typical of undifferentiated pleomorphic sarcoma (see fig. 12-16). Immunostaining is necessary to specifically diagnose leiomyosarcoma.

Right: In the epithelioid variant, polygonal cells are sometimes binucleated, with eccentric nuclear placement. Immunostaining is required to differentiate this from epithelioid melanoma and other epithelioid forms of sarcoma (left, right: Papanicolaou stain).

spindle, and bizarre shapes), two or more nuclei per cells, coarse chromatin, macronucleoli, and variable amounts of misshapen cytoplasm, and often lose any semblance of regular linear parallel organization (fig. 12-29) (61,63,65). Cellular necrosis and mitotic figures are more likely to be found in high-grade leiomyosarcoma. The myxoid form is easily confused with myxofibrosarcoma, while the epithelioid variant is mistakable for melanoma, carcinoma, and the epithelioid variant of other sarcomas (fig. 12-29, right).

Adult-Type Rhabdomyoma

FNA cytopathology of *adult-type rhabdomyoma* shows large polygonal cells distributed in loose clusters and as single cells, with a clean background. The abundant finely granular cell cytoplasm displays parallel arrays of cross-stria-

tions in some, but not all, cells (66). Enlarged cell nuclei (compared to normal skeletal muscle) are round to oval, with a single obvious round nucleolus. The nuclei are sometimes located eccentrically within the cell (67), and multiple nuclei per cell may be seen (fig. 12-30). Unlike sarcolemmal nuclei of mature skeletal muscle, these lack the characteristic linear and orderly arrangement at the myofiber periphery.

The "spider cell" morphology seen in tissue sections is lost in smears since cytoplasmic vacuoles are randomly scattered within the cytoplasm when present. If the cross-striations are not readily apparent, aspirates may be confused with granular cell tumor (67,68). Cells of rhabdomyoma, however, are larger, have discrete cell borders, and lack the coarse granules of granular cell tumor.

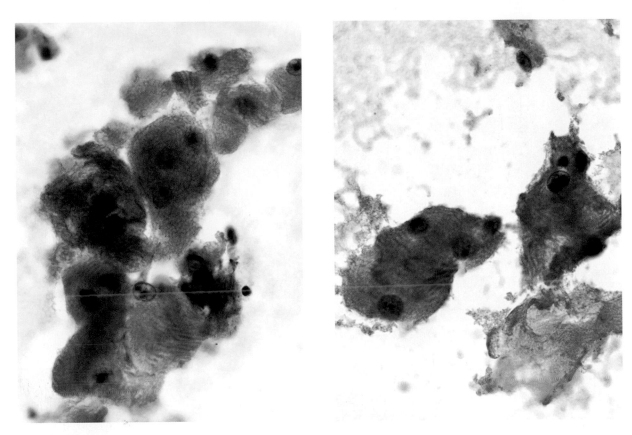

Figure 12-30

ADULT-TYPE RHABDOMYOMA

Enlarged nuclei with single discrete nuclei are randomly arranged within the cell cytoplasm, unlike mature skeletal muscle. Nonuniform cross striations are noticeable in these two examples (left, right: Papanicolaou stain).

Rhabdomyosarcoma

Smears of *rhabdomyosarcoma* are highly cellular, with small to intermediate-sized, singly dispersed cells and cells in crowded aggregates, similar to any aspirate of a malignant small round cell tumor. Round to oval, minimally pleomorphic, hyperchromatic nuclei possess dense chromatin, generally indistinct nucleoli, minimally visible cytoplasm, focal nuclear molding, and numerous bare nuclei (fig. 12-31). Intranuclear inclusions and spindle-shaped cells are less common in most aspirates (69,70). Differentiating rhabdomyoblasts possess a modest amount of cytoplasm and may display binucleation or multinucleation and cytoplasmic vacuoles, but cytoplasmic cross-striations are rare (70).

The characteristic tadpole or ribbon shape of differentiating rhabdomyoblasts is recognized in only a minority of aspirates. Mitoses and individual cell necrosis are variably present in an otherwise clean smear background; in those cases with sufficient cytoplasmic glycogen, smear cytoplasmic debris may lead to a so-called tigroid background. This feature is nonspecific as it is also recognized in Ewing sarcoma.

It is not usually possible to discern the two major rhabdomyosarcoma subtypes, embryonal and alveolar, cytologically. Nonetheless, a specific cytologic diagnosis of the alveolar type is possible with ancillary FISH testing for the *FOXO1* gene rearrangement (71,72). The differential diagnosis includes other malignant small round cell tumors: extraosseous Ewing sarcoma, desmoplastic small round cell tumor, lymphoblastic lymphoma, poorly differentiated synovial sarcoma, and mesenchymal chondrosarcoma. Many of these neoplasms are identified with the use of ancillary immunochemistry and flow cytometry to analyze this category of neoplasms (73).

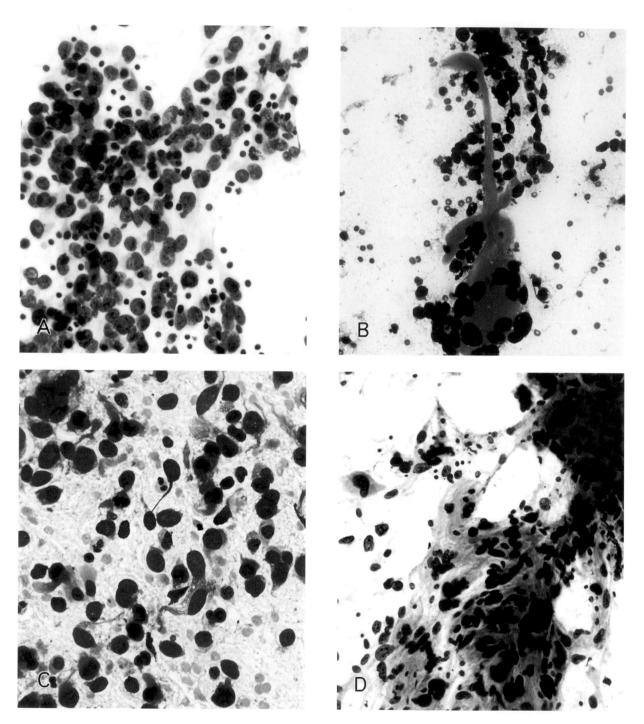

Figure 12-31

RHABDOMYOSARCOMA

A: The alveolar variant shows a hypercellular population of malignant small rounded nuclei with minimal cytoplasm. Small dots in the background are individually necrotic (apoptotic) cells, not lymphocytes.

B: The alveolar variant shows myogenic differentiation with the acquisition of much more cytoplasm and multinucleation.

C: The embryonal variant shows some malignant cells with unipolar cytoplasmic tails producing a "tadpole" shape.

D: The pleomorphic variant has the typical appearance of a high-grade undifferentiated sarcoma (A,D: Papanicolaou stain; B,C: Romanowsky stain).

PERIPHERAL NERVOUS SYSTEM TUMORS

Benign Nerve Sheath Tumors (Neurofibroma and Schwannoma)

Some authors believe a distinction between *schwannoma* and *neurofibroma* is not possible cytologically, and it is best to diagnose them as benign nerve sheath tumors (74). In general, neurofibroma aspirates are much less cellular than schwannoma aspirates. Smears, however, show a wide spectrum in cellularity, with cases unsatisfactory due to insufficient cells not uncommon as a consequence of cystic change or hyalinization within the tumor, or because severe pain during the aspiration prematurely ends the procedure (75).

Both neoplasms have spindle cells in both myxofibrillary/collagenous microfragments and as scattered single forms; the latter are often stripped bare nuclei while the former are embedded in a cell syncytium. In schwannoma, both parallel and random arrangements of nuclei are present, but well-developed palisading is not common, and Verocay body formation is unusual (fig. 12-32) (75). Rounded, plump oval nuclei exist along with spindle cells; isolated nuclear enlargement, pleomorphism, and intranuclear inclusions are more typical of "ancient" schwannoma. Cells may have pale ill-defined borders and wispy or ropy cytoplasmic processes in both schwannoma and neurofibroma. Spindle-shaped nuclei are often smooth. Neurofibromas usually have irregular nuclear outlines described as buckled, wavy, fishhook, or serpiginous (fig. 12-33) (76).

The smear background for both neoplasms lacks vascularity, necrosis, and mitotic figures, but a semitransparent myxoid stroma is possible in either tumor. Nondiagnostic fluid is aspirated in schwannomas with cystic degenerative change. Of course, a fibrous capsule or perivascular hyalinization cannot be evaluated in smears. A helpful, but not pathognomonic clinical clue for those pathologists performing their own FNA is the sharp stinging/radiating pain (Tinel sign) that some patients experience during the aspiration procedure.

With schwannoma, the major differential diagnostic problem is distinction from spindle cell sarcoma. In many instances, the lower cellularity, lack of mitotic figures, and presence of necrotic cells coupled with imaging studies are sufficient to avoid this error. Cellular schwannoma, however, is a major pitfall because of highly cellular microfragments combined with nuclear pleomorphism (77). Acquiring cells to construct a cell block is extremely useful in this regard to detect the strong S-100 protein staining of this variant of schwannoma.

Granular Cell Tumor

Smears of *granular cell tumor* are often moderately cellular or hypocellular due to the desmoplastic response induced in surrounding tissue. This fibrosis typically precludes extracting a large number of cells with a fine needle. Polygonal and epithelioid cells are distributed in loose syncytia with frayed, indistinct cell borders, and as single cells (78).

The key to cytologic recognition lies in the impressive coarse granularity of the nonvacuolated, nonpigmented cell cytoplasm (79). The granularity is evenly dispersed throughout the cytoplasm, and is much better seen in alcohol-fixed smears (fig. 12-34). In some R-stained aspirates this granularity is difficult to appreciate. The cell nuclei are spherical to oval, with discrete, sometimes enlarged, single nucleoli; bare nuclei are common due to cell fragility (81,82). With the exception of extracellular granular material, the smear background is clean and a vascular pattern is absent.

The degree (coarseness) of the cytoplasmic graininess in a well-made smear is usually greater than that seen in aspirates of other tumors in the differential diagnosis such as adult rhabdomyoma, clear cell sarcoma, epithelioid sarcoma, and alveolar soft part sarcoma. It is also more common for the cells of granular cell tumor to aggregate in a loose syncytium rather than disperse as individual cells, a feature more appropriate for these other tumors. The histiocytic cells in aspirates of fat necrosis and granulomatous reactions are vacuolated, without coarse granularity. The reniform configuration of epithelioid histiocytes seen in granulomas is absent in granular cell tumor.

Perineurioma

Too few cases of soft tissue (extraneural) *perineurioma* have been encountered to make dogmatic statements. The few reported cases and our own experience show smears of moderate to

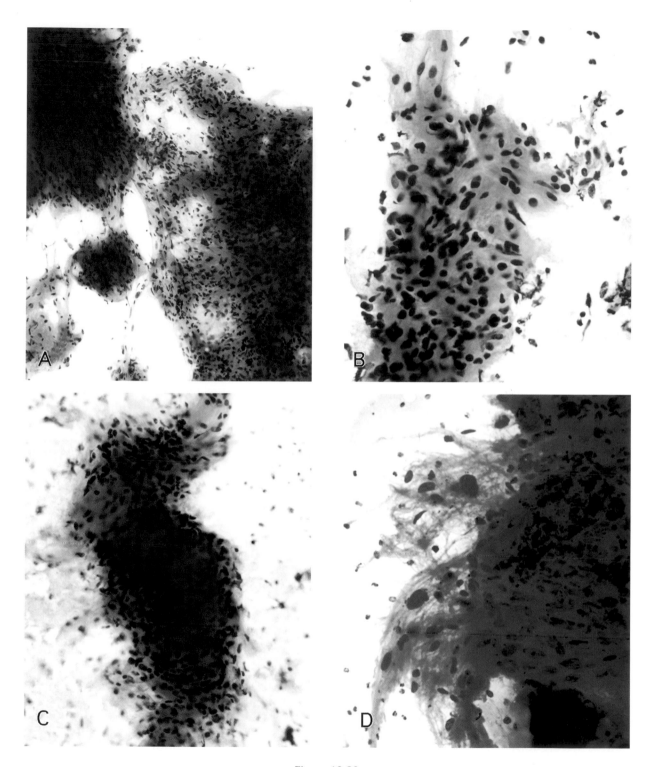

Figure 12-32

SCHWANNOMA

A: Two hypercellular 3-dimensional fragments can easily be mistaken for sarcoma.
B: Oval and spindled nuclei are inset in a fibrous syncytium.
C: Linear-shaped Verocay body shows an acellular center with nuclear palisading on either side.
D: Isolated marked nucleomegaly typical of "ancient" change (A–C: Papanicolaou stain; D: Romanowsky stain).

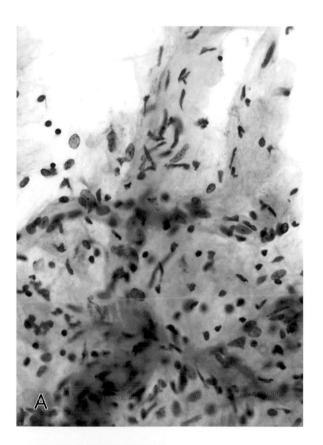

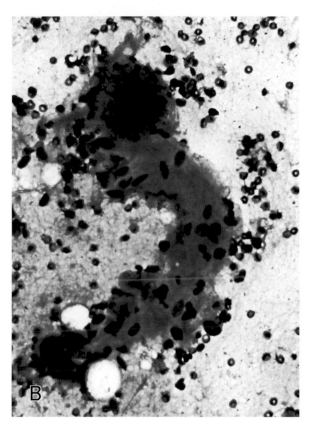

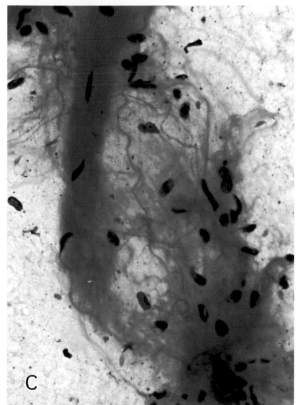

Figure 12-33

NEUROFIBROMA

A: A modestly cellular cluster shows myxoid change; wavy nuclei are noticeable (upper left) (Papanicolaou stain).

B: Nuclei are set in a collagenous fiber.

C: Curved and buckled spindle-shaped nuclei display bipolar thin undulating cytoplasmic processes in a myxoid stroma (B,C: Romanowsky stain).

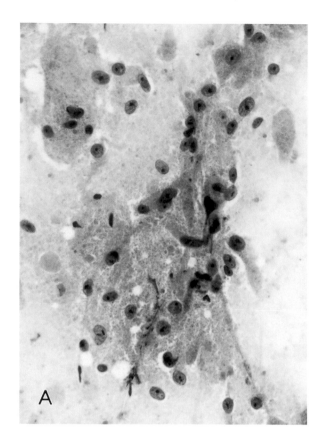

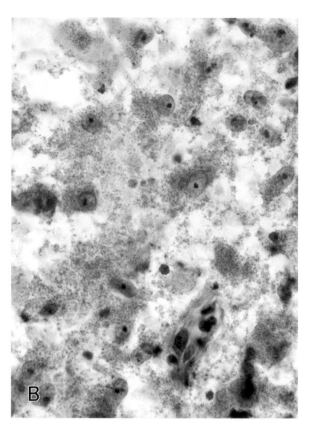

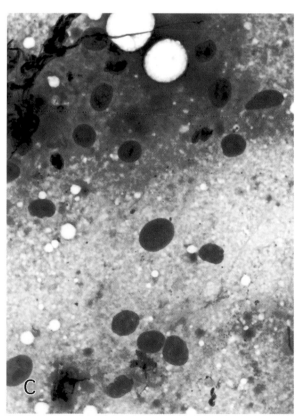

Figure 12-34

GRANULAR CELL TUMOR

A,B: A cellular syncytium displays easily recognizable coarse cytoplasmic granules both intracellularly and extracellularly (Papanicolaou stain).

C: Granularity is imperceptible. Discrete, enlarged nucleoli are seen with both preparations (Romanowsky stain).

high cellularity, with a paucicellular sclerosing variant (82). Discrete microfragments of slight myxoid stroma lacking an obvious vascular pattern contain small spindled cells in a loose, random arrangement with dispersed bare nuclei. Fragments of mature adipose tissue and singly scattered lipocytes are also present. The cells have elongated or oval pale nuclei of uniform size with smooth nuclear contours, evenly dispersed chromatin, and indistinct nucleoli. Only a small amount of finely granular cytoplasm is present, however, cytoplasmic processes are often lengthy and coiled (fig. 12-35). Smears lack background necrosis and cytologically atypical cells (82,83).

The myxofibrillar nature of the cell microaggregates is similar to that seen in benign nerve sheath tumors, but the serpentine contour of the cell nuclei of schwannoma/neurofibroma is absent. Nonetheless, immunochemistry is needed for a definite diagnosis.

Malignant Peripheral Nerve Sheath Tumor

The principal cytologic feature of *malignant peripheral nerve sheath tumor* (MPNST) is marked spindle cell hypercellularity arranged in aggregates and as single forms. Pale and hyperchromatic spindle cells show variable anisonucleosis of serpentine, rounded, and oval nuclei, depending on tumor differentiation (84,85). Well-differentiated MPNST aspirates show similar-sized nuclei with overlapping and slight to moderate contour irregularity, but not the accentuated serpiginous shapes seen in most examples of neurofibroma. This undulating nuclear quality is replaced in poorly differentiated examples with nucleomegaly, multinucleation, and obvious pleomorphism. The nuclear to cytoplasmic ratio is high and the cell cytoplasm is nonvacuolated (86). The nucleoli are indistinct in well-differentiated examples, but visible in less differentiated examples (fig. 12-36). Mitotic figures, individual cell necrosis, and the cytopathologic features described for undifferentiated pleomorphic sarcoma are seen in high-grade MPNST.

From a purely morphologic standpoint, MPNST closely mimics monophasic synovial sarcoma and other spindle and pleomorphic sarcomas, and without immunophenotyping a specific diagnosis is reached in less than 50 percent of cases (84,86). Knowledge that the neoplasm has arisen from a nerve or in a patient with neurofibromatosis 1 (NF1) is the most useful piece of information to allow for a specific diagnosis.

VASCULAR TUMORS

Lymphangioma

Aspirates of *lymphangioma* yield translucent, straw-colored fluid unless contaminated by blood, and thus are best submitted for cytocentrifugation rather than conventional smears. Lymphangioma is more common in infants and children, but occasionally seen in adults. The number of cells is variable, and consists almost entirely of small mature lymphocytes, with a fraction of centrocytes, centroblasts, and histiocytes set in a clean or proteinaceous background (fig. 12-37) (87). Unlike branchial cleft cyst or epidermal inclusion cyst, lymphangioma lacks any cells with squamous differentiation.

Hemangioma

Most aspirates of *hemangioma* result in the procurement of blood but few if any cells, resulting in a nondiagnostic smear. Since the FNA technique rarely is able to capture an intact vessel larger than a capillary, it is not used to recognize the multitude of histologic variants of hemangioma (capillary, cavernous, arteriovenous, spindle cell, epithelioid, glomeruloid). The mere presence of capillaries is not diagnostic of hemangioma.

Because of their tightly packed nature and minute lumens, aspirates of juvenile capillary hemangiomas may result in cellular aspirates composed of small rounded and polygonal cells with high nuclear to cytoplasmic ratios (88). These may be so cellular, particularly in newborns and young infants, that the potential exists to confuse these with malignant small round cell tumors of childhood. Intramuscular and spindle cell hemangiomas may contain bland polygonal and spindle cells with unipolar and bipolar cytoplasmic processes, smooth nuclei, and small nucleoli resembling reactive fibroblasts in a smear rich with blood (fig. 12-38) (89).

Angiosarcoma

Conventional *angiosarcoma* varies in cellularity. This is often dependent on the amount of blood aspirated, which does not correlate with

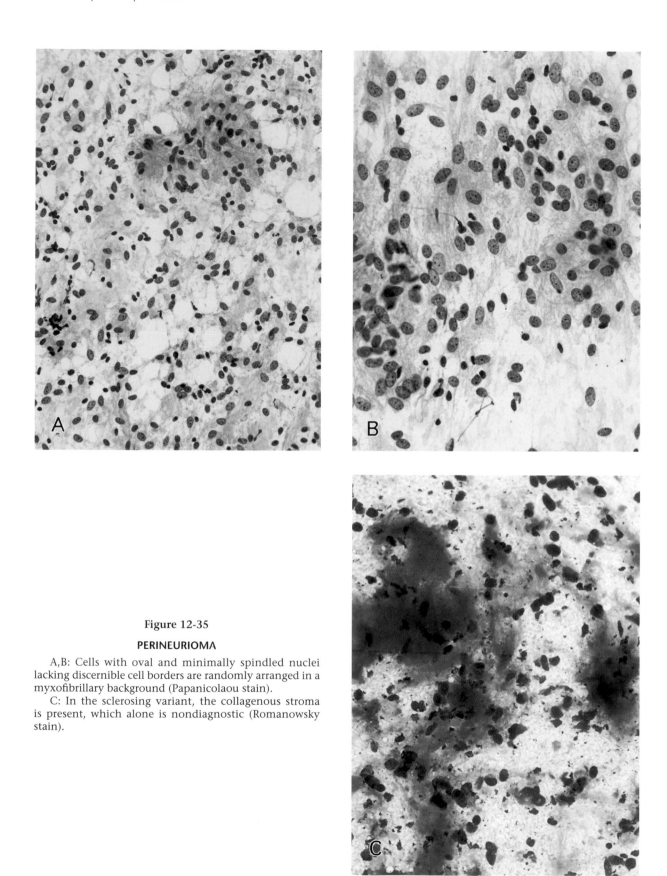

Figure 12-35

PERINEURIOMA

A,B: Cells with oval and minimally spindled nuclei lacking discernible cell borders are randomly arranged in a myxofibrillary background (Papanicolaou stain).

C: In the sclerosing variant, the collagenous stroma is present, which alone is nondiagnostic (Romanowsky stain).

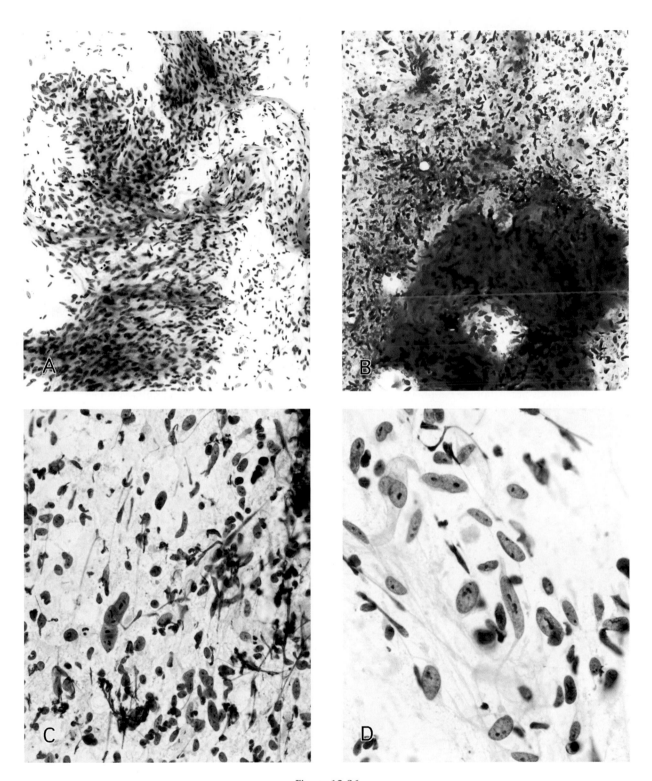

Figure 12-36

MALIGNANT PERIPHERAL NERVE SHEATH TUMOR

A,B: Hypercellular 3-dimensional microfragments are surrounded by dissociated bland-appearing spindle cells.

C,D: Randomly scattered abnormally enlarged cells retain their spindle configuration and cytoplasmic processes but exhibit coarse chromatin and enlarged misshapen nucleoli (A,C,D: Papanicolaou stain; B: Romanowsky stain).

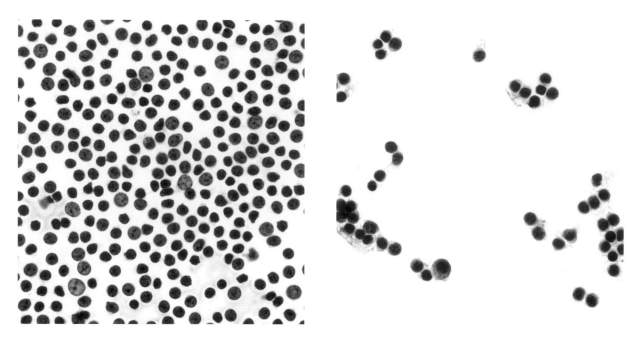

Figure 12-37

LYMPHANGIOMA

A heterogenous population of lymphocytes is present. The cellularity in these two examples is varied (left, right: Romanowsky stain).

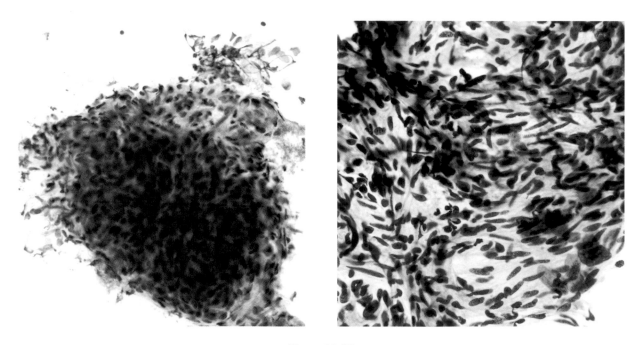

Figure 12-38

HEMANGIOMA

Left: An intramuscular hemangioma shows a nodule of spindle cells, presumably fibroblasts and endothelial cells, in a bloody aspirate.

Right: This spindle cell hemangioma had only a few clusters of uniform spindle cells. Most of the smears in both examples contained blood only (left, right: Papanicolaou stain).

any specific soft tissue neoplasm. Paucicellular smears are common due to the bloody dilution of diagnostic cells (90–92). A heterogeneous-appearing spindle and polygonal cell population is sorted into tight 3-dimensional aggregates, loosely cohesive groups, and single cells. The nuclei show moderate to marked anisonucleosis and coarse chromatin with variable number and size of nucleoli, and vary from fusiform to oval and rounded (fig. 12-39A,B) (91,93). Multinucleated giant cells may be seen.

The cell cytoplasm is usually modest and finely granular, with occasional hemosiderin deposits and microvacuoles. The morphologic features suggesting vascular formation, such as intracytoplasmic vacuoles with or without red cells, erythrophagocytosis, or microacinar formation, are unusual and nonspecific. Of course, anastomosing vascular channels are not appreciated in smears. Necrosis and background inflammatory cells, particularly neutrophils, are variable and may be absent (90,92).

The epithelioid variant has large, relatively monotonous cells arranged singly, or less frequently, in loose clusters. The presence of polygonal shapes with a large amount of finely granular cytoplasm, occasional binucleation, and single nucleoli is the dominant feature in this variant; spindle cells are infrequent (fig. 12-39C). Some cells contain delicate "bleb-like" cytoplasmic vacuoles, and some have a "rhabdoid" appearance (92).

Epithelioid hemangioendothelioma is easily confused with epithelioid angiosarcoma (fig. 12-40) (94). Epithelioid hemangioma, in contrast, typically contains a heavy infiltrate of lymphocytes and eosinophils. Because of the nonspecificity of angiosarcoma aspirates and the inability to reliably identify an anastomosing vascular pattern, a specific diagnosis requires either immunochemical confirmation using a cell block or a separate tissue biopsy.

MYXOID AND CHONDRO-OSSEOUS TUMORS AND TUMOR-LIKE LESIONS

Intramuscular Myxoma/Soft Tissue Ganglion/Juxta-articular Myxoma

Intramuscular myxoma, soft tissue ganglion, and *juxta-articular myxoma* are described together since their cytopathology is almost identical,

with a few exceptions (95,95a). The gross appearance in nearly all aspirates is that of viscous, gelatinous material with the texture and stringy quality of egg whites. In most cases it is clear but can be light yellow, and the material has a tendency of to plug the needle (95–97). This tacky material spreads like clear film with a glossy finish. The R-stain nearly always produces a slide in which the material is easily visible to the naked eye, and varies from light lavender to a vibrant magenta depending on the thickness of the material. Smears contain a copious amount of myxoid stroma that is semitransparent rather than opaque. This finely granular matrix smears as a smooth film that often folds over itself in a pleated fashion. In Papanicolaou-stained smears the stroma may show "cracking" artifact. Only small clusters or widely scattered mucinous macrophages exist in this matrix (fig. 12-41). These display a rounded smoothly contoured nucleus, no visible nucleolus, and sometimes, fine vacuolation. Delicate wisps of cytoplasm give some cells a spindle or stellate configuration. No cytologic atypia, multinucleated giant cells, mitotic figures, or cellular necrosis is present.

In addition to a myxoid stroma and muciphages, aspirates of intramuscular myxoma contain strips of benign skeletal muscle, occasional aggregates of mature adipose tissue, and bland isomorphic spindle cells (95,97). The ability to appreciate the lobular character of intramuscular myxoma, evaluate its border with surrounding skeletal muscle, identify the presence of cysts or the subtle (usually delicate) collagenous fibers that intermingle with the copious stroma, all features seen in a tissue section, is not possible with smears.

Myositis Ossificans

Due to its bony matrix, the FNA of *myositis ossificans* may feel gritty during the actual procedure, and a bony shell may prevent a satisfactory number of cells for interpretation. The zonation phenomenon seen in histologic specimens is absent. Aspirates are of variable cellularity: most are moderately cellular, with cells scattered mainly as single cells and fewer as loose clusters. Most cells are embedded in irregular clumps of dense metachromatic-staining stroma that varies in size and typically has a fibrillar, indistinct border (98,99).

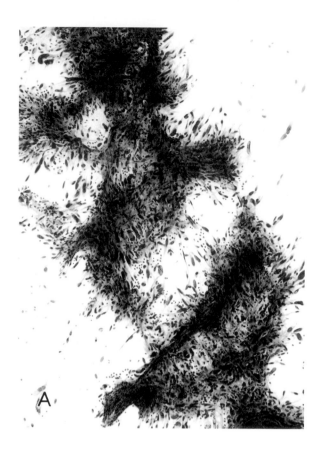

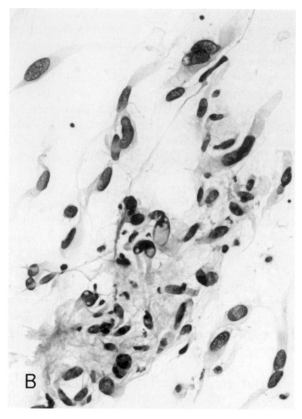

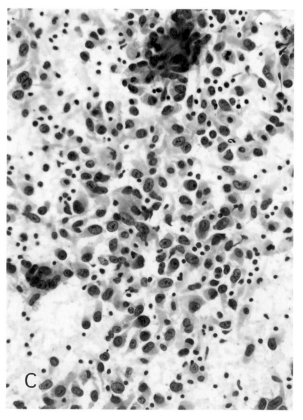

Figure 12-39

ANGIOSARCOMA

A,B: Hypercellular clusters and singly dispersed spindled/ pleomorphic cells are indistinguishable from a high-grade undifferentiated pleomorphic sarcoma.

C: The polygonal cells of the epithelioid variant are of similar size, with minimal anisonucleosis and discrete nucleoli (Papanicolaou stain).

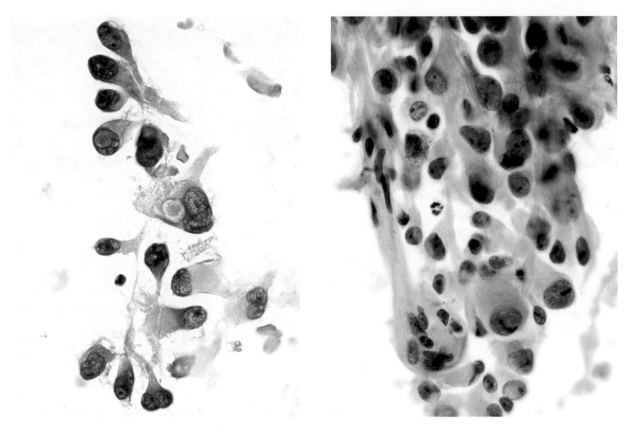

Figure 12-40

EPITHELIOID HEMANGIOENDOTHELIOMA COMPARED TO EPITHELIOID ANGIOSARCOMA

Both epithelioid hemangioendothelioma (left) and epithelioid angiosarcoma (right) show enlarged primarily epithelioid cells and some spindle cells with large rounded nuclei and abundant cytoplasm. The intranuclear inclusion and intracytoplasmic vacuole in the image of epithelioid hemangioendothelioma although suggestive, are not pathognomonic (left, right: Papanicolaou stain).

The cells are round to oval, with short cytoplasmic tapering and a feathery edge. They often display osteoblast-like features, having eccentrically placed bland, euchromic nuclei, single sometimes enlarged nucleoli, and a perinuclear zone of cytoplasmic clearing (fig. 12-42) (100). Multinucleated cells are uncommon.

Radiographic imaging is extremely helpful for diagnosing this lesion. The gritty character of myositis ossificans is unusual in other pseudosarcomatous soft tissue masses. The opaque nature of the background stroma should not to be confused with the more transparent myxoid background of nodular fasciitis or myxoid neoplasms.

Extraskeletal Myxoid Chondrosarcoma

Aspirates of *extraskeletal myxoid chondrosarcoma* have a background of thin to opaque myxoid/chondromyxoid stroma that is most obvious in R-stained slides where it appears as a dark magenta; it also visible, however muted, in P-stained smears (101–104). In most cases, the stroma is a solid film, but also exists as discrete inspissated fragments that may have a frayed, fibrillar or smooth edge. The cellularity ranges from very high to large stroma-only hypocellular zones. The multilobulated pattern that is present in tissue sections is absent in smears, but the arrangement of cells into solitary linear and intersecting lace-like cords of one to several cells in thickness or as flat aggregates imitates the histologic pattern.

In some smears, the cell clusters have rounded lobular or ball-like shapes, with sharp cell borders, whereas in others, the cells loosely trail away from the cluster center as single cells. Monotony is the rule, with cells having rounded and oval shapes with a minor population of spindle cells.

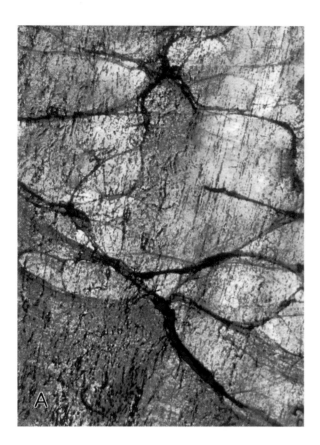

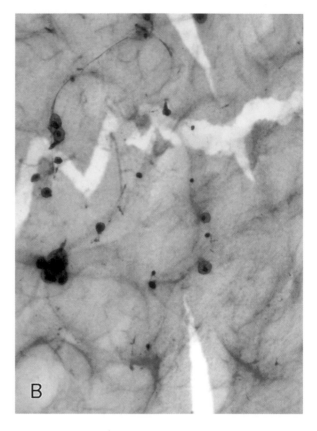

Figure 12-41

MYXOMA

A: An almost acellular smear contains folds and pleats of copious myxoid stroma (Romanowsky stain).

B: Single muciphages are scattered within the stroma, which may exhibit artificial cracking due to its thickness (Papanicolaou stain).

C: Pieces of normal skeletal muscle are surrounded by stroma in this intramuscular example (Papanicolaou stain).

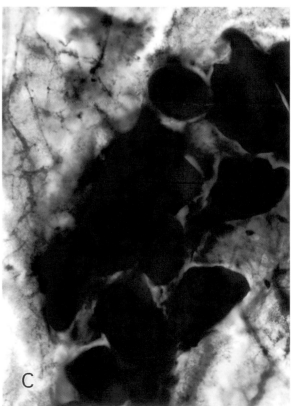

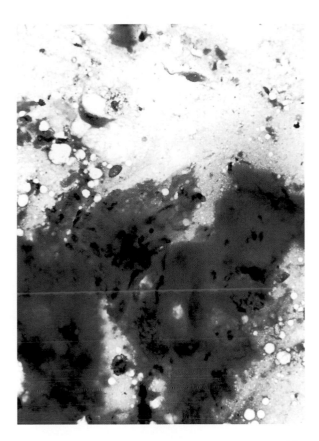 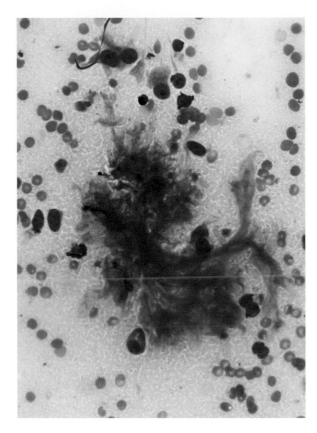

Figure 12-42

MYOSITIS OSSIFICANS

Left: A thick osteocollagenous stromal fragment is infiltrated and surrounded by banal spindle cells.
Right: A more delicate fibrillar piece of stroma is mixed with osteoblast-like cells (left, right: Romanowsky stain).

The cell nuclei show evenly dispersed chromatin, a modest amount of cytoplasm (sometimes semitransparent with a Papanicolaou stain), and nucleoli that range from barely discernible to large (fig. 12-43). Nuclear grooves and intranuclear inclusions are infrequent. Cytoplasmic vacuoles are rare, and are sometimes seen in a perinuclear fashion creating a "lacunar" appearance. Slides are devoid of necrosis, inflammation, and obvious vascularity. FISH testing for the *EWSR1* gene rearrangement has been successfully applied to FNA specimens, allowing for an unequivocally specific diagnosis (101).

Chordoma

Although a tumor of bone, FNA of *chordoma* usually is done for a soft tissue mass, particularly a mass in the paraspinal region or buttock. Air-dried, R-stained slides highlight a copious, brightly colored myxoid stroma that sometimes is so thick and abundant that it obscures cells. The opaque and fibrillar stroma interdigitates and weaves between individual cells and among groups of cells that show moderate to marked anisonucleosis (53,105). The cells are in lobulated tight clusters, isolated single forms, or, sometimes, in incompletely formed trabecular cords.

The most common cell type has a single rounded or polygonal nucleus, an obvious nucleolus, and a moderate amount of cytoplasm (fig. 12-44). Nuclear pleomorphism, binucleation, multinucleation, intranuclear cytoplasmic inclusions, and cytoplasmic vacuoles are common (106). Small nonvacuolated cells are interspersed among these larger ones. It is common to see cells embedded within discrete fragments of stroma that obscure their cytoplasmic characteristics. Physaliphorous cells, characterized by one or several nuclei surrounded by large coarse cytoplasmic vacuoles at

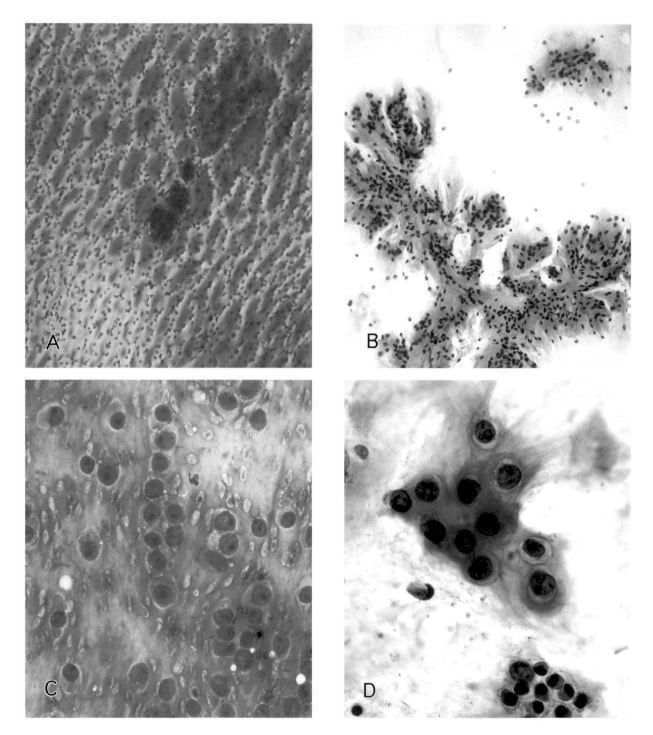

Figure 12-43

EXTRASKELETAL MYXOID CHONDROSARCOMA

A: Small tight clusters of rounded cells are set in an abundant myxoid stroma (Romanowsky stain).

B: The cells are arranged in short branching cords with less noticeable and more fibrillar stroma (Papanicolaou stain).

C: Haphazardly dispersed as well as linear profiles of epithelioid cells exhibit single, slightly enlarged nucleoli (Romanowsky stain).

D: Rounded cells with circumferential lightly stained cytoplasm and distinct borders are set in chondromyxoid stroma, imparting a "lacunar" look to the image (Papanicolaou stain).

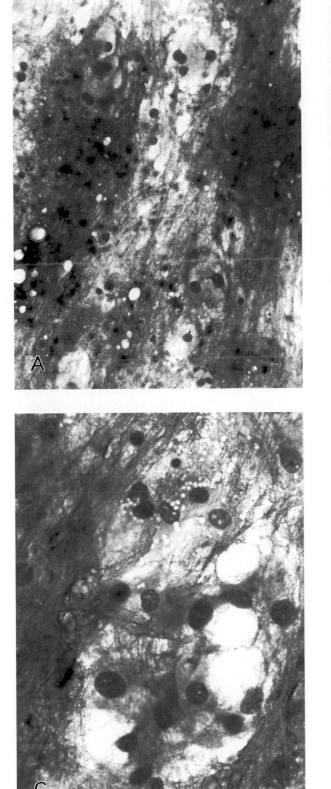

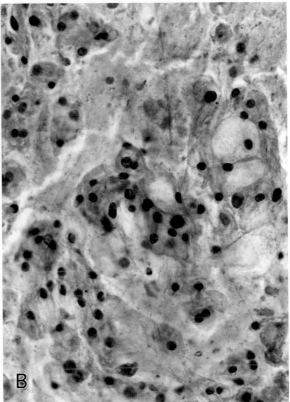

Figure 12-44

CHORDOMA

A: Large cells are partially hidden by a copious myxoid stroma (Romanowsky stain).

B: Cells in vague lobules and having enormous amounts of cytoplasm create a low nuclear to cytoplasmic ratio. Rounded nuclei and multiple nuclei per cell are common (Papanicolaou stain).

C: Common also are multiple small vacuoles per cell and single large univacuolated cells (Papanicolaou stain).

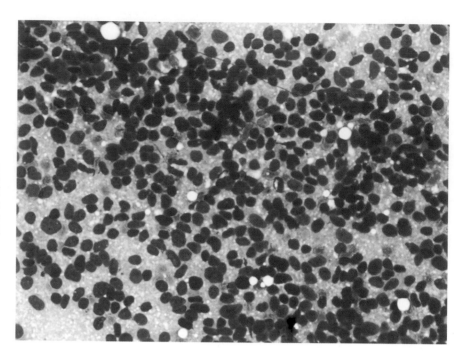

Figure 12-45

MESENCHYMAL CHONDROSARCOMA

Rounded and oval cells with meager cytoplasm are arranged in a solid sheet. The absence of a chondroid stroma precludes a diagnosis from this image, which is typical of a malignant small round cell tumor (Romanowsky stain).

the cell periphery, are large and not particularly common in some series (107), but this may be a function of not using R-stained smears (106).

Extraskeletal Mesenchymal Chondrosarcoma

Due to the paucity of differentiated chondroid foci, aspirates of *mesenchymal chondrosarcoma* are populated primarily by cells typical of the malignant small round cell tumor category. Highly cellular smears contain compact clusters and single cells. Cells have a minimum amount of cytoplasm, rounded to oval nuclei, finely granular chromatin, and indistinct nucleoli (fig. 12-45). When present, a metachromatic staining matrix is a clue to the correct diagnosis (108). Like Ewing sarcoma, a second population of degenerating cells having smaller pyknotic, markedly hyperchromatic nuclei is often present.

UNCLASSIFIED AND MISCELLANEOUS SOFT TISSUE TUMORS

Synovial Sarcoma

On a case-by-case basis, most spindle cell sarcomas are not separable from one another using conventional smears alone, and thus require accompanying ancillary immunophenotyping, cytogenetic analysis, or FISH for a specific diagnosis. In contrast, aspiration cytopathology is generally an excellent method for confirming specific locally recurrent and/or metastatic spindle cell sarcomas.

Synovial sarcoma serves as a paradigm for spindle cell malignancies characterized by cell monotony. FNA slides contain a rich cell yield dispersed as single cells and in thick, tightly aggregated clusters having multiple cell layers that may be so thick that individual cells cannot be seen within these aggregates (fig. 12-46A–D) (109–111).

The cells are uniform, rounded to spindle-shaped and intermediate-sized, with oval to oblong monotonous nuclei. These have evenly dispersed chromatin, inconspicuous to absent nucleoli, and smooth contours combined with scant nonvacuolated cytoplasm. Although some have described the nuclei as hyperchromatic, this is not necessarily the case in R- or P-stained smears. Stripped nuclei are common and unless a necrotic focus is seen, there is minimal background stroma. A background vascular network is appreciated in a minority of cases.

The biphasic variant of synovial sarcoma (gland formation) is difficult to appreciate on smears since these glandular structures, which remain intact in tissue sections, are often disrupted by the FNA technique. Nonetheless, an acinar arrangement of cells with nuclear palisading is suggestive of the biphasic form (fig. 12-46E,F). Mitoses are less commonly seen in aspirates or smears than in tissue sections.

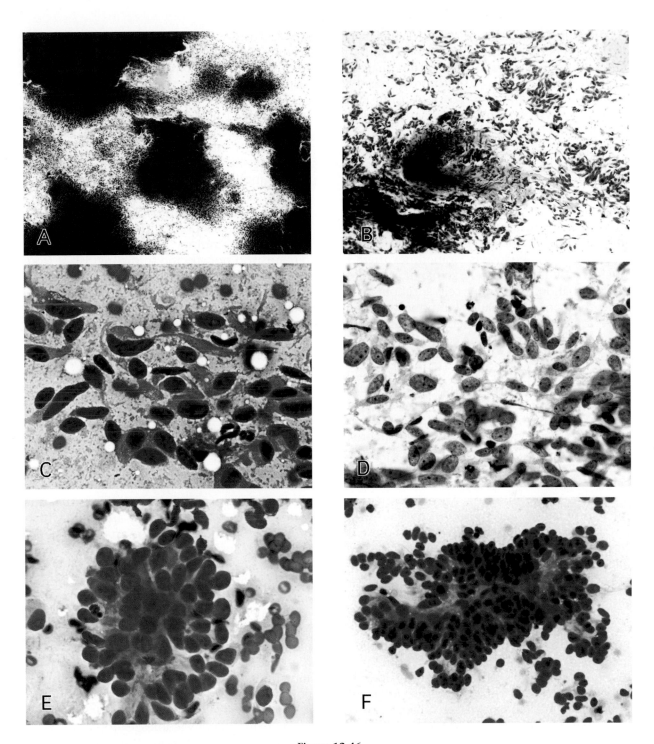

Figure 12-46

SYNOVIAL SARCOMA

A: Many thick, hypercellular, 3-dimensional fragments are seen. This degree of cellularity is nearly always indicative of a malignant process (Papanicolaou stain).

B: Cells have a monotonous spindle shape and are in clusters and single forms (Papanicolaou stain).

C,D: Oval and spindled nuclei display both smooth and irregular contours with small almost indistinct nucleoli (C: Papanicolaou stain; D: Romanowsky stain).

E,F: Biphasic synovial sarcoma with a glandular arrangement (E,F: Romanowsky stain).

The differential diagnosis includes malignant peripheral nerve sheath tumor, cellular solitary fibrous tumor, low-grade leiomyosarcoma, and the rare fibrosarcoma. A specific diagnosis of synovial sarcoma is now possible using FISH for the synovial sarcoma translocation in FNA specimens (112,113).

Extraosseous Ewing Sarcoma/Primitive Neuroectodermal Tumor Family

As expected for nearly all neoplasms that fall into the malignant small round cell tumor category, *Ewing sarcoma* has highly cellular aspirates that contain single isolated cells with a minority in loose clusters. Sometimes there is nuclear molding, and rarely, acinar or pseudorosette formation. Isomorphic cells are about 2 to 3 times the diameter of mature lymphocytes. These have rounded to oval nuclei, evenly dispersed chromatin, indistinct nucleoli, and minimal visible cytoplasm (114). Cytoplasmic vacuoles or blebs are variably present (fig. 12-47). In a logistic regression analysis study of small round cell neoplasms (115), cytoplasmic vacuolization and scant cytoplasm were the most helpful features in the identification of Ewing sarcoma. Bare nuclei are common, but binucleated or multinucleated cells are rare (116). Due to high cell turnover, a second population of smaller apoptotic cells exhibiting various degrees of nuclear pyknosis, and hyperchromasia is present. If enough cytoplasmic glycogen is present, the smear background may show a lacy "tigroid" background. When cells with this morphology are positive for the t(11:22)(q24;q12) translocation, a specific diagnosis is possible (40).

A wide differential diagnosis accompanies any case of putative Ewing sarcoma due to its primitive, undifferentiated morphology. Entities to consider include rhabdomyosarcoma, desmoplastic small round cell tumor, blastic forms of non-Hodgkin lymphoma, mesenchymal chondrosarcoma, and poorly differentiated synovial sarcoma. Only with the application of ancillary immunochemistry, FISH, cytogenetics, and/or flow cytometry are these other entities distinguished.

Epithelioid Sarcoma

Most reports of *epithelioid sarcoma* describe moderate to highly cellular smears with single cells, loosely clustered cells, and tight 3-dimen-sional clusters, but with no particular pattern. Despite its name, epithelioid cells are mixed with spindle cells having pale cytoplasmic tails, and occasional pale perinuclear zones cells (117). The nuclear shapes range from monomorphic rounded nuclei to more anaplastic forms with misshapen macronucleoli (118); these are mixed with mitotic figures and, sometimes, multinucleated cells. These pleomorphic cells have a moderate to copious amount of dense cytoplasm (fig. 12-48). When the necrotic zones are aspirated, the smear background shows degenerating neutrophils and cellular debris.

The cytopathology of epithelioid sarcoma remains too nonspecific to distinguish it from epithelioid variants of malignant peripheral nerve sheath tumor, metastatic carcinoma, melanoma, leiomyosarcoma, and angiosarcoma that may mimic this neoplasm (79). Immunophenotyping is required to separate these other neoplasms. Unlike tissue specimens, however, where a benign granulomatous process may be confused with epithelioid sarcoma, this is not the case cytologically (119). The nodular pattern of epithelioid sarcoma seen in tissue is missing from aspirate smears, as is a zonal phenomenon.

Alveolar Soft Part Sarcoma

Smears of *alveolar soft part sarcoma* are variably cellular, but may be very hypocellular due to the bloody nature of many aspirates, which dilutes the smear. The cells are arranged in loose syncytial groups as well as single forms, but not in thick 3-dimensional clusters as is typical of many sarcomas with an epithelioid morphology. Only rarely are cells in a pseudoalveolar or acinar arrangement as discerned in tissue. Cell fragility is common, and leads to cytoplasmic detachment resulting in many large, rounded, bare nuclei in an amorphous granular, sometimes striated, background. When intact, polygonal cells harbor an enormous amount of fine to coarsely granular cytoplasm with a variable number of vacuoles. Cytoplasmic clear cell change is uncommon (120). The large nuclei are nearly always rounded and smoothly surfaced, but of similar size and contain easily visible single circular macronucleoli (fig. 12-49). These are placed centrally or eccentrically within the cell, and may be coupled with mirror-image nuclei. Fibrillar metachromatic

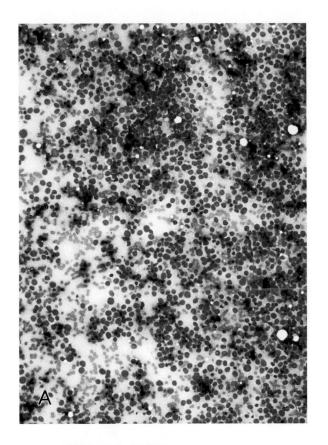

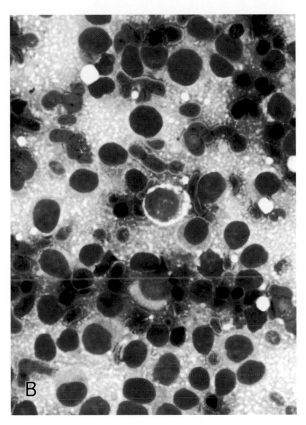

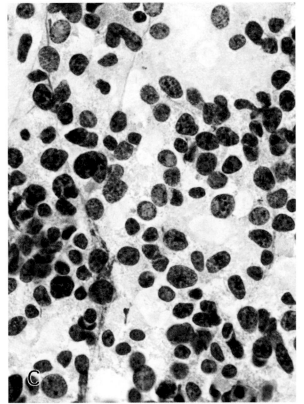

Figure 12-47

EWING SARCOMA

A: A monotonous sheet of malignant small rounded cells is indistinguishable from mesenchymal chondrosarcoma (see fig. 12-45) and rhabdomyosarcoma (see fig. 12-31) (Romanowsky stain).

B,C: The fine cytoplasmic vacuoles sometimes seen in this R-stained smear are lost in Papanicolaou-stained preparations (C). A delicate lace-like cytoplasmic network in seen in B.

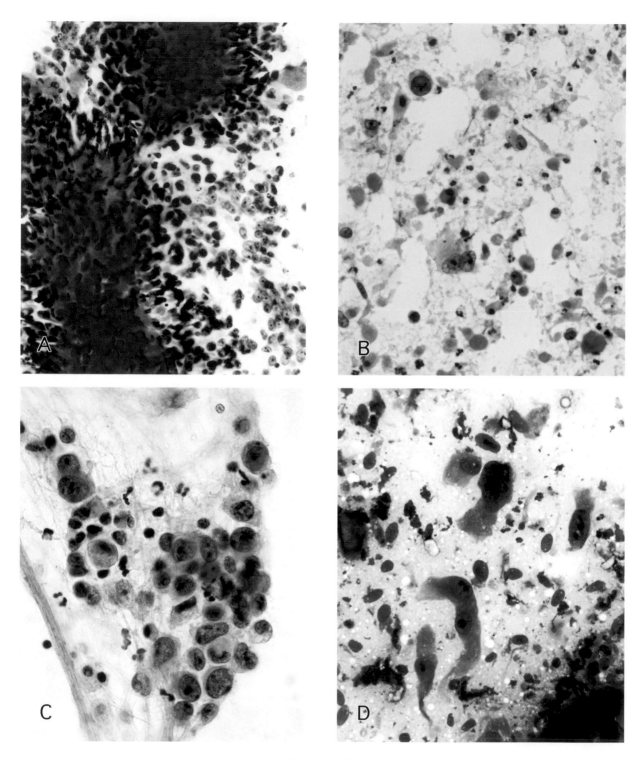

Figure 12-48

EPITHELIOID SARCOMA

A: There is a hypercellular 3-dimensional fragment of epithelioid cells.
B: Some epithelioid cells have mirror-image nuclei; background necrotic cell debris is present.
C: Epithelioid cells imitate those of other sarcomas with an epithelioid morphology.
D: Anaplastic cells with macronucleoli are common (Papanicolaou stain except D).

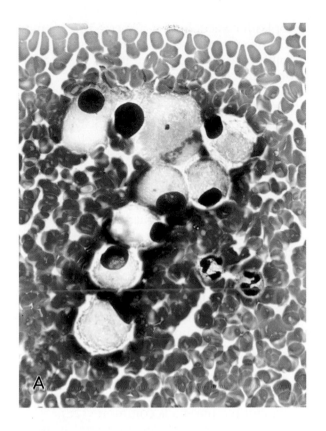

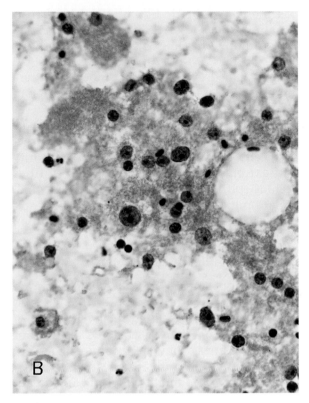

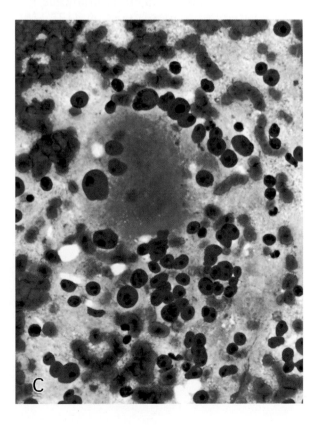

Figure 12-49

ALVEOLAR SOFT PART SARCOMA

A,B: Due to cell fragility, bare nuclei are scattered within a granular or striated background (A: Papanicolaou stain; B: Romanowsky stain).

C: A markedly enlarged single nucleolus (Romanowsky stain).

basement membrane-like material is seen in R-stained slides (121,122). Mitotic figures are uncommon. The cells may contain periodic acid–Schiff (PAS)-positive, diastase-resistant needle-shaped cytoplasmic crystals, but these are typically less obvious and infrequently observed in aspirates.

The differential diagnosis includes any sarcoma or nonsarcomatous neoplasm with epithelioid cells that demonstrate relative uniformity and extremely large nucleoli. Major entities include epithelioid sarcoma, clear cell sarcoma, melanoma, paraganglioma, metastatic carcinoma (especially clear cell renal carcinoma), and granular cell tumor.

Clear Cell Sarcoma

Aspiration smears of *clear cell sarcoma* are highly cellular, with cells scattered singly and in loose groups. The cells are relatively monotonous epithelioid forms with some fusiform or reniform shapes. They are intermediate-sized, with fine nuclear chromatin, a single enlarged nucleolus or 2 to 3 smaller nucleoli, and eccentric nuclear placement producing a plasmacytic appearance in many. Little variation in nuclear size is appreciated and the nuclear contours are smooth. A moderate amount of finely granular, pale cytoplasm with well-defined cell borders may contain small and large vacuoles (fig. 12-50). Melanin pigment is rare (123–125). Binucleated and multinucleated cells are seen, but it is rare to find osteoclast-type giant cells with more than 10 nuclei per cell. The smear background is usually clean, but cases with cytoplasmic vacuoles may exhibit a lacy, frothy appearance reminiscent of the "tigroid" background seen in seminoma and other neoplasms containing glycogen-filled cytoplasm. The pseudoalveolar pattern recognizable in tissue sections is lost in smears.

The epithelioid variant of malignant melanoma is the entity most easily confused with clear cell sarcoma. Melanoma, however, usually displays a much greater degree of cellular anaplasia, with more frequent mirror-image nuclei and intranuclear inclusions. Both may display cytoplasmic vacuoles, be dispersed in a single cell (dissociated) pattern, and be amelanotic. Pleomorphic giant cells are much more common in melanoma smears.

Clear cell sarcoma may be confused with giant cell tumor of tendon sheath. The single cell pattern of bland cells with spherical nuclei is common to both. The differences include larger, more obvious nucleoli in clear cell sarcoma, and more numerous multinucleated giant cells with greater than 5 nuclei per cell in giant cell tumor of tendon sheath. Granular cell tumor differs by having much coarser cytoplasm and lacking the vacuoles and discrete cell membranes that are common to clear cell sarcoma.

Metastatic Malignant Melanoma

Metastatic malignant melanoma mimics the entire spectrum of soft tissue cytology, including spindle cell, epithelioid, signet ring cell, small cell, and pleomorphic tumors. Smears are highly cellular, with cells more often individually dispersed, but also in loose aggregates. A pure dissociated cell pattern mirroring that seen in malignant lymphoma is common (126).

The most frequently encountered form of melanoma is composed of epithelioid cells, but a wide variety of shapes is possible (127,128). The characteristic "cytomorphologic signature" of epithelioid melanoma includes eccentric (plasmacytoid) nuclear positioning, mirror-image binucleation/multinucleation, macronucleoli, and one or more intranuclear cytoplasmic inclusions. Spindle cell nuclei may display moderate to marked nuclear pleomorphism or appear cytologically bland and monotonous. Most cells have a moderate to sometimes abundant amount of finely granular cytoplasm, which may be vacuolated. Pigment varies from absent, to a fine cytoplasmic stippling, to large coarse deposits.

With a clinical history, a diagnosis of metastatic melanoma is generally made with little difficulty because of the aforementioned cytomorphology. Melanin, of course, when present in the malignant cells, is diagnostic.

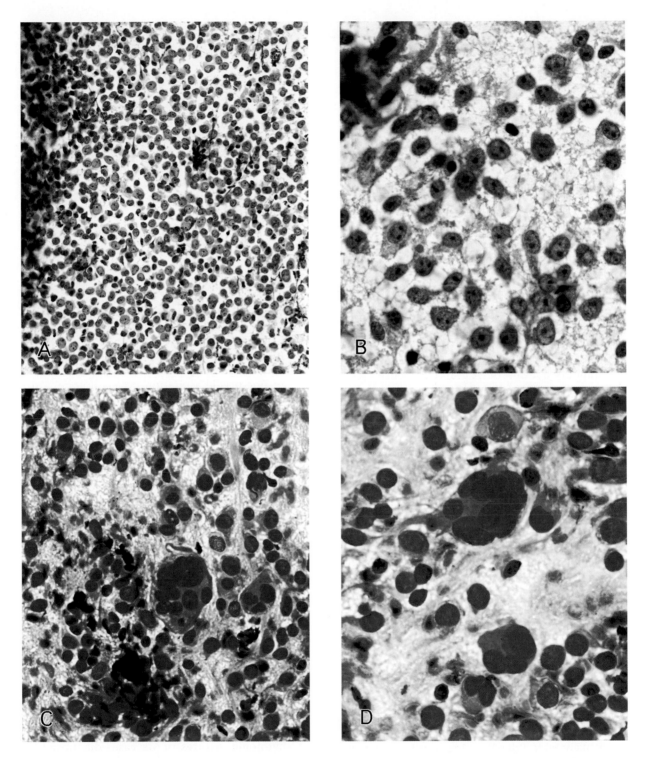

Figure 12-50

CLEAR CELL SARCOMA

A: There is a monolayer of plasmacytoid-appearing cells with single visible nucleoli and no background stroma (Papanicolaou stain).

B: Macronucleolated cells have an epithelioid quality; cytoplasmic clearing is rare (Romanowsky stain).

C,D: Scattered multinucleated cells may be misinterpreted as giant cell tumor of tendon sheath (C,D: Romanowsky stain).

REFERENCES

Introduction

1. Kasraeian S, Allison DC, Ahlmann ER, Fedenko AN, Menendez LR. A comparison of fine-needle aspiration, core biopsy, and surgical biopsy in the diagnosis of extremity soft tissue masses. Clin Orthop Relat Res 2010;468:2992-3002.
2. Ng VY, Thomas K, Crist, M, Wakely PE Jr, Mayerson J. Fine needle aspiration for clinical triage of extremity soft tissue masses. Clin Orthop Relat Res 2010;468:1120-1128.
3. Qian X. Soft Tissue. In: Cibas ES, Ducatman BS, eds. Cytology: diagnostic principles and clinical correlates, 3nd ed. Philadelphia, Saunders Elsevier; 2009:452.
4. Akerman M, Rydholm A, Persson BM. Aspiration cytology of soft-tissue tumors. The 10-year experience at an orthopedic oncology center. Acta Orthop Scand 1985;56:407-412.
5. Willen H, Akerman M, Carlen B. Fine needle aspiration (FNA) in the diagnosis of soft tissue tumours: a review of 22 years experience. Cytopathology 1995;6:236-247.
6. González-Cámpora R. Fine needle aspiration cytology of soft tissue tumors. Acta Cytol 2000;44:337-343.
7. Wakely PE Jr, Kneisl JS. Soft tissue aspiration cytopathology. Cancer 2000;90:292-298.
8. Kilpatrick SE, Ward WG, Cappellari JO, Bos GD. Fine-needle aspiration biopsy of soft tissue sarcomas. A cytomorphologic analysis with emphasis on histologic subtyping, grading, and therapeutic significance. Am J Clin Pathol 1999;112:179–188.
9. Khalbuss WE, Teot LA, Monaco SE. Diagnostic accuracy and limitations of fine-needle aspiration cytology of bone and soft tissue lesions: a review of 1114 cases with cytological-histological correlation. Cancer 2010;118:24–32.
10. Palmer HE, Mukunyadzi P, Culbreth W, Thomas JR. Subgrouping and grading of soft-tissue sarcomas by fine-needle aspiration cytology: a histopathologic correlation study. Diagn Cytopathol 2001;24:307-316.

Fibroblastic, Myofibroblastic, and Fibrohistiocytic Tumors

11. Wakely PE Jr, Price WG, Frable WJ. Sternomastoid tumor of infancy (fibromatosis colli): diagnosis by aspiration cytology. Mod Pathol 1989;2:378-381.
12. Owens CL, Sharma R, Ali SZ. Deep fibromatosis (desmoid tumor): cytopathologic characteristics, clinicoradiologic features, and immunohisto-chemical findings on fine-needle aspiration. Cancer 2007;111:166-172.
13. Sharma S, Mishra K, Khanna G. Fibromatosis colli in infants. A cytologic study of eight cases. Acta Cytol 2003;47:359-362.
14. Dalén BP, Meis-Kindblom JM, Sumathi VP, Ryd W, Kindblom LG. Fine-needle aspiration cytology and core needle biopsy in the preoperative diagnosis of desmoid tumors. Acta Orthop 2006;77:926-931.
15. Wong NL, Di F. Pseudosarcomatous fasciitis and myositis; diagnosis by fine-needle aspiration cytology. Am J Clin Pathol 2009;132:857-865.
16. Dahl I, Åkerman M. Nodular fasciitis: a correlative cytologic and histologic study of 13 cases. Acta Cytol 1981;25:215-223.
17. Wong NL. Fine needle aspiration cytology of pseudosarcomatous reactive proliferative lesions of soft tissue. Acta Cytol 2002;46:1049-1055.
18. Plaza JA, Mayerson J, Wakely PE Jr. Nodular fasciitis of the hand: a potential diagnostic pitfall in fine-needle aspiration cytopathology. Am J Clin Pathol 2005:123:388-393.
19. Stanley MW, Skoog L, Tani EM, Horwitz CA. Nodular fasciitis: spontaneous resolution following diagnosis by fine-needle aspiration. Diagn Cytopathol 1993;9:322-324.
20. Vera-Alvarez J, García-Prats MD, Marigil-Gómez M, Abascal-Agorreta M, López-López JI. Elastofibroma dorsi diagnosed by fine needle aspiration cytology. Acta Cytol 2008;52:264-266.
21. Domanski HA, Carlén B, Sloth M, Rydholm A. Elastofibroma dorsi has distinct cytomorphologic features, making diagnostic surgical biopsy unnecessary: cytomorphologic study with clinical, radiologic, and electron microscopic correlations. Diagn Cytopathol 2003;29:327-333.
22. Pisharodi LR, Cary D, Bernacki EG Jr. Elastofibroma dorsi: diagnostic problems and pitfalls. Diagn Cytopathol 1994;10:242-244
23. Ali SZ, Hoon V, Hoda S, Heelan R, Zakowski MF. Solitary fibrous tumor. A cytologic-histologic study with clinical, radiologic, and immunohisto-chemical correlations. Cancer 1997;81:116-121.
24. Clayton AC, Salomão DR, Keeney GL, Nascimento AG. Solitary fibrous tumor: a study of cytologic features of six cases diagnosed by fine-needle aspiration. Diagn Cytopathol 2001;25:172-176.
25. Dusenbery D, Grimes MM, Frable WJ. Fine needle aspiration cytology of localized fibrous tumor of pleura. Diagn Cytopathol 1992;8:444-540.

26. Bishop JA, Rekhtman N, Chun J, Wakely PE Jr, Ali SZ. Malignant solitary fibrous tumor: cytopathologic findings and differential diagnosis. Cancer Cytopathol 2010;118:83-89.

27. Klijanienko J, Caillaud JM, Lagacé R. Fine-needle aspiration of primary and recurrent dermatofibrosarcoma protuberans. Diagn Cytopathol 2004;30:261-215.

28. Domanski HA, Gustafson P. Cytologic features of primary, recurrent, and metastatic dermatofibrosarcoma protuberans. Cancer 2002;96:351-361.

29. Domanski HA. FNA diagnosis of dermatofibrosarcoma protuberans. Diagn Cytopathol 2005;32:299-302.

30. Piao Y, Guo M, Gong Y. Diagnostic challenges of metastatic spindle cell melanoma on fine-needle aspiration specimens. Cancer 2008;114:94-101.

31. Wakely PE Jr, Frable WJ. Fine needle aspiration biopsy cytology of giant cell tumor of tendon sheath. Am J Clin Pathol 1994;102:87-90.

32. Iyer VK, Kapila K, Verma K. Fine-needle aspiration cytology of giant cell tumor of tendon sheath. Diagn Cytopathol 2003;29:105-110.

33. Jakowski J, Mayerson J, Wakely PE Jr. Fine-needle aspiration biopsy of the distal extremities: a study of 141 cases. Am J Clin Pathol 2010; 133:224-231.

34. Beal M, Mayerson J, Wakely PE Jr. Fine-needle aspiration cytology of giant cell tumor of soft tissue (soft tissue giant cell tumor of low malignant potential). Ann Diagn Pathol 2003;7:365-369.

35. Kim NR, Han J. Primary giant cell tumor of soft tissue. Report of a case with fine needle aspiration cytologic and histologic findings. Acta Cytol 2003;47:1103-1106.

36. Lindberg GM, Maitra A, Gokaslan ST, Saboorian MH, Albores-Saavedra J. Low grade fibromyxoid sarcoma: fine-needle aspiration cytology with histologic, cytogenetic, immunohistochemical, and ultrastructural correlation. Cancer 1999;87:75-82.

37. Domanski HA, Mertens F, Panagopoulos I, Akerman M. Low-grade fibromyxoid sarcoma is difficult to diagnose by fine needle aspiration cytology: a cytomorphological study of eight cases. Cytopathology 2009;20:304-314.

38. Berardo MD, Powers CN, Wakely PE Jr, Almeida MO, Frable WJ. Fine-needle aspiration cytopathology of malignant fibrous histiocytoma. Cancer 1997;81:228-237.

39. Klijanienko J, Caillaud JM, Lagacé R, Vielh P. Comparative fine-needle aspiration and pathologic study of malignant fibrous histiocytoma: cytodiagnostic features of 95 tumors in 71 patients. Diagn Cytopathol 2003;29:320-326.

40. Fleshman R, Mayerson J, Wakely PE Jr. Fine needle aspiration biopsy of high grade sarcoma: a report of 107 cases. Cancer 2007;111:491-498.

41. Kilpatrick SE, Cappellari JO, Bos GD, Gold SH, Ward WG. Is fine-needle aspiration biopsy a practical alternative to open biopsy for the primary diagnosis of sarcoma? Experience with 140 patients. Am J Clin Pathol 2001;115:59-68.

42. Colin P, Lagacé R, Caillaud JM, Sastre-Garau X, Klijanienko J. Fine-needle aspiration in myxofibrosarcoma: experience of Institut Curie. Diagn Cytopathol 2010;38:343-346.

43. Layfield LJ, Liu K, Dodge RK. Logistic regression analysis of myxoid sarcomas: a cytologic study. Diagn Cytopathol 1998;19:355-360.

44. Kilpatrick SE, Ward WG. Myxofibrosarcoma of soft tissues: cytomorphologic analysis of a series. Diagn Cytopathol 1999;20:6-9.

Lipomatous Tumors

45. Lemos MM, Kindblom LG, Meis-Kindblom JM, et al. Fine-needle aspiration characteristics of hibernoma. Cancer 2001;93:206-210.

46. Chen X, Yu K, Tong GX, Hood M, Storper I, Hamele-Bena D. Fine needle aspiration of pleomorphic lipoma of the neck: report of two cases. Diagn Cytopathol 2010;38:184-187.

47. Åkerman M, Rydholm A. Aspiration cytology of lipomatous tumors: a 10-year experience at an orthopedic oncology center. Diagn Cytopathol 1987;3:295-302.

48. Thirumala S, Desai M, Kannan V. Diagnostic pitfalls in fine needle aspiration cytology of pleomorphic lipoma. A case report. Acta Cytol 2000;44:653-656.

49. Rigby HS, Wilson YG, Cawthorn SJ, Ibrahim NB. Fine needle aspiration of pleomorphic lipoma: a potential pitfall of cytodiagnosis. Cytopathology 1993;4:55-58.

50. Shattuck M, Victor TA. Cytologic features of well-differentiated sclerosing liposarcoma in aspirated samples. Acta Cytol 1988;32:896-901.

51. Domanski HA, Carlén B, Jonsson K, Mertens F, Akerman M. Distinct cytologic features of spindle cell lipoma. A cytologic-histologic study with clinical, radiologic, electron microscopic, and cytogenetic correlations. Cancer 2001;93:381-9.

52. Maitra A, Ashfaq R, Saboorian MH, Lindberg G, Gokaslan ST. The role of fine-needle aspiration biopsy in the primary diagnosis of mesenchymal lesions: a community hospital–based experience. Cancer 2000;90:178-85.

53. Wakely PE Jr. Myxomatous soft tissue tumors: correlation of cytopathology and histopathology. Ann Diagn Pathol 1999;3:227-242.

54. Walaas L, Kindblom LG. Lipomatous tumors: a correlative cytologic and histologic study of 27 tumours examined by fine needle aspiration cytology. Hum Pathol 1985;16:6-18.

55. Szadowska A, Lasota J. Fine needle aspiration cytology of myxoid liposarcoma: a study of 18 tumors. Cytopathology 1993;4:99-106.

56. Klijanienko J, Caïllaud JM, Lagacé R. Fine-needle aspiration in liposarcoma: cytohistologic correlative study including well-differentiated, myxoid, and pleomorphic variants. Diagn Cytopathol 2004;30:307-312.

57. Elwood H, Parwani A, Cai G. Fine-needle aspiration biopsy of myxoid liposarcoma metastatic to the liver: cytomorphologic and cytogenetic features. Diagn Cytopathol 2007;35:734-737.

58. Kapila K, Ghosal N, Gill SS, Verma K. Cytomorphology of lipomatous tumors of soft tissue. Acta Cytol 2003;47:555-562.

59. Dey P. Fine needle aspiration cytology of well-differentiated liposarcoma. A report of two cases. Acta Cytol 2000;44:459-462.

60. Nagira K, Yamamoto T, Akisue T, et al. Reliability of fine-needle aspiration biopsy in the initial diagnosis of soft-tissue lesions. Diagn Cytopathol 2002;27:354-361.

61. González-Cámpora R, Muñoz-Arias G, Otal-Salaverri C, et al. Fine needle aspiration cytology of primary soft tissue tumors. Morphologic analysis of the most frequent types. Acta Cytol 1992;36:905-917.

62. Geethamani V, Savithri R, Suguna BV, Niveditha SR. Cytomorphology of dedifferentiated liposarcoma of the subcutis of the upper back with axillary lymph node metastasis: a case report. Acta Cytol 2010;54:333-336.

Myogenic Tumors

63. Tao LC, Davidson DD. Aspiration biopsy cytology of smooth muscle tumors. A cytologic approach to the differentiation between leiomyosarcoma and leiomyoma. Acta Cytol 1993;37:300-308.

64. Barbazza R, Chiarelli S, Quintarelli GF, Manconi R. Role of fine-needle aspiration cytology in the preoperative evaluation of smooth muscle tumors. Diagn Cytopathol 1997;16:326-330.

65. Klijanienko J, Caillaud JM, Lagacé R, Vielh P. Fine-needle aspiration of leiomyosarcoma: a correlative cytohistopathological study of 96 tumors in 68 patients. Diagn Cytopathol 2003;28:119-125.

66. Vuong PN, Neveux Y, Balaton A, et al. Adult-type rhabdomyoma of the palate. Cytologic presentation of two cases with histologic and immunologic study. Acta Cytol 1990;34:413-419.

67. McGregor DK, Krishnan B, Green L. Fine-needle aspiration of adult rhabdomyoma: a case report with review of the literature. Diagn Cytopathol 2003;28:92-95.

68. Domanski HA, Dawiskiba S. Adult rhabdomyoma in fine needle aspirates. A report of two cases. Acta Cytol 2000;44:223-226.

69. Klijanienko J, Caillaud JM, Orbach D, et al. Cyto-histological correlations in primary, recurrent and metastatic rhabdomyosarcoma: the Institut Curie's experience. Diagn Cytopathol 2007;35:482-487.

70. de Almeida M, Stastny JF, Wakely PE Jr, Frable WJ. Fine-needle aspiration biopsy of childhood rhabdomyosarcoma: reevaluation of the cytologic criteria for diagnosis. Diagn Cytopathol 1994;11:231-236.

71. Das K, Mirani N, Hameed M, Pliner L, Aisner SC. Fine-needle aspiration cytology of alveolar rhabdomyosarcoma utilizing ThinPrep liquid-based sample and cytospin preparations: a case confirmed by FKHR break apart rearrangement by FISH probe. Diagn Cytopathol 2006;34:704-706.

72. Kilpatrick SE, Bergman S, Pettenati MJ, Gulley ML. The usefulness of cytogenetic analysis in fine needle aspirates for the histologic subtyping of sarcomas. Mod Pathol 2006;19: 815-819.

73. Gautam U, Srinivasan R, Rajwanshi A, Bansal D, Marwaha RK. Comparative evaluation of flow cytometric immunophenotyping and immunocytochemistry in the categorization of malignant small round cell tumors in fine-needle aspiration cytologic specimens. Cancer 2008;114:494-503.

Peripheral Nervous System Tumors

74. Resnick JM, Fanning CV, Caraway NP, Varma DG, Johnson M. Percutaneous needle biopsy diagnosis of benign neurogenic neoplasms. Diagn Cytopathol 1997;16:17-25.

75. Domanski HA, Akerman M, Engellau J, Gustafson P, Mertens F, Rydholm A. Fine-needle aspiration of neurilemoma (schwannoma). A clinicocytopathologic study of 116 patients. Diagn Cytopathol 2006;34: 403-412.

76. Klijanienko J, Caillaud JM, Lagacé R. Cytohistologic correlations in schwannomas (neurilemmomas), including "ancient," cellular, and epithelioid variants. Diagn Cytopathol 2006; 34:517-522.

77. Henke AC, Salomao DR, Hughes JH. Cellular schwannoma mimics a sarcoma: an example of a potential pitfall in aspiration cytodiagnosis. Diagn Cytopathol 1999;20:312-316.

78. Liu K, Madden JF, Olatidoye BA, Dodd LG. Features of granular cell tumor on fine needle aspiration. Acta Cytol 1999;43:552-557.

79. Wakely P Jr. Epithelioid/granular soft tissue lesions: correlation of cytopathology and histopathology. Ann Diagn Pathol 2000;4:316-328.
80. McCluggage WG, Sloan S, Kenny BD, Alderdice JM, Kirk SJ, Anderson NH. Fine needle aspiration cytology (FNAC) of mammary granular cell tumour: a report of three cases. Cytopathology 1999;10:383-389.
81. Gibbons D, Leitch M, Coscia J, et al. Fine needle aspiration cytology and histologic findings of granular cell tumor of the breast: review of 19 cases with clinical/radiologic correlation. Breast J 2000;6:27-30.
82. Lee LH, Bos GD, Marsh WL, Wakely PE Jr. Fine-needle aspiration cytology of sclerosing perineurioma. Ann Diagn Pathol 2004;8:80-86.
83. Housini I, Dabbs DJ. Fine needle aspiration cytology of perineurioma. Report of a case with histologic, immunohistochemical and ultrastructural studies. Acta Cytol 1990;34:420-424.
84. Klijanienko J, Caillaud JM, Lagacé R, Vielh P. Cytohistologic correlations of 24 malignant peripheral nerve sheath tumor (MPNST) in 17 patients: the Institut Curie experience. Diagn Cytopathol 2002;27:103-108
85. McGee RS Jr, Ward WG, Kilpatrick SE. Malignant peripheral nerve sheath tumor: a fine-needle aspiration biopsy study. Diagn Cytopathol 1997; 17:298-305.
86. Gupta K, Dey P, Vashisht R. Fine-needle aspiration cytology of malignant peripheral nerve sheath tumors. Diagn Cytopathol 2004;31:1-4.

Vascular Tumors

87. Bosch-Príncep R, Castellano-Megías VM, Alvaro-Naranjo T, Martínez-González S, Salvadó-Usach MT. Fine needle aspiration cytology of a cervical lymph node lymphangioma in an adult. A case report. Acta Cytol 1999;43:442-446.
88. Hilborne LH, Glasgow BJ, Layfield LJ. Fine-needle aspiration cytology of juvenile hemangioma of the parotid gland: a case report. Diagn Cytopathol 1987;3:152-155.
89. Powers CN, Berardo MD, Frable WJ. Fine-needle aspiration biopsy: pitfalls in the diagnosis of spindle-cell lesions. Diagn Cytopathol 1994;10:232-240.
90. Liu K, Layfield LJ. Cytomorphologic features of angiosarcoma on fine needle aspiration biopsy. Acta Cytol 1999;43:407-415.
91. Klijanienko J, Caillaud JM, Lagacé R, Vielh P. Cytohistologic correlations in angiosarcoma including classic and epithelioid variants: Institut Curie's experience. Diagn Cytopathol 2003;29:140-145.
92. Wakely PE Jr, Frable WJ, Kneisl JS. Aspiration cytopathology of epithelioid angiosarcoma. Cancer 2000;90:245-251.

93. Boucher LD, Swanson PE, Stanley MW, Silverman JF, Raab SS, Geisinger KR. Cytology of angiosarcoma. Findings in fourteen fine-needle aspiration biopsy specimens and one pleural fluid specimen. Am J Clin Pathol 2000;114:210-219.
94. Sharma SG, Aron M, Kapila K, Ray R. Epithelioid hemangioma: morphological presentation on aspiration smears. Diagn Cytopathol 2006; 34:830-833.

Myxoid, Chondro-osseous Tumors

95. Wakely PE Jr. Myxomatous soft tissue tumors: correlation of cytopathology and histopathology. Ann Diagn Pathol 1999;3:227-242.
95a. Wakely PE Jr, Bos GD, Mayerson J. The cytopathology of soft tissue myxomas: ganglia, juxta-articular myxoid lesions and intramuscular myxoma. Am J Clin Pathol 2005;123: 858-865.
96. Dodd LG, Layfield LJ. Fine-needle aspiration cytology of ganglion cysts. Diagn Cytopathol 1996;15:377-381.
97. Caraway NP, Staerkel GA, Fanning CV, Varma DG, Pollock RE. Diagnosing intramuscular myxoma by fine-needle aspiration: a multidisciplinary approach. Diagn Cytopathol 1994;1: 255-261.
98. Dodd LG, Martinez S. Fine-needle aspiration cytology of pseudosarcomatous lesions of soft tissue. Diagn Cytopathol 2001;24:28-35.
99. Wakely PE Jr, Almeida M, Frable WJ. Fine-needle aspiration biopsy cytology of myositis ossificans. Mod Pathol 1994;7:23-25.
100. Rööser B, Herrlin K, Rydholm A, Akerman M. Pseudomalignant myositis ossificans. Clinical, radiologic, and cytologic diagnosis in 5 cases. Acta Orthop Scand 1989;60:457-460.
101. Jakowski J, Wakely PE Jr. Cytopathology of extraskeletal myxoid chondrosarcoma: a report of 8 cases. Cancer 2007;111:298-305.
102. Niemann TH, Bottles K, Cohen MB. Extraskeletal myxoid chondrosarcoma: fine-needle aspiration biopsy findings. Diagn Cytopathol 1994;11:363-366.
103. Kilpatrick SE, Ward WG, Bos GD. The value of fine-needle aspiration biopsy in the differential diagnosis of adult myxoid sarcoma. Cancer 2000;90:167-177.
104. Bjerkehagen B, Dietrich C, Reed W, et al. Extraskeletal myxoid chondrosarcoma: multimodal diagnosis and identification of a new cytogenetic subgroup characterized by t(9;17) (q22;q11). Virchows Arch 1999;435:524-530.
105. Wakely PE Jr, Geisinger KR, Cappellari JO, Silverman JF, Frable WJ. Fine needle aspiration cytology of soft tissue: chondromyxoid and myxoid lesions. Diagn Cytopathol 1995;12:101-105.

106. Walaas L, Kindblom LG. Fine-needle aspiration biopsy in the preoperative diagnosis of chordoma: a study of 17 cases with application of electron microscopic, histochemical, and immunocytochemical examination. Hum Pathol 1991;22:22-28.

107. Kay PA, Nascimento AG, Unni KK, et al. Chordoma: cytomorphologic findings in 14 cases diagnosed by fine needle aspiration. Acta Cytol 2003;47:202-208.

108. Trembath DG, Dash R, Major NM, Dodd LG. Cytopathology of mesenchymal chondrosarcomas: a report and comparison of four patients. Cancer 2003;99:211-216.

Unclassified and Miscellaneous Soft Tissue Tumors

109. Ryan MR, Stastny JF, Wakely PE Jr. The cytopathology of synovial sarcoma: a study of six cases, emphasizing architecture and histopathologic correlation. Cancer 1998;84:42-49.

110. Kilpatrick SC, Teot LA, Stanley MW, Dodd LG. Fine-needle aspiration biopsy of synovial sarcoma. A cytomorphologic analysis of primary, recurrent, and metastatic tumors. Am J Clin Pathol 1996;106:769-775.

111. Klijanienko J, Caillaud JM, Lagacé R, Vielh P. Cytohistologic correlations in 56 synovial sarcomas in 36 patients: the Institut Curie experience. Diagn Cytopathol 2002;27:96-102.

112. Srinivasan R, Gautam U, Gupta R, Rajwanshi A, Vasistha RK. Synovial sarcoma: diagnosis on fine-needle aspiration by morphology and molecular analysis. Cancer 2009;117:128-136.

113. Åkerman M, Ryd W, Skytting B; Scandinavian Sarcoma Group. Fine-needle aspiration of synovial sarcoma: criteria for diagnosis: retrospective reexamination of 37 cases, including ancillary diagnostics. A Scandinavian Sarcoma Group study. Diagn Cytopathol 2003;28:232-238.

114. Silverman JF, Berns LA, Holbrook CT, Neill JS, Joshi VV. Fine needle aspiration cytology of primitive neurocctodcrmal tumors. A report of these cases. Acta Cytol 1992;36:541-550.

115. Layfield LJ, Liu K, Dodge RK. Logistic regression analysis of small round cell neoplasms: a cytologic study. Diagn Cytopathol 1999;20:271-7.

116. Guiter GE, Gamboni MM, Zakowski MF. The cytology of extraskeletal Ewing sarcoma. Cancer 1999;87:141-148.

117. Lin O, Olgac S, Zakowski M. Cytological features of epithelioid mesenchymal neoplasms: a study of 21 cases. Diagn Cytopathol 2005;32:5-10.

118. Lemos MM, Chaves P, Mendonça ME. Is preoperative cytologic diagnosis of epithelioid sarcoma possible? Diagn Cytopathol 2008;36:780-786.

119. Kitagawa Y, Ito H, Sawaizumi T, et al. Fine needle aspiration cytology of primary epithelioid sarcoma. A report of 2 cases. Acta Cytol 2004;48:391-396.

120. Wakely PE Jr, McDermott JE, Ali SZ. Cytopathology of alveolar soft part sarcoma: a report of 10 cases. Cancer 2009;117:500-507.

121. Shabb N, Sneige N, Fanning CV, Dekmezian R. Fine-needle aspiration cytology of alveolar soft-part sarcoma. Diagn Cytopathol 1991;7:293-298.

122. López-Ferrer P, Jiménez-Heffernan JA, Vicandi B, González-Peramato P, Viguer JM. Cytologic features of alveolar soft part sarcoma: report of three cases. Diagn Cytopathol 2002;27:115-119.

123. Creager AJ, Pitman MB, Geisinger KR. Cytologic features of clear cell sarcoma (malignant melanoma) of soft parts: a study of fine-needle aspirates and exfoliative specimens. Am J Clin Pathol 2002;117:217-224.

124. Almeida MM, Nunes AM, Frable WJ. Malignant melanoma of soft tissue. A report of three cases with diagnosis by fine needle aspiration cytology. Acta Cytol 1994;38:241-246.

125. Caraway NP, Fanning CV, Wojcik EM, Staerkel GA, Benjamin RS, Ordóñez NG. Cytology of malignant melanoma of soft parts: fine-needle aspirates and exfoliative specimens. Diagn Cytopathol 1993;9:632-638.

126. Perry MD, Gore M, Seigler HF, Johnston WW. Fine needle aspiration biopsy of metastatic melanoma: a morphologic analysis of 174 cases. Acta Cytol 1986;30:385-396.

127. Murali R, Doubrovsky A, Watson GF, et al. Diagnosis of metastatic melanoma by fine needle biopsy: analysis of 2,204 cases. Am J Clin Pathol 2007;127:385-397.

128. Morrison C, Young DC, Wakely PE Jr. Cytopathology of malignant melanoma in conventional and liquid-based smears. Am J Clin Pathol 2002;118:435-441.

Index*

*In a series of numbers, those in boldface indicate the main discussion of the entity.

M

N